IUD	Intrauterine (contraceptive) device	POA	Power-of-attorney
IVP	Intravenous pyelogram	POP	Progestin only pill
JRA	Juvenile rheumatoid arthritis	PPI	Proton pump inhibitor
JVD	Jugular venous distention	PSA	Prostate-specific antigen
KOH	Potassium hydroxide	PT	Posterior tibialis (pulse); physical therapy
KUB	Kidney-ureter-bladder (X-ray examination)	PTCA	Percutaneous transluminal coronary angioplasty
LA	Left atrial	PTSD	Posttraumatic stress disorder
LABA	Long-acting beta agonist	PTT	Partial thromboplastin time
LAMA	Long-acting muscarinic agonist	PUD	Peptic ulcer disease
LBBB	Left bundle branch block	PUVA	Psoralen plus ultraviolet A (light therapy)
LDH	Lactate dehydrogenase	PVC	Premature ventricular contraction
LDL	Low-density lipoprotein	PVR	Postvoid residual
LFT	Liver function test	RA	Rheumatoid arthritis
LH	Luteinizing hormone	RCA	Right coronary artery
LMP	Last menstrual period	RF	Rheumatoid factor
LOC	Level of consciousness	RLS	Restless legs syndrome
LSB	Left sternal border	ROM	Range of motion
LSIL	Low-grade squamous intraepithelial lesion	RMSF	Rocky Mountain Spotted Fever
LV	Left ventricular	RPR	Rapid plasma reagin (test for syphilis)
LVH	Left ventricular hypertrophy	RSV	Respiratory syncytial virus
MCH	Mean corpuscular hemoglobin	S/S	Signs and symptoms
MCV	Mean corpuscular volume	SABA	Short-acting beta agonist
MDI	Metered dose inhaler	SAMA	Short-acting muscarinic agonist
MDR-TB	Multi-drug-resistant tuberculosis	SBE	Subacute bacterial endocarditis
MI	Myocardial infarction	SCA	Sickle cell anemia
MRSA	Methicillin-resistant staphylococcus aureus	SGLT$_2$	Sodium-glucose cotransporter-2 inhibitor (diabetes medication)
MS	Multiple sclerosis	SIL	Squamous intraepithelial lesion
MVP	Mitral valve prolapse	SLE	Systemic lupus erythematosus
N/V	Nausea and vomiting	SLR	Straight leg raise
NAAT	Urine test for gonorrhea and chlamydia	SNRI	Selective norepinephrine reuptake inhibitor
NAFLD	Nonalcoholic fatty liver disease	SOB	Shortness of breath
NASH	Nonalcoholic steatohepatitis	SSRI	Selective serotonin reuptake inhibitor
NSAID	Nonsteroidal antiinflammatory drug	STI	Sexually transmitted infection
NYHA	New York Heart Association	SVT	Supraventricular tachycardia
O&P	Ova and parasites	T4	Thyroxine
OA	Osteoarthritis	TB	Tuberculosis
OB	Occult blood	TCA	Tricyclic antidepressant
OC	Oral contraceptive	TIA	Transient ischemic attack
OCD	Obsessive-compulsive disorder	TIBC	Total iron-binding capacity
OD	Overdose	TMJ	Temporomandibular joint
OE	Otitis externa	TMP-SMZ	Trimethoprim-sulfamethoxazole (Bactrim)
OGC	Oral glucocorticoid	TSH	Thyroid-stimulating hormone
OHA	Oral hypoglycemic agent	TTP	Thrombotic thrombocytopenic purpura
OME	Otitis media with effusion	U/S	Ultrasound
OSA	Obstructive sleep apnea	UCG	Urine chorionic gonadotropin (pregnancy test)
OTC	Over-the-counter	UGI	Upper gastrointestinal (X-ray examination)
PAD	Peripheral arterial disease	URI	Upper respiratory (tract) infection
PCOS	Polycystic ovarian syndrome	UTI	Urinary tract infection
PE	Pulmonary embolism	V/D	Vomiting and diarrhea
PEF	Peak expiratory flow	V/Q	Ventilation perfusion (ratio)
PFT	Pulmonary function test	VDRL	Venereal Disease Research Laboratories (test for syphilis)
PHN	Postherpetic neuralgia	VLDL	Very-low-density lipoprotein
PID	Pelvic inflammatory disease	VT	Ventricular tachycardia
PMI	Point of maximal impulse	WNL	Within normal limits
PMR	Polymyalgia rheumatica		
PMS	Premenstrual syndrome		
PND	Paroxysmal nocturnal dyspnea; postnasal drainage		

Practice Guidelines for Family Nurse Practitioners

SIXTH EDITION

Practice Guidelines for Family Nurse Practitioners

KAREN FENSTERMACHER, MS, RN, FNP-BC
Family Nurse Practitioner
Carthage, Missouri

BARBARA TONI HUDSON, MSN, RN, FNP-BC
Family Nurse Practitioner
Walnut Grove, Missouri

ELSEVIER

Elsevier
3251 Riverport Lane
St. Louis, Missouri 63043

Notice

Previous editions copyrighted 2020, 2015, 2004, 2000, 1997.

Executive Content Strategist: Lee Henderson
Director, Content Development: Ellen Wurm-Cutter
Senior Content Development Specialist: Kathleen Nahm
Publishing Services Manager: Deepthi Unni
Project Manager: Kamatchi Madhavan
Designer: Bridget Hoette

Printed in India

Last digit is the print number: 9 8 7 6 5 4 3 2

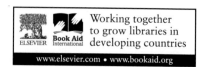

Working together
to grow libraries in
developing countries

www.elsevier.com • www.bookaid.org

Tamika Dowling, DNP, FNP-C, PCCN
Nurse Practitioner, Faculty, Urgent Care
 Nurse Practitioner, Business Owner,
 Advent Health, Orlando,
 Florida

Jessica Gonzalez, DNP, NP-C, DCNP
Family Nurse Practitioner, Dermatology
 Nurse Practitioner, Christus St. Vincent
 Hospital, Santa Fe, New Mexico

Yvette Lowery, DNP, MSN/Ed, FNP-C, CEN, CCRN, PCCN
Family Nurse Practitioner, North Florida
 Regional Medical Center, Jacksonville,
 Florida

Matthew Rodgers, MSN, APRN, FNP-C
Advanced Practice Registered Nurse,
 PrimeCare Medical Clinic, Searcy,
 Arkansas

ACKNOWLEDGMENTS

My thanks first to God, without whose help I would not be where I am now. Also, thank you to the nursing and NP colleagues and NP students who have challenged me with their questions and encouraged me with their comments.

Karen

My thanks to my family (David and Cody) for their support with the amount of time spent on this edition; they have been very supportive. My colleagues have challenged me and expanded my abilities in being able to make information easily understandable.

Toni

We have been very blessed over the years to have many collegial relationships with physicians, nurse practitioners, and physician assistants whom we worked with, consulted with, and referred to—too many to name individually, but we thank you all! We are also blessed to have earned the trust of our patients, and we have learned much from them.

We also thank the staff at Elsevier for all their help; our book would not be what it is without their input.

Karen and Toni

Practice Guidelines for Family Nurse Practitioners is a quick-reference book for practicing and student nurse practitioners in a variety of disciplines. Although not intended as a textbook, it is an excellent resource, providing protocols for treatment options for patients of varied ages in varied settings.

For ease of use, the expanded Table of Contents includes a list of the topics plus figures, tables, and boxes for each chapter. Chapters 1 through 3 contain complete and detailed histories and physical examinations of adult, pediatric, and geriatric patients. Focused exams are included for each body system. Specialized physical examinations are included for sports physicals, child abuse and assessing functional status in geriatrics. Chapter 4 covers laboratory and diagnostic pearls; Chapter 14 discusses pain.

Chapters 5 through 17 (other than Chapter 14) are written in an easy-to-read and accessible format according to body systems. Common diseases are covered, including signs and symptoms, diagnostic methods, drug therapies, and treatment and adjunctive therapies. Some conditions (e.g., cognitive impairment, anemia, and diabetes) have been expanded. Updated national standard guidelines are used where available (e.g., asthma, diabetes, hypertension, Pap smears); new content has been added on unintentional weight loss, jaundice, fever of unknown origin, and restless legs. As new features to this edition, within each chapter the topics are listed alphabetically, not-to-be-missed conditions are now in **_bold, italic_** font with a blue square icon (■) in the margin, and all referrals are in **_bold, italic_** font with urgent referrals identified with a red triangle icon (▲) and non-urgent referrals identified with a gold circle icon (●) in the margin.

Special chapters include geriatric evaluation, pediatrics, and psychiatric conditions. There is also a section on the care of wounds resulting from vascular disease or peripheral pressure. Pain management guidelines have been expanded.

Appendices A–D provide information about dietary sources of different nutrients, a peak flow chart, and acetaminophen and ibuprofen dosing charts.

Karen Fenstermacher
Barbara Toni Hudson

CONTENTS

9   **Abdominal Conditions   264**

10 Gynecologic Conditions   308

13 Musculoskeletal Conditions 386

CHAPTER 1

Adult Assessment

INTRODUCTION

I. The following guidelines assume that the patient is in a stable condition. The order should be modified as the patient's condition warrants.

II. In cases of acute illness, the initial focus is on the affected and related body systems, with emphasis on the history of the present illness (HPI).

III. The Focused Exams include more specific details.

HISTORY

I. Patient profile
   A. Marital status and relationship with spouse
   B. Phone number(s), including name and number of who can be contacted if needed; email address, if desired
   C. Living arrangements
      1. With whom?
      2. Where (e.g., an apartment or home, homeless)?
   D. Education, occupation, and current employment
   E. Adequacy of finances and health insurance
   F. Transportation (e.g., has a vehicle or relies on friend/family member or taxi)

II. Chief complaint (CC)
   A. State in the patient's own words
   B. Note if the patient's actions agree with or contradict the stated CC

III. History of the present illness (HPI)
   A. Chronic condition(s) visit: focus on how the patient has been doing
      1. Current treatment and changes
      2. Review any home monitoring results (e.g., blood pressure or blood glucose readings)
   B. Acute illness: focus on the specific reason for the visit
      1. Try to obtain a clear account of the patient's CC, including what treatments have been tried before (what worked and what did not)
      2. Focus on affected and related body systems, with regard to the following:
         (a) Onset (e.g., when, where)
         (b) Characteristics (e.g., description of the quality of discomfort, radiation, associated symptoms such as N/V)
         (c) Course (e.g., length of the event, alleviating or aggravating factors)
         (d) What does the patient think is wrong?
      3. Also note pertinent negative responses (e.g., absence of cough or fever)

IV. Past medical history (PMH)
   A. Significant childhood and adult illnesses; surgeries (including gender transition), hospitalizations, or Emergency Department visits: any changes since last seen (including Urgent Care or other hospital system visit(s) not part of the currently used electronic health record [EHR])

B. Current medications and treatments, including over-the-counter (OTC) preparations, oral contraceptives (OCs), inhalers, eye drops, herbal supplements or vitamins, and customs (e.g., home remedies, cultural treatments)

C. Immunization status, including influenza, pneumococcal vaccine(s), shingles vaccines (Zostavax, Shingrix), COVID-19 vaccines, and tuberculosis (TB) test. See www.cdc/gov/vaccines or the Shots Immunizations app for the current immunization schedules

D. Allergic reactions or sensitivities to medications, including what occurs when the medicine is taken (common side effects such as nausea are often perceived as an allergy)

E. Street drug, alcohol, and tobacco use (specific types, amounts, and routes; include vaping)

V. Family history (FH)

A. FH is important for the identification of risk factors; gather information about grandparents, parents, and siblings

B. Focus on cardiovascular disease, diabetes mellitus (DM), cancer, autoimmune diseases, peripheral vascular disease (PVD), seizure disorders, asthma, and psychiatric disorders

C. The phrase "significant FH" indicates that several family members from different generations have had a specific disease

VI. Psychosocial history

A. Dietary and rest patterns

B. Types and frequency of exercise

C. Spiritual assessment
1. Faith or beliefs and the importance and influence in the patient's life
2. Involvement in a religious/spiritual community and if it is a source of support to the patient

D. Depression screening (if indicated)

VII. Review of systems (ROS)

A. Chronic conditions(s) visit: questions pertaining to affected body systems and current treatments (i.e., possible medications side effects)

B. Acute illness visit: questions about various body systems to obtain any additional information to help arrive at an accurate diagnosis

C. Also see Focused Examinations, later in this chapter

PHYSICAL EXAMINATION

I. General observations

A. General appearance
1. Grooming and dressing, facial expressions, symmetry of movement
2. *Not to be missed*
   (a) *Appears acutely ill/toxic appearing*
   (b) *Signs of dehydration (e.g., dry mucous membranes, tachycardia, dizziness)*
   (c) *Cyanosis or pallor*
   (d) *Shortness of breath (SOB) or use of accessory muscles to breathe*
   (e) *Drooling* (consider epiglottitis; see Chapter 16)

B. Vital signs (VS): temperature, pulse, respiration, blood pressure (BP) (including postural VS with dizziness or syncope), weight, height, and body mass index (BMI)
1. Postural VS changes: initially determine the VS with the patient lying quietly; next have the patient sit (and then stand, if indicated), and within 2 min of position change(s), recheck the VS. With postural changes, one or more of the following will happen:
   (a) ≥20 mmHg drop in systolic BP or ≥10 mmHg drop in diastolic BP

■ = *not to be missed;* ▲ = *urgent referral*

       (b) Increase in heart rate of > 30 bpm

       (c) Patient becomes symptomatic (e.g., dizzy)

    2. A low diastolic BP (<65 mmHg) implies decreased peripheral resistance or aortic valve regurgitation (which is significant, even if the heart sounds are not loud).

  C. Skin inspection

    1. Color and turgor

    2. *Not to be missed*

       (a) *Fingernail clubbing*

       (b) *Suspicious or unusual lesions*

Focused Examinations

EYES

   I. Emphasis on HPI and ROS

    A. Change in vision (e.g., blurred or double vision or visual field deficit in one or both eyes) or sudden, painless, total or near total loss of vision in one eye

    B. Possible injury (e.g., "something in my eye," tanning without protective eye wear)

    C. Photophobia

    D. Headache

  II. PMI

    A. Glaucoma

    B. History of eye surgery (e.g., cataracts or retinal surgery, laser surgery)

    C. Wears contacts or glasses

 III. Examination (also see Chapter 6, Common Eye Conditions)

    A. Check for the best visual acuity, if indicated: right eye, left eye, and both eyes (note with/without corrective lenses).

     1. Distance (e.g., Snellen chart)

     2. Newsprint (document how far away it is held to read; e.g., 6 inches)

     3. Counting fingers

     4. Hand motion

     5. Light perception

     6. No light perception

    B. External: observe lid symmetry.

    C. Pressure: gently press on closed eyes for symmetry.

    D. Check for pupil reactivity: shine light first in the unaffected eye (both pupils should constrict) and then in the affected eye; if pupils dilate, the optic nerve in the affected eye is not working (see Marcus Gunn pupil, Table 1.1).

    E. Anterior: examine the conjunctiva, sclera, and cornea; fluorescein staining is used to detect injuries to the surface of the cornea (e.g., abrasion, foreign body). This is done easily with minimal discomfort and is a good tool for determining further care and/or referral for care.

     1. Make sure the patient is not wearing a contact lens.

     2. Instill 1 to 2 local anesthetic eye drops. *Do not let patient touch eyes for the next 60 min;* this can injure the cornea because the corneal reflex is now absent.

       (a) If anesthetic eye drops give immediate relief, the problem is most likely caused by surface pain.

       (b) If pain remains, the pain is most likely deep in the eye itself (more serious).

■ = *not to be missed*

TABLE 1.1 ■ Eye Signs

Eye Sign	Characteristics	Pathology
Normal findings	Pupils 3–4 mm, symmetric, round, and reactive to light and accommodation Palpebral fissure 8–12 mm and symmetric	
Adie pupil	Unilateral, large pupil Sluggish constriction to prolonged light exposure Direct light reflex absent	Post viral infection Loss of parasympathetic reactions
Anisocoria	Unequal pupil size Reactive to light and accommodation	May be a normal variant if the difference is <1 mm Compression of CN III (e.g., aneurysm, cerebral herniation)
Argyll Robertson pupil	Pupils smaller than normal in dim light Minimal dilation, often unequal Pupils may appear irregular Visual disturbance	Neurosyphilis, viral encephalitis Lesion in midbrain DM
Dysconjugate gaze	Inability to follow a moving finger in all eye fields Deviation of eye Lack of gaze coordination	Space-occupying lesion Neuromuscular disorders (e.g., MS) Frontal lobe dysfunction (dementia or trauma) DM
Marcus Gunn pupil	Pupils equal, with positive direct light reflex Pupil dilates when direct light is moved from the intact eye to the eye with the abnormal pupil	Optic nerve involved (e.g., with multiple sclerosis)
Nystagmus*	Involuntary, oscillating eye movements May occur at rest or during eye field examination May be vertical or lateral	May be associated with strain secondary to poor lighting Side effect of certain drugs (e.g., phenytoin, alcohol, barbiturates) Bilateral nystagmus may indicate myasthenia gravis
Ptosis	Palpebral fissure <5 mm Asymmetric	CN III palsy Myopathy Neuromuscular disorders (e.g., myasthenia gravis) Atonic eyelid muscles Inflammatory lesion of the eyelid

* Marked nystagmus on lateral gaze or any nystagmus on vertical gaze suggests a peripheral or central nervous system (CNS) lesion.
CN, cranial nerve; *DM*, diabetes mellitus; *MS*, multiple sclerosis.

3. Put a drop of saline on a fluorescein paper and touch the paper to the inner lower eyelid. The conjunctiva will turn orange immediately (if it does not, remoisten the fluorescein strip and touch to eye again). Have the patient open and close the eyes a few times.
4. Using a cobalt blue pen light, inspect the cornea and under the eyelids; if there is an injury or foreign object (FO), the dye will enhance the area. Possible findings:
   (a) "Ice rink sign": scratches on the cornea from blinking due to FO in the upper eyelid
   (b) Dendrite appearance: possibly herpes zoster or other virus

  (c) Abrasions seen at the 3 and 9 o'clock positions on the cornea are common with contact lens wearers

  (d) Isolated dots across the cornea from poorly fitted contact lenses or dry eyes

 (e) Lesion(s) located in the central vision (over the pupil) will decrease visual acuity and depth perception (may not be seen with the dye, but patient will report this during exam)

 5. After examination, irrigate the eye(s) with saline solution until clear and reevaluate in the same manner; injury or FO will be seen.

 6. If an abrasion is noted, refer to Corneal Abrasion, in Chapter 6, CORNEAL INJURIES/ABNORMALITIES.

 7. Remind patient to not touch eye if the anesthetic drops are used; an eye patch may be needed if concern for touching is present.

  (a) Explain to patient that orange drainage may be present after "blowing the nose" for the next hour; this is due to dye running down tear ducts.

  (b) Anesthetic eye drops are for examination purposes only and not for continued relief; do not send home with patient.

F. Eversion of upper eyelid is an important tool for inspecting under the upper lids for injury, FO, or swelling (see Fig. 1.1).

G. Peripheral visual fields: sit/stand at eye level directly in front of the patient to check peripheral field vision.

H. Alignment

 1. Have the patient look straight ahead toward the light—the light reflection should be symmetric.

 2. Test extraocular muscles (EOMs).

I. Perform ophthalmoscopy, if possible (see Table 1.2).

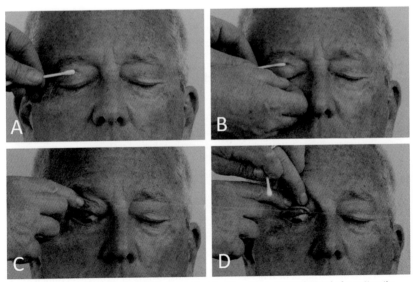

Fig. 1.1 Eyelid eversion technique. (A) With the patient looking down, place the end of a cotton tip applicator in the center of the upper eyelid fold. (B) Grab the eyelashes of the upper lid with the other hand. (C) Gently pull the eyelashes slightly outward and upward until the upper lid everts over the cotton tip applicator, and then remove the applicator. (D) To fully reveal the tarsal conjunctiva, gently pull back the eyelashes at the nasal aspect of the lid margin with a finger of the other hand. When finished, gently pull the eyelashes of the upper lid outward and downward until the lid flips back to its normal position. (From Efron, N. (2019). *Contact lens complications* (4th ed.). Philadelphia: Elsevier.)

TABLE 1.2 ■ Ophthalmologic Examination

Finding	Characteristics	Possible Causes
Normal	Yellow-white disc Well-defined disc margins Arteries (smaller) enter and veins (larger) leave at the optic disc	
Papilledema	Edema of the optic disc: unilateral if inflammatory (may have a sudden loss of vision in the inflammatory state); usually bilateral if noninflammatory Impaired visual acuity in the chronic stage	Lesions that increase intracranial pressure Encephalopathy Optic artery aneurysm or cavernous sinus thrombosis Guillain-Barre syndrome
Optic atrophy	Decreased vision Optic disc white or gray-white The cup may be absent	Optic neuritis Neurosyphilis Trauma to the orbit Toxins or poisons Diabetes mellitus

     IV. Examination findings *not to be missed*
        A. *Nystagmus, strabismus*
        B. *Red eye(s)*
        C. *Foreign body in eye*
        D. *Retinal artery occlusion* (e.g., sudden, painless, total or near total loss of vision in one eye); also, see Chapter 6, PRACTICE PEARLS FOR EYES
    V. *Referral*
        A. *To ED with foreign body in eye that cannot be removed*
        B. *To ED or ophthalmologist*
           1. *Immediately with sudden, painless, total or near total loss of vision*
           2. *Urgently with acute onset eye pain, diminished visual acuity, and photophobia*

HEAD, EARS, NOSE, AND THROAT (HENT)

    I. Emphasis on HPI and ROS
        A. Onset and changes (e.g., new or chronic, worsening or more constant)
        B. Associated symptoms
           1. Fever, nausea/vomiting (N/V), or diarrhea, loss of taste/smell, cough
           2. Possible exposure to contagious illness (e.g., influenza, COVID-19, strep throat)
           3. Fatigue, tachycardia or palpitations, thinning hair
    II. PMH (as indicated by chief complaint)
        A. Seasonal or perennial allergies, including if treatments are PRN (as needed) or routine
        B. Recurrent sinus issues
        C. Gastroesophageal reflux disease (GERD)
        D. Tinnitus
        E. Vertigo
        F. Hard of hearing or deaf or wears hearing aids; history of recurrent cerumen impaction
        G. Hair loss
        H. History of head injuries
   III. Examination
        A. Inspect the face and head (includes noticing hair patterns and irregularities from past head injury)

■ *= not to be missed;* ▲ *= urgent referral*

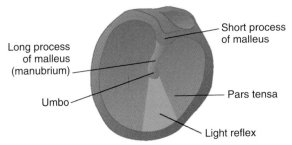

Fig. 1.2 Right tympanic membrane. (From Black, J., & Hawks, J. H. (2009). *Medical-surgical nursing* (8th ed.). Philadelphia: Elsevier.)

B. Ears
   1. Palpate the auricle and tragus.
   2. Perform otoscopy (Fig. 1.2).
   3. Administer appropriate hearing tests: Weber test, Rinne test (Fig. 1.3), and 5-foot whisper.
   4. If the patient is hard of hearing, ask the patient to hum.
      (a) Conductive defect: hum is louder in the affected ear.
      (b) Sensorineural defect: hum is louder in the unaffected ear.
C. Nose: examine the nasal septum and nares for mucosal color, polyps, perforations, and presence of swelling
D. Oropharynx: inspect the lips, gums, teeth, tongue, buccal mucosa, uvula, and pharynx
   1. Determine the "grade" of tonsils.
      1+: barely extend beyond the tonsillar pillars
      2+: extend halfway to the uvula
      3+: touch the uvula
      4+: tonsils touch each other
   2. Note the presence of partial plates, full dentures, caries, if any.
E. Palpation
   1. Over sinuses (e.g., over maxillofrontal areas, mastoids, C2) for pain or pressure
   2. Neck for lymph nodes (Fig. 1.4) or thyroid abnormalities
IV. Examination findings ***not to be missed***
   A. Ears
      1. ***Redness, bulging, perforation, retraction, or decreased mobility of tympanic membrane (TM)***
      2. ***Bullae on TM (mycoplasma infection)***
      3. ***Pain on palpation of the auricle or tragus***
   B. Oropharynx
      1. ***Peritonsillar abscess*** (see Chapter 6, PHARYNGITIS)
      2. ***Exudative pharyngitis***
      3. ***Palatine petechiae***
      4. ***Postnasal drainage***
   C. Neck
      1. ***Lymphadenopathy with or without tenderness*** (Fig. 1.4 and Table 1.3)
      2. ***Thyroid abnormalities***
V. ***Referral***
   A. ***To ENT or ED urgently with peritonsillar abscess***
   B. ***To ENT with recurrent ear or sinus infections***

■ = *not to be missed;* ● = *non-urgent referral;* ▲ = *urgent referral*

Rinne	Weber	Hearing Status
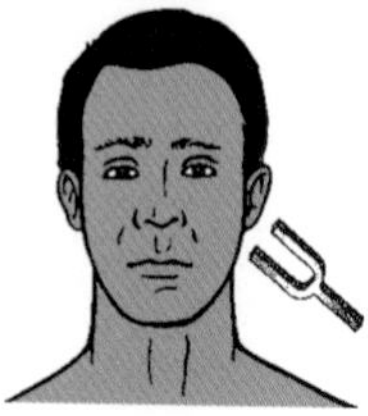 Air conduction > bone conduction	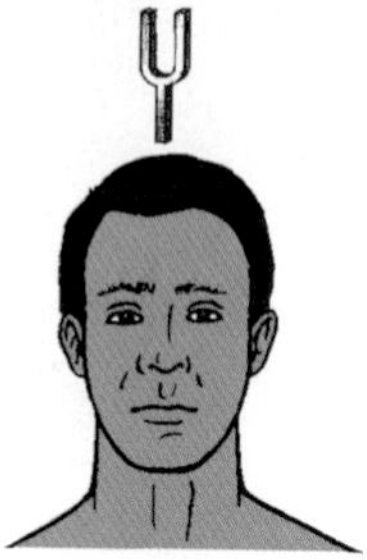 Sound equal to both ears	Either no hearing loss or symmetric hearing loss
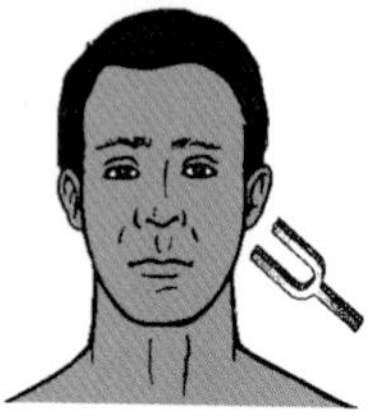 Air conduction > bone conduction	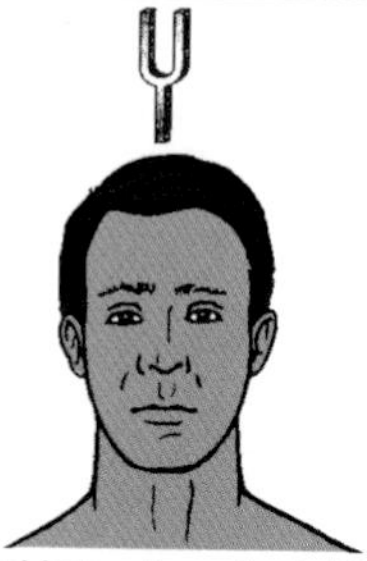 Sound lateralizes to right ear	Sensorineural hearing loss in left ear
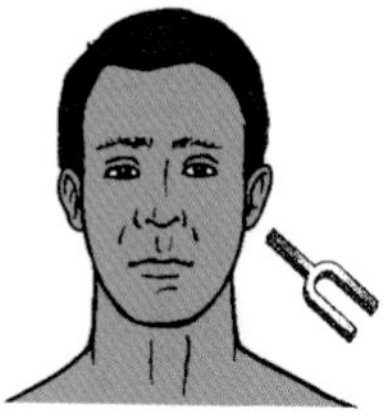 Bone conduction > air conduction	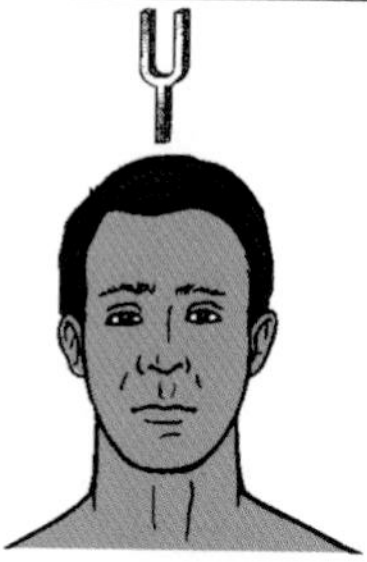 Sound lateralizes to left ear	Conductive hearing loss in left ear
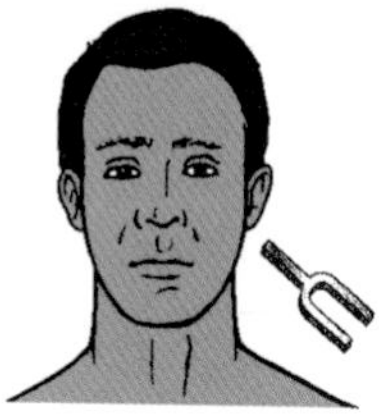 Bone conduction > air conduction	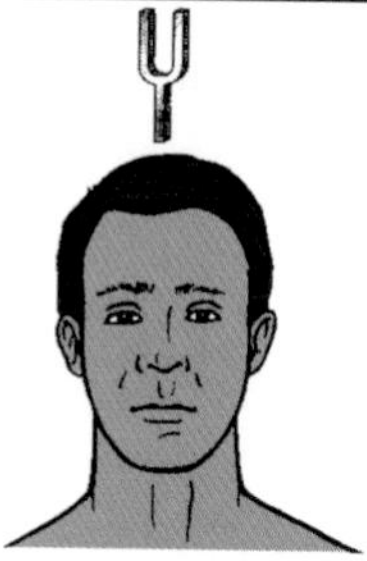 Sound lateralizes to right ear	Severe sensorineural hearing loss in left ear

Fig. 1.3 Rinne and Weber tests.

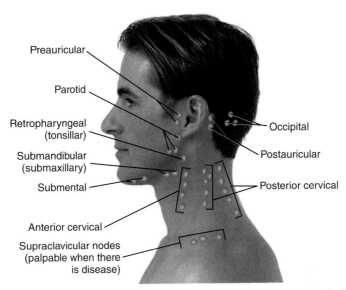

Fig. 1.4 Lymph nodes of the head and neck. (From Seidel, H. M., Stewart, R. W., Ball, J. W., Dains, J. E., Flynn, J. A., Solomon, B. S., & Stewart, R. W. (2011). *Mosby's guide to physical examination* (7th ed.). Philadelphia: Elsevier.)

TABLE 1.3 ■ **Common Causes of Lymphadenopathy**

Auricular Anterior: viral conjunctivitis, trachoma Posterior: scalp infection, rubella	**Axillary** Breast cancer or infection Upper extremity infection	**Cervical (unilateral), Submandibular** Buccal cavity infection Pharyngitis (may be bilateral) Nasopharyngeal tumor Thyroid cancer
Cervical (bilateral) Mononucleosis (especially posterior nodes) Toxoplasmosis pharyngitis	**Epitrochlear** Syphilis (bilateral) Hand infection (unilateral)	**Hilar area (unilateral or bilateral)** Sarcoidosis Lymphoma Bronchogenic cancer Tuberculosis Fungal infection (e.g., histoplasmosis, coccidioidomycosis)
Inguinal Syphilis, genital herpes Lymphogranuloma venereum chancroid Lower extremity or local infection	**Supraclavicular** Right: cancer (pulmonary, mediastinal, or esophageal) Left: cancer (intraabdominal, renal, testicular, or ovarian)	**Any area** Cat scratch fever Hodgkin's disease, leukemia Metastatic cancer Sarcoidosis

RESPIRATORY

I. Emphasis on HPI and ROS
   A. SOB, dyspnea, orthopnea, wheezing, and nocturnal dyspnea
   B. Fever (when, how high?)
   C. Cough, sputum, and hemoptysis
   D. Sore throat, sneezing, congestion
   E. Earache

II. PMH
   A. Asthma (include ED visits and hospitalizations)
   B. Bronchitis or COPD
   C. Pneumonia or TB
   D. COVID-19 infection (when; did all symptoms resolve?)
   E. Frequent strep throat or ear infections
   F. Sleep apnea; use of CPAP or BiPAP machine
   G. Occupational exposure and tobacco use (current or past use of any type, including vaping)
   H. Chest trauma or spontaneous pneumothorax
   I. Last influenza or pneumonia vaccine, COVID-19 vaccines (if any); TB test

III. FH
   A. Asthma
   B. Chronic airway disease

IV. Examination (include cardiovascular and abdominal examinations in case of respiratory complaints)
   A. Observe the chest for AP and lateral diameter and deformities.
   B. Auscultate the anterior and posterior chest and right lateral chest (Fig. 1.5).
      1. For symmetry of breath sounds throughout all lung fields
      2. Listen for bronchial, bronchovesicular and vesicular breath sounds, as well as abnormal breath sounds
         (a) Crackles: fine, crackle sounds that can be associated with fluid in the airways or with fibrosis
         (b) Rhonchi: coarser sounds, as with someone who needs to cough; often clears with cough
         (c) Stridor: high-pitched inspiratory sound associated with laryngeal spasm
         (d) Wheeze: low-pitched inspiratory or expiratory sound associated with bronchospasm or pulmonary congestion
   C. Examine the chest, including respiratory excursion, and perform bronchophony, egophony, and whispered pectoriloquy, if indicated.
   D. Percuss posterior lung fields for symmetry and normal/abnormal sounds.
   E. Percuss diaphragmatic excursion and palpate for vocal fremitus, if indicated.
   F. Examine capillary refill in the nail beds; also examine the fingernail beds for shape (e.g., clubbing).

V. Examination findings *not to be missed*
   A. *Fingernail clubbing, capillary refill >3 sec*
   B. *Cyanosis*
   C. *SOB or use of accessory muscles to breathe, prolonged expiration*
   D. *Hypoxemia (pulse ox <90%)*
   E. *Tachypnea at rest and/or hypotension and tachycardia*
   F. *Abnormal, absent, or decreased breath sounds (e.g., crackles, rhonchi, stridor, wheeze) or abnormal percussion*

■ = *not to be missed*

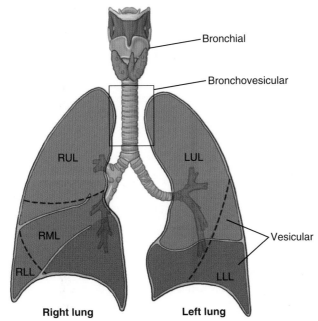

Fig. 1.5 Lung lobes and breath sounds. (From Bontrager, K. (2009). *Textbook of radiographic positioning and related anatomy* (7th ed.). Philadelphia: Elsevier.)

    1. *Dullness indicates consolidation* (e.g., pneumonia, pleural effusion)

    2. *Hyperresonance* (consider emphysema or pneumothorax)

  G. *Unequal inspiration/expiration contours of the right and left sides of the chest*

  H. *Pleural friction rub*

  VI. *Referral: emergency transfer to ED with acute respiratory distress*

CARDIOVASCULAR

  I. Emphasis on HPI and ROS

    A. Cardiac (e.g., chest pain, palpitations, dysrhythmias, tachycardia, cyanosis, cough, exertional dyspnea, orthopnea, nocturnal dyspnea, edema, dizziness, syncope, diaphoresis)

    B. Vascular (e.g., phlebitis, intermittent claudication, skin color changes, cold or painful extremities)

  II. PMH

    A. Rheumatic fever; COVID-19 infection (when; did all symptoms resolve?)

    B. Murmurs, mitral valve prolapse (MVP)

    C. Ischemic heart disease (e.g., angina, MI, stent placement, PTCA, heart surgery)

    D. Dysrhythmia (e.g., atrial fibrillation)

    E. Hypertension (HTN)

    F. Heart failure (HF)

    G. Deep venous thrombosis (DVT)

    H. Venous stasis (including presence/absence of ulcers)

    I. Prior peripheral vascular surgery (stent or "bypass")

    J. Dyslipidemia

    K. cerebral vascular accident (CVA) or transient ischaemic attack (TIA)

■ = *not to be missed;* ▲ = *urgent referral*

    L. DM

    M. Gallbladder disease, peptic ulcer

    N. Marfan syndrome

    O. Women with a history of breast cancer (some treatments are cardiotoxic)

III. FH

    A. Sudden death of a family member before 50 yr of age

    B. Coronary artery disease (CAD) or cardiomyopathy

    C. HTN

    D. Raynaud disease or other peripheral vascular disease (PVD)

    E. DM

IV. Examination (include respiratory and abdominal examinations in case of cardiovascular complaints)

    A. Palpate the precordium

    B. Auscultation (Fig. 1.6)

        1. Using both the bell and the diaphragm, listen over the precordium with the patient seated upright and leaning forward, in the supine position, and in the left lateral position.

        2. Listen for S_1 and S_2 (including splits); to identify S_1, time it with the carotid pulse (see also **V. Examination findings *not to be missed*,** below).

        (a) Split S_1 is usually normal; best heard in the tricuspid area

        (b) S_2 findings

            (i) Split S_2 is physiologic (normal) if it resolves with deep expiration (i.e., it is "blown away").

            (ii) Paradoxical split S_2: consider left bundle branch block (LBBB) or aortic stenosis.

            (iii) ***Loud S_2 means increased peripheral resistance, regardless of BP measurement; requires aggressive treatment.***

        3. Listen over the carotid arteries, abdominal aorta, and renal and femoral arteries.

    C. Inspect the neck (with the head of the bed at a 45-degree angle) for carotid and internal jugular venous pulsations and jugular venous distention (JVD).

    D. Palpation

        1. Check the carotid pulses (individually).

        2. Check the abdomen for hepatojugular reflux and aortic pulsation.

        3. Check the peripheral pulses for rate, rhythm, and amplitude (Fig. 1.7).

        4. Check the lower extremities for edema.

        (a) Nonpitting edema: consider lymphatic obstruction or hypothyroidism.

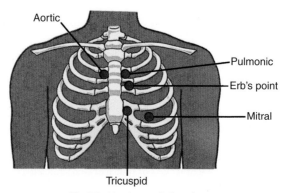

Fig. 1.6 Heart auscultation sites.

▨ = not to be missed

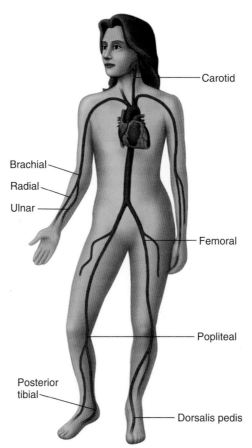

Fig. 1.7 Peripheral pulses. (From Harkreader, H., Hogan, M., & Thobaben, M. (2007). *Fundamentals of nursing* (3rd ed.). Philadelphia: Elsevier.)

      (b) Pitting edema: consider right-sided HF, cirrhosis, renal disease, or venous insufficiency (edema may be asymmetric with venous insufficiency); press with fingertips firmly on area of edema for 5 sec.

        1+: Mild pitting, slight indentation; rapid return to normal

        2+: Moderate pitting (4 mm deep); rebounds in a few seconds

        3+: Deep pitting (6 mm deep); takes 30 sec to resolve

        4+: Very severe pitting (8 mm deep); takes >30 sec to resolve

  V. Examination findings *not to be missed*

      A. *Chest pain indicating possible MI, pulmonary embolism (PE), or aneurysm* (see Table 8.5)

      B. *Dyspnea on exertion*

      C. Jugular veins (see IV., C above)

         1. *JVD elevated >2 cm above the clavicle* (would mean a pressure of >7 cm because the clavicle is approximately 5 cm above the right atrium)

         2. *Visible jugular veins that do not collapse with inspiration* (Kussmaul sign)

      D. *Change in the usual heart rhythm or rate or blood pressure*

■ = *not to be missed*

       E. Abnormal heart sounds
- 1. *New or worsening murmur* (see Chapter 8, HEART MURMURS, Table 8.12)
- 2. *S_3 or S_4* (see unnumbered figure with Chapter 8, HEART MURMURS)
- 3. *Fixed split S_2* (consider atrial septal defect)
- 4. *Clicks* (consider mitral valve prolapse [MVP])
- 5. *Opening snap* (consider mitral valve stenosis)
- 6. *Friction rubs* (consider pericarditis)

       F. Palpation
- 1. *Thrills, heaves (left ventricular [LV] dysfunction: apical; right ventricular [RV] or left atrial [LA] dysfunction: parasternal)*
- 2. *Displacement of point of maximal impulse (PMI)*
- 3. *Widened aortic pulsation >2.5 cm* (consider abdominal aortic aneurysm)
- 4. *Hepatomegaly*
- 5. *Exaggerated, widened femoral pulse* (consider femoral aneurysm)
- 6. *Absence of peripheral pulse(s)*

       G. **Bruits, especially new ones:** record presence or absence (presence may indicate renal artery stenosis or abdominal aortic aneurysm)

       H. *Swelling and pain in one leg only*

    VI. *Referral*
- A. *Emergency transfer to ED with*
  - 1. *Chest pain of cardiac origin (e.g., suspected MI or new angina)*
  - 2. *Suspected aortic dissection*
  - 3. *Pulmonary embolism*
  - 4. *New or refractory HF*
  - 5. *Acute arterial insufficiency*
- B. *To Cardiologist: symptomatic childhood or adult murmurs*

ABDOMINAL

    I. Emphasis on HPI (also see Chapter 9, ABDOMINAL PAIN, if indicated) and ROS
- A. Location (see Fig. 9.1 and Table 9.1 for pain sites)
- B. Onset and changes (e.g., worsening, more constant)
- C. Characteristics (e.g., sharp, crampy, dull)
- D. Associated symptoms (e.g., nausea, vomiting, diarrhea)
- E. Presence or absence of appetite and fever; unexpected weight loss or gain
- F. Review of 24-h dietary intake and presence of similar symptoms in the patient's family

    II. PMH
- A. Usual elimination patterns
- B. Ulcer or gallbladder disease
- C. Irritable bowel syndrome or inflammatory bowel disease
- D. Abdominal operations (open and laparoscopic)
- E. Women: date of last menstrual period (LMP), type of contraception used
- F. Recent travel or exposure to known sick individuals

    III. FH of GI tract disorders

    IV. Examination (include respiratory and cardiovascular examinations in case of abdominal complaints)
- A. Inspection
  - 1. For contours, scars, striae
  - 2. Have the patient raise their head and shoulders off the table; look for localized abdominal swelling (possible hernia or mass)

■ = not to be missed; ● = non-urgent referral; ▲ = urgent referral

       3. For engorged veins (consider hepatic cirrhosis or inferior vena cava obstruction)

       4. For abdominal distention (consider ascites or abdominal tumor)

  B. Auscultate for bowel sounds

  C. Percussion

     1. Liver and splenic borders

     2. Other areas as necessary

     3. Costovertebral angle tenderness (CVAT): the patient must sit for this test

  D. Palpation

     1. Light for generalized tenderness

     2. Deep

       (a) For masses, palpable or tender liver or spleen border, for width of aorta

       (b) For rebound tenderness or guarding

     3. Inguinal nodes

  E. Rectal examination (if indicated)

     1. Check for rectal masses, fecal retention, abnormal prostate

     2. Consider obtaining stool sample for occult blood

V. Examination findings *not to be missed*

  A. *"Acute abdomen"* (also see Chapter 9, ABDOMINAL PAIN)

  B. *Pulsating mass or aorta > 2.5 cm*

  C. *Hernia*

  D. *Hepatosplenomegaly (whether tender or not), abdominal distention* (consider ascites or abdominal tumor)

  E. *Engorged veins* (consider cirrhosis or inferior vena cava obstruction)

  F. *Abnormal bowel sounds*

     1. *High pitched, tinkling* (consider intestinal obstruction)

     2. *Decreased or absent* (consider paralytic ileus or peritonitis)

  G. *New bruits*

  H. *Palpable inguinal lymph nodes* (consider infection or malignancy, Table 1.3)

  I. *Pregnancy*

  J. *Purple striae indicative of Cushing syndrome* (see Chapter 15)

VI. *Referral*

  A. *Transfer to ED with symptoms suggestive of an acute abdomen or aortic aneurysm*

  B. *Patients with an initial diagnosis of hepatic cirrhosis or Cushing disease*

  C. *Any abdominal bruit* (may obtain appropriate ultrasound first)

  D. *Rectal mass or inguinal lymphadenopathy*

GENITOURINARY (MALE)

I. Emphasis on HPI and ROS

  A. Penile pain, discharge, or abnormal lesions

  B. Pain or swelling of scrotum/testicles

  C. Difficulty with urination, increased frequency or abnormal stream

  D. Difficulty with intercourse (e.g., ejaculation, pain, erection)

  E. Abnormal discoloration or lesions in the "boxer area"

II. PMH

  A. Prostatitis, benign prostatic hyperplasia (BPH), sexually transmitted infections (STIs) (which ones and last treated), genital warts

  B. Urinary stream difficulties and/or nocturia, incontinence

  C. Sexual dysfunction

  D. Penile or testicular injuries or infections

■ = *not to be missed;* ▲ = *urgent referral*

  E. Circumcision, phimosis
  F. Gynecomastia
  G. genitourinary (GU)-related surgeries (e.g., for injuries, trauma, prostate) or treatments
III. FH
  A. Genital cancers
  B. Low testosterone
  C. Osteoporosis
  D. Abnormal sexual development
IV. Examination (should include general observation for secondary sexual characteristics)
  A. Penis
   1. Skin around base of penis for nits or lice
   2. Skin lesions, pain or deformity of the penis (e.g., induration in ventral surface could indicate urethral stricture)
   3. Note location of urethra and any redness or discharge
   4. If uncircumcised, retract the foreskin and note any lesions (e.g., syphilitic chancre); be sure to replace foreskin
  B. Scrotum and testicles
   1. Inspect scrotum for contour, note any abnormal swelling; transilluminate if needed. Lift up scrotum and inspect the posterior surface.
   2. Note symmetry of scrotal sac; normally the left testis is slightly longer than the right. If the right is significantly longer than the left, suspect situs inversus or renal cell cancer and obtain renal ultrasound (U/S).
   3. Gently palpate testis, noting size and any lumps, swelling, or tenderness.
   4. If area of swelling is noted in supine position, listen with stethoscope over the area for bowel sounds (this indicates a hernia); in supine position, the mass may resolve.
  C. Hernias
   1. Inspect inguinal and femoral areas for bulges; ask patient to bear down or strain and note any bulges.
   2. Manually check for inguinal hernias: ask patient to bear down to see if a bulge/hernia is felt.
V. Examination findings *not to be missed* and *referral to urologist*
  A. *Phimosis, balanitis, epispadias*
  B. *Peyronie's disease, suspected urethral stricture*
  C. *Undescended testicle or right testis lower than left*
  D. *Painless nodule on testicle*
  E. *Hydrocele, varicocele*
  F. *Large or painful hernias*
  G. *Abnormal lesions, inguinal lymphadenopathy* (see Table 1.3)
VI. *Referral to ED with sudden onset testicular pain* see **Chapter 11, Common Disorders in Men, TESTICULAR TORSION)**

GENITOURINARY (FEMALE)

 I. Emphasis on HPI and ROS
  A. Menstrual history (age at menarche, last menstrual period (LMP), age at menopause)
  B. Sexual history
   1. Age at first intercourse, number of sexual partners
   2. STIs (which ones and last treated), genital warts
  C. Obstetric history (number of pregnancies, live births, abortions/miscarriages)
  D. Use of contraception (ask: "What do you do to prevent pregnancy?")

■ = *not to be missed;* ● = *non-urgent referral;* ▲ = *urgent referral*

II. PMH
    A. Date of last Pap smear and results; history of abnormal Pap smears
    B. Menopausal symptoms, dyspareunia, vaginal discharge, lesions
    C. Urinary incontinence
    D. Last mammogram (and bone mineral density (BMD), if indicated)
    E. Gallbladder disease
    F. Heart disease
    G. Varicose veins
    H. Nutritional history

III. FH
    A. Breast or reproductive tract cancer
    B. Heart disease, HTN
    C. DM
    D. Osteoporosis
    E. Thyroid problems

IV. Examination
    A. Breast (if patient has concerns, e.g., lump, pain, nipple discharge)
      1. Inspect for skin redness, dimpling, or puckering; specifically, inspect while the woman:
        (a) Places her hands on her hips and shrugs her shoulders backward
        (b) Presses her palms together over her head
      2. Palpate breasts and axillary, supraclavicular, and epitrochlear nodes (with patient supine)
    B. Urethra: check for discharge and erythema
    C. External genitalia
      1. Inspect hair pattern and observe for lesions
      2. Determine the presence and condition of the hymen
      3. Perineal support: spread the labia and have the patient "bear down"; inspect for drainage and rectocele or cystocele
    D. Palpate Bartholin, urethral, and Skene glands for pain, swelling, drainage
    E. Perform vaginal examination
      1. Insert a speculum to visualize the cervix and vaginal walls (lubricate speculum if needed with warm water; may use K-Y jelly if not obtaining Pap smear).
      2. Inspect vaginal walls for color, discharge, rugae and lesions.
      3. Inspect cervix
        (a) For color, parity, lesions, discharge, friability
        (b) Note the cervical os for size and position and any lesions
      4. Obtain indicated cultures and Pap smear
        (a) Gonorrhea/Chlamydia (GC/CT) culture can also be done with the Pap smear.
        (b) GC/CT culture can also be done with a swab or with a urine specimen.
        (c) Perform a wet prep, if indicated (see the following section, "How to do a wet prep").
    F. How to do a wet prep
      1. Items needed: three cotton-tipped applicators; two capped test tubes, one with 1–2 mL of saline and one with 1–2 mL of potassium hydroxide (KOH) solution; nitrazine paper; two slides with slide covers.
      2. Obtain specimens from the lateral wall of the vagina; place one of the applicators in each of the test tubes.
      3. Use third applicator to check vaginal pH with nitrazine paper (normal is <5).
      4. Perform a "whiff" test by smelling the applicator in the KOH tube; the result is considered positive if there is an "amine" or fishy odor.

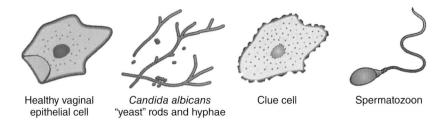

Healthy vaginal   *Candida albicans*   Clue cell   Spermatozoon
epithelial cell   "yeast" rods and hyphae

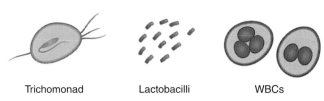

Trichomonad   Lactobacilli   WBCs

Fig. 1.8   Microscopic findings for wet prep.

     5. If pH is normal and whiff is negative, no further testing may be needed for bacterial vaginosis (BV).
     6. Microscopic evaluation
        (a) Prepare the slides: using the applicator, place a few drops from the saline tube on one slide and top with a slide cover; repeat with the KOH tube applicator on the other slide.
        (b) View under high power to look for (Fig. 1.8):
           (i) Saline slide: epithelial cells, white blood cells (WBCs), clue cells, lactobacilli, or trichomoniasis
           (ii) KOH slide: yeast buds and hyphae
   G. Bimanual examination (palpation)
     1. Cervix for contour, smoothness, cervical motion tenderness
     2. Uterus for size, shape, position, and consistency (Fig. 1.9)
     3. Adnexa for size, presence of masses, and tenderness; if unable to palpate, document such (it is often difficult to palpate adnexa in larger women)
  V. Examination findings *not to be missed*
    A. *Skin lesions, abnormal discharge*
    B. *Cervical motion tenderness* (consider pelvic infection or inflammation)
    C. *Enlarged or tender uterus*
    D. *Adnexal fullness or tenderness*
    E. *Breast mass or nipple discharge*
    F. *Lymphadenopathy in axilla, supraclavicular or epitrochlear areas* (see Table 1.3)
 VI. *Referral*
    A. *To ED: abdominal pain with suspected ectopic pregnancy* (may/may not have spotting)
    B. *To OB/GYN urgently: suspected malignancy* (e.g., uterine, ovarian, vulvar)

◼ = *not to be missed;* ▲ = *urgent referral*

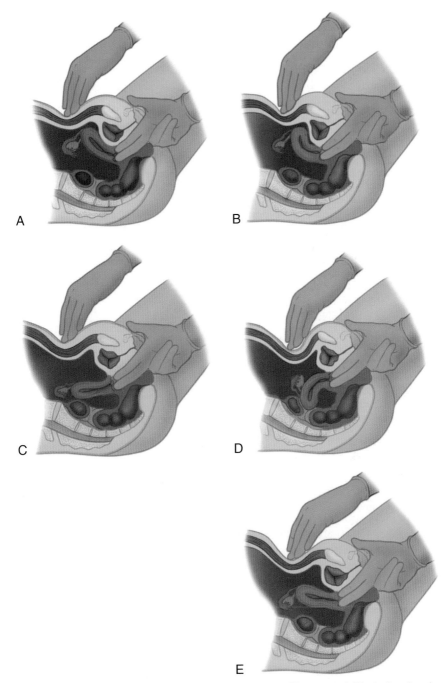

Fig. 1.9 Cervix and uterus positions. (A) Anteverted; (B) anteflexed; (C) retroverted; (D) retroflexed; and (E) midposition. (From Seidel, H. M., Stewart, R. W., Ball, J. W., Dains, J. E., Flynn, J. A., Solomon, B. S., & Stewart, R. W. (2011). *Mosby's guide to physical examination* (7th ed.). Philadelphia: Elsevier.)

MUSCULOSKELETAL

   I. See Chapter 13 for specific joint examinations.

  II. For overall MS examination

     A. Inspect joints for redness, increased heat, ROM

     B. Examine the back for abnormal curvatures and document if present

     C. Observe gait

  III. May be combined with neurological system

NEUROLOGICAL
(MAY BE INTEGRATED WITH THE REST OF THE EXAMINATION)

   I. Focus on HPI and ROS

     A. Dizziness, vertigo, loss of consciousness

     B. Vision or hearing changes, tinnitus

     C. Fever, sinus drainage, allergy symptoms

     D. Nausea or vomiting

     E. Headache (also see Chapter 12, HEADACHES)

     F. Paresthesias or numbness in extremities

     G. Confusion or mental status changes (also see Chapter 17, COGNITIVE IMPAIRMENT/DEMENTIA)

  II. PMH

     A. Past CVA or TIA(s)

     B. HTN

     C. DM

     D. Diagnosis of cognitive impairment or dementia

     E. Migraine or cluster headaches

     F. Past head injuries or intracranial surgery

  III. FH

     A. CVA

     B. HTN

     C. DM

     D. Migraine headaches

  IV. Examination

     A. Cognitive status (for further evaluation, see Chapter 17, COGNITIVE IMPAIRMENT/DEMENTIA)

       1. Evaluate for orientation to person, place, and time.

       2. Determine judgment and problem-solving abilities: ask, "If you smell smoke in the house, what do you do?"

       3. Test abstract thinking: ask the patient to explain a proverb such as "A stitch in time saves nine."

       4. Evaluate affect: behaviors that may signify depression or mood lability (see Chapter 3, Fig. 3.1 for an example).

     B. Language

       1. Test verbal abilities—namely, speech patterns, fluency, and content (Table 1.4).

       2. Test the ability to write and copy.

       3. Check gestures and the ability to follow serial and three-step commands; for example, ask the patient, "Hold up your right hand, stick out your tongue, and close your eyes."

TABLE 1.4 ■ **Speech Disturbances: Characteristics and Pattern**

Speech Disturbance	Characteristics
Fluent aphasia (Wernicke area)	Lacks content Unable to comprehend spoken words and phrases Unable to repeat or name objects
Nonfluent aphasia (Broca area)	Slow, scanning speech Intact comprehension Impaired writing ability Inability to verbally express thoughts
Global aphasia (both Broca and Wernicke areas)	Nonfluent speech Unable to comprehend, read, or write Unable to name objects

    4. Check whether the patient has appropriate recognition skills (i.e., the ability to name common objects).

    5. Check reading ability and comprehension.

C. Vision

    1. See EYE section for description of visual acuity examination.

    2. Ophthalmologic examination (Tables 1.1 and 1.2).

D. Sensory: head and neck

    1. Always test right and left separately.

    2. Check tactile ability: ask the patient to identify the body part being touched.

    3. Test auditory ability: Rinne and Weber tests (see Fig. 1.3) and sound comprehension.

E. Motor

    1. Gait and any assistive devices (e.g., walker, quad cane)

    2. Test muscle strength

       (a) Upper extremities: shoulder abduction, elbow and wrist flexion and extension

       (b) Lower extremities: hip and knee flexion and extension, ankle dorsiflexion, and plantar flexion

    3. Grading scale for motor (muscle) strength:

       5 = normal

       4 = weak but able to resist the examiner

       3 = moves against gravity but cannot resist the examiner

       2 = moves but unable to resist gravity (passive range of motion (ROM) only)

       1 = has muscle contraction but limited or no joint motion

       0 = no movement

F. Cranial nerve (CN) examination (Table 1.5)

    1. Central nervous system (CNS) lesions cause contralateral facial weakness below the eyes (the forehead is spared).

    2. Peripheral CN VII lesions may cause complete facial weakness (including the forehead).

G. Coordination

    1. Ability to perform rapid alternating movements—have the patient alternately pronate and supinate the hand against a stable surface (e.g., a table or patient's own thigh).

    2. Finger-to-nose: ask the patient to touch their nose and the examiner's finger alternately with rapid repetition; observe for accuracy and tremor.

TABLE 1.5 ■ Cranial Nerve Examination

Cranial Nerve	Type and Function	Tests	Abnormal Findings
Olfactory	Sensory: Smell	Do not use ammonia Test each nostril separately with alcohol preparation, mint, and coffee	Obstructive nasal passage Lesions of the frontal lobe, pituitary uncus, or hippocampal gyrus
▲ Optic	Sensory: Central and peripheral vision	Snellen chart Newspaper print Color vision Count fingers in peripheral fields Ophthalmoscopic examination	**Amaurosis (loss of vision); refer immediately** Cataracts Cortical blindness Papilledema Optic atrophy
Oculomotor	Motor: Pupillary constriction Eyelid elevation	Pupil size, symmetry, shape, and accommodation	Ptosis Nonreactive pupil Anisocoria Optic nerve lesions
Trochlear	Motor: Eye movements	Follow a finger or object in all planes (EOMs)	Nystagmus* Diplopia Dysconjugate gaze
Trigeminal	Sensory and motor: Tongue and facial sensation Corneal reflex	Pinprick to face with eyes closed Have the patient open and close the jaw Corneal reflex (use a drop of saline)	Loss of sensation, paresthesia, or pain Deviation of jaw Lack of blink reflex
Abducens	Motor: Lateral eye movement	(Test with CN III and IV)	
Facial	Sensory and motor: Facial expression Salivary and lacrimal glands Taste	Have the patient wrinkle the forehead, grimace, raise eyebrows, smile, and frown Taste: sweet, sour, and bitter substances to the anterior tongue	Asymmetry of face Deviation of mouth Weakness of forehead Inability to close eyes Loss of taste Excessive tearing
Acoustic[†]	Sensory: Hearing Equilibrium	Rinne and Weber tests Whisper Ticking watch Equilibrium	Unilateral deafness Tinnitus Lateralization Vertigo, dizziness, or ataxia
Glossopharyngeal	Sensory and motor: Taste on the posterior tongue Gag or swallow	Taste: sweet, sour, and bitter substances to the posterior tongue Gag and swallow	Loss of taste Loss of gag or swallow Dysphagia
Vagus	Sensory and motor: Gag or swallow	Inspect the soft palate Uvula in the midline Stimulate the pharyngeal wall Voice quality	Loss of voice or hoarseness Deviation of uvula Coughing and choking
Accessory	Motor: Fluid movement of the head and neck in flexion, extension, and rotation	Palpate trapezius and sternocleidomastoid muscles Have the patient turn the head against resistance Have the patient shrug the shoulders against resistance	Paralysis or weakness Atrophy Spasticity

▲ = *urgent referral*

Continued

TABLE 1.5 ■ Cranial Nerve Examination—cont'd

Cranial Nerve	Type and Function	Tests	Abnormal Findings
Hypoglossal	Motor: Tongue movement	Have the patient move the tongue side to side Observe for symmetry and rhythmicity	Spastic paralysis Deviation from the midline Dysarthria Spastic speech

* Marked nystagmus on lateral gaze or any nystagmus on vertical gaze suggests a peripheral or CNS lesion.
† Ask the patient to hum if he or she has decreased hearing: if the hum is louder in the affected ear, this would be a conductive defect; if the hum is louder in the unaffected ear, this indicates a sensorineural defect.
CN, cranial nerve; *EOMs,* extraocular muscles.

3. Heel-to-shin: have the patient place his or her heel on the opposite knee and slide the heel down the shin to the foot; observe for accuracy and tremor.
4. Romberg test: have the patient stand with the feet together and eyes open for 20–30 sec and then with eyes closed for 20–30 sec (there should be minimal, if any, swaying). Then check pronator drift: while continuing to stand with eyes closed, have the patient raise the arms straight forward with the palms up and hold for 30 sec (both arms should remain in position); then gently press down on each wrist and the arm should return to the previous position.

H. Gait
1. Ask the patient to walk forward on heels and backward on tiptoes.
2. Observe tandem gait (ability to walk a straight line, as if on a tightrope).

I. Sensory: peripheral
1. Compare right and left sides with the patient's eyes covered or closed
2. Definitions
   (a) Hyperesthesia: excessively sensitive to touch
   (b) Paresthesia: sensations without stimulation from the examiner
3. Evaluate the patient's ability to discern the following:
   (a) Vibration: use a tuning fork on the distal interphalangeal (DIP) joints of both thumbs and both big toes.
   (b) Light touch: use a wisp of cotton.
   (c) Stereognosis: patient recognizes an item placed in the hand (e.g., a quarter).
   (d) Two-point discrimination: touch the patient in various places at the same time using sharp and dull objects and note any differences; if felt on only one side, CNS sensory deficit is present on the opposite side of the brain.
   (e) Temperature: blow gently on the patient's skin (medial wrist is best) with lips apart (warm) and lips pursed (cool); may also use very warm and cold water in test tubes.

J. Reflexes (also see figure on next page)
1. Assess for symmetry.
2. Check for deep tendon reflexes (DTRs): the joint being tested should be at approximately 90 degrees and fully relaxed.
3. In patients with altered level of consciousness (LOC) or possible CVA or paralysis, the following reflexes may also be checked:
   (a) Abdominal: stroke the skin above and below the umbilicus; normally, the umbilicus moves toward the side stimulated.
   (b) Plantar: stroke the sole of the foot from the heel to the big toe with a blunt object; normally, the toes flex; a positive (abnormal) Babinski sign occurs when the big toe moves up and the toes fan out.
4. Comparison of central and peripheral nervous system lesions (Table 1.6).

TABLE 1.6 ■ **Distinguishing Central and Peripheral Lesions**

	Upper Motor Neuron (central nervous system)	Lower Motor Neuron (peripheral)
Deep tendon reflexes	Increased	Decreased
Muscle tone	Increased	Decreased
Atrophy	Not usually	Yes
Fasciculations	No	Yes
Babinski reflex	Present	Absent

	Reflex	*Level*	*Normal Response*
	Biceps, A	C5–C6	Elbow flexion
	Triceps, B	C7	Elbow extension
	Brachioradialis, C	C6–C7	Wrist flexion
	Patellar, D	L3–L4	Knee extension
	Achilles, E	S1	Foot extension

Scoring: 0, absent; 1+, weak; 2+, normal; 3+, exaggerated; 4+, clonus.

■   **V.** Examination findings *not to be missed*
■   A. *Cognitive or mental status changes*
■   B. *Speech disturbances* (Table 1.4)
■   C. *Inability to write* (agraphia)
■   D. *Inability to read, if the patient previously able to read* (alexia)
■   E. *Inability to execute volitional activity* (apraxia)
■   F. *Inability to complete coordination tests*
        G. Gait abnormalities
■   1. *Staggering, unsteady, wide-based* (ataxia)
■   2. *Spasticity or bradykinesia*
■   3. *Shuffling or Parkinson-like gait*
■   4. *Foot drop*
    VI. *Referral*
▲   A. *To ED via ambulance with suspected CVA or TIA*
●   B. *To Neurologist with gait abnormalities, inability to perform the coordination tests, or new tremor*

SPORTS PHYSICAL EXAMINATION

I. Goals of the examination include the following:
    A. To identify problems carrying risks of life-threatening complications during participation (e.g., hypertrophic cardiomyopathy)
    B. To maximize safe participation in sports

■ = *not to be missed;* ● = *non-urgent referral;* ▲ = *urgent referral*

   C. To identify conditions requiring a treatment plan (e.g., HTN)

   D. To identify and treat old musculoskeletal injuries

   E. To identify and treat conditions that can interfere with performance (e.g., exercise-induced bronchospasm)

   F. To remove unnecessary restrictions on participation

II. The emphasis of history and examination is on cardiovascular, respiratory, and musculoskeletal systems. The medical history is the most sensitive and specific part of the examination for detecting possible condition(s) that would restrict or exclude participation.

   A. Each school or organization will have an evaluation form to be completed for sports participation.

      1. The history section is completed by the athlete or parent/guardian; the provider reviews this with the athlete and writes comments on any positive answers.

      2. The history section includes questions about symptoms/signs suggesting possible serious medical conditions.

      3. The physical examination section is completed by the provider (or providers if the examination is completed by more than one person).

   B. For the history of past injuries, ask about the following:

      1. Previous exclusion from sports for any reason

      2. Length of time lost from participation

      3. Current sequelae of the injury

      4. Any loss of consciousness or amnesia after a head injury

   C. Most children and teens with chronic medical conditions can participate in sports at some level after evaluation and treatment. (see IV. Referral for conditions requiring a treatment plan, later in this section).

   D. The cardiovascular history questions are aimed at identifying conditions that predispose to sudden death. Sudden cardiac death (SCD) is disproportionately more common in males. Cardiovascular conditions that predispose individuals to SCD are rare and difficult to treat.

III. Physical examination is directed by the form used; components listed below are included for evaluation, because if present, further evaluation is required.

   A. Musculoskeletal

      1. Pain or restriction of movement with full neck ROM

      2. Asymmetric shoulder height

      3. Swelling of any extremity

      4. Limited shoulder ROM

      5. Asymmetry or loss of motion with elbow ROM (especially if the student is involved in throwing sports)

      6. Inability to "duck walk"

      7. Inability to hop five times on each foot without ankle pain or instability

   B. Cardiovascular

      1. Vital signs ("normal" range depends on the age of the athlete; some states also have guidelines)

      2. Ideal body weight (<85th percentile)

      3. ECG if an FH of atrial fibrillation, SCD, or arrhythmia is present, or if the athlete has a history of tachycardia that does not resolve with rest

   C. Concussions

      1. The return to play plan for each athlete should be personalized, gradual, and progressive; a provider with experience in evaluating and managing sports-related concussion should make the final decision.

2. Although most athletes will be able to return to play within a month, the full progression may take days, weeks, or even months.
3. Worrisome signs of possible permanent brain injury include the following:
   (a) Prolonged recovery time
   (b) Shorter intervals between concussions
   (c) Progressively less force needed to cause a concussion
4. Providers may check for current guidelines at www.cdc.gov/concussion/clinicain.html. Consider SCAT5 form for assessment of concussions.

IV. *Referral:* **athletes with the following symptoms or conditions should be evaluated by a specialist before participation in sports activities:**
   A. *Cardiac*
      1. HTN (see Table 2.3)
      2. Undiagnosed systolic heart murmur louder than grade 2/6
      3. Any bruits
      4. Complaints of dyspnea on exertion, fatigue, atypical or angina chest pain, presyncope or syncope (especially during or immediately following exertion), palpitations, lightheadedness; these can be symptoms of hypertrophic cardiomyopathy (formerly called idiopathic hypertrophic subaortic stenosis [IHSS]), coronary artery anomalies, dysrhythmias, or Wolff-Parkinson-White syndrome
      5. Personal history or FH of Marfan syndrome
      6. FH of death from heart problems or of sudden death before 50 yr of age (including drowning or unexplained car accident)
   B. *Musculoskeletal*
      1. Restriction/limitation of joint ROM or painful ROM of joint; inability to "duck walk"
      2. Down syndrome with atlantoaxial instability
      3. Cerebral palsy or muscular dystrophy
   C. *Neurologic*
      1. History of head or spinal trauma, craniotomy
      2. Severe or repeated concussions, including the following:
         (a) Persistent symptoms lasting 21 days or longer after injury
         (b) Repeated concussions that occur with less force and/or are associated with more intense symptoms or more cognitive dysfunction
      3. Poorly controlled seizure disorder
   D. *Miscellaneous*
      1. Loss of an eye or the best vision in the good eye is worse than 20/40
      2. History of detached retina, previous eye surgery, or serious eye injury
      3. Absent kidney or testicle
      4. Enlarged liver or spleen
      5. Malignancy
      6. Organ transplant recipient
      7. Sickle cell disease
      8. Bleeding disorders
      9. Uncontrolled DM
      10. Pregnancy
      11. Eating disorders (e.g., anorexia nervosa or bulimia)
V. Conditions requiring a treatment plan before or during exercise
   A. Exercise-induced bronchoconstriction
   B. HTN
VI. Return to play after recovery from COVID-19 illness or following a positive test

---

■ = *not to be missed;* ● = *non-urgent referral*

A. There are currently no evidence-based guidelines available to help direct decisions; however, there are recommendations from authorities experienced in sports medicine.
 1. Refrain from exercise for
  (a) Asymptomatic: 3 days after positive test
  (b) Mild illness: 3 days after symptom onset and symptoms resolved
  (c) Moderate illness/CV symptoms: at least 5 days after symptom onset and symptoms resolved
 2. All athletes with moderate or severe illness should have a clinical evaluation before returning to activity.
B. The period of inactivity can result in a degree of "detraining." This must be kept in mind with any recommendations for return to play.
C. The following steps can be used to help guide return to play decisions. They are based on the severity of the COVID-19 infection/illness and the presence of high-risk, comorbid cardiac disease. They also assume the athlete is at least 5 days from the symptom onset.
 1. Asymptomatic or mild disease
  (a) No ongoing signs or symptoms (S/S): gradual return to play with periodic reassessment
  (b) If athlete has S/S (other than loss of taste/smell), continued rest for 4–6 wk from symptom onset
   (i) At reassessment, if all S/S are resolved, the athlete can start gradual return to play with periodic reassessment.
   (ii) With persistent S/S ***referral*** **to cardiologist and/or pulmonologist (concern for myocarditis, possible pulmonary embolism (PE) or pneumonia, residual pulmonary injury).**
 2. Moderate or severe illness or presence of high-risk, comorbid cardiac disease: obtain ECG, high-sensitivity troponin and echocardiogram; ask, "Are signs consistent with myocarditis?"
  (a) Yes: ***Referral*** **to cardiology**
  (b) No: Are there ongoing S/S?
   (i) Yes: continued rest for 4–6 wk from symptom onset; if still persistent S/S at recheck, ***referral*** **to cardiologist and/or pulmonologist (concern for myocarditis, possible PE or pneumonia, residual pulmonary injury).**
   (ii) No: gradual return to play with periodic reassessment.
D. As the athlete is returning to sports activities, monitor for "red flag" signs or symptoms that may indicate possible myocarditis or PE; if present, the athlete needs to be seen urgently by a provider or at the ED.
 1. Chest pain or palpitations
 2. Breathlessness beyond what would be expected during recovery from exercise
 3. S/S of possible blood clot or PE: tachycardia, dyspnea at rest, swollen leg
E. There is no consensus on how long to take to progress from recovery and rest to light and then moderate and then intense activity, and finally to normal training and full play.
 1. The American Academy of Pediatrics (AAP) recommends:
  (a) Younger than 12 yr of age: progress back to sports and PE classes as tolerated
  (b) Children over 12 yr of age and adolescents: gradual return to play once cleared by a provider, the athlete is at least 3–5 days without symptoms and has no cardiac or respiratory symptoms with ADLs. The return to play should be

---

▲ = *urgent referral*

over at least 7 days. If the patient has not participated in consistent physical activity for >1 mo:
  (i) Start at 25% of usual volume and intensity of activity
  (ii) Increase volume and intensity by 10% weekly until reaching desired level
  2. Strength training resumption: see guidelines from the National Strength and Conditioning Association (NSCA) and/or the Collegiate Strength and Conditioning Coaches Association (CSCCa) of the United States.
VII. Performance-enhancing substances
  A. Advise patients/parents that OTC supplements are not regulated and may be contaminated with substances that can be harmful or are banned by the World Anti-Doping Agency (WADA). Also, the supplement label may list the chemical name or the plant from which it comes, making it difficult to determine if the supplement is safe.
  B. Amino acids: no evidence that they improve performance or increase lean body weight more than regular food.
  C. Caffeine (especially in the form of "energy drinks" or "shots")
    1. Found to increase endurance and reaction times and to delay fatigue.
    2. Doses of 250 mg/day can cause insomnia, tachycardia, nervousness, GI complaints (each energy drink contains 50–500 mg caffeine).
    3. Caffeine withdrawal can cause fatigue and headaches, which may adversely affect the competing athlete.
  D. Creatine
    1. It has been shown to improve performance in sports involving short intervals of high-intensity effort (e.g., football, rugby, racquet sports); its effects on endurance sports are inconsistent.
    2. Up to 30% of people do not respond to creatine supplements.
    3. Because the potential long-term effects are not known, it is not recommended for adolescence use.
  E. Dietary antioxidants
    1. Have not consistently shown to decrease muscle damage or soreness in acute exercise.
    2. Includes beetroot juice and substances such as quercetin, resveratrol, vitamins E and C, N-acetylcysteine, and glutathione.
  F. Guarana
    1. Commonly included in energy drinks and supplements.
    2. There are no controlled research studies on its effects on athletes.
  G. Nitrates
    1. Present in whole vegetables and vegetable juices; also found in supplements.
    2. May be beneficial in a high-intensity event lasting 4–8 min (e.g., sprint cycling, rowing, swimming), especially in less fit athletes; it is not as effective in highly trained athletes.
    3. Athlete should ensure than any nitrate-containing supplement uses only the inorganic form of nitrate (nitrites can be toxic).
    4. Because oral bacteria are involved in nitrate metabolism, the athlete should avoid using antibacterial mouthwashes and chewing gum.
  H. Tart cherry juice
    1. Produces antiinflammatory and antioxidant effects.
    2. May decrease muscle soreness and improve recovery times; may improve performance in endurance sports.

CHAPTER 2

Pediatric Assessment

INTRODUCTION

I. The goals of pediatric assessment are as follows:
   A. To record and monitor overall growth and development from birth through late adolescence.
   B. To verify attainment of age-related milestones.
   C. To identify problems with the patient's psychosocial maturity and/or problem-solving abilities.
   D. To note any deviations or problems that the parent/caregiver has identified.
   E. To identify any genetic anomalies and seek appropriate referral when necessary.

II. The assessment should always consist of identifying normal patterns of development; if illness is main focus, consider pattern in symptoms.

III. The approach to pediatric assessment depends on the goal of the encounter: is this a well-child checkup or illness visit?
   A. Identifying the problem is the most difficult issue; the infant/toddler cannot say specifically what the problem is in words, and many times the caregiver also cannot identify the presenting problem; however, as the patient matures, the problems are easier to identify.
   B. Always try to establish a rapport with both the caregiver and the patient; pediatric assessment relies heavily on the trust between the caregiver, pediatric patient, and practitioner.
   C. Always assume a calm, matter-of-fact attitude; children can sense uncomfortableness or nervousness.

IV. Assessment findings may vary with each visit, depending on the stage of growth and development exhibited by the patient.

V. Inspection is the most important clue; your eyes and ears are the best tools for assessment.

HEALTH HISTORY

I. Patient profile
   A. Document the patient's name, age, birth date, sex, ethnic background, and cultural and religious practices of child and/or family at the time of the visit.
   B. Name of the physician/pediatrician, dentist, or other health care provider involved with the patient's care.
   C. Identify current living arrangements/situation (e.g., lives with parent[s] or foster care).
   D. Home environment (exposure to smoke, alcohol, drugs, or unsafe practices).
   E. Leisure activities and physical activity; amount of time spent watching television or playing computer or video games.
   F. Habits such as smoking, drug use, nail biting, temper tantrums, or hair pulling/twisting.

G. Patient should be assessed for depression, suicide, and alcohol/drug abuse with appropriate screening at least annually; examples are:
   1. Modified Patient Health Questionnaire (PHQ)-9 for adolescents for depression
   2. CRAFFT for adolescents for substance use
   3. SAD PERSONS for suicide; elementary and middle school

II. Chief complaint or reason for the visit
   A. Try to elicit the patient's and caregiver's reason for the visit; is this a well-child exam, personal, or illness-related visit?
   B. The caregiver may have other reasons for seeking health care besides the scheduled visit; this may be related to sensitive, personal reasons for both the caregiver and the patient.

III. History of present illness
   A. A well-child visit focuses on growth and development, assessing developmental milestones, nutritional habits, and safety in the home and during outside activities, as well as the immunization status and current medications, including over-the-counter (OTC) and herbal products.
   B. An episodic illness examination focuses on the specific reason for the visit.

IV. Review of the past medical history is important at all visits
   A. Prenatal history
      1. Health during pregnancy (e.g., hypertension [HTN], edema, gestational diabetes, thyroid disorder)
      2. Any history of drug, alcohol, or tobacco use
      3. Obstetric history of this and previous pregnancies (e.g., gravida, para, ectopic pregnancy, or abortions)
   B. Birth and neonatal history, including any difficulty with delivery
      1. Apgar score (if known)
      2. Preterm birth, and gestational age at delivery
      3. Intensive care admission and reason
      4. O_2 for any length of time, and reason for O_2
      5. Hearing/vision screenings performed at birth, and what were the results?
      6. First hepatitis B immunization given?
      7. Any immunizations given at birth, results of any laboratory tests at birth
   C. Note growth, social and personal development
      1. Have developmental milestones been achieved on time (Table 2.1)?
      2. At what age was the patient toilet trained; if toilet trained, does the patient have accidents and are they continent at night?
      3. Any phobias, nightmares, walking in sleep
      4. Grade and performance in school; any behavior problems at school?
      5. Type of discipline; problems identified at home, school, or in social settings
      6. Attention span and perceived hyperactivity
   D. Past illnesses/injuries
      1. Any childhood illnesses/injuries; if so, what were they and how were they treated?
      2. Past hospitalizations/surgeries
      3. Past blood or blood product transfusions

V. Family history (FH) and dynamics
   A. Composition of the family
   B. Congenital abnormalities or illnesses identified in the family; any history of consanguinity (i.e., sexual relations with a first-degree relative)

TABLE 2.1 ■ Developmental Milestones

Age	Motor Development	Language/Cognitive Development	Social and Emotional Development
Birth– 1 mo	Kicks legs, flails arms, raises head when prone	Cries when hungry, angry, or uncomfortable; presence of rhythmic suck-swallow pattern	Becomes quiet with caregiver's contact
2 mo	Holds head steady when pulled into sitting position	Starts making sounds other than crying; smiles	Reacts to bottle or breast
3 mo	Makes crawling movement; uses arms to start propping self up; visually tracks through the midline	Continues with more different sounds; sustained cooing for up to 20 s; smiles spontaneously; more curious about surroundings	Keeps one hand on the bottle or breast while feeding; begins to recognize and smile at parents
4 mo	Holds hands together, grasps toy	Squeals, laughs, and coos; shows interest in surroundings	Recognizes the caregiver by sight and voice and acts excited when the caregiver is around
5 mo	Rolls over stomach to back; reaches for objects	Orients to sounds	Smiles when the caregiver makes noises
6 mo	Rolls over back to stomach; begins to transfer objects from hand to hand	Babbles; plays with sounds (e.g., blows bubbles and raspberries); recognizes caregiver's voice from a stranger's	Shows likes and dislikes; beginning of "stranger anxiety"
7–8 mo	Sitting without support; bears some weight on legs; transfers objects and will let go of objects at times when asked	Responds to name	"Stranger anxiety" continues
9–10 mo	Pulls to stand; three-finger pincer grasp; able to stand longer toward end of 10 mo; starts to creep on hands and knees	Imitates sounds, begins "mama" and "dada"; understands single words such as "bye bye"	"Stranger anxiety"; begins to play "pat a cake"; cries when objects are taken away
11–12 mo	Gets into sitting position with little help; walks with one hand held, starts "cruising"; two-finger pincer grasp and will release toy when asked	Uses "mama," "dada" specifically for the caregiver; speaks one word (e.g., "no"); knows object permanence	Comes when called; imitates actions; cooperates with dressing
15 mo	Walks backward; has independent locomotion; throws things; stacks two items	Develops 18 sounds; knows objects have purpose	Helps to undress self; feeds self finger foods
18 mo	Descends/ascends stairs with help; throws ball over the hand	Knows 10–50 words, 2–3 body parts; uses echolalia and jargon which peaks at 18 mo	Partially feeds self; undresses self and tries to redress self; enters into the "terrible twos," throws tantrums and becomes more stubborn
2 yr	Runs well; goes up stairs with alternating feet; uses utensils to eat	2–3-word sentences that are understandable, understands more concepts, begins to put puzzles together; copies vertical and horizontal lines; builds tower of three blocks	Refers to self as "I"; may start toilet training; attaches to toys; feeds self

Continued

TABLE 2.1 ■ Developmental Milestones—cont'd

Age	Motor Development	Language/Cognitive Development	Social and Emotional Development
3 yr	Stands on one foot for <1 min; starts trying to ride tricycle; holds sippy cup with one hand Rule of 3: 3 yr, 3 ft, 33 lbs; height 3–4 inches/yr; weight 4–5 lbs/yr	300–500-word vocabulary; speech is mostly understandable but may have some phonologic issues; magical thinking; egocentric; knows age, sex, and full name; asks questions; copies circle	Uses toilet but needs help to wipe, stays dry during the day and mostly at night; washes hands by self; puts on shoes, partially dresses self; starts to interact with others of age and has imaginary friends
4 yr	Climbs well; hops on one foot; cuts across paper	Vocabulary of 1500 words, uses 6–8-word sentences and knows plurals; knows primary colors; copies cross, draws person with 2–4 body parts; uses scissors	Can tell a story; responds to two-part commands; toilets independently but may still have "accidents" at night; brushes teeth with supervision; has cooperative play with peers
5 yr	Swings; prints first name; skips, hops on alternate feet	Copies triangle and square, draws person with body parts; counts up to 10 items; knows four colors	Responds to three-part commands; begins school separation
6 yr	Somersaults; ties shoes, buttons shirt	Copies diamond; knows most of own body parts	Cooperative play, social and friendly

C. Interaction between the patient and caregiver, patient's interactions with siblings and playmates, patient's interactions with authority figures
D. Parental satisfaction with the patient's behavior
E. Is the patient in a daycare, in a public or private school, or home-schooled?
VI. Nutritional status
   A. Bottle- or breast-fed, number of feedings per day, and amount ingested
      1. Less than 1 yr of age: bottle- or breast-fed for how long, length of each feeding
      2. Greater than 1 yr of age: when was cow's milk or other supplement started (e.g., soy, goat, or other milk); is it whole milk or its equivalent?
   B. Does the infant seem satisfied after bottle- or breast-feeding?
   C. Types of foods offered and how much the patient eats daily
   D. Does the child eat with the rest of the family or alone?
   E. Current weight and height and any gain or loss over the past year
   F. Food allergies and what symptoms are elicited
   G. Any pica habits and describe what things are eaten
VII. Sleep habits
   A. Where does the infant/child sleep; in what position is the infant placed for sleeping purposes?
   B. Does the patient sleep all night?
      1. Does the patient sleepwalk, and is there a safety plan for the child?
      2. Does the patient have nightmares/night terrors?
      3. Does the patient snore, how loudly and how often (e.g., every night, few times a week)?
   C. Is there a safety plan in case of fire or other disasters?

VIII. Medication history
    A. Use of any OTC, herbal, prescribed, or illicit medications; does the patient like to take medications, and is this a risk at home? Does the patient take vitamin/fluoride supplements?
    B. Allergies to any medications or environmental pollens/chemicals; what reactions occur?
    C. Immunization history and any problems with immunizations; obtain written immunization record (see www.cdc.gov/vaccines for recommendations for current immunization schedules or Shots immunization app for current and catch-up routine)

Guidelines for Comprehensive Assessment

GENERAL OBSERVATIONS

    I. The overall physical examination for pediatrics is the same as that for adults, although there are some variations specific to pediatrics that are addressed at the following site: www.aap.org/periodicityschedule.
    II. The practitioner may need to change the order of examination and may not be able to perform the entire examination in one visit.
        A. Initially, when first touching the patient, always touch nonthreatening body areas first, such as the head/hair, legs, or feet.
        B. If child is uncooperative, examine pertinent body areas (e.g., heart, lungs, and ears) first because children do not remain quiet for very long.
        C. Use puppets or stuffed animals as distraction (with any age), and allow them to hold objects during examination.
        D. Suggested examination techniques:
            1. Infant on exam table
            2. Preschooler on the parent's lap
            3. Older child on exam table
            4. Adolescent alone in room, if possible
  III. Note that any discrepancies between the history and physical findings should alert the examiner to the possibility of neglect/abuse and should be investigated further.
  IV. The examination begins when the practitioner enters the room; during the "warming up" period the practitioner can assess the child's behavioral patterns and interaction with the caregiver and surroundings.
        A. Assess the overall health status, general symmetry of movement, speech patterns, and nutritional status (see Tables 2.1 and 2.2).
        B. Note the patient's attention to sounds and sights and overall curiosity about the environment.
        C. Observe the patient for unusual characteristics that might indicate genetic abnormalities.
        D. Focus on normal, healthy body parts and perform traumatic procedures last (e.g., eye, ear, nose, throat [EENT], genitalia, painful areas).
        E. Plot height, weight, and head circumference (when appropriate) on a standardized chart at each visit or more often if an abnormality is noted (see Table 2.2).
            1. Use the same chart at each visit for consistency and to easily monitor growth progress.
            2. Measure the head circumference above the eyebrows, above the pinnae, and over the occipital prominence.
            3. Use the same weight scale (if possible) at each visit; if weighing an infant, remove all clothes except for the diaper (weigh the diaper and subtract the diaper weight when entering the weight in the chart).

TABLE 2.2 ■ **Stages of Growth and Development**

Age	Normal Growth Rate	Special Considerations
Birth–12 mo	Birth length: 9–11 inches/yr Birth weight: doubles by 6 mo, triples by 12 mo, quadruples by 24 mo	Rapid, highly variable rate of growth; "catch up" and "catch down" growth ***Refer if height or weight falls >2 standard deviations on growth chart within 2 mo*** Nutritional factors should be monitored closely Observe for **failure to thrive** for any reason Infants should be weighed and measured at every visit (minimum twice yearly) and more often if deviation is noted
12–36 mo	Height: 3–5 inches/yr Average weight gain: approximately 5 lbs/yr from 2 yr to adolescence	Growth rate declines from the neonatal period Between 18 and 24 mo, the growth "channel" (percentile on growth chart) is established Growth patterns and velocity established by 36 mo Weight and height should be performed at least once a year
3–puberty	Height: 2–2.5 inches/yr Weight gain: approximately 5 lbs/yr	Can calculate "mid-parental height" to establish the baseline for height potential. This is only an estimate: add the mother's and father's heights, then add 5 inches for boys or subtract 5 inches for girls, and then divide by 2 Linear growth stabilizes; ***changes in growth velocity signal potential growth or health disorder*** Weight and measurements should be performed at least once a year
Adolescence	Growth rate: rapid and highly variable Onset of pubertal growth spurt: average age is 10 yr for girls and 12.5 yr for boys Weight gain: approximately 5–10 lbs/yr	***Refer precocious puberty (occurring before 8 yr of age)*** Menarche occurs approximately 2 yr after breast buds appear Girls must weigh at least 88–90 lbs before menarche will occur Once puberty begins, growth plates start to close, which stabilizes height ***Refer if puberty is delayed beyond 15 yr of age for boys and girls***

    F. Start screening for underweight patients at the first office visit and obesity in patients 2 yr of age and older.
       1. Underweight is defined as body mass index (BMI) ≤5th percentile for child's age and sex.
       2. Obesity is defined as BMI ≥95th percentile for child's age and sex; severe obesity is defined as BMI ≥99th percentile for child's age and sex.
       3. Plot on growth chart to monitor progress; monthly office weights may be required to monitor progress.
       4. Try to seek out the cause of weight problem.
       5. Recommend comprehensive behavioral programs directed at good nutrition, adequate activity/exercise, and meal preparation for the patient and the family.
    G. Always obtain temperature, pulse, and respiration (TPR) (if febrile and younger than 2 yr of age, recommend rectal temperature) at each visit (Table 2.3).

⬤ = *non-urgent referral;* ■ = *not to be missed*

TABLE 2.3 ■ Vital Signs: Approximate Normal Findings

Age	RR	HR	BP
0–2 mo	30–60	80–170	70–92/52–65
2–12 mo	20–30	80–150	91–109/53–67
1–3 yr	25–35	80–130	95–105/56–68
3–5 yr	22–32	70–120	99–110/55–70
5–11 yr	20–30	70–110	97–118/60–76
12–18 yr	16–22	65–100	110–130/65–85

BP, blood pressure; *HR*, heart rate; *RR*, respiratory rate.

H. Blood pressure
  1. Check blood pressure (BP) for all patients older than 3 yr of age at every visit, especially if
     (a) Obese
     (b) Taking medications that could ↑ BP
     (c) Have current renal disease or diabetes mellitus (DM)
     (d) Congenital heart defects
  2. Normal BP defined as <90th percentile
  3. Stages of HTN
     (a) Stage 1 (confirmed at three different visits): SBP and/or DBP ≥ 95th percentile
     (b) Stage 2: SBP and/or DBP ≥95th percentile + 12 mmHg
  4. If "white coat syndrome" is suspected, check BP more often; if using home monitoring to evaluate BP, make sure the cuff is checked with the office cuff.
  5. You cannot diagnose elevated BP with home monitoring alone or single office visit.
  6. Children may need more extensive evaluation or referral to specialist with either primary or secondary HTN (see Chapter 16, HYPERTENSION).

Focused Examinations

INTEGUMENTARY

  I. Emphasis on history of present illness (HPI)
     A. History of or currently has seasonal allergies, eczema, asthma or dry patches
     B. Episodes of itching on skin that are worse at night or chronic itching
     C. Change in texture, pigmentation, or fingernail/toenail growth
     D. History of lice, scabies, or bed bug infestation in the past or currently
     E. Any unusual bleeding or bruising
  II. Evaluate primarily with clinical inspection
     A. Vascular findings
        1. Variations in color, including cyanosis or a ruborous color of the extremity(s)
        2. Ecchymosis, petechiae, "stork bite(s)," hemangiomas
     B. Birthmarks, color changes with position, or variations in skin color (e.g., vitiligo or tinea versicolor)
     C. Eczematous changes, areas of excoriation from scratching
     D. Palmar creases and hair whorls
     E. Hair, fingernails, and toenails for discolorations; unusual growth patterns, and any interdigital excoriations

   III. Some areas may also involve palpation
- A. Lesions such as moles, nevi, milia, or warts
- B. Characteristic rashes of possible communicable diseases
- C. Skin plasticity, sensation, turgor, and any unusual odors
- D. Marks or discolorations suggestive of abuse occur on areas of body not likely to be bruised (e.g., eyes, ears, cheeks, neck, inner arms, upper inner thighs, genitals, and buttocks), and may be identified by the presence of patterned bruises (e.g., paddle or handprint), numerous scars, or evidence of past or present "cutting"

   IV. *Not to be missed*
- A. *Cyanosis, pallor, and erythema*
- B. *Viral rash, impetigo, and dermatitis*
- C. *Unusual patterned bruising or fractures in non-weight-bearing infants/children, which could indicate abuse*
- D. *Unusual spots, stains, nevi, or supernumerary nipples*
- E. *Jaundice*
- F. *Umbilicated papular lesions or vesicular lesions (consider molluscum contagiosum or herpes virus [see Chapter 5, Figs. 5.18 and 5.16])*
- G. Any vascular, soft tissue, or pigmented lesions noted in midline of head, neck, or back

HEAD, EARS, EYES, NOSE, AND THROAT (HEENT)

   I. Emphasis on HPI
- A. Head: abnormal hair growth/loss; H/A, dizziness, syncope, or loss of consciousness
- B. Eyes: color of eyes, changes in vision or squinting during distance vision (possible need for glasses), crossed eyes, eye injuries; any familial eye diseases
- C. Ear, nose, and throat (ENT): ear infection, perception of hearing, response to loud noises, speech development, runny nose, mouth breathing and snoring, nosebleeds
- D. Teeth: age of eruptions and number of teeth, cavities, extractions, abscesses, and dental visits (Fig. 2.1)

   II. The head should be observed for
- A. Overall symmetry, and placement of facial parts, including facial expressions and attention
- B. Inspect for scaling/crusting, dilated scalp veins
- C. Observe and inspect hair patterning, color consistency, and amount of hair
- D. Skull should be observed for:
  1. Size (e.g., microcephaly, macrocephaly), shape (e.g., rounded or flattened), appearance of cranial suture lines (e.g., craniosynostosis)
  2. Prominence of scalp veins (increased intracranial pressure [ICP])

   III. Observe and palpate for overriding suture lines or softening of the occipital/parietal bones (craniotabes); this may be normal up to 4 mo of age.

   IV. Palpation of fontanelles for normal (slightly soft) or any flattening or bulging
  1. More accurate if the infant is quiet
  2. Posterior fontanelle closes by 8 wk of age
  3. Anterior fontanelle closes between 10 and 24 mo of age
  4. May palpate a slight pulsation in a normal infant

   V. Eyes may be better visualized in dim light because this will encourage the infant to open eyes and look around.
- A. At 2–6 wk of age, an infant should be able to follow light.

■ = *not to be missed*

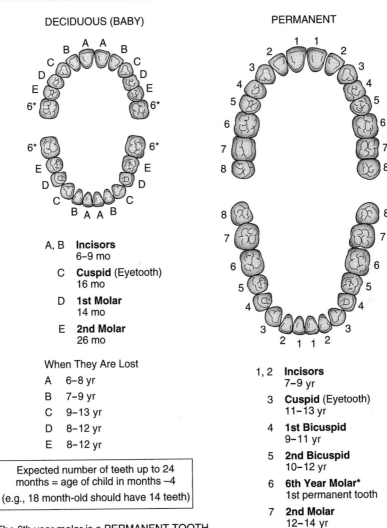

DECIDUOUS (BABY)

PERMANENT

A, B **Incisors**
6–9 mo

C **Cuspid** (Eyetooth)
16 mo

D **1st Molar**
14 mo

E **2nd Molar**
26 mo

When They Are Lost

A   6–8 yr
B   7–9 yr
C   9–13 yr
D   8–12 yr
E   8–12 yr

Expected number of teeth up to 24
months = age of child in months –4
(e.g., 18 month-old should have 14 teeth)

* The 6th year molar is a PERMANENT TOOTH.
It is not shed, nor does it replace a baby tooth.
It is there for a lifetime!

1, 2 **Incisors**
7–9 yr

3 **Cuspid** (Eyetooth)
11–13 yr

4 **1st Bicuspid**
9–11 yr

5 **2nd Bicuspid**
10–12 yr

6 **6th Year Molar***
1st permanent tooth

7 **2nd Molar**
12–14 yr

8 **3rd Molar** (Wisdom)
16–20 yr

Fig. 2.1   Dental chart.

B. At 3–5 mo of age, an infant should have coordinated eye movement and regards faces and other interesting objects.

C. Note abnormal appearance of pupils and document if asymmetrical; note any nystagmus at rest or with movement. With abnormal findings, *referral to pediatric ophthalmologist is indicated.*

D. Note tearing, redness of sclera or tear ducts, and any plugging of tear ducts.

E. Note presence or absence of corneal light reflex (test for strabismus, an ocular muscle tone imbalance that can lead to blindness if not corrected).

● = non-urgent referral

  F. Note presence or absence of red reflex (abnormal reflex could indicate cataracts or intraocular lesions).

  G. Assess vision by the ability to fix and grasp or follow objects without difficulty (patient should be able to do this when less than 3 yr of age).

  H. Vision testing charts are available for children older than 3 yr of age, including Allen picture cards, "E" chart, Sheridan-Gardiner geometric designs, and Snellen charts.

  I. Perform the cover-uncover test, test extraocular movements (EOMs), and assess pupillary response to light and accommodation.

  J. Perform fundoscopic examination, if possible; observe the macula, optic disc, and retinal background and veins/arteries.

VI. Ears

  A. Ears should be evaluated for size, shape, and placement on the head.

  B. Ears are considered low set if they are below a line drawn from the lateral angle of the eye to the external occipital protuberance (Fig. 2.2). This is often associated with urinary tract disorders and mental retardation.

  C. To best visualize the tympanic membrane (TM), use the following techniques:

   1. For infants: pull the auricle backward and downward

   2. For older children: pull the auricle backward and upward

  D. Observe the TM for mobility, color, and intactness (see Chapter 1, Fig. 1.2); evaluate for wax or foreign objects.

  E. Hearing should be assessed at birth via auditory brain stem testing (usually done before discharge from hospital); question the caregiver about the test results; hearing can be tested in the office by making a loud, unexpected noise or ringing a bell and observing for a startle reflex; absence of the startle reflex may indicate hearing deficits.

  F. Infants localize sounds by 6–8 mo of age, know several words by 12 mo of age, and can articulate short sentences by 2 yr of age (see Table 2.1).

  G. ***Refer a school-age child*** without a physical reason for failure to hear any frequency ≥25 dB on an audiometer or if the parent or teachers identify problems. Ask the parent/caregiver if the television must be very loud for the child to hear or if there are problems with discipline (this can indicate hearing deficit).

  H. Language skills correspond to hearing abilities; evaluate speech quality and development (see Table 2.1).

VII. Nose should be examined for occlusion or discharge, especially unilateral nasal discharge.

  A. Observe for flaring and distress and for presence of "allergic salute" line.

  B. Observe the nasal septum and the color of the nasal mucosa (e.g., bogginess, polyps).

  C. Palpate the sinus areas: frontal, maxillary, ethmoid, and sphenoid.

   1. Maxillary and ethmoid sinus cavities are present at birth but very small.

   2. The frontal sinus develops between 2 and 4 yr of age but is rarely a site of infection until 6–10 yr of age.

   3. The sphenoid sinus is rarely a site of infection until 5–8 yr of age.

VIII. Mouth

  A. Oropharynx examination of a toddler

   1. Have the infant/child sit with their back against the caregiver's chest, facing the practitioner, and ask the caregiver to give the infant/child a big "hug," encircling the upper torso and arms with the caregiver's arm. Have the caregiver use the other arm to hold the forehead, which will secure the head fairly well for tongue blade examination.

⬤ *= non-urgent referral*

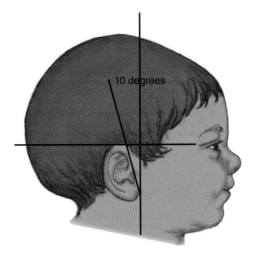

Normal alignment

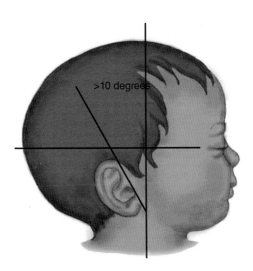

Low-set ears and
deviation in alignment

Fig. 2.2 Normal and low-set ears. (From James, S. R., Nelson, K. A., & Ashwill, J. W. (2007). *Nursing care of children: principles and practice.* Philadelphia: Elsevier.)

    2. The infant/child will usually open the mouth to "scream" and the practitioner can get a very good look during this time and do any swabs that are needed; gag reflexes can also be evaluated at this time.
  B. Examine the lips and buccal mucosa for lesions, moistness, and fissures; check the hard and soft palates for intactness, any unusual nodules, and clefting.
  C. Evaluate the tongue for appearance, movement, and color; if possible, observe the infant sucking on a bottle or breast for the strength of the suck reflex.

D. Evaluate the teeth (see Fig. 2.1) for number and condition; ask about eruption history.

E. Appearance or absence of tonsils, tonsil size, color, and color of exudate.

IX. Neck/lymph nodes

A. Have the child move neck in all range of motion (ROM) to determine any limitations or pain.

B. Inspect and palpate all neck muscles for symmetry, and observe any abnormal positioning of the head secondary to a spasm (e.g., torticollis).

C. Inspect tracheal position, palpate the thyroid, and identify any cysts or lymph nodes in the neck.

D. Palpate the lymph nodes (see Chapter 1, Fig. 1.4) for size, mobility, and consistency.

E. Lymph nodes enlarge more often in children than adults because of infection above the site of the lymph node; this should resolve with warm, moist compresses and antibiotics.

X. *Not to be missed*

A. *Abnormal facies, paralysis, or abnormal facial expressions* (consider congenital abnormality)

B. *Abnormally shaped skull or craniotabes after 4 mo of age* (consider birth trauma, rickets, or syphilis)

C. *Sunken fontanelle, dry tear ducts, and no wet diapers* (consider dehydration)

D. *Nystagmus, strabismus, amblyopia, presence of cloudy pupils* (consider blindness, ocular muscle deformity, or cataracts)

E. *Loss of red reflex or light reflex*

F. *Unresponsiveness to surrounding noises; lacking speech* (consider deafness)

G. *Nasal obstructions, snoring, or unilateral orifice discharge*

H. *Dental malocclusions, cavities, or missing teeth*

I. *A single persistent enlarged lymph node* (consider cancer/lymphoma)

J. *An enlarged or nodular thyroid*

K. *Nuchal rigidity* (consider infection or cervical trauma)

XI. *Referral to appropriate specialist, depending on the finding(s).*

RESPIRATORY SYSTEM

I. Emphasis on HPI

A. Does the patient sleep well at night and have normal energy during the day?

B. Does patient take naps, number of naps per day?

C. Does the patient snore?

D. Has the patient had numerous colds or other severe respiratory illnesses?

E. Does the patient take a flu shot every year?

F. Does the patient have asthma or coughing with activity; any dyspnea on exertion (DOE); can patient keep up with peers in physical activities?

II. Inspect the chest for:

A. Shape, size, movement.

B. The chest is usually rounded until the child is older; if an older child continues to have a rounded chest wall, suspect an underlying pulmonary disease (e.g., cystic fibrosis)

C. The shape of the chest is usually symmetric

■ = not to be missed; ● = non-urgent referral

  1. Asymmetric abnormalities include pectus excavatum (funnel chest) and pectus carinatum (bird chest).

  2. Sternal nodules may signal vitamin D deficiency (rickets).

 D. Observe respiratory rate, use of accessory muscles (e.g., retractions), and pattern of breathing

  1. Infants are abdominal "breathers" (lungs do not fully mature until approximately 8 yr of age).

  2. Infants may have periods of apnea of up to 15 sec.

 E. Nipple placement, nipple discharge, or any supernumerary nipples

 F. Unusual markings, masses

III. Auscultate all lung fields (see Chapter 1, Fig. 1.5) for equal breath sounds, abnormal breath sounds, and upper airway extraneous noises; palpate for vocal fremitus, if indicated.

 1. Increased fremitus due to consolidation (e.g., pneumonia or solid tumor)

 2. Decreased fremitus due to increased airspace (e.g., asthma, chronic obstructive pulmonary disease [COPD] or increased fluid outside lung space)

IV. Infants are obligatory nasal breathers until approximately 6 mo of age; nares and adenoids may swell because of allergies or exposure to smoke. Ask about snoring and unilateral nasal discharge.

V. Nasal sounds can be heard throughout the lung fields in infants but are usually louder in the upper lobes because of the size of the infant and the proximity of the bronchial tree to the chest wall.

VI. *Not to be missed*

 A. *Grunting, nasal flaring, and stridor (respiratory syncytial virus [RSV], bronchiolitis; urgent referral to ED)*

 B. *Persistent wheezing/coughing or fever* (consider gastric reflux, pneumonia, or asthma)

 C. *Inability to clear secretions, failure to thrive, or unusual postures to assist breathing* (consider cystic fibrosis or pulmonary fibrosis)

VII. *Referral to pediatric pulmonologist* if suspecting cystic fibrosis or pulmonary fibrosis.

CARDIOVASCULAR SYSTEM

 I. Emphasis on HPI

  A. Cardiopulmonary: chest pain or shortness of breath (SOB) with activity, unusual posture during activity, cyanosis, tachycardia

  B. Can the child keep up with peers during play?

  C. Any cardiac abnormalities at birth

  D. Any change in color of skin with activity, or at rest; any unusual posturing to assist with breathing (e.g., squatting)

 II. Observe the child's activity level, and ask about response to exercise; observe for any unusual posturing during activity and skin color at rest and during activity.

 III. Auscultation for the rhythm, rate, and location of heart sounds (see Chapter 1, Fig. 1.6).

  A. S_3: caused by turbulence of rapid left ventricle filling; it may be normal in children and is heard at the apex or along the lower left sternal border.

  B. S_4: abnormal and indicates decreased ventricular compliance (e.g., heart failure [HF]).

  C. Murmurs (see Chapter 8, Table 8.12)

   1. Should be identified in relation to the intensity, location, and radiation of sounds especially with any change in position.

■ = *not to be missed;* ● = *non-urgent referral;* ▲ = *urgent referral*

      2. All new murmurs should be initially evaluated by a pediatric cardiologist.

      3. All murmurs greater than grade 3/6 should be followed annually by a pediatric cardiologist and/or echocardiogram.

IV. Palpate pulses (see Chapter 1, Fig. 1.7) for strength, quality, and symmetry in the bilateral upper and lower extremities.

V. Palpation of point of maximal impulse (PMI)

    A. Best felt: at the fourth intercostal space in a child younger than 7 yr of age; at the fifth intercostal space in a child older than 7 yr of age

    B. Lower PMI may indicate cardiac enlargement

    C. Bounding PMI may indicate anemia, fever, or fear

■ **VI.** *Not to be missed*

■   A. *Unusual posture during activity, decrease in stamina, and/or any pathologic murmurs* (congenital heart defects)

■   B. *Poor growth or feeding, fever, excessive sweating, or cardiomegaly* (consider anemia, myocarditis, or HF)

■   C. *Delayed or absent femoral pulses*

      1. May have pulse differences between arms and legs, with pinker upper extremities and more cyanotic lower extremities.

      2. Measure BP in both arms and legs; if the pressure in arms is >20 mmHg over that in legs, consider coarctation of the aorta (CoA).

▲ **VII.** *Referral to pediatric cardiologist* with any of the above abnormalities.

ABDOMINAL SYSTEM

I. Emphasis on HPI

    A. Any extreme fluctuations in weight, changes in appetite

    B. Does patient eat with the family or alone?

    C. Any changes in stooling, emesis, or urination

    D. Any complaints of belching, burping, acid brash

II. Observe for any peristaltic waves in infants (as caused by pyloric stenosis)

III. Inspect shape, muscular integrity, umbilicus, and any unusual skin markings

    A. Vascular skin markings (e.g., hemangiomas) are common but prominent veins over the abdominal wall may indicate chronic liver or renal disease.

    B. The shape is usually rounded and protuberant in infants; this slowly resolves, becoming more scaphoid with age and mobility.

    C. Diastasis recti is common and can be elicited in infants when sitting up; it is not noticeable when lying flat. This usually resolves with age and surgery is only considered if a hernia should develop.

    D. Observe the umbilicus for any hernias or exudates.

      1. Hernias are not uncommon in infants, toddlers, and young children; can be elicited by having the child tense abdominal muscles or raise his or her head off the bed; usually resolve without treatment.

■   2. The umbilical cord usually separates by 1 wk after birth; *if still present after 3 wk, suspect infection, immunodeficiency, or congenital malformations.*

      3. Exudates from the umbilicus may be caused by a foreign object; clean the area well and inspect for debris.

IV. Auscultate for bowel sounds and bruits

■ *= not to be missed;* ▲ *= urgent referral*

A. Bowel sounds can be referred across the abdomen in infants/children; listen for 30–60 sec if no sounds are heard initially.
  1. *Absent bowel sounds may be due to peritonitis or appendicitis.*
  2. *High pitched, tinkling sounds may be due to obstruction.*
B. Listen over the aorta and other large abdominal vessels (bruits are usually easier to hear because of less abdominal fat occluding sounds).
V. Palpate the abdomen with the child's hand over the practitioner's and have the child press down on your hand; this gives the child some control over the examination and will decrease "ticklishness."
  A. Palpate all quadrants (see Chapter 9, Fig. 9.1) both lightly and deeply for tenderness, rebound, and guarding; check the liver, kidney, and spleen for size.
    1. In infants and younger children, the liver may be felt 1–3 cm below the rib edges; in older children, the liver should not be felt below the rib edges.
    2. Palpate the spleen with the child lying on the right side with knees drawn up; palpate just under the intercostal margin while the child is taking a deep breath; *if you suspect splenomegaly or injury, DO NOT PALPATE.*
  B. An easy way to test for rebound or guarding pain is to have the child "blow up their belly" to touch your hand.
VI. *Not to be missed*
  A. *Projectile vomiting* (consider pyloric stenosis)
  B. *Painless abdominal mass, hematuria* (consider Wilms tumor)
  C. *Rigid abdomen with pain, unusual bulging noted with or without pain, drainage from the umbilicus, or a fissure in the umbilicus* (consider hernia or cancer)
VII. *Referral*
  A. *To ED if patient is unstable (e.g., diaphoretic, hypotensive and/or lethargic)*
  B. *To pediatric surgeon if suspecting pyloric stenosis*
  C. *To pediatric oncologist if suspecting Wilms tumor or cancer*

GENITOURINARY SYSTEM

I. Emphasis on HPI
  A. If toilet trained, the age when continent during both day and night
  B. Any enuresis, dysuria or hematuria, urinary continence
  C. Menstrual history, sexual activity, use of contraception/condoms
  D. Is patient circumcised and if so, at what age; any problems with cleanliness?
  E. Sexual maturity (see Tanner staging, Box 2.1)
  F. Have there been any abnormal growth patterns and any asymmetric growth in body?
  G. Intake of unusual amounts of fluids, heat/cold intolerance, or purplish skin striae
II. Take a "matter-of-fact" approach to the examination
III. Observe the placement of nipples (widespread nipples may be indicative of genetic anomalies [e.g., Turner syndrome]); observe for normal development of the breast tissue and note any discharge
IV. Genitalia
  A. Male exam
    1. If <5 yr of age: examine with him in a "tailor sit" position to avoid testicular retraction (cremasteric reflex); observe for presence of testicle(s), urethral position, penis size and shape, and circumcision.

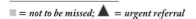

■ = *not to be missed;* ▲ = *urgent referral*

BOX 2.1 ■ Tanner Sexual Maturity Rating

Pubic Hair

1. Sparse, slightly darker hair along the labia and at the base of the penis
2. Hair darker, coarser, curlier; spreading over the entire pubis
3. Hair thick and dark like adult; covering the pubis but not on thighs
4. Adult type and quantity; also on medial thighs

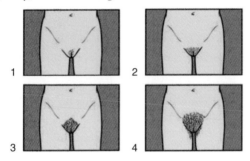

Breasts

1. Elevation of only the nipple
2. Breast bud; small mound of breast and nipple develop; areola widens
3. Breast and areola grow, but the nipple is flush with the breast surface
4. Areola and nipple form a second mound over the breast
5. Mature breast; only the nipple projects

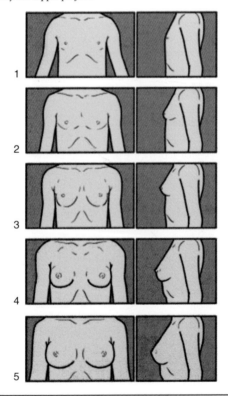

BOX 2.1 ■ Tanner Sexual Maturity Rating—cont'd

Genitals
1. Same size and proportion as early childhood
2. Testes and scrotum begin to enlarge; scrotum reddens and changes texture
3. Testes and scrotum continue to grow; penis longer
4. Testes almost fully grown; scrotum darker; penis larger and broader (glans develops)
5. Adult size and shape

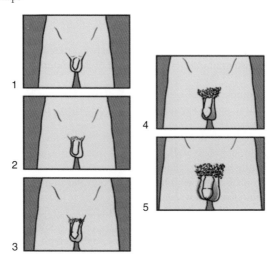

(Adapted from Engel, J. K. (2006). *Mosby's pocket guide to pediatric assessment* (5th ed.). St. Louis: Elsevier; Blackwell, J. M. (1962). *Growth at adolescence.* Oxford, England: Blackwell Publishing Ltd.)

2. If >5 yr of age: examine him either standing or lying, observe for urethral position, penis size and shape, circumcision, testis development and can gently palpate for hernia, if indicated (for adolescents, see Chapter 1, GENITOURINARY (MALE)).

B. Female exam
1. Examine a girl while she is in the "hands and knees" position or butterfly position (e.g., supine with the plantar aspect of the feet touching and legs relaxed outward).
2. Observe for hymenal injuries, imperforate hymen, extruding vaginal masses, or labial adhesions (see Chapter 16, Gynecological Disorder, LABIAL ADHESIONS).

V. Anal area
A. Assess anal area for any masses, fissures, or bleeding
B. Elicit anal wink by gently stroking the perianal tissue with a finger or sharp object
1. If normal, this will cause visible puckering to the external anal sphincter.
2. Lack of response suggests defect in sensory or motor nerve roots.

VI. Assess sexual maturity using Tanner staging (see Box 2.1)

VII. *Not to be missed*
   A. *Abnormal genitourinary (GU) bleeding, hematuria, hypospadias, abnormal curvature of penis (Peyronie's disease)*

■ = *not to be missed*

      B. *Early or delayed puberty*
      C. *Breast or vaginal masses or structural defects, labial adhesions; undescended testicle(s) or masses*
  VIII. *Referral to pediatric specialist*, depending on the problem(s).

MUSCULOSKELETAL SYSTEM

    I. Emphasis on HPI
      A. Are there any issues with weakness, balance and coordination or swelling of joints?
      B. Unusual gait, foot deformities
      C. Any complaints of back pain and where is pain located?
      D. Any past history of injuries (e.g., fracture or dislocations) or surgeries?
   II. Spine
      A. Observe contours of the spine for scoliosis (see Chapter 16, SCOLIOSIS).
      B. The cervical spine should have full extension, flexion, rotation, and lateral movements.
        1. A 10-degree flexion restriction is noted if one finger breadth is noted between the chin and chest wall; atlantoaxial instability is a concern (this is seen more frequently in Down syndrome).
        2. Torticollis is noted with lateral restriction and shortening of muscles forcing the head into lateral movement.
      C. The spine should have full mobility, and the child should be able to bend forward and touch hands on the floor easily without bending the knees.
      D. Observe the overall shape, contour, tone, and strength of the muscles in the back; there should be equal movements bilaterally.
      E. Observe for sacral dimpling or tufts of hair in the pilonidal area.
      F. Palpate the spine and paravertebral muscles for pain or spasm.
  III. Gait
      A. Assess gait as the patient navigates the room; watch for symmetry, ability to turn and stop, and smoothness of these actions.
      B. Try to observe the patient in the anatomical position from all sides, front and back.
        1. Abnormalities observed might include spinal deviation, limb alignment and length, limited ability to fully extend arms and knees, abnormalities in feet.
        2. Observe for limping (see Chapter 16, LIMPING CHILD) and when it occurs (e.g., walking, running, turning, stopping).
   IV. Arms
      A. Inspect all joints for swelling, redness, and pain with movement; offer items to grasp and hold against resistance.
      B. Palpate all upper extremity joints for pain and ROM (active, passive, and against resistance; see Chapter 13).
   V. Legs
      A. In the standing position, observe the shape and alignment of the legs (from hip to feet), both individually and bilaterally.
      B. Observe for bilateral in-toeing (pigeon-toed), which means that the foot turns inward while walking or running; can be considered a congenital condition and usually corrects itself with growth. *If this condition is unilateral, painful, and grossly asymmetric, referral to an orthopedist is recommended.*

  ■ = *not to be missed;* ● = *non-urgent referral*

VI. Hips should be evaluated in regard to flexion, extension, internal and external rotation, and abduction and adduction.

    A. Perform the Barlow-Ortolani test to detect hip dislocation; observe buttock creases.

    B. Hip flexion should be 100 degrees; hip extension should show the leg to be flat on bed.

    C. Hip internal rotation should be approximately 35 degrees; external rotation should be approximately 45 degrees.

    D. Knees should be evaluated for full extension, with the posterior popliteal fossa touching the bed, and flexion, with the knees flexed to approximately 120 degrees.

    E. Evaluate for varus and valgus alignment.

        1. Genu varum (bowlegs) can be physiologic younger than 2 yr of age and usually resolves with continued ambulation; is bilateral and seen with in-toeing and waddling. The child usually appears "clumsy" when ambulating.

        2. Genu valgum (knock knees) may be physiologic and will resolve by 6 yr of age. *Referral to an orthopedist* if the deformity is unilateral and/or painful.

    F. To evaluate leg length discrepancy, have the child stand and observe the iliac crest and gluteal folds, which should be even; if there is any asymmetry, there may be leg length discrepancy. *Referral to an orthopedist* if the discrepancy is >2 cm or if it causes pain or difficulty with mobility.

VII. Ankles/feet should be assessed for ankle ROM, soles of feet, and foot alignment.

    A. Pes planus (i.e., flat foot) is common in infants/toddlers until the arch develops in childhood with walking; this is nonpainful and associated with pronation.

    B. The child may appear to be "flat footed" until approximately 3 yr of age, when the fat pad starts to resolve.

VIII. *Not to be missed*

    A. *Fractures or evidence of healed fractures in infants/toddlers*

    B. *Swollen, red, and hot joints; poorly healing open wounds over bony areas* (consider arthritic conditions)

    C. *Unusual growths on bone, scoliosis, unexplained fractures, muscle mass atrophy, or abnormal masses or "pits" in the spinal column* (consider spinal cord anomalies)

    D. *Abnormal gait and/or pain in the hip joints, unusual protuberance over the joints* (consider hip dysplasia, cancer, or cerebral palsy)

    E. *Delayed growth and development*

    F. *Ataxia, muscle atrophy, and abnormal reflexes* (consider cerebral palsy)

IX. *Referral to appropriate specialist*, depending on the problem(s).

NEUROLOGIC SYSTEM

    I. Emphasis on HPI

        A. Headaches, dizziness, fainting

        B. Brain injuries at birth or later in life, any hypoxic episodes, seizures, ataxia

        C. Learning problems, attention span, sleep disturbances

        D. Caregivers' perception of activity (e.g., hyperactivity or hypoactivity)

        E. Any problems with depression, mood changes, suicidal thoughts (see Chapter 17, DEPRESSION, Major Depression [pediatrics])

    II. The practitioner should make observations related to:

        A. Cerebral function

            1. Mental status, appearance, behavior

            2. Language and social and emotional responses (see Table 2.1)

        B. Mobility and limb symmetry

■ = *not to be missed;* ● = *non-urgent referral*

    C. Gait disturbances

    D. Abnormality in balance, coordination, and neuromuscular development

  III. Cranial nerves (CNs) (also see Table 1.5)

    A. CN I: olfactory sense appears at approximately 5–7 mo of age

    B. CN II, III, IV, VI: optic nerves

       1. Fundoscopic for optic disc, macula, and veins; evaluate pupil size and PERRLA (pupils, equal, round, reactive to light and accommodate).

       2. Test peripheral vision by having the patient focus on the parent, and then bring the object into the visual range from the side and evaluate when the patient looks toward it.

       3. Monitor for nystagmus at rest and with EOM.

       4. Blink reflex is not strong at birth and starts to develop at approximately 3–4 mo of age and is fully developed by 12 mo of age.

    C. CN V: test sensation of face; chewing or sucking strength, ability to clench teeth and corneal reflex.

    D. CN VII: observe for facial symmetry, movement and sucking or taking in foods; taste is more difficult in younger children because they do not understand different tastes but may relate to "good" or "bad" taste.

    E. CN VIII: check hearing by making a loud noise and watching for a reaction; older children may be tested with whispering and having them say what was whispered.

    F. CN IX, X: gag reflex can be checked when examining the throat; CN X controls uvula and palate movement when saying "ah" (the uvula will deviate to the unaffected side if there is vagal nerve dysfunction).

    G. CN XI: watch for symmetry in shrugging shoulders and in turning head against resistance to evaluate the strength of the sternocleidomastoid muscle.

    H. CN XII: tongue movement can be evaluated by watching the tongue and evaluating sucking strength.

  IV. Motor examination (see Table 2.1)

    A. Watching a patient walk or run assists with evaluation of cerebellar function for balance and coordination; testing passive ROM evaluates motor strength and identifies any abnormalities of tone.

       1. Patient should be able to stand on one foot without help by 4–6 yr of age.

       2. Patient should be able to tandem walk by 4 to 6 yr of age.

    B. Test pronator drift by having the patient (starting at 3 to 4 yr of age) extend their arms with eyes open and palms up, then have the patient close the eyes and watch the extended arms for drifting. Try to press down on the arms while extended; this is a good test for assessing strength in the upper extremities.

    C. Test proprioception with Romberg test (between 3 and 4 yr of age): have the patient stand with eyes closed and evaluate the ability to stand without swaying/falling.

  V. Sensory examination distinguishes between different levels of touch, vibration, and position; test higher function by asking the patient to note objects (that would be familiar to their age) through touch with eyes closed.

  VI. Reflexes should be tested from birth according to age (Table 2.4); after 5 yr of age, reflexes should be the same as in adults; any time reflexes are found to be abnormal, ***refer to pediatric neurologist.***

  VII. Developmental screening should be performed at a minimum of 9, 18, and 30 mo of age, using appropriate tools to screen for motor, speech, and cognitive development (e.g., Early Language Milestone Scale-2 [0–36 mo of age], Early Motor Pattern Profile

---

⬤ = *non-urgent referral*

TABLE 2.4 ■ **Normal Primitive Reflexes**

Reflex	Definition	Disappears by Age
Rooting	When the cheek is stroked, the head turns toward the stimulus Tests tactile reflexes and proprioception	3–4 mo
Moro	With sudden movement of the body from the neutral position to the lower position, arms flail outward and are then brought into body; hands will open and the infant will usually cry out Tests general level of excitability	6 mo
Palmar grasp	Flexion of fingers, fisting when an object is placed in an open hand **Considered abnormal if the response is asymmetric or is absent before 2–3 mo** Tests tactile reflexes and proprioception	3–5 mo
Tonic neck reflex (fencer's position)	The head is turned to the side while the rest of the body lies flat on table; normal response is extension of the arm and leg on the side that the head is turned and flexion of the opposite arm and leg **Considered abnormal if the response is not symmetric**	6–7 mo
Parachute response	The infant is suspended horizontally with the face down and is quickly brought down toward the floor (make sure that the infant is held securely). Normal response is arms extended and hands open Tests symmetry of movement	8–9 mo
Stepping response	Stepping occurs when the sole of the foot is placed on the table; infant appears to be walking	4–5 mo
Babinski sign	Positive sign is dorsiflexion of the great toe and fanning of other toes after firm stroking of the plantar aspect of the foot **Abnormal if asymmetric response** Tests pyramidal tract dysfunction	Can be normal until 1 yr of age; usually disappears by the time the toddler starts walking
Clonus	**Maintaining dorsiflexion of the foot after stimulation or having sustained clonus after checking reflexes is ALWAYS abnormal**	

[6–12 mo of age], Checklist for Autism in toddlers [CHAT; 18–24 mo of age], and CAPUT scale [3–36 mo of age]).
- **VIII.** *Not to be missed*
  - A. *Hydrocephaly, macrocephaly, microcephaly*
  - B. *Headaches* (benign intracranial hypertension)
  - C. *Uncontrolled, inconsolable crying* (consider increased ICP)
  - D. *Seizure* (consider trauma or disease process)
  - E. *Loss of use of extremities, abnormal mass, or pitting in the spinal column* (consider neural tube deformity)
- **IX.** *Referral to ED or pediatric specialist, depending on suspected problem(s) and patient's condition.*

■ *= not to be missed;* ● *= non-urgent referral*

CHILD ABUSE

I. Definition: nonaccidental, purposeful physical, emotional, or sexual abuse directed at a minor child.

II. All health care providers are mandated reporters and are obligated to notify authorities or HOT-LINE for child sexual and physical abuse.

III. Physical abuse is defined as nonaccidental trauma and is usually committed by family members, caretakers, or other people in the family setting; occurs in daycare settings; also seen with "bullying" in school settings.

IV. A high level of suspicion is needed to recognize risk factors that contribute to child abuse. This is of utmost importance for the practitioner because this may be the patient's first entry into the health care system.

   A. Risk factors identified in the family setting that contribute to abuse may include the following:
      1. Number of children in household younger than 3 yr of age (infants are at the highest risk because of complete reliance on the caregiver for all physical needs)
      2. Family patterns of violence
      3. Poverty or very low socioeconomic status
      4. Lack of parenting skills due to immaturity and poor coping skills
      5. Lack of extended family support
      6. Single-parent status and social isolation
      7. Financial difficulties
      8. Drug or alcohol abuse or overuse

   B. Risk factors associated with the child's physical abilities
      1. Mental or developmental delays/disability resulting in different physical appearance from peers
      2. Hearing or visual difficulty of any degree of severity (e.g., wearing hearing aids or glasses)
      3. Small size without developmental delays
      4. Immunodeficiency diseases (e.g., AIDS) or musculoskeletal disorders (e.g., cerebral palsy)

   C. Risk factors related to physical settings other than the home
      1. Large daycare, preschool, or primary school settings with poor monitoring systems for intervention in cases of physical violence
      2. Multiple family settings
      3. Having a distance to walk home after school (e.g., either in urban or rural settings)
      4. Frequent stays in shelters

V. Types of abuse vary from minor to major, with some leading to death

   A. Neglect of basic needs or education, or abandonment by the caregiver

   B. Emotional abuse involves caregivers detachment from the child's needs; unrealistic expectations and angry outbursts over insignificant actions/issues

VI. Patient behaviors indicative of emotional abuse

   A. Withdraws from physical touch or exhibits aggressive behaviors if approached by the caregiver or others in the family; may exhibit same behaviors with noncaregivers in other settings

   B. May "cling" to the caregiver and exhibit terror if separated from the caregiver (this is not as bothersome if the child is 6–18 mo of age and exhibits "stranger separation")

   C. Somatic complaints of soreness while moving without obvious bruising

   D. Wears inappropriate clothing for the weather

VII. Caregiver behaviors indicative of emotional abuse of the child
  A. Yelling at inappropriate times and more often than necessary
  B. Refusing to touch or look at the child when needed
  C. Verbally belittling, shaming, ridiculing, or threatening the child
VIII. Suspect physical abuse in case of the following:
  A. Repeated visits to a health care facility for injuries that do not coincide with the provided stories or there are questionable causes for injury or condition
  B. Any injuries that occur in nonhigh-impact areas of the body, such as the face, eyes, ears, cheeks, head (especially sides), chest, genital area, buttocks, upper arms, or thighs
  C. Any patterned marks (e.g., hands, buckles, broom handles), especially if the child names the object
  D. Soft tissue injuries such as burns, bruising, lacerations, or bite marks, especially if the story does not fit with the injury (e.g., water burns from pulling hot water off the stove should involve the chest and abdomen, not feet or buttocks)
  E. Multiple fractures in the rib area, fractures in various stages of healing, or femur fractures in a nonambulatory infant; also history of fractures
IX. Sexual abuse
  A. Defined as any adolescent or adult in a position to force or coerce a child into unwanted sexual activity, which could be touching, forcible penetration into orifices, or pornography; is usually more subtle and the child may present with the following:
    1. Complaints of dysuria or pain in the genital area
    2. Vaginal discharge, bleeding, itching, or swelling
    3. Rectal pain with or without itching
    4. Acting out sexually in inappropriate ways
  B. If sexual abuse is suspected, the child should be interviewed by a forensic interviewer and practitioner to ensure adequate documentation.
  C. If the practitioner is concerned for the child's welfare, the authorities should be notified immediately and the child can be sent to the hospital for their protection.
  D. This should be discussed and considered at every encounter.

Geriatric Assessment

- The goal is maintaining and enhancing the daily functioning of the elderly patient; normal changes of aging are often complicated by chronic and/or acute illnesses.
- The clinical presentation of a health problem in an elderly patient often appears in an atypical manner and may mimic many different illnesses.
- For a comprehensive assessment, include the following parameters of health:
  - Visual and auditory perception
  - Nutrition
  - Social and psychologic assessment
  - Gait and balance; ability to perform activities of daily living (ADLs)
- For the most effective assessment:
  - Make sure the room is well lit; do not stand in front of a bright light or window
  - Minimize background noise as much as possible
  - When addressing the patient, use the last name (unless the patient requests otherwise)
  - Sit level with the patient during the interview
  - Note if patient is or is not a reliable historian

HEALTH HISTORY*

    I. Chief complaint

        A. Complaints may be numerous

        B. Help patients identify which complaint is personally of greatest concern to them

   II. History of present illness (HPI)

  III. Self-rated health (elderly patients often see themselves as healthier than practitioners do)

  IV. Past medical history (PMH)

        A. Ask the patient specifically about reported illnesses and which provider gave that diagnosis

        B. Ask about past blood transfusions or medical infusions

        C. Medication history is extremely important (including pain medications, laxatives, eye medicines, over-the-counter [OTC] sleep aids, and cold or allergy medicines); have the patient or family bring ALL of the patient's current prescriptions and OTC medications, and herbal products/vitamins in their bottles at the time of the visit

    V. Patient profile

        A. Marital status and relationship with spouse

        B. Children/grandchildren (e.g., relationship and frequency of contact with them; obtain their telephone numbers if patient wants you to share information with them. Be sure that the patient has signed the HIPAA form allowing information to be shared)

        C. Living arrangements

            1. With whom?

            2. Where (e.g., an apartment or home, assisted living facility)?

            3. What type of heating and cooling system is used at home?

* Only additions to a normal health history are listed here

D. Support systems (e.g., family, friends, faith organization, community services)

E. Recent losses, including pets

F. Education, occupation, and retirement or current employment

G. Adequacy of finances and health insurance

H. Transportation: when was the patient's last driving test and where do they drive; or if the patient does not drive, who drives for them?

I. Typical daily activities (if indicated)

VI. Nutrition

A. Determine if the diet is adequate, and if the patient is at risk for malnutrition. Consider asking about the previous day's food intake; has the patient's weight been stable?

B. Screening tools are available to identify older adults at risk for poor nutrition; two commonly used ones include the following:

1. SCREEN II (Seniors in the Community: Risk Evaluation for Eating and Nutrition): 17-item tool (there is also an 8-item version available)

2. MNA (Mini Nutritional Assessment) or MNA-SF (Mini Nutritional Assessment-Short Form)

C. Conditions associated with malnutrition include chronic alcoholism, chronic myocardial or pulmonary diseases, cognitive disorder or depression, malabsorption syndromes, and polypharmacy (see VIII. Safety, C, below).

VII. Sleep patterns

A. What time does the patient go to bed and get up?

B. What medication(s)—if any—do they take for sleep?

C. How often do they wake at night and for how long? What wakes them?

D. Is the sleep restful? Do they nap during the day?

VIII. Safety

A. See ASSESSING FUNCTIONAL STATUS, III. Functional Assessment at the end of this chapter.

B. Does the patient have concerns about possible abuse or neglect?

C. "Deprescribing" unnecessary medications

1. It is very common that a patient will see one or more specialists. This can lead to polypharmacy (i.e., use of multiple medications that have potential to harm and/ or are unnecessary), often because each provider prescribes for the condition(s) they treat. Compounding the problem is the fact that all of the providers may not be using the same electronic health record (EHR), so they may not know all medications being taken.

2. Patients especially at risk for polypharmacy are older than 62 yr of age with

(a) Multiple diagnoses

(b) Multiple prescribers or pharmacies (e.g., local and mail-in)

(c) Self-treatment using OTC medications

(d) A history of hospitalizations

(e) Long-term care residents

3. Possible consequences of polypharmacy

(a) Adverse medication events (which can lead to additional medication(s) being prescribed if the adverse event is misinterpreted as a new medical condition)

(b) Nonadherence

(c) Increased cost and mortality; individualize the medication regimen, matching the patient's condition and the goals of care (e.g., is the medication appropriate, given the patient's other medical conditions and expected life expectancy?)

(d) Functional impairment (due to medication interactions or patient prescribed more than one medication from same class)

4. Deprescribing is a process to identify unnecessary, inappropriate, or duplicate medications and stop them.
   (a) Reconcile all medications (see IV, C above); for each medication, determine which are actually being taken and how (i.e., dose and how often).
   (b) Identify which ones may be inappropriate, harmful, or unneeded; also consider those that are not working, that lack an indication, or that the patient may want to stop because of unwanted side effects. Helpful tools are:
       (i) *http://anticholinergicscales.es/calculate* (Anticholinergic Burden Calculator); start with level 3 category medications
       (ii) Beers Criteria list (can be found through the American Geriatrics Society [AGS])
       (iii) *https://deprescribing.org/*
       (iv) *http://medstopper.com/*
   (c) To help the patient "buy in" to stopping medications (Rx, OTC, herbal)
       (i) Discuss potential or real adverse effects of the medications and the potential benefits of deprescribing (e.g., less risk of hospitalization, improved quality of life, functional gains).
       (ii) Point out medications that do not have a clear indication or significant benefit clinically.
       (iii) Consider stopping or tapering off just one medication at a time; assure patient you will monitor for worsening conditions or withdrawal.
       (iv) Discuss nonpharmacological (e.g., lifestyle) changes that can be effective and are safer (e.g., weight loss of 5%–10% body weight and reduced sodium intake can lower blood pressure).

Focused Examinations

◼ *Note: If there are discrepancies between the history answers and physical findings, consider hidden problems such as falls or abuse.*

INTEGUMENTARY SYSTEM

I. See Table 3.1 for physiologic changes and abnormal findings.
II. Additional questions to ask:
   A. What changes have you noted in your skin's condition over the last few years?
   B. Has there been any delayed wound healing?
   C. Have you had any new or changing skin lesions, itching, or pain?
   D. Do you have a history of diabetes mellitus (DM) or peripheral vascular disease (PVD)?
   E. Have you received either of the shingles vaccines (Zostavax or Shingrix)?

PRACTICE PEARLS FOR INTEGUMENTARY SYSTEM

- Elderly patients are at a higher risk of ulcer formation because of decreased turgor and subcutaneous fat.
- With skin changes, remember to ask about a history of allergies or atopy, work history, and environmental exposure (including sun).
- The incidence of herpes zoster peaks in people 50–70 yr of age, and postherpetic neuralgia occurs more frequently in people >70 yr of age.
- Current recommendations for shingles vaccine (Shingrix): two injections, with the second dose 2–6 mo after the first one; recommended for all people >50 yr of age. This should be given even if the person received the Zostavax vaccine previously.
- Signs of neglect can include poor grooming and bedsores.

◼ = *not to be missed*

TABLE 3.1 ■ Physiologic Changes and Abnormal Findings: Integumentary System

Physiologic Changes	Clinical Correlation	*Not to Be Missed*
Loss of elasticity	Wrinkles	*Abnormal skin lesions (e.g., actinic keratosis, skin cancers)*
Loss of elastin, collagen, sub-q fat	Paper-thin skin prone to breakdown and injury	*Dehydration Hypothermia*
Decreased sweat and oil glands	Dry skin and pruritus Difficulty in regulating body temperature, especially with changes in environmental temperatures	*Pruritus due to renal or hepatic disease, diabetes mellitus, hyperthyroidism, drug allergy, iron deficiency anemia, parasitic infections Heat stroke*
Increased vascular fragility	Senile purpura	*Bruising, purpura, or abrasions secondary to falls or abuse*
Slower epidermal growth rate	Slower wound healing	
Hair turns gray or white and feels thin and fine	Potential effect on self-esteem	
Hair distribution changes	"Male pattern" baldness Decreased axillary and pubic hair Women may develop bristly facial hair and/or have hair thinning in the frontal and vertex areas of the scalp	*Localized hair loss due to peripheral vascular disease Diffuse alopecia due to hypothyroidism, iron deficiency, hypoproteinemia*
Nails grow more slowly and develop longitudinal ridges	Nails prone to splitting	*Nails that are thickened or overgrown, causing pain with shoes or with walking*

SENSORY SYSTEM

I. See Table 3.2 for physiologic changes and abnormal findings.

II. Additional questions to ask:

A. Do you have any difficulty climbing steps or driving?

B. When was your eye last exam?

1. When were you last tested for glaucoma? If you have glaucoma, how do you manage the eye drops?

2. Do you have macular degeneration?

3. Do you have cataracts or have you had cataract surgery?

C. Do you have any problem with night vision?

D. Do your eyes feel dry or burning? How do you manage this?

E. Have you noticed a change in your hearing or taste? For example, can you hear a fire alarm or the phone ringing?

F. Have you noticed any burns, bruises, or cuts that you do not know how they occurred?

G. The degree of pain in elderly patients may not accurately reflect the seriousness of the underlying condition.

■ = *not to be missed*

TABLE 3.2 ■ **Physiologic Changes and Abnormal Findings: Sensory System**

Physiologic Changes	Clinical Correlation	Not to Be Missed
Eye skin loses elasticity	Wrinkling and drooping (may cause decreased vision or visual defects) May have ectropion or entropion	
Distorted depth perception	Incorrect assessment of height of curbs and steps	*Falls due to other conditions (e.g., stroke or arrhythmia)*
Changes in retina, choroid, and skin	Decreased visual acuity Visual fields narrow Slower light-to-dark adaptation (patient needs more light to see)	*Macular degeneration* *Diabetes mellitus (DM)*
Increased intraocular pressures	Increased incidence of glaucoma	*Glaucoma*
Lens turns yellow and loses elasticity	Decreased visual acuity (may affect safe driving) Color vision may be impaired (blue, green, violet)	*Cataract*
Decreased tear production	Dry or burning eyes	
Cilia in ear canal become coarse and stiff	May cause cerumen buildup Harder to hear consonants and to localize sound	*Impaired hearing due to cerumen impaction*
Gradual sensorineural hearing loss, starting in the 50s	Difficulty hearing whispered words or in a noisy background	*Social isolation due to hearing loss* *Hearing loss due to Paget disease, ototoxic medications, vascular or mass lesions; if no obvious cause for loss of hearing, referral to ENT*
Decreased number of olfactory nerve fibers	May have decreased sense of smell (which may affect appetite, leading to possible weight loss)	*Potential hazard if the patient cannot detect harmful odors* *If acute loss of smell, consider tumor*
Altered taste sensation	Possible weight loss or gain May have edema due to increased salt intake	*Zinc deficiency* *Medications that may affect taste* *DM neuropathy*
Reduced tactile sensation	Decreased ability to sense pressure, pain, and temperature	*Vascular diseases* *DM* *Neurological disorder* *Burns*

RESPIRATORY SYSTEM

I. See Table 3.3 for physiologic changes and abnormal findings.

II. Additional questions to ask:

A. Do you have any SOB or fatigue with your normal activities?

B. What is your usual level of physical activity?

C. Do you use O_2: at night, with activity, or all the time?

D. Do you use CPAP or BiPAP? If so, how is it working?

E. For patients with chronic obstructive pulmonary disease (COPD): How are you getting along each day? Has your weight changed? When was your last respiratory infection and hospitalization?

■ = *not to be missed;* ● = *non-urgent referral*

TABLE 3.3 ■ **Physiologic Changes and Abnormal Findings: Respiratory System**

Physiologic Changes	Clinical Correlation	Not to Be Missed
Rib cage less mobile	Commonly results in an increased AP diameter May obscure heart and lung sounds Less vigorous cough	*Thorax changes due to COPD* *Decreased breath sounds due to effusion, atelectasis, pneumonia, COPD*
Decreased lung tissue elasticity	Decreased vital capacity Increased residual volume Increased work of breathing with exercise May have difficulty with PFT and using inhalers	*SOB or crackles due to HF, COPD, or pneumonia* *Deconditioning*
Ciliary atrophy	Change in mucociliary movement	*Pulmonary infection*

COPD, chronic obstructive pulmonary disease (COPD); *HF,* heart failure.

    F. Where do you sleep at night? If not in a bed, why not?
    G. Vaccines
        1. Have you received one or both pneumonia vaccines?
        2. Did you get COVID-19 vaccines/booster(s)? Which one?
        3. Do you get a yearly flu shot?

PRACTICE PEARLS FOR RESPIRATORY SYSTEM

- Elderly patients may not have respiratory signs and symptoms until late in the course of a disease (e.g., patients with pneumonia may have a decreased level of responsiveness, confusion, poor appetite, or evidence of falls). With dehydration, the patient may not have a cough.
- Using a stethoscope with a pediatric diaphragm may be helpful for patients with prominent ribs.
- The most common respiratory complaint is dyspnea; the cause may be cardiac, respiratory, metabolic, mechanical, or hematologic.
- Rales (or crackles) are the most common physical finding; the cause may be age-related fibrotic changes, infection, or cardiac or pulmonary disorders.
- An annual low-dose chest computed tomography (CT) scan to check for lung cancer is recommended in men and women age 50–77 yr, with a history of more than 20 pack-years of smoking (either currently or who quit within the past 15 yr). Stop screening at age 80 yr or when patient has not smoked for 15 yr or has a limited life expectancy.
- Current recommendations for pneumonia vaccines for all people > 65 yr of age:
  - Received Pneumovax 23 (PPSV23) only: 1 dose of PCV20 at least 1 yr after PPSV23 completes the series.
  - No previous pneumoccal vaccine: 1 dose of PCV20 completes the series.
  - Received PCV13 or PCV15 only: 1 dose of PPSV23 ≥1 yr after PCV13 or 15 completes the series.

CARDIOVASCULAR SYSTEM

    I. See Table 3.4 for physiologic changes and abnormal findings.
    II. Additional questions to ask:
        A. Do you get dyspneic with activity? Is it increasing?
        B. Do you ever experience edema?
        C. Have you ever experienced dizziness or syncope?
        D. If you have heart failure (HF), how often do you use OTC NSAID medicines such as ibuprofen?

■ = *not to be missed*

TABLE 3.4 ■ Physiologic Changes and Abnormal Findings: Cardiovascular System

Physiologic Changes	Clinical Correlation	Not to Be Missed
Atherosclerosis and arteriosclerosis	Increased incidence of HTN and CHD Pedal pulses may be difficult to palpate	*HTN secondary to anemia or hyperthyroidism* *Changes indicating PVD* *Aneurysms*
Decreased compliance of left ventricle	S_4 may be audible and is not worrisome	*Increased fatigue; exercise intolerance*
Decreased sensitivity of baroreceptors	Valsalva maneuver may cause a sudden drop in BP	*Falls secondary to postural hypotension* *Volume depletion* *Postural hypotension secondary to the use of medication*
ECG changes may include the following: Decreased precordial QRS voltage ST- and T-wave changes Prolonged PR and QT intervals (QRS remains normal) Ectopic (extra) heartbeats	PACs are not associated with increased cardiac risk Isolated PVCs can be seen in healthy older individuals	*ECG changes secondary to ischemia, injury, or infarction* (see Chapter 8, Table 8.6)
Heart valves thicken	Increased incidence of murmurs, especially aortic stenosis and mitral regurgitation	*Pathologic murmur* (see Chapter 8, Table 8.12)
Decreased number of pacemaker cells	Slower or irregular heart rate	*Atrial fibrillation*

BP, blood pressure; *ECG,* electrocardiogram; *PVD,* peripheral vascular disease.

PRACTICE PEARLS FOR CARDIOVASCULAR SYSTEM

- Systolic murmurs are common in elderly people and frequently indicate aortic stenosis.
- Although S4 can be normal or with HTN, S3 warrants investigation for other signs of HF.
- Check BP while the patient is lying, sitting, and standing to evaluate for orthostatic hypotension; wait 2 min between position changes to allow baroreceptors to compensate; evaluate further if systolic BP drops ≥20 mmHg and/or diastolic BP drops ≥10 mmHg or the pulse increases >30 bpm.
- Chest pain is not always present with severe disease or even with myocardial infarction (MI).
- Edema may be caused by HF, protein malnutrition, PVD, venous varicosities, or lymphatic obstruction.
- Elderly patients may develop postprandial hypotension: systolic BP drops ≥20 mmHg within 75–120 min after a meal.
- For men 65–75 yr of age who have ever smoked: one-time abdominal U/S to check for abdominal aortic aneurysm (AAA) is recommended.

GASTROINTESTINAL SYSTEM

  I. See Table 3.5 for physiologic changes and abnormal findings.
  II. Additional questions to ask:
    A. Have you lost any teeth? Do you have partial plate(s) or dentures?
    B. Are you able to care for your teeth or dentures?

■ = *not to be missed*

TABLE 3.5 ■ **Physiologic Changes and Abnormal Findings: Gastrointestinal System**

Physiologic Changes	Clinical Correlation	Not to Be Missed
Dental enamel thins and gums begin to recede	Tooth and gum decay Tooth loss may lead to malocclusion	**Insufficient nutrition** **Periodontal disease** **Poorly fitting dentures**
Decreased saliva production	Dry mouth Increased susceptibility to injury and infection Decreased ability to digest foods	**Dry mouth due to medications or systemic disease** **Dysphagia** **Aspiration due to decreased food clearance from throat**
Delayed esophageal emptying	Occasional discomfort if food stays longer in the esophagus	**GERD or hiatal hernia** **Barrett esophagus** **Medication reaction or side effect** **Dysphagia due to esophageal stricture, tumor, or central nervous system dysfunction**
Decreased gastric acid secretion	May delay absorption of certain vitamins and minerals (e.g., iron, calcium, vitamin B12) and medications	**Pernicious anemia** **Gastric cancer**
Decrease in liver size with concomitant decrease in albumin production	May have significant effect on drug metabolism	**Drug toxicity: fewer albumin-binding sites result in more "free" drug (e.g., digoxin, warfarin)**
Decreased muscle tone and atrophy of mucosa	May contribute to constipation, esophageal spasm, diverticulosis, incontinence	**Bowel changes due to tumors, dehydration, loss of defecation reflex**

C. Can you chew all types of food? Do you have any problems with swallowing or choking? Do you have trouble with any foods?

D. How do you obtain groceries and prepare your meals?

E. Do you eat alone or share meals with others?

F. What did you eat yesterday for meals and snacks?

G. How often do your bowels move? Do you take anything for constipation or diarrhea?

H. Have you lost any weight in the last year? (with loss ≥5% usual body weight in the past 3 mo, consider malnutrition or cancer).

PRACTICE PEARLS FOR GASTROINTESTINAL SYSTEM

- Abdominal pain
  - Abdominal pain in elderly patients can be a vague symptom of a serious or life-threatening disease—*do not take this lightly.*
  - With abdominal pain, obtain an ECG to rule out MI.
  - With significant pain, especially after eating (often in absence of clinical findings), consider intestinal ischemia; history of cardiovascular disease suggests vascular involvement.
  - Abdominal pain associated with confusion and shoulder pain may be observed with lower lobe pneumonia.
  - Because of diminished muscle mass, an elderly patient may not have a rigid abdomen with peritoneal irritation.

Continued

■ = *not to be missed*

PRACTICE PEARLS FOR GASTROINTESTINAL SYSTEM—CONT'D

- Elderly people are prone to constipation.
  - Try increased fiber (foods and/or bulk-forming laxative, e.g., Metamucil, FiberCon) and fluid intake first; if not enough, add MiraLAX and then stool softener plus laxative.
  - Heat together and drink: 4 oz prune juice + 4 oz apple juice + pat of butter.
  - Mix together 2 c. bran cereal (e.g., All-Bran or bran flakes) + prune juice 1 c. + applesauce (to give desired consistency); eat 1–2 T. one to two times a day; store remainder in refrigerator.
  - If an enema is needed, use plain water or mineral oil. Avoid Fleets enema (high risk of electrolyte disturbance), and soap suds enema (may cause rectal damage).
  - If applicable, stop or lower the dose of any anticholinergic medication they are taking.
- Elderly patients also can have anorexia or bulimia.
  - To improve appetite, try mirtazapine (Remeron) 7.5–15 mg at bedtime (hs), or doxepin (Sinequan) 25–50 mg at bedtime (hs).
  - Avoid megestrol acetate (Megace) and high calorie supplements (have not been found to be helpful).
- Malnutrition can be a sign of neglect.

MUSCULOSKELETAL SYSTEM

I. See Table 3.6 for physiologic changes and abnormal findings.

II. Additional questions to ask:
  A. Have you noticed any weakness in the past year?
  B. Have you noticed an increase in falls or stumbling?
  C. Do you use anything to help you get around (e.g., cane)?
  D. How often and for how long do you exercise? What type of activity?

TABLE 3.6 ■ Physiologic Changes and Abnormal Findings: Musculoskeletal System

Physiologic Changes	Clinical Correlation	Not to Be Missed
Loss of muscle mass and muscle strength (lower extremities more than upper extremities)	Decreased ROM, gait changes	*Accelerated changes due to immobility* *Increased falls*
Tendons shrink	Decreased ROM Gait changes	*Decreased ROM due to fractures, OP, inflammation, or contractures* *Falls or increased fall risk*
Deterioration of joint cartilage	May lead to pain and limited movement Gait changes Osteoarthritis	*Pain due to fracture* *Bursitis* *"Frozen" joint* *Falls or increased fall risk*
Decreased bone mass and osteoblastic activity	Osteoporosis Postural changes (e.g., kyphosis) Decrease in height	*Fracture* *Gait and posture changes*

■ = *not to be missed*

PRACTICE PEARLS FOR MUSCULOSKELETAL SYSTEM

- Inspect muscles for atrophy and bones for any deformities; muscle tone is evaluated by passively moving each limb to feel for any rigidity.
  - Increased tone: marked resistance or spasms
  - Decreased tone: no or minimal resistance
- ESR and alkaline phosphatase levels rise in elderly people.
- Pain and stiffness are the most common musculoskeletal complaints in elderly people.
- A change in gait may result from deconditioning or from a musculoskeletal or neurological cause.
- Muscle weakness is not a normal aging process; look for a cause (e.g., diabetes mellitus (DM), hypokalemia, or thiamine deficiency due to alcohol abuse).
  - Evaluate by having the patient stand from sitting in a chair; if the patient must use his or her arms, there is muscle weakness.
  - Falls may be an early sign of an underlying illness.
- Fracture(s) can be a sign of abuse or of a new-onset or progressing problem with gait/balance.

GENITOURINARY SYSTEM

    I. See Table 3.7 for physiologic changes and abnormal findings.

   II. Additional questions to ask:

      A. Males

         1. Do you have difficulty urinating: hesitancy, weaker force of stream, or dribbling?

         2. How many times at night do you get up to urinate?

         3. Do you have any urinary incontinence?

      B. Females

         1. Have you noticed any bleeding since menopause?

         2. Do you have any vaginal itching, burning, or dryness, or bleeding, or pain with intercourse?

         3. Do you feel any pressure in the genital area or have any urinary frequency and/or incontinence?

TABLE 3.7 ■ Physiologic Changes and Abnormal Findings: Genitourinary System

Physiologic Changes	Clinical Correlation	*Not to Be Missed*
Males		
Decreased testosterone levels	Slower and less intense sexual response	*Impotence*
Decrease in the size and firmness of testicles		
Decrease in scrotal muscle tone	Less rugae in scrotal skin and contents hang lower	
Prostatic hypertrophy	Urinary frequency, hesitancy, change in stream	*Prostate cancer* (see Chapter 11) *UTI due to difficulty emptying the bladder*
Females		
Decreased estrogen levels	Vaginal dryness and fragility Narrowing of the vagina UTI symptoms without infection Cessation of menses	*UTI* *Incontinence* (see Chapter 11, Box 11.1) *Palpable ovaries* *Postmenopausal bleeding*

Continued

■ = *not to be missed*

TABLE 3.7 ■ **Physiologic Changes and Abnormal Findings: Genitourinary System—cont'd**

Physiologic Changes	Clinical Correlation	Not to Be Missed
Decreased elasticity of pelvic ligaments		**Cystocele** (see Chapter 11, INCONTINENCE) **Uterine prolapse**
Atrophy of breast tissue	Breasts become more pendulous	**Breast cancer**
Both sexes		
Loss of glomeruli and reduced renal mass	Decreased kidney function; may need to modify medication doses	**eGFR less than 60 mL/h** (see Chapter 11, CHRONIC KIDNEY DISEASE)
Reduced bladder muscle tone	Decreased bladder capacity may lead to increased nocturia or urge to urinate only when the bladder is full	**Nocturia due to BPH, renal insufficiency, HF, or DM**

DM: diabetes mellitus; *HF:* heart failure; *UTI,* urinary tract infection.

PRACTICE PEARLS FOR GENITOURINARY SYSTEM

- With nocturia, ask when diuretics are taken and what the fluid intake is before bedtime.
- Prostate cancer screening with PSA is not recommended in men over age 70 yr or with a life expectancy <10 yr. In men 50–69 yr of age, the decision to screen is made on an individual basis.
- With impotence, look for a cause; it may be psychologic, physiologic, or pharmacologic (see Chapter 11, ERECTILE DYSFUNCTION).
- With decreased renal function and use of ACE inhibitors, do not use NSAIDs.
- With signs of trauma to the anogenital area, consider significant vulvovaginal atrophy or sexual abuse.
- Try to limit overactive bladder (OAB) medications, especially in a patient with poor cognition. Try other measures first (e.g., decrease caffeine, limit fluids before hs, bladder training).

ENDOCRINE/IMMUNE SYSTEMS

   I. See Table 3.8 for physiologic changes and abnormal findings.
  II. Additional questions to ask if the patient has diabetes:
    A. How often do you check your blood sugar?
    B. Do you ever have low blood sugar spells (e.g., feeling weak, sweaty)?
    C. What was your last A1c?
    D. If using an injectable medication, what difficulties (if any) do you have with the injections, and do you prepare the insulin for injections (possible vision problems)?
    E. Do you have any numbness or tingling in your feet? Do you feel your feet when you stand up?

■ = *not to be missed*

TABLE 3.8 ■ **Physiologic Changes and Abnormal Findings: Endocrine/Immune Systems**

Physiologic Changes	Clinical Correlation	Not to Be Missed
Decreased hormone secretion and diminished tissue sensitivity to hormones	Stresses, such as surgery or trauma, may increase mortality	
Fibrosis of thyroid gland	Hypothyroidism signs and symptoms	*Myxedema*
Decreased basal metabolic rate	Increased incidence of obesity and altered carbohydrate tolerance	*Diabetes mellitus*
Defects in temperature regulation	Reduced sweating Fever not always present with infection	*Infection*
Decreased number of T cells and T-cell function	Delayed hypersensitivity reactions Increased incidence of infections Increased prevalence of autoimmune disorders	*Reactivation of latent infections* *Autoimmune disorders*
Increased IgA and decreased IgG levels	Increased prevalence of infection	
Decreased activity in the renin-angiotensin-aldosterone system		*Hyperkalemia*

PRACTICE PEARLS FOR ENDOCRINE/IMMUNE SYSTEMS

- Atypical presenting symptoms of diabetes mellitus (DB) in elderly people include altered mentation, behavior changes, sleep disturbances, incontinence, weight loss, anorexia, and falls.
- Earlier warning signs of DM may include shin spots and recurrent skin infections (especially yeast infections).
- Any changes in eye appearance or heart rate warrant evaluation for a thyroid problem.
- Infections
  - The usual symptoms of infection (e.g., fever, chills, leukocytosis, and tachycardia) may be blunted or absent in elderly patients.
  - The most common atypical signs and symptoms of infection include failure to thrive and changes in mental status, activity, appetite, or weight.
  - Pneumonia and influenza are the most common causes of death.
  - *Overlooked sites* of infection include teeth, the lining of the heart, feet, and gastrointestinal tract.
- Encourage a yearly influenza vaccine. See Practice Pearls for Respiratory System for pneumococcal vaccine recommendations.

NEUROLOGICAL SYSTEM

I. See Table 3.9 for physiologic changes and abnormal findings.

II. Additional questions to ask:

A. Have you noticed any dizziness (lightheadedness—not vertigo)? If so:

1. Does it seem associated with changes in position (e.g., turning over in bed or getting up or down)?

2. Is it associated with a decrease in hearing?

B. Have you noticed any changes in memory or mental functioning? Have you gotten lost in familiar surroundings (e.g., driving to the grocery store or home)?

C. Have you noticed any muscle weakness or tremors?

D. Have you had any sudden vision changes (e.g., halos, lines, or colors) or brief blindness?

■ = *not to be missed*

TABLE 3.9 ■ Physiologic Changes and Abnormal Findings: Neurological System

Physiologic Changes	Clinical Correlation	Not to Be Missed
Loss of neurons and nerve fibers	Decreased Achilles tendon reflex	*Falls*
Slower impulse conduction between neurons	Slower reaction time and decreased vibratory sensation Decreased pain sensation	*Falls or injuries (e.g., burns)* *Changes due to PVD, CNS disease, or neuropathies*
Atrophy of brain	Loss of completion of activities or memory loss	*Subdural hematoma*
Modest decline in short-term memory	Benign loss, usually involving more trivial events	*Mild cognitive impairment* *Dementia* *Delirium* *Depression* *Medication-related cause* (see Beers list for inappropriate medications for the elderly; can be accessed online) *Patient unable to safely set up own medications or remember what has been taken*
Changes in the sleep-wake cycle	More or less time sleeping May have nightmares	*Sleep changes due to dementia, depression, medications, sleep deprivation*

CNS, Central nervous system; *PVD,* peripheral vascular disease.

PRACTICE PEARLS FOR NEUROLOGICAL SYSTEM

- Because there are few significant neurological changes associated with aging, most neurological decline is evidence of a disease process.
- Mental (cognitive) status can be evaluated during the history and examination, using the Short Portable Mental Status Questionnaire (Box 3.1); also consider a brief screening tool for depression (Fig. 3.1, Patient Health Questionnaire [PHQ]-9 scale). Current guidelines do not support screening *asymptomatic* elderly patients for dementia.
- With changes in consciousness (e.g., confusion, lethargy), check for urinary tract infection (UTI) and pneumonia.
- Sensory testing is crucial in elderly patients. Test distal arms and legs bilaterally for both light touch and pain.
- The most common peripheral neuropathies are caused by type 2 diabetes mellitus (DM), alcohol abuse (thiamine deficiency), and vitamin B12 deficiency.
- Tremors should be evaluated.
- Dizziness may be caused by problems with the eyes or ears or with the cardiovascular, musculoskeletal, or neurological systems.
- Gait evaluation is essential in most elderly patients (see Table 3.10 for Tinetti balance and gait evaluation).
- For insomnia, try mirtazapine (Remeron) 7.5 mg, trazodone (Desyrel) 25 mg, or melatonin 3–6 mg at bedtime (hs).

FALLS

I. Assessment tools can be used for initial evaluation and to monitor clinical changes over time. However, the U.S. Preventive Services Task Force (USPSTF) recommends against automatically performing the risk assessment for all community-dwelling adults, noting a small likelihood of benefit for interventions targeted to identified risks.

■ = *not to be missed*

II. Timed "Up and Go" test
   A. This is a reliable, valid, and practical test of balance and gait speed.
   B. To perform, time the patient as he or she rises from a standard armchair, walks 10 ft, turns 180 degrees, returns to the chair, and sits down again.
   C. The score is the number of seconds taken to complete the test; a freely mobile person can complete it in <10 sec. Further evaluation is required if the test is not completed in 20 sec.
III. Tinetti balance and gait evaluation (see Table 3.10)
   A. Assesses musculoskeletal and neurological disorders that increase the risk of falls
   B. Requires no equipment other than a hard, armless chair
   C. Administered in 5–15 min in the clinical setting by observing actual function
   D. Activity-based test that asks the patient to perform tasks such as sitting and rising from a chair, turning, and bending. Scoring:
   <19 = high fall risk
   19–24 = medium fall risk
   25–28 = low fall risk

PRACTICE PEARLS FOR FALLS

- Must include evaluation of balance and gait problems; gait disturbances in elderly people are a risk factor for future cardiovascular diseases and dementia.
- Performed as part of an annual examination, as well as when there appears to be a change in the patient's health status.
- May be critical to include a home visit to assess both the patient and the environment for prevention and safety.
- Elderly people often do not understand negative commands well; for example, say, "please stay in bed (chair)" rather than "please do not get out of bed (chair)."
- Risk factors for falls in elderly people
  - Cardiovascular
    - Arrhythmias
    - Blood pressure fluctuation (e.g., orthostatic hypotension)
    - Cerebrovascular accident (CVA)
  - Musculoskeletal
    - Arthritis
    - Joint weakness
    - Preexisting orthopedic conditions
    - Poor conditioning or inactivity
  - Neurological
    - Dementia
    - Cognitive impairment (even mild to moderate), especially executive dysfunction (see Chapter 17, COGNITIVE IMPAIRMENT)
    - Parkinson disease
    - Multiple sclerosis (MS)
    - Vision and/or hearing loss
  - Urinary or bladder problems
  - Environmental
    - Wet or slippery surfaces
    - Cluttered paths (e.g., throw rugs, poor furniture arrangement)
    - Poor lighting
    - Inadequate footwear (e.g., wearing socks without shoes)
    - Inadequate supervision
  - Medications
    - Especially sedatives, hypnotics, benzodiazepines, antidepressants, anticholinergics
    - Recent dose changes or additional medication(s)
    - Poor adherence to medications

TABLE 3.10 ■ Tinetti Balance and Gait Evaluation

Balance Tests

Instructions: Seat the subject in a hard, armless chair. Test the following maneuvers and select the number that best describes the subject's performance in each test; add up the scores at the end.

1. Sitting balance	Leans or slides in the chair	0
	Steady, safe	1
2. Arises	Unable without help	0
	Able, uses arms to help	1
	Able without using arms	2
3. Attempts to arise	Unable without help	0
	Able, requires >1 attempt	1
	Able to rise, 1 attempt	2
4. Immediate standing balance (first 5 sec)	Unsteady (swaggers, moves feet, trunk sway)	0
	Steady but uses walker or other support	1
	Steady without walker or other support	2
5. Standing balance	Unsteady	0
	Steady but wide stance (medial heels >4 in apart) or uses cane, walker, or other support	1
	Narrow stance without support	2
6. Nudging (with the subject's feet as close together as possible, push lightly on the sternum with the palm of the hand 3 times)	Begins to fall	0
	Staggers, grabs, catches self	1
	Steady	2
7. Eyes closed (same position as in the previous exercise)	Unsteady	0
	Steady	1
8. Turning 360 degrees	Discontinuous steps	0
	Continuous steps	1
	Unsteady (grabs and staggers)	0
9. Sitting down	Unsafe (misjudged distance, falls onto chair)	0
	Uses arms or not a smooth motion	1
	Safe, smooth motion	2
	Balance score	**/16**

Gait Tests

Instructions: Subject stands with the examiner, walks down the hallway or across the room, first at the "usual" pace, then back at a "rapid, but safe" pace (using usual walking aids).

1. Initiation of gait (immediately after told to "go")	Any hesitancy or multiple attempts to start	0
	No hesitancy	1
2. Step length and height		
Right swing foot	Does not pass left stance foot with a step	0
	Passes left stance foot	1
	Right foot does not clear the floor completely with a step	0
	Right foot completely clears the floor	1

TABLE 3.10 ■ **Tinetti Balance and Gait Evaluation—cont'd**

Gait Tests

	Left swing foot	Does not pass right stance foot with a step	0
		Passes right stance foot	1
		Left foot does not clear the floor completely with a step	0
		Left foot completely clears the floor	1
3.	Step symmetry	Right and left step length not equal (estimate)	0
		Right and left step length appear equal	1
4.	Step continuity	Stopping or discontinuity between steps	0
		Steps appear continuous	1
5.	Path (observe excursion of the left or right foot over about 10 ft of the course)	Marked deviation	0
		Mild/moderate deviation or uses walking aid	1
		Straight without walking aid	2
6.	Trunk	Marked sway or uses walking aid	0
		No sway but flexion of knees or back, or spreads arms out while walking	1
		No sway, no flexion, no use of arms, and no use of walking aid	2
7.	Walking stance	Heels apart	0
		Heels almost touching while walking	1
		Gait score	**/12**
		Balance score (from previous page)	**/16**
		Total (gait + balance)	**/28**

(From Tinetti, M. E (1986). Performance-oriented assessment of mobility problems in elderly patients. *Journal of the American Geriatrics Society, 34*(2), 119–126.)

Assessing Functional Status

I. Functional ability must be the focus when providing care to elderly people; this includes evaluating cognition and depression, ADLs, and gait.

II. Cognitive and emotional status (see Practice Pearls for Cognitive and Emotional Status, below)

A. Additional questions to ask:

1. Do you have a living will or advanced directives, or have you designated a Power of Attorney (POA) for health care choices?
2. Have you thought about end-of-life decisions (e.g., CPR or code status)?
3. Do you have a will or a financial POA?
4. What gives your life meaning and value?
5. Are you part of a spiritual or religious community?
6. Do you have friends or family that you communicate with regularly? How often and in what way (e.g., by phone, by computer, in person)?

B. Assessment tools

1. Short Portable Mental Status Questionnaire (SPMSQ) (see Box 3.1)

   (a) Test detects intellectual impairment in elderly people.

   (b) The score can be adjusted to reflect education.

Patient Health Questionnaire (PHQ-9)

Name: _____   **Date:** _____

Over the last *2 weeks,* how often have you been bothered by any of the following problems? *(use "✓" to indicate your answer)*

	Not at all	Several days	More than half the days	Nearly every day
1. Little interest or pleasure in doing things	0	1	2	3
2. Feeling down, depressed, or hopeless	0	1	2	3
3. Trouble falling or staying asleep, or sleeping too much	0	1	2	3
4. Feeling tired or having little energy	0	1	2	3
5. Poor appetite or overeating	0	1	2	3
6. Feeling bad about yourself, or that you are a failure, or have let yourself or your family down	0	1	2	3
7. Trouble concentrating on things, such as reading the newspaper or watching television	0	1	2	3
8. Moving or speaking so slowly that other people could have noticed. Or the opposite—being so fidgety or restless that you have been moving around a lot more than usual	0	1	2	3
9. Thoughts that you would be better off dead, or of hurting yourself	0	1	2	3

Add columns: [_____] + [_____] + [_____]

(Healthcare professional: For interpretation of TOTAL, please refer to accompanying scoring card.)   Total: [_____]

10. If you checked off *any problems,* how *difficult* have these problems made it for you to do your work, take care of things at home, or get along with other people?	Not difficult at all _____ Somewhat difficult _____ Very difficult _____ Extremely difficult _____

Fig. 3.1   PHQ-9 Patient Depression Questionnaire.

PHQ-9 Patient Depression Questionnaire

For initial diagnosis:

1. Patient completes PHQ-9 Quick Depression Assessment.
2. If there are at least 4 ✓s in the shaded section (including Questions #1 and #2), consider a depressive disorder. Add score to determine severity.

Consider Major Depressive Disorder

- If there are at least 5 ✓s in the shaded section (one of which corresponds to Question #1 or #2)

Consider Other Depressive Disorder

- If there are 2–4 ✓s in the shaded section (one of which corresponds to Question #1 or #2)

Note: Since the questionnaire relies on patient self-report, all responses should be verified by the clinician, and a definitive diagnosis is made on clinical grounds taking into account how well the patient understood the questionnaire, as well as other relevant information from the patient.

Diagnoses of Major Depressive Disorder or Other Depressive Disorder also require impairment of social, occupational, or other important areas of functioning (Question #10) and ruling out normal bereavement, a history of a Manic Episode (Bipolar Disorder), and a physical disorder, medication, or other drug as the biological cause of the depressive symptoms.

To monitor severity over time for newly diagnosed patients or patients in current treatment for depression:

1. Patients may complete questionnaires at baseline and at regular intervals (eg, every 2 weeks) at home and bring them in at their next appointment for scoring, or they may complete the questionnaire during each scheduled appointment.
2. Add up ✓s by column. For every ✓: Several days = 1; More than half the days = 2; Nearly every day = 3
3. Add together column scores to get a TOTAL score.
4. Refer to the accompanying **PHQ-9 Scoring Box** to interpret the TOTAL score.
5. Results may be included in patient files to assist you in setting up a treatment goal, determining degree of response, as well as guiding treatment intervention.

Scoring: add up all checked boxes on PHQ-9

For every ✓ Not at all = 0; Several days = 1;
More than half the days = 2; Nearly every day = 3

Interpretation of Total Score

Total Score	Depression Severity
1–4	Minimal depression
5–9	Mild depression
10–14	Moderate depression
15–19	Moderately severe depression
20–27	Severe depression

Fig. 3.1, Cont'd

BOX 3.1 ■ Short Portable Mental Status Questionnaire

What is the date today (month/day/year)?
What day of the week is it?
What is the name of this place?
What is your telephone number? (If no telephone, what is your street address?)
How old are you?
When were you born (month/day/year)?
Who is the current president of the United States?
Who was the president just before him?
What was your mother's maiden name?
Subtract 3 from 20 and keep subtracting 3 from each new number all the way down.

Scoring
0–2 errors = intact
3–4 errors = mild intellectual impairment
5–7 errors = moderate intellectual impairment
8–10 errors = severe intellectual impairment
Allow one more error if the subject had no grade school education.
Allow one fewer error if the subject had education beyond high school.

_____

(From Pfeiffer, E. (1975). A short portable mental status questionnaire for the assessment of organic brain deficit in elderly patients. *Journal of the American Geriatrics Society, 23*(10), 433–441.)

PRACTICE PEARLS FOR COGNITIVE AND EMOTIONAL STATUS

- Provide a quiet, private environment.
- Ensure that the patient has the necessary aids (e.g., glasses or a hearing aid).
- Develop a rapport with the patient before beginning assessment.
- Assessing the cognitive and emotional status can create anxiety for the patient; interspersing assessment questions throughout the interview or examination can reduce stress.
- Consider medications (e.g., anticholinergics) with delirium, cognitive impairment, or falls.
- Consider abuse with an overbearing caretaker, new-onset depression- or dementia-like behavior, failure to pay bills, or abrupt changes in finances.

    2. See Chapter 17, COGNITIVE IMPAIRMENT for assessment of mild cognitive impairment and dementia.
    3. Patient Health Questionnaire (PHQ-9) scale (Fig. 3.1)
       (a) Completed by the patient directly or by interviewing the patient.
       (b) Short form has nine questions; can be completed in a few minutes.
III. Functional assessment
    A. Refers to the ability to perform necessary or desirable ADLs. Changes in the functional status (e.g., unable to bathe independently) should prompt further evaluation and possible intervention.
    B. Physical examination and identification of disease(s) do not sufficiently define the functional ability of the patient.

TABLE 3.11 ▦ **The Vulnerable Elders Survey**

Domain	Score
Age:	
75–85 yr	1
>85 yr	3
Self-rated health:	
Good, very good, and excellent	0
Fair and poor	1
Activities of daily living (ADLs)/instrumental activities of daily living (IADLs):	
Needs assistance with:	
Bathing or showering	1
Shopping	1
Money management	1
Transfer	1
Light housework	1
Difficulty in special activities:	
Kneeling, bending, and stooping	1
Performance of housework (e.g., scrubbing the floor)	1
Reaching out and lifting upper extremities above the shoulder	1
Lifting and carrying 10 lbs	1
Walking quarter of a mile	1
Writing or handling and grasping small objects	1

A score of ≥3 indicates a vulnerable elder.
(From Saliba, D., Elliot, M., Rubenstein, L. Z., Solomon, D. H., Young, R. T., Kamberg, C. J., & Wenger, N. S. (2001). The Vulnerable Elders Survey: a tool for identifying vulnerable older people in the community. *Journal of American Geriatric Society, 49*(12), 1691–1699.)

C. Assessment tools
1. Activities of Daily Living Index Evaluation Forms
   (a) Valid measure of ADLs
   (b) Completed by the interviewer in approximately 3–4 min
   (c) Helps to identify ADLs with which the patient needs assistance (e.g., through rehabilitative therapy, adaptive devices, or personal care assistance)
2. The Vulnerable Elders Survey (VES) 13 Scale (see Table 3.11)
   (a) Can be self-administered or administered by nonmedical personnel in <5 min.
   (b) Identifies community-dwelling elderly at an increased risk of functional decline or death over a 5-yr period.
   (c) Use at repeated visits to monitor for decline in condition.

Laboratory and Diagnostic Pearls

Laboratory Pointers

INTRODUCTION

I. Patient education: prelab instructions
   A. Encourage patient to drink at least 8 oz of water before the tests; may drink all the noncaloric liquids desired (easier to obtain blood).
   B. Do not eat anything for 8 hr before labs are drawn (while not all tests require fasting, it is easier for the patient to remember if all are performed in the same way).
   C. May take medications at regular times.
II. A normal test *does not* mean a healthy patient.
III. With abnormal lab results, *first* consider fluid status or medications (prescription, OTC, herbal).
IV. With dehydration
   A. CBC: all cell lines (RBC, WBC, platelets) increase
   B. UA: specific gravity increases and ketones often present
   C. Chemistries: sodium increased, BUN/creatinine ratio >10

CHEMISTRIES

I. Amylase and lipase
   A. A perforated ulcer is accompanied by increased amylase but not lipase.
   B. Although pancreatitis is a common cause of elevations, there are many other causes; however, lipase elevated >3× the normal has 98% sensitivity for pancreatitis.
II. BUN: the liver produces ammonia from protein breakdown, which results in nitrogen; this is then transformed into urea, which is excreted by the kidneys. BUN can reflect liver or kidney dysfunction.
   A. Increased BUN
      1. Renal failure: creatinine will also be high
      2. Dehydration, GI bleeding, and high-protein diet: creatinine is normal
   B. Decreased BUN
      1. With GI bleeding, BUN decreases within 24 hr of bleeding cessation; monitor BUN daily, and if it increases, consider recurrent bleeding even if not clinically apparent
      2. Starvation (inadequate protein intake), liver failure (inadequate production of urea), and overhydration
   C. BUN/creatinine ratio = 10 normally
      1. If <10, consider renal failure
      2. If >10, consider prerenal azotemia; if > 36, consider UGI bleed
III. Cardiac enzymes may be helpful if positive, but if within normal limits, they do *not* rule out MI (serial tests are needed).

IV. Hypercalcemia
  A. Likely causes: hyperparathyroidism or some type of cancer
  B. Recheck serum calcium to verify it is elevated; if this test is also high, then obtain free (ionized) calcium and a serum PTH (parathyroid hormone).
   1. If both calcium and PTH are elevated, *referral to endocrinologist.*
   2. If calcium is elevated but PTH is low, check PTH-related peptide (PTH-RP); if it is elevated, consider computed tomography (CT) abdomen and chest (looking for lung or kidney cancer) and *referral to oncologist (may be urgent, depending on patient's condition).*
V. Hypokalemia
  A. With hypokalemia, also check magnesium, calcium, and phosphorus; a serum magnesium or phosphate <1 mg/dL is life-threatening
  B. Signs and symptoms
   1. Weakness: skeletal (e.g., weak muscles and voice); cardiac (e.g., HF); smooth muscle (e.g., nausea, ileus)
   2. Metabolic: insulin resistance, hepatic encephalopathy, urinary concentrating defect
   3. ECG: prolonged Q-T and/or presence of U wave
  C. Classification

Class	Serum K+ (mEq/L)
Mild	3.0–3.5
Moderate	2.5–3.0
Severe	2.0–2.5

  D. There is an obligate renal loss of 40 mEq K^+ daily; if the patient is NPO, consider adding KCl to IV fluids
VI. Hyponatremia
  A. A change in serum sodium levels reflects serum osmolality; if it occurs quickly, the patient can experience neurological symptoms (e.g., H/A, confusion, drowsiness, restless and irritable, dizziness), so correct hyponatremia/hypernatremia over the time period you think it has occurred. *Transfer to ED, if symptomatic.*
  B. With hyponatremia
   1. Check *serum* osmolality
    (a) *Serum* osmolality >300 mOsm/kg: hyperglycemia (DKA or hyperosmolar hyperglycemic state [HHS]); recent TURP or hysteroscopy with absorption of irrigation solutions
    (b) *Serum* osmolality <280 mOsm/kg: thiazides, severe liver or heart disease
   2. Check *urine* osmolality in patients with edema (e.g., peripheral or pulmonary edema, ascites) or with signs of hypovolemia (e.g., hypotension, postural hypotension) or low circulating blood volume (e.g., HF, cirrhosis).
    (a) Increased *urine* osmolality (>285 mOsm/kg): dehydration, high-protein diet, hypernatremia, hyperglycemia, SIADH
    (b) Decreased *urine* osmolality (<280 mOsm/kg): DI, excess fluid intake, renal insufficiency, glomerulonephritis
   3. If not recently done, also check liver function tests and calcium, CBC, TSH and 8 a.m. cortisol level.

HEMATOLOGY (CBC)

I. General recommendations
  A. All cell lines (RBC, WBC, and platelets) increase with hemoconcentration (e.g., dehydration).
  B. If two of three cell lines are abnormal (elevated or decreased), repeat CBC in 24 to 48 hr; if still abnormal without a known cause (e.g., dehydration with infection), consider *referral to a hematologist (may be urgent, depending on patient's condition).*
  C. With abnormal RBC, WBC, or platelet counts, recheck CBC along with peripheral smear (gives a direct cell count and identifies any atypical cells).
II. Platelets
  A. Normal platelet appearance does not mean that they function normally.
  B. With abnormal platelet count, repeat CBC with peripheral smear; *if still abnormal, referral to a hematologist.*
    1. Thrombocytosis (>450,000/µL): recheck in ≤1 wk
      (a) Types
        (i) Reactive: commonly caused by infection, after surgery, cancer, anemia
        (ii) Chronic myeloproliferative: essential thrombocythemia, polycythemia vera, CML
        (iii) Mild increase in platelet count: consider dehydration, chronic hypoxia (COPD, chronic carbon monoxide poisoning in a patient who smokes)
      (b) Is often associated with vasomotor symptoms (e.g., H/A, chest pain, pain/burning in toes, lightheadedness) and thrombotic or bleeding complications (less likely with reactive thrombocytosis)
    2. Thrombocytopenia (<150,000/µL)
      (a) Recheck platelet count
        (i) With 100,000–150,000/µL: in 1–2 mo
        (ii) With 75,000–100,000/µL in an asymptomatic, nonbleeding patient: in 1–2 wk
        (iii) With <75,000/µL: in no more than 1 wk
      (b) Bleeding risk
        (i) 50,000–80,000/µL: may have petechiae (or be asymptomatic)
        (ii) 20,000–50,000/µL: bleeding risk increased
        (iii) <20,000/µL: highest risk for bleeding (may have spontaneous bleeding at counts of <10,000/µL)
      (c) Possible causes
        (i) NSAID use does not usually cause a platelet count of <50,000/µL
        (ii) Idiopathic thrombocytopenic purpura (or immune thrombocytopenia; ITP)
        (iii) Drug related: condition usually resolves within 1 wk after drug cessation; ask about quinine-containing herbal products (e.g., cinchona, quina, Peruvian bark)
        (iv) Viral: HIV, hepatitis C, CMV, rickettsial diseases
        (v) Less common: liver disease with hypersplenism, myelodysplastic syndrome, and alcohol-induced coagulopathy
III. RBCs (see also ANEMIA, later in this chapter)
  A. RBCs
    1. Primary cell responsible for carrying oxygen to all tissues and organs

---

● = *non–urgent referral;* ▲ = *urgent referral*

    2. Any change/decrease in size, shape, or number of RBCs will affect the ability of the RBC to carry oxygen

B. H&H
    1. Hemoglobin (Hgb) is the O_2-carrying component of RBC.
    2. Hematocrit (Hct) is the percentage of RBCs in blood volume; normally, $Hgb \times 3 = Hct$ (if not, consider lab error).
    3. With CKD, baseline H&H is ~10/30; if normal or lower, there is an additional problem (e.g., "normal" H&H with dehydration).
    4. If H&H counts are abnormal, repeat CBC along with peripheral smear; if still abnormal, ***consider hematology referral.***

C. Abnormal-looking RBCs
    1. Size is denoted by MCV, which notes the average size of RBC and can help to classify type of anemia.
      (a) MCV 80–100 fL (normocytic) can be seen with anemia of chronic disease (ACD) and autoimmune anemias. It can also reflect a combination macrocytic and microcytic anemia, since the MCV is an average size of RBC.
      (b) MVC >105 fL (macrocytic) could be related to
        (i) Vitamin deficiency
        (ii) Bone marrow depression or cell division
        (iii) Alcoholism, liver disease
      (c) MCV <77 fL (microcytic) related to
        (i) Acute blood loss
        (ii) Iron deficiency anemia (IDA) or ACD
    2. Shape
      (a) Schistocytes, helmet-shaped cells: fragmented RBCs due to destruction within vessels (e.g., with TTP, DIC) or defective prosthetic valve
      (b) "Tear-drops": thalassemia, iron deficiency, other anemias
      (c) Spherocyte: autoimmune hemolytic anemia, hereditary spherocytosis
      (d) Target cells: presence of many target cells in peripheral smear highly suggests sickle disease
      (e) Basophilic stippling: heavy metal poisoning (e.g., lead, arsenic), thalassemia, hemoglobinopathies
    3. If RBCs look abnormal, repeat CBC along with peripheral smear; if still abnormal, ***consider hematology referral.***

D. Reticulocytes are immature RBCs produced in the bone marrow and can help evaluate the functional response to anemias or other processes (e.g., cancer, chemotherapy).

E. Red cell distribution (RDW) looks at variations in RBC width (presence of variance is called "anisocytosis").
    1. Elevated RDW indicates nutritional deficiency (e.g., iron [Fe], folate or B12).
    2. When compared with MCV, it can assist in classifying anemia further:
      (a) Normal RDW with
        (i) Low MCV: anemia of chronic disease (ACD), thalassemia
        (ii) Normal MCV: acute blood loss, ACD, renal disease
        (iii) Elevated MCV: aplastic anemia, liver disease, chemotherapy, alcoholism
      (b) Elevated RDW with
        (i) Low MCV: IDA, sickle cell anemia (SCA), thalassemia
        (ii) Normal MCV: early IDA, folate or B12 deficiency, SCA, chronic liver disease

---

● = *non-urgent referral*

   (iii) Elevated MCV: vitamin deficiency, thyroid or liver disease, hemolytic
         anemia, myelodysplastic disease
F. Iron studies
   1. Serum Fe level is the iron bound to transferrin and thus able to bind to Hgb and
      carry O_2.
      (a) Elevated Fe: consider pernicious anemia, thalassemia, lead poisoning, exces-
          sive iron intake, and hemochromatosis
      (b) Decreased Fe: consider IDA, CKD, cancer, thyroid disease
   2. Ferritin is the storage protein for iron and correlates with total body stores of iron
      (good test for IDA).
   3. TIBC measures the blood's capacity to bind iron with transferrin.
      (a) Increased: consider IDA, blood loss, liver disease, currently taking COCs
      (b) Decreased: consider hemochromatosis, thalassemia, hyperthyroidism, ACD
G. B12 level: if low, deficiency is present; consider obtaining methylmalonic acid level
   (MMA), and if MMA is elevated, this is confirmatory for B12 deficiency.
H. Lactate dehydrogenase (LDH) is used to identify destruction of RBCs; if elevated,
   this indicates hemolytic anemias or other destructive processes.
IV. WBC
A. The normal neutrophil (seg) to lymphocyte (lymph) ratio is 60:40; the percentage of
   segs may be elevated with infection, even with a normal total WBC count; reverse
   ratio indicates lymphocytosis.
B. "Shift to the left" (i.e., >5 bands [immature WBCs]) can occur with increased, normal, or decreased WBC counts and indicates infection.
C. Leukocytosis: WBC count *generally* >11,000 mm^3; the reference range is age-specific.
   1. "Greatly" elevated WBC count (e.g., >30,000 mm^3) with lymphadenopathy: sus-
      pect leukemia or lymphoma.
   2. Stress can increase WBC count to 20,000–25,000 mm^3, with resolution within
      <24 hr; this is more common in children.
   3. Lymphocytosis
      (a) In patients >50 yr of age, asymptomatic lymphocytosis often indicates
          chronic lymphocytic leukemia. ***Referral to a hematologist.***
      (b) Lymphocytosis *plus* anemia, thrombocytopenia, or neutropenia suggests can-
          cer; ***referral to a hematologist or to ED, depending on patient's condition overall.***
D. Leukopenia: WBC generally <4000 mm^3 in adults; age-specific ranges in children
   1. Decreased WBC with increased lymphocytes: viral infection, pertussis
   2. In an immunosuppressed patient with neutropenia and any fever >100.4°F with-
      out a clear cause, ***treat as a medical emergency and refer or transfer to ED*** (consider
      sepsis until proven otherwise)
E. Eosinophilia: consider allergies or helminth parasitic infection.

LAB TESTS FOR ARTHRALGIAS

I. Antinuclear antibody (ANA)
A. Negative test (<1:80) excludes systemic lupus erythematosus (SLE) in 95% of the
   cases
B. Positive test
   1. Titer (≥1:160) is more likely a true result, but can still be false positive with
      chemo, cancer, some medications (e.g., INH, procainamide, hydralazine).

▲ = *urgent referral*

2. Positive titer alone is not diagnostic of SLE.

3. ***Referral to a rheumatologist*** because the positive titer must be verified with other tests; tell the patient, "The test shows inflammation in the blood, but other tests need to be performed."

II. C-reactive protein (CRP)

   A. It is not known what level is truly normal or clinically innocuous; serial tests are best.

      1. Used to guide management of RA.

      2. Elevated levels are definitely linked to ACS but *not* to stable angina.

      3. Increases with high-fat meal or foods sweetened with high-fructose corn syrup.

   B. High-sensitivity CRP (hs-CRP) only means that the results were determined using an assay to measure very low levels of CRP (i.e., <0.3 mg/L).

   C. Hs-CRP >10 mg/L: often rheumatic cause, infection, or inflammation; recheck in 2 wk.

   D. CRP changes more quickly than ESR as the patient's condition worsens or improves.

III. Erythrocyte sedimentation rate (ESR or sed rate)

   A. Increased with anemia, inflammation, infection, obesity, cancer; may exhibit mild to moderate increase with significant psychosocial stress.

      1. Elevated ESR with negative RA and ANA: suspect cancer.

      2. If >100 mm/h, consider infection (33%), cancer, inflammation (e.g., temporal arteritis, polymyalgia rheumatica [PMR]), nephrotic syndrome (a common cause is diabetic nephropathy).

   B. If symptoms improve but ESR remains high, consider additional causes of inflammation (e.g., temporal arteritis) or need for more aggressive treatment.

   C. ESR changes more slowly than CRP, as the patient's condition worsens or improves.

IV. Rheumatoid arthritis (RA) factor

   A. 80% sensitive in RA.

   B. False-positive results can occur in chronic infections and other chronic inflammatory conditions.

V. Uric acid

   A. Not the only criteria used to diagnose gout; it can be used to monitor the response to medications such as allopurinol.

   B. Also, is often monitored in CKD.

LIVER TESTS (SEE ALSO CHAPTER 9, LIVER DISEASE)

I. *Biliary enzymes* (e.g., alkaline phosphatase, bilirubin, and GGT) are increased in cholestatic conditions (obstruction either within the liver itself or affecting the bile duct [e.g., gallstone, pancreatic mass]).

   A. If alkaline phosphatase is the only elevated liver test, it often indicates an infiltrative process (e.g., tumor mass). To confirm that it is from the liver, obtain a GGT level (GGT is usually elevated in liver disorders but not in bone disorders).

   B. If GGT is the only elevated liver test, it may indicate excessive alcohol use.

   C. Bilirubin

      1. Total bilirubin: function of Hgb breakdown; reflects the liver's ability to dispose of Hgb; increases with obstructive jaundice, stones, or damaged liver cells.

      2. Increased total bilirubin with normal direct bilirubin: consider hemolytic anemia or transfusion reaction.

● = *non-urgent referral*

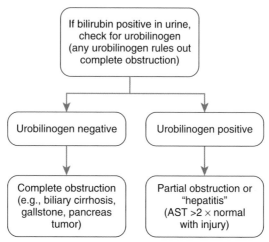

Fig. 4.1   Bilirubin in urine.

    3. Bilirubin >3.5 mg/dL results in jaundice, which indicates an obstruction in the bile duct area. Because no bilirubin should be excreted renally (normally goes out in the bowel), check urinalysis for bilirubinuria (Fig. 4.1).

II. *Hepatocellular enzymes* measure the severity of hepatocellular inflammation (also see Chapter 9, PRACTICE PEARLS FOR LIVER DISEASE). They do not reflect how well the liver functions and may actually be normal in patients with advanced cirrhosis.

    A. ALT: more specific to the liver and less to the heart, muscle, and kidney.

    B. AST: present in tissues with high metabolic activity and increased with liver disease, tumor, MI, heat stroke.

       1. With elevated levels, first consider **A**lcohol-**S**tatins-**T**ylenol (common causes).

       2. AST >1000 IU/L is often due to infection or toxins (e.g., medications, herbs, poisons); if it occurs within the first 24 hr of illness, there is a high likelihood that the patient will not survive.

    C. If AST and ALT levels are elevated but are <3 times the normal, stop alcohol and all OTC medications and supplements; recheck labs in 2 wk (e.g., CMP, hepatitis panel, CBC, PT/INR, lipids). If still elevated, consider abdominal U/S to check for NAFLD, cirrhosis, etc. May consider *referral to gastroenterologist*, depending on test results.

    D. AST/ALT ratio

       1. Normally ~1

       2. Helps to differentiate ETOH-induced liver damage from infectious hepatitis.

         (a) ALT > AST = infectious hepatitis

         (b) AST > ALT = alcohol-related damage (usually 3:1 to 8:1)

       3. If >1, consider medications, viruses, autoimmune hepatitis, hemochromatosis, Wilson disease, α-1-antitrypsin deficiency, NAFLD, a fast food–heavy diet.

III. *Liver function tests* evaluate hepatocellular function. These tests plus albumin are included as part of the Child-Pugh score to estimate cirrhosis mortality.

    A. PT/INR (INR is a standardized way to report PT): prolonged with liver disease, causing inadequate production of certain clotting factors.

● = *non–urgent referral*

  B. Albumin: controls osmotic pressure, which maintains fluid in blood vessels.
      1. Decreased: leads to edema (e.g., in cirrhosis, liver failure, and malnutrition; also in
          nonhepatic acute and chronic illnesses)
      2. Increased: may indicate dehydration
IV. Miscellaneous
  A. Medications commonly associated with drug-induced liver injury include acetamin-
      ophen, anabolic steroids, NSAIDs (especially diclofenac), amiodarone, valproic acid,
      isoniazid, rifampin, and azathioprine.
  B. *Any* medication can increase enzymes in susceptible people; people with liver
      disease or cirrhosis are at no higher risk than the general population to develop
      medication-related enzyme changes.
  C. Medication adjustments
      1. Most medications do not need dose adjustments until liver function is >90%
          impaired (e.g., patient has cirrhosis with jaundice or bleeding varices).
      2. Monitor highly protein-bound medications (e.g., phenytoin, warfarin) because
          low albumin levels may increase side effects.
      3. The patient may also have renal failure, along with the hepatic failure.
  D. Always check TSH level; hypothyroidism may cause a mild increase in liver enzymes.
V. *Referral to a gastroenterologist/hepatologist*
  A. With unexplained, persistent elevations of ALT and AST >2 times the upper limit
      of normal (ULN) or alkaline phosphatase >1.5 times ULN
  B. Patients being considered for liver biopsy

MISCELLANEOUS TESTS

  I. Indicate on the order if the following tests are being ordered for screening or diagnostic
      reasons (especially with Medicare):
  A. Lipids, blood glucose
  B. PSA, Pap smear, HPV, chlamydia, gonorrhea, syphilis, HIV
  C. HCV, HBsAg
  D. Fecal occult blood (guaiac or immunoassay), Cologuard
 II. A1c (elevated)—also see Chapter 15, Diabetes, MONITORING, II
  A. Marker for accelerated ASCVD: every 1% increase in A1c increases the risk of CV
      events by 20% overall and CV mortality by 24% (males) and 28% (females).
  B. Increases the risk of HF after MI.
III. Pulse oximetry (ox): noninvasive measurement of arterial O_2 saturation
  A. There is no defined abnormal level because there is no defined threshold of tissue
      hypoxia. It is most helpful to know the patient's usual level, but "reasonable" *abnormal*
      values could be as follows:
      1. Resting pulse ox ≤95%
      2. Exercise *desaturation* ≥5% (should increase with exercise)
  B. Possible causes of low values
      1. COPD most common cause of hypoxia
          (a) Only 10%–20% of patients with COPD retain CO_2
          (b) Baseline O_2 sat in COPD is 88%–90%
      2. Hypoventilation
          (a) CNS depression (e.g., drug OD, ischemic lesion impacting respiratory center)
          (b) Obesity

● = *non-urgent referral*

(c) Neurological (e.g., ALS, Guillain-Barre)
(d) Musculoskeletal (e.g., myasthenia gravis, muscular dystrophy, kyphoscoliosis)
(e) Severe hypothyroidism

URINE TESTS

   I. Urine specific gravity and *serum* sodium are the only tests that reliably vary with hemo-dilution and hemoconcentration (see Table 4.1 for urinalysis findings).

  II. Positive ketones: very nonspecific; consider dehydration first but also low-carb diet. Diabetic ketoacidosis (DKA) is diagnosed with *serum* ketones.

 III. Urine culture

     A. Clean-catch urine culture recommended with suspected UTI: it confirms infection and guides antibiotic use

     B. *Positive results* (from clean-catch specimen)

       1. Asymptomatic patient: >100,000 CFU/mL

       2. Symptomatic patient: 100–100,000 CFU/mL

     C. In patients with chronic Foley catheter use, *do not* obtain UA with C&S unless patient is symptomatic (e.g., fever, hematuria, decreased LOC), because they will usually be colonized but not infected; *this includes* a follow-up UA after treatment for a UTI

TABLE 4.1 ■ **Urinalysis Findings**

Normal Findings	Abnormal Findings	Significance
Appearance: Clear, straw-yellow color	Colorless/pale	Diabetes insipidus, alcohol, increased fluid intake, water intoxication related to psychiatric medications
	Red or brown	Blood, porphyrin Foods: beets, rhubarb, food color Medications: sulfisoxazole, phenytoin, cascara, chlorpromazine, rifampin, senna
	Orange	Decreased oral intake, urobilinogen, fever Medications: phenazopyridine (Pyridium), sulfa, nitrofurantoin Foods: carrots, rhubarb
	Blue or green	*Pseudomonas* Medications: amitriptyline, methylene blue Vitamin B complex
	Brown or black	Hemorrhage, melanin, bilirubin, methemoglobin, myoglobin Medications/foods: cascara, senna, iron
	Cloudy	Bacteria, pus, prostatic fluid, semen
	Milky	Pyuria, dyslipidemia
	Foamy	Cirrhosis, bilirubin, bile, hepatitis, obstructive liver disease, proteinuria
Odor: Aromatic	Ammonia Foul Mousy Fruity	Urea breakdown, increased nitrites Bacteria Phenylketonuria DM, starvation or extreme dieting, anorexia, bulimia

TABLE 4.1 ▪ **Urinalysis Findings—cont'd**

Normal Findings	Abnormal Findings	Significance
pH: 4.6–6.5	<4.6	Acidosis, high-protein diet, severe diarrhea/vomiting, severe COPD, renal stones Medications: metformin
	6.5–8	Bacteriuria, UTI, metabolic alkalosis Medications: neomycin, sulfa, potassium citrate
Specific gravity (reflects renal concentrating ability): 1.005–1.030	<1.005	Diabetes insipidus, increased oral intake Medications: diuretics
	>1.030	Decreased oral intake, dehydration, fever, excess vomiting/diarrhea, iodine dye, DM
Protein: Negative	Positive If >2+, get 24-hr urine for protein and creatinine clearance	Trace/1+: consider exercise and recheck early morning specimen Pyelonephritis, glomerulonephritis (1+ to 2+), bladder cancer, UTI, HF, myeloma, fever, lead poisoning, toxemia, DM, nephrosis (3+ to 4+) Medications: barbiturates, sulfa, neomycin
Glucose: Negative	Positive	DM, CVA, anesthesia, extreme stress Medications: ASA, cephalosporin, vitamin C, epinephrine
Ketone: Negative	Positive	High-protein diet, decreased oral intake, heat exhaustion, early diabetic ketoacidosis, fever, hyperthyroidism
Bilirubin: Negative	Positive	Hepatitis, cirrhosis, obstructive gallbladder disease
Urobilinogen: <2 mg/dL	>2 mg/dL	Can be due to normal bile metabolism (also see Fig. 4.1), HF, hyperthyroidism Medication: neomycin
Leukocyte esterase: Negative	Positive	Infection
Nitrite: Negative	Positive	Infection
Blood: Negative	Positive	Kidney stones, cancer, infection, menses, transfusion reaction, trauma, Foley catheterization, polycystic kidneys; unexplained hematuria in young Black patients is often caused by sickle trait Medications: anticoagulants
Microscopic Findings		
RBCs: <2/HPF	>2/HPF >3/HPF: repeat UA; if 2 tests abnormal, evaluate further	Renal disease, kidney stones, cancer, UTI, strenuous exercise, trauma to GU tract Medications: ASA, warfarin sodium
WBCs: <4/HPF	>4/HPF	UTI, interstitial cystitis, AGN, fever, SLE, strenuous exercise, TB, analgesic abuse
Epithelial cells: <5/HPF	>5/HPF	Usually indicates contaminated specimen
Hyaline casts: <5/HPF	10–30/HPF	Strenuous exercise, HF, fever, HTN, AGN
RBC cast: None	>2/HPF	AGN, renal cancer, SBE, vasculitis, GABHS, malignant HTN
WBC cast: None	>2/HPF	Kidney inflammation (possible pyelonephritis, acute tubular necrosis)
Bacteria: None	>5/HPF	UTI

IV. Proteinuria
   A. From urinalysis or urine dipstick: see Table 4.1
   B. From a 24-hr urine specimen
      1. Minimal (<0.5 g/day): exercise or concentrated urine in a healthy person; fever, cystitis, polycystic kidneys
      2. Moderate (0.5–3 g/day): mild DM nephropathy, chronic glomerulonephritis
      3. Marked (>3 g/day): lupus nephritis, AGN, severe DM nephropathy, amyloid disease
V. Albumin/creatinine ratio (ACR): CKD diagnosis if >17 mg/g (males) or >25 mg/g (females).
VI. Polyuria: determine if nocturia is present and if the frequent voiding is large or small volume.
   A. Nocturia validates that there is polyuria
   B. Urine voiding volume
      1. Large amounts: consider renal or endocrine cause
         (a) Renal (impaired ability to concentrate the urine): hypokalemia, hypercalcemia
         (b) Endocrine: DM or diabetes insipidus
      2. Small amounts: UTI problem (e.g., cystitis, prostatitis)

Radiology Pointers

   I. Carotid Doppler: 80%–99% stenosis with/without symptoms indicates severe stenosis; **surgeon consultation recommended.**
   II. Chest X-ray (CXR): changes indicating pneumonia may lag 3 days behind clinical diagnosis (i.e., CXR may appear normal but the patient has signs/symptoms of pneumonia). This is also why follow-up CXR is performed 1–4 wk after finishing therapy.
   III. Contrast medium
      A. Gastrografin: an oral contrast that does no harm if it enters the peritoneal cavity (e.g., with bowel or stomach perforation)
      B. Barium: an oral contrast that is contraindicated with suspected acute abdomen
      C. When patient takes metformin
         1. With eGFR >30 mL/min: *no need* to stop medication before or after the exam
         2. With eGFR <30 mL/min (the radiology department may have a different protocol):
            (a) Emergent cases—stop medication for 48 hr *after* exam
            (b) Nonemergent cases—hold medication for 48 hr *before and after* exam
            (c) Recheck renal function after 48 hr, *before restarting* the medication
   IV. CT/MRI scans (also see Table 4.2)
      A. With renal insufficiency, order CT of the abdomen and/or pelvis with and without ORAL contrast only.
      B. MRI scans of the spine are performed without contrast unless the patient has a history of cancer, has had surgery in the area of the spine within 2 yr, or has infection.
      C. MRI scans of an extremity or joint are usually performed without contrast; contrast is indicated to rule out soft tissue mass or osteomyelitis.
      D. For pediatric patients: consider U/S before ordering CT or MRI.
   V. Pelvic with transvaginal U/S recommendations
      A. Suspected pelvic mass
      B. Suspected ectopic pregnancy, early pregnancy of <9 wk, or with abnormal uterine bleeding (to check uterus and endometrial lining)
   VI. PET scan: blood glucose needs to be <250 mg/dL to prevent false-positive test (hyperglycemia causes greater intake of the injection material)

● = *non-urgent referral*

TABLE 4.2 ■ CT and MRI Scans

Condition Considered	Test Ordered (With [w/] or Without [w/o] Contrast*)	Notes
Head/Brain		
Acute H/A or suspected acute stroke	CT brain w/o	Contrast only if indicated after first scan
Chronic H/A, especially with mental status changes (consider mass, bleed, hydrocephalus)	CT brain w/ and w/o OR MRI brain w/ and w/o	MRI brain *never* with contrast only
Seizures	MRI brain w/o	Radiology may have an MRI seizure protocol
Known aneurysm or strong FH of aneurysm	MRI brain w/o OR MRA head w/o (often both done)	MRI brain *never* with contrast only MRA head *never* done with contrast
Pituitary/sella pathology	MRI w/ and w/o	MRI brain *never* with contrast only Radiology may have an MRI pituitary protocol
Sinus	Limited CT sinus	Usually done w/o
Facial trauma	CT facial bones	
Neck		
Mass or lump in neck	CT soft tissue of neck w/	U/S of neck if thyroid or parotid suspected
Salivary stone suspected	CT neck w/ and w/o	
Chest		
PE suspected	CTA chest w/ or CT with pulmonary angiography	Radiology may have a CT-PE protocol
Any other pathology (including possible aneurysm)	CT chest w/	
Abdomen/Pelvis**		
AAA (abdominal aortic aneurysm) suspected	CT angiography (CTA) abd/pelvis w/	
Acute abdomen/LLQ pain	CT abd/pelvis w/ IV *and* oral contrast	
RLQ pain (suspected appendicitis)	CT abd/pelvis w/	U/S recommended first in pediatric patients
Mass/tumor suspected	CT abd/pelvis w/ IV *and* oral contrast	
Hematuria Possible kidney stone(s)	CT abd/pelvis w/o	Radiology may have kidney stone protocol
Kidney/adrenal pathology	CT abd w/ and w/o IV contrast	
Bladder pathology	CT pelvis w/ IV *and* oral contrast	
RUQ pain (possible gallbladder)		U/S recommended first May need HIDA scan also
Pancreatic mass/LUQ pain	CT abd/pelvis w/ and w/o IV *and* oral contrast	Radiology may have pancreas protocol
Pelvic fracture (seen on plain X-rays)	CT pelvis w/o	

Continued

TABLE 4.2 ■ CT and MRI Scans—cont'd

Condition Considered	Test Ordered (With [w/] or Without [w/o] Contrast*)	Notes
Spine		
Any area w/ acute trauma	CT w/o	Plain films first
Any painful area w/o acute trauma	MRI w/o, *unless* infection suspected, <2yr after surgery of spine, or Hx of any cancer; then MRI w/ and w/o	
Possible spinal lesion (abnormal plain X-ray)	MRI w/o	
Wounds (Lower Extremities)		
Diabetic foot ulcer	Suspect osteomyelitis: MRI w/ With decreased circulation but not immediate intervention: CTA or MRA	Plain films first Nuclear bone scan is alternative to MRI but not as accurate
Pressure injury/ulcer	Suspect osteomyelitis: MRI w/	Plain films first Nuclear bone scan is alternative to MRI but not as accurate

* IV contrast, unless noted otherwise.
** Abdominal and/or pelvic CT: *oral contrast* if the suspected problem is in the gut, *IV contrast* if the suspected problem is vascular.

Clinical Conditions

ANEMIA

   I. Anemia is a sign of a disease, not a disease without a cause.
  II. Definition: decrease in RBCs, Hgb, and HCT; generally defined lab values may vary
    A. Infants/children: Hgb <11 g/dL or Hct <33%
    B. Women: Hgb <12 g/dL or Hct <35%
    C. Men: Hgb <13 g/dL or Hct <41%
 III. Causes of anemia
    A. Blood loss
       1. Emergent blood loss through trauma, acute GI bleed, surgery
       2. Slower continuous losses with menorrhagia, GI microbleeds (e.g., polyps, gastric mucosa irritation)
    B. Increased destruction of RBCs
       1. Hemolysis
       2. Autoimmune disease
    C. Decreased production of RBCs
       1. Inability to absorb certain nutrients (i.e., iron, B12, folate)
       2. Bone marrow disorder resulting in lack of production
       3. Inadequate production due to decreased use of iron and/or shortened life span of RBCs, usually from malignancy or chronic illness
 IV. Signs and symptoms
    A. Anemias of *all causes*
       1. *Early* signs (Hgb ~10 g/dL)
         (a) Easily fatigued, weakness, pallor to skin and conjunctiva
         (b) Mild-to-moderate orthostatic changes (e.g., tachycardia, tachypnea, dizziness)

2. *Later* signs (Hgb ≤10 g/dL)
   (a) Early signs progress in intensity
   (b) Pallor in hand creases and circumoral pallor
   (c) Systolic murmur (either at rest or with movement); new-onset venous hum
   (d) Brittle hair, spoon-shaped nails (koilonychias)
   (e) Pica (usually ice-related)
   B. Related to *vitamin deficiency* (e.g., B12, folate)
   1. Glossitis, stomatitis
   2. Confusion, decreased cognition and ability to care for self
   3. Diminished position sense, shuffling gait
   4. Symmetric numbness and tingling in hands, legs or feet; restless leg syndrome (RLS)
V. Diagnostic testing for all type anemias
   A. Lab tests
   1. CBC, CMP, CRP, homocysteine level, reticulocyte count
   2. Fe, ferritin, TIBC (these three may be available as an iron panel), folate and B12 levels, methylmalonic acid (MMA; more sensitive test for B12 deficiency), LDH (marker of hemolysis)
   3. Consider RBC smear/pathology
   B. For women ≥50 yr of age
   1. Perform pelvic exam, Pap smear, test stool for occult blood; obtain transvaginal and pelvic US; breast exam and mammogram
   2. If all normal, consider EGD/colonoscopy
   C. For men, obtain EGD and/or colonoscopy and PSA
VI. Anemia related to decreased production of RBCs
   A. ACD (usually normocytic/hypochromic; see Box 4.1) secondary to chronic inflammation, infection, organ failure, senescence, or cancer
   1. Signs, symptoms, diagnostic testing (see IV and V, above)
   2. Treatment is aimed at identifying and controlling the underlying cause; may need iron supplements (see VII, Iron-deficiency anemia, below), oxygen therapy, or transfusions
   B. Myelodysplastic anemia is caused by bone marrow dysfunction that affects the production of RBCs, platelets, and/or granulocytes; more common in the elderly and can be a precursor to leukemias (see Box 4.2)
   1. Signs and symptoms particular to myelodysplastic anemia
   (a) May have more petechiae, ecchymosis and bleeding from mouth/nose
   (b) Exercise intolerance, dizziness, recurrent infections with fever, cough, UTIs
▲ 2. *Referral to hematologist for evaluation.*

BOX 4.1 ■ Laboratory Findings With Anemia of Chronic Disease

Test	*Finding*
RBC	Decreased
Hgb	Mildly decreased
MCV	Normal to decreased
Reticulocyte count	Normal to decreased
RDW	Normal to increased
Iron	Low (11–27 μg/dL)
Ferritin	Normal to decreased
TIBC	Normal to increased
CRP	Increased

▲ = *urgent referral*

BOX 4.2 ■ Laboratory Findings With Myelodysplastic Anemia

Test	Finding
RBC	Decreased
Hgb	Decreased
MCV	Increased >100 fL
Reticulocyte count	Decreased
RDW	Normal to increased
Platelets	Decreased
WBC	Decreased
LDH	Increased

BOX 4.3 ■ Laboratory Findings With Iron Deficiency

Test	Finding
RBC	Decreased
Hgb	Decreased
MCV	Decreased
Reticulocyte count	Normal to decreased
RDW	Increased
Platelets	Increased
Iron	Decreased
TIBC	Increased
Ferritin	Decreased

VII. Iron-deficiency anemia (microcytic, hypochromic) (see Box 4.3)
   A. Risk factors
      1. Children 1–5 yr of age on milk diet or non–iron-fortified diets; increased risk with lead exposure
      2. Adolescents on fad diets
      3. Impoverished; elderly; pregnant or menstruating women
      4. Chronic ASA/NSAID users
      5. All cancers
      6. Resulting from some types of bariatric surgery
   B. Signs/symptoms and evaluation (see IV and V, above)
   C. Treatment
      1. All ages
         (a) Therapy is taken for a minimum of 3 mo and then continued for 2–3 mo after Hgb and ferritin levels have returned to normal.
         (b) Recheck CBC and iron studies after 1–2 mo of therapy and then q6mo for a year.
      2. Adults
         (a) Begin OTC ferrous sulfate 1 tab daily for most patients (giving 2 tabs every other day does not limit GI side effects; giving 1 tab every other day will take up to twice as long to correct the iron deficiency).
         (b) Slow Fe tablets are time released and may be better tolerated.
         (c) Giving vitamin C 200 mg or 8 oz of orange juice with iron supplement enhances absorption of the iron by about 10%.

       (d) Take the iron tablets 1–2 hr after the following:
          (i) Foods: tea, coffee, milk, and eggs
          (ii) Medications: antacids, H2 blockers, PPIs, bisphosphonates, levothyroxine
       (e) Consider stool softener (docusate 100 mg) 1–2 caps once or twice daily along with the iron replacement.

  3. Children <12 yr of age
       (a) Screening for anemia at 12 and 24 mo of age with CBC (or H/H)
       (b) Limit cow's milk to about 20 oz/day
       (c) Evaluate diet; increase servings of iron-rich foods with each meal (see Appendix A)
       (d) Ferrous sulfate 3–6 mg/kg elemental iron daily between meals with orange juice or vitamin C supplement
         (iii) May cause temporary staining of teeth, rinse well, or brush after dose
         (iv) Monitor for constipation

  4. Adolescents
       (a) Screening for girls at ~12 yr of age (if menses have started) and then annually after menses; boys once and annually if heavily involved in sports
       (b) Ferrous sulfate 1 tablet daily; slow Fe tablets are time released and may be better tolerated
       (c) Encourage 3 servings per day of iron-rich foods (see Appendix A)
       (d) Monitor for GI effects (e.g., constipation or gastric pain)

VIII. Vitamin deficiency anemia (macrocytic/hyperchromic anemia; see Box 4.4)
  A. Risk factors
    1. Total or partial gastrectomy or bariatric surgery, gastric cancer
    2. Alcoholism
    3. Elderly or impoverished patients
    4. Vegans with no B12 or folate supplements
    5. Autoimmune disease (e.g., thyroid disorder, vitiligo)
  B. Signs/symptoms and lab tests (see IV and V, above)

BOX 4.4 ■ Laboratory Findings With Vitamin Deficiency

Test	Finding
RBC	Normal
WBC	Decreased
Platelets	Decreased
Hgb	Normal to slightly decreased
MCV	Increased (>105 fL suspect alcoholism; >115 fL suspect pernicious anemia)
Reticulocyte count	Decreased
Platelets	Decreased
LDH	Increased
B12 level	Decreased with B12 deficiency; normal with folate deficiency
MMA	Increased with B12 deficiency; normal with folate deficiency
Folate	Decreased with both B12 and folate deficiency
Homocysteine	Increased with both folate and B12 deficiency

C. Treatment
1. B12/folate deficiency may need lifetime replacement; with a reversible cause, may need temporary supplementation
2. Initial replacement—give one of the following:
   (a) Cyanocobalamin 1000 mcg daily IM for 5 days, then weekly for 4 wk, then monthly
   (b) Cyanocobalamin nasal (Nascobal) 500 mcg/spray in one nostril every week (often given to maintain remission after vitamin deficiency is corrected with IM B12)
   (c) Cyanocobalamin oral 1000 mcg daily (must have intact intrinsic factor)
3. Folate replacement: folic acid 1 mg/day
D. Recheck CBC and vitamin levels in 12 wk.

IX. Treatment of acute blood loss anemia
A. Acute blood loss will require emergent care and probably admission for further work-up and transfusion(s)
B. Posthospitalization care will involve
1. Iron supplementation (see VII C, Iron-deficiency anemia, Treatment, above).
2. Addition of iron-rich foods with each meal (see Appendix A).
3. Monitor CBC and Fe monthly until stable, then annually for at least a year.

X. Anemias secondary to overdestruction or poor synthesis of RBCs
A. Thalassemia minor (see Box 4.5)
1. There are usually other family members with unexplained (or diagnosed) anemia.
2. Anemia is similar to IDA, with a chronic microcytic anemia and mild IDA symptoms with elevated iron levels, and is usually *unresponsive* to iron supplementation.
3. Treatment
   (a) No iron supplementation
   (b) Monitor for worsening anemia (decreasing Hgb, fatigue, tachycardia)
4. *Referral*
   (a) *To hematologist for evaluation and treatment*
   (b) May need *referral to gynecologist* if women is still menstruating, as this can be a source of continued blood loss
B. SCA (see Box 4.6)
1. Autosomal recessive inherited disease with an abnormally shaped RBC that limits ability to carry oxygen; cannot pass through distal small capillaries, thus causing pain and hypoxia.

BOX 4.5 ■ Laboratory Findings With Thalassemia

Test	Finding
RBC	Normal to slightly increased with unusual red cell morphology
Hgb	Mildly decreased (10–12 mg/dL)
MCV	Decreased
Reticulocyte count	Decreased
RDW	Normal to elevated
Iron	Increased
Ferritin	Normal to increased
TIBC	Normal

● = *non-urgent referral*

BOX 4.6 ■ Laboratory Findings With Sickle Cell Anemia	
Test	*Finding*
RBC	Decreased
Hgb	Decreased (8–10 mg/dL)
MCV	Mildly to moderately decreased
Reticulocyte count	3–4 times the upper normal limit
RDW	Increased
Platelets	Increased
WBC	Increased
LDH	Increased

2. Patient can have SCA disease or trait
   (a) Predominantly found in Black individuals and people of Mediterranean and Central African descent; can be found in some mixed race people
   (b) Screening is performed at birth
3. Signs and symptoms
   (a) General to anemias (see IV, earlier in chapter)
   (b) Specific to SCA: intermittent crises of hypoxia, pain in chest and joints, SOB
   (c) Increased risk for CVA, MI, bleeding into organs
4. Additional points of care for anemia
   (a) Keep immunizations up to date
   (b) Increase fluid intake and educate regarding dehydration
   (c) Maintain adequate weight and nutritional status
5. *Referral to hematologist specializing in SCA*

FEVER OF UNDETERMINED ORIGIN

I. Definition: a prolonged febrile illness without an established diagnosis, in spite of a thorough evaluation; fever >101°F
   A. Adult: occurring several times over at least 3 wk
   B. Children: occurring at least once a day for ≥8 days
II. Most common causes of undetermined fever include
   A. Infections (common infections include TB, cat scratch disease, Epstein-Barr virus, cytomegalovirus, HIV; other possible infections include typhoid fever, malaria, and amoebic abscesses)
   B. Cancer, especially
      1. Hematologic (e.g., leukemia, Hodgkin's lymphoma)—adult and children
      2. Renal cell, breast or colon cancer; metastases especially to the brain or liver—adult
   C. Connective tissue diseases (e.g., vasculitis, RA, giant cell arteritis; in children, also SLE)
   D. Some patients recover completely with no cause identified; other patients will have recurring fevers that defy diagnosis
III. History and laboratory evaluation
   A. Adult
      1. Evaluation may be outpatient or inpatient, depending on how ill the patient is.
      2. A detailed history and physical examination are usually unrevealing; besides commonly asked history questions (see Chapter 1), also ask patient about:
         (a) Travel in the past 6 mo, especially out of the country

● = *non-urgent referral*

(b) Animal exposure including pets, occupational, living on a farm, and wild animals

(c) History of immunosuppression or current HIV status

(d) Drug use or toxin exposure

(e) Tick bites, exposure to mosquitos; skin rashes

(f) Consumption of game meat or raw meat or shellfish

(g) Unexpected or unexplained weight loss

3. Diagnostic testing includes:

(a) CBC with differential; possible peripheral smear

(b) CMP, LDH

(c) Hepatitis A-B-C panel (if the liver tests are abnormal)

(d) ESR and CRP

(e) Urinalysis with microscopic examination and C&S

(f) Blood cultures times 3 (recommended to draw each from different sites, with hours between each set)

(g) HIV antibody and HIV viral load (in high-risk patients)

(h) TB skin test or interferon-gamma release assay

(i) CXR, PA, and lateral

(j) Depending on patient's symptoms, may also order CT abdomen and/or chest

(k) Other tests are considered, based on patient's symptoms and H&P

B. Children

1. Indications for hospitalization

(a) Ill-appearing

(b) Progressive symptoms or clinical deterioration

(c) Need to observe the patient in a controlled setting or perform procedures best done in the hospital

2. Besides usual history questions, ask about the following:

(a) Fever

(i) How was it assessed (i.e., by touch or with what type of thermometer)?

(ii) Was the fever confirmed by someone other than the caregiver?

(iii) What are the pattern, duration, and height of the fevers?

(iv) Are there prodrome symptoms before the fever (e.g., fatigue, H/A)?

(v) Does it respond to antipyretics?

(b) Travel in the past 6 mo, especially out of the country

(c) Animal exposure including pets, occupational, living on a farm, and wild animals

(d) Tick bites, exposure to mosquitos; skin rashes

(e) Consumption of game meat or raw meat or shellfish

(f) Contact with infected or ill persons (FUO in children is often caused by an unusual presentation of a common illness)

(g) Unexpected or unexplained weight loss

3. Diagnostic testing includes:

(a) CBC with differential and peripheral smear

(b) CMP

(c) ESR and CRP (if normal, FUO likely not due to infection or inflammation)

(d) Aerobic and anaerobic blood cultures

(e) HIV antigen and antibody

(f) Possible strep screen

(g) TB skin test or interferon-gamma release assay

(h) CXR, PA, and lateral

IV. Physical examination (noting the presence or absence of the findings listed below)
  A. General appearance of illness or stress; vital signs; note any weight loss
  B. Head and neck
    1. Conjunctivitis (consider Kawasaki disease)
    2. Pharyngitis, strawberry tongue, cracked lips, oral ulcers (consider strep pharyngitis, Kawasaki disease, inflammatory bowel disease)
    3. Sinus congestion, tender sinuses to percussion
    4. Thyroid (e.g., enlarged or tender)
    5. Lymphadenopathy—localized or generalized (see Table 1.3)
    6. If >50 yr of age, palpate temporal arteries for tenderness
    7. Infant: palpate fontanelles
  C. Skin
    1. Generalized rash (e.g., raised, flat)
    2. Petechiae and/or purpura (consider Rocky Mountain spotted fever); blotchy, salmon-pink rash (consider juvenile idiopathic arthritis)
    3. Subcutaneous nodules, erythema nodosum (consider juvenile idiopathic arthritis, vasculitis, SLE, inflammatory bowel disease)
    4. Malar rash (consider SLE)
    5. Skin peeling on hands and feet (consider Kawasaki disease)
  D. Cardiac
    1. Bradycardia or tachycardia (consider typhoid, SLE)
    2. New-onset murmur (consider infective endocarditis)
    3. New-onset HTN (consider vasculitis)
    4. Pericardial rub (consider SLE)
  E. Abdominal
    1. Generalized abdominal pain; right upper quadrant pain (consider gallbladder or liver)
    2. Hepatosplenomegaly (consider cat scratch fever, brucellosis, malaria, leukemia, lymphoma)
    3. Suprapubic tenderness, positive CVAT (consider UTI, especially pyelonephritis)
  F. Genitourinary
    1. Testicular pain (consider cancer, leukemia, vasculitis, brucellosis)
    2. Breast cancer
  G. Musculoskeletal: joint tenderness/swelling (consider osteomyelitis, septic arthritis, juvenile RA, SLE)
  H. Neurological (assessing for meningeal irritation)
    1. Conduct mental status examination (can be included during rest of exam)
    2. Brudzinski's and Kernig's signs and/or focal deficits
V. Referral
  ▲ A. Adult—*Referral may be urgent, depending on the patient's condition.*
    1. *To surgeon if a biopsy is indicated* (e.g., liver mass, lymphadenopathy, possible temporal arteritis)
    2. *To infectious disease doctor* (e.g., positive test for typhoid fever, malaria, or TB)
    3. *To hematologist with abnormal CBC not attributed to infection, or if fevers continue without diagnosis*
  ▲ B. Children—*Refer to pediatric specialist (e.g., infectious diseases, rheumatology, hematologist-oncologist) if there is no diagnosis after the initial evaluation; may be urgent, depending on the patient's condition.*

⎯⎯⎯⎯⎯⎯⎯⎯

● = *non-urgent referral;* ▲ = *urgent referral*

WEIGHT LOSS (UNINTENTIONAL)

I. Definition: weight loss is clinically relevant if more than 5%–10% of body weight is lost over 3–6 mo, although smaller amounts may be significant in the frail elderly.

   A. Unintentional weight loss can be associated with moderate to severe protein-calorie malnutrition (PCM), nutritional deficiency, and/or organ failure.

   B. It is common in elderly and impoverished people in all age groups if availability of food is limited.

   C. When associated with malnutrition, it is identified by

      1. Insufficient energy intake

      2. Weight loss and a BMI below $21\,kg/m^2$

      3. Loss of muscle mass in the arms, legs, buttocks, and face; loss of subcutaneous fat in the face, orbits, triceps; and of fat over the ribs

      4. Localized or generalized fluid accumulation in the distal extremities and genital area; this may mask weight loss

      5. Diminished functional ability seen in weak hand grip strength and the inability to perform activities of daily living (ADLs).

II. Causes

   A. Malignancy of any type (especially GI, pancreatic, lung, lymphoma, renal, and prostate) and cancer treatments

   B. Nonmalignant causes

      1. Gastrointestinal disease

         (a) PUD, malabsorption (e.g., celiac disease), ulcerative colitis (UC)

         (b) Hepatitis, liver disease

      2. Cardiopulmonary disease, secondary to HF, COPD, and restrictive diets related to treatment

      3. Endocrinopathies

         (a) Hyperthyroidism, DM

         (b) Adrenal insufficiency

      4. Infectious processes

         (a) HIV, TB, hepatitis C

         (b) Helminths

      5. Neurologic processes

         (a) Parkinson disease, CVA, dementia

         (b) Vitamin B and zinc deficiency

      6. Psychologic illness

         (a) Depression, bipolar states

         (b) Eating disorders (anorexia nervosa)

         (c) Alcoholism, drug abuse

      7. Social issues

         (a) Poverty, inability to procure food (e.g., transportation)

         (b) Isolation and financial difficulty (inability to afford proper foods)

         (c) Excessive exercise and weight-loss programs

      8. Medication effects

         (a) Altered taste/smell

         (b) Anorexia

         (c) Dry mouth

         (d) Dysphagia

         (e) N/V

       9. Drugs of abuse
- (a) Alcohol (many patients are not hungry because of consuming most of their calories from alcohol).
- (b) Cocaine use, amphetamine use, and withdrawal from chronic marijuana use can cause anorexia.
- (c) Heavy tobacco use can lead to weight loss.

III. Signs and symptoms
- A. Unexplained fevers or night sweats and chronic infections
- B. Chronic or exertional fatigue, weakness altering ADLs, dyspnea
- C. Dysphagia, gum disease, poor dentition
- D. Indigestion, dysphagia, GERD, abdominal pain
- E. Change in stool patterns with constipation or diarrhea (including steatorrhea)
- F. Early satiety, loss of appetite
- G. Physical inability to feed self
- H. Heart palpitations, short of breath

IV. History questions
- A. Question about changes in caloric intake, numbers of meals per day and per week
- B. Has there been a significant weight-loss episode? When and how much weight was lost?
- C. Have there been changes in clothing size?
- D. Questionnaires (as applicable)
  1. PHQ9 for depression
  2. CAGE for alcoholism
  3. SLUMS (or preferred dementia test) for mental status
  4. ESP (Eating disorder Screen for Primary care)

V. Physical exam
- A. General appearance and overall affect/attitude
  1. Record weight and BMI (BMI <21 kg/m^2 increases the risk for mortality). If patient is not able to be weighed, can use middle upper arm circumference (MUAC); MUAC <22 cm (women) or 23 cm (men) is abnormal.
  2. Record VS, including orthostatic blood pressure/heart rate.
  3. Note loss of tissue mass in face and/or extremities.
- B. Head and neck
  1. Dentition/dentures (e.g., poorly fitting dentures, cavities, or broken teeth)
  2. Periodontal disease
  3. Glossitis or stomatitis
  4. Thyromegaly, lymphadenopathy (see Table 1.3)
  5. Exophthalmos
- C. Cardiac
  1. Heart rate and rhythm, new-onset murmurs, or worsening previous murmurs
  2. Heaves or thrills
- D. Abdomen
  1. Abdominal girth, masses, pain
  2. Ascites
- E. Gynecologic
  1. Breast examination for masses or obvious abnormality
  2. Pelvic examination for uterine or other masses, Pap smear (if indicated)
- F. Neurologic
  1. Peripheral neuropathy
  2. Dementia, depression, mania
  3. Any functional deficits related to CVA

VI. Laboratory/radiologic testing (based on findings)

    A. CBC, CMP (looking for anemia or organ failure)

    B. TSH, PTH (looking for thyroid and parathyroid dysfunction)

    C. CRP/ESR (looking for infectious/inflammatory processes)

    D. Vitamin B12, folate, zinc, and vitamin D deficiency

    E. Urinalysis, urine hCG (if patient is of childbearing age)

    F. FOBT if no colonoscopy within past 5–10 yr (looking for occult blood in stool; colonoscopy is not indicated, as colon cancer without obstruction or extensive metastases does not usually cause weight loss)

    G. CXR (looking for HF, COPD, lung disease or mass)

    H. US RUQ of pelvis; CT chest/abdomen/pelvis (looking for masses or occult diseases)

    I. EGD, if patient complains of early satiety (looking for masses, malignancy)

    J. Mammogram and Pap smear

VII. Treatment (based on findings)

    A. *Referral to appropriate specialist if indicated, including to dentist if dentures or teeth are causing problems.*

    B. If initial history and exam are normal, 3 mo of watchful waiting is preferable; consider shorter interval with progressive weight loss.

    C. Assess for depression and cognitive impairment at least every 6–12 mo.

    D. Dietary

        1. All patients (if possible) should be evaluated by a dietitian and given recommendations for dietary changes.

        2. Remove restrictions from diet and offer high-calorie foods (even if patient has DM).

            (a) Assure the meals and foods meet the patient's tastes (i.e., ethnic or regional preferences), if at all possible.

            (b) Can increase fat content by adding olive oil or butter in preparation of sauces, vegetables, grains, and pastas.

        3. Increase frequency of meals with appropriate-sized portions and between-meal snacks based on patient preferences and physical ability; offer dietary supplements between meals (not with meals).

        4. Daily multivitamin and mineral supplement

        5. Consider if patient needs assistance with

            (a) Shopping or meal preparation (consider Meals on Wheels, also)

            (b) Feeding

    E. Medications

        1. Review all medications and stop those that might cause a problem (including those used to treat dementia).

        2. Medications that may enhance appetite (use as a trial for 1 mo and then reassess):

            (a) Mirtazapine (Remeron) 7.5 mg hs (off label; higher doses may cause drowsiness)

            (b) Megestrol (Megace) 40 mg/mL susp: 10–20 mL daily (monitor elderly patients for edema, worsening HF, DVT, and muscle weakness); usually reserved for cancer/HIV patients

            (c) Dronabinol (Marinol) 2.5 mg 1–2 times daily, may increase up to 20 mg/day (can have significant CNS side effects in elderly patients)

● = *non-urgent referral*

CHAPTER 5

Skin Conditions

Disorders Causing Inflammation

ACNE

I. A disorder involving chronic inflammation with open and closed comedones (blackheads and whiteheads) and can present with pustules, papules, and nodules
   A. Probably involving an increase in androgenic hormones.
   B. Usually occurs in adolescents and has a familial tendency.
   C. May disrupt lifestyle because of appearance of the skin.

II. Age-specific acne
   A. Neonatal and infantile (up to 12 mo of age) acne are more common in males. Typically closed comedones are noted on forehead, nose, and cheeks; usually caused by androgen excess; usually resolve by 3–4 mo of age. If severe, this could be linked to endocrine disorders.
   B. Mid-childhood acne (1–7 yr of age) is not common because of decreased circulating androgens; *the patient should be referred to pediatric endocrinologist.*
   C. Preadolescent (11–17 yr of age)
      1. Common sign of maturation
      2. Usually comedones with "T zone" distribution (forehead and central face)
      3. Few inflammatory lesions
      4. No workup unless concern for glandular abnormality such as polycystic ovary syndrome (PCOS)

III. Variants of acne may be caused by the following
   A. Pressure, friction, or rubbing (e.g., acne beneath the hatband)
   B. Some oil-based cosmetics or OTC acne creams; acne usually resolves when cosmetics are not used
   C. Overuse of topical steroids; when the steroid is stopped, acne will resolve

IV. Grades of acne (treatment should be reassessed every 1–3 mo)
   A. Grade I (mild): few comedones or mixed appearance, no erythema, and few papules; limited skin involvement to one body area
      1. Wash skin once or twice daily using hands to avoid trauma, not a cloth or buff puff; do not rub the skin.
      2. Avoid harsh soaps; use OTC acne wash such as Neutrogena acne wash, Dove, or Cetaphil; pat skin dry; do not rub skin.
      3. Start with benzoyl peroxide (BP) in the morning for 4 wk (Table 5.1).
      4. If no improvement, add a retinoid at bedtime (see Table 5.1).
         (a) Start with a low dose and gradually increase as needed.
         (b) Use in entirely affected area (not just spots).
      5. If response is inadequate after 4 wk, change to topical antibiotic or combination antibiotic with topical retinoid or benzoyl peroxide (see Table 5.1).

● = *non-urgent referral*

TABLE 5.1 ■ Topical Acne Medications

Moisturizers	Benzoyl Peroxide (BP)	Retinoids	Antimicrobials	Combinations
Cetaphil	Benzoyl peroxide (BP) generic 2.5%–5% cream, gel, lotion, wash, pad (higher % cause more irritation and are not more effective)	Retin-A (tretinoin)	Cleocin T (Clindamycin gel, lotion, solution 1%)	Epiduo gel (adapalene + BP 0.1%/2.5%) Epiduo forte gel (adapalene + BP 0.3%/2.5%)
Purpose		Differin* (adapalene)	Erythromycin gel, solution, pad 2%	Ziana gel (clindamycin + tretinoin 1%/0.025%)
Neutrogena		Azelex (azelaic acid)	Amzeeq foam (Minocycline 4%)	Benzamycin gel (erythromycin + BP 3%/5%)
Clinique		Tazorac (tazarotene)†	Aczone gel (Dapsone gel 5%, 7.5%)	Duac gel (clindamycin + BP 1%/5%)
		Aveeno Clear complexion (salicylic acid)	Klaron (Sulfacetamide lotion 10%)	
		Aklief (trifarotene)† cream 0.005%	Winlevi cream (Clascoterone 1%) Can use in male/female >12yr of age for short term use	

* Adapalene: OTC 1% gel; Rx 1% and 3% cream.
† Contraindicated with pregnancy; caution with child-bearing age.

6. Apply a topical antibiotic cream, gel, or solution in the morning and a retinoid at night; always use a moisturizer over the retinoid at night and a moisturizer in combination with a sunscreen in daytime.

B. Grade II (moderate) acne: moderate amount of comedones with increasing papular and pustular lesions, and mild-to-moderate erythema

1. Treatment is the same as with grade I acne, but add an oral antibiotic 1–2 times daily until lesions start to resolve; the patient may need daily dosing until the condition is resolved. Oral antibiotics may be needed intermittently to control outbreaks (see Table 5.2).

2. Maintenance antibiotics are same as those listed previously, except that dosing is daily; a patient could take antibiotics for years
   (a) Antibiotics should not be taken alone, continue topical therapy.
   (b) Antibiotics should be used for 1–3 mo or until acne improves then continue with topical therapy; antibiotics can be restarted with flare-ups.

3. Consider dapsone (Aczone) topical
   (a) Use pea-sized amount in thin layer to acne bid.
   (b) Reassess in 12 wk.
   (c) Use in > 12 yr of age.

4. If androgen excess is the predominant cause of acne, for the female patient consider oral contraceptives or spironolactone 25–100 mg daily. For male or female patient >12 yr of age, consider Clascoterone 1% (Winlevi) topical cream (see Table 5.1).

TABLE 5.2 ■ Oral Antibiotics for Acne

Drug	Dosages	Cautions
Tetracycline	Adolescent*: 125–250 mg bid for 1 wk, then daily Adult: 125–250 mg bid	May cause sun sensitivity; GI distress Always use a sunscreen Take on empty stomach Contraindicated in pregnancy
Doxycycline	Adolescent*: 2.2 mg/kg/day Adult: 50–100 mg qd-bid	May cause sun sensitivity; GI distress Always use a sunscreen
Minocycline IR	Adolescent* and adult: 50–100 mg qd-bid	Superior to tetracyclines for moderate-to-severe non-nodular acne May cause sun sensitivity
Minocycline ER	Adolescent* and adult: 1 mg/kg 12 wk (round to nearest available dose)	Always use a sunscreen May cause dizziness or vertigo Give with food
Azithromycin	Adolescent* and adults: 250 mg 3 times a wk, up to 3 mo	
TMP-SMZ DS	Adolescents* and adults: 1 tab qd-bid	May cause sun sensitivity Use only if unable to take tetracyclines or macrolides
Sarecycline (Seysara)	≥9 yr of age, daily × 12 wk 33–54 kg: 60 mg 55–84 kg: 100 mg 85–136 kg: 150 mg	For mod-severe inflammatory lesions Caution with child-bearing age of both female and male Contraindicated in pregnancy

* Adolescent is defined as a person 11–17 yr of age.

5. Skin of color (i.e., non-Caucasian) will scar more easily and have increased de-pigmentation and may require more aggressive treatment with combinations of benzoyl peroxide, retinoids with antibiotics, or oral antibiotics.
      6. *Referral to a dermatologist if response is poor.*
   C. Grade III (severe): pustular, nodular, and cystic lesions, and erythema
      1. Treatment aimed at avoiding scarring or disfigurement.
      2. Oral antibiotics plus topical retinoids plus benzoyl peroxide.
      3. Add OC hormonal therapy or spironolactone 25–100 mg daily (for females), or clascoterone cream (Winlevi) (for males or females >12 yr of age).
      4. *Referral to a dermatologist for consideration of isotretinoin (Accutane) and other therapies if needed.*

PRACTICE PEARLS FOR ACNE

- Therapies for acne are time-consuming and involve commitment of the person to a daily regimen of care; resolution is very slow, and continual reinforcement is needed.
- Always obtain a detailed history of the patient's symptoms, including all OTC and prescription drugs used and the use of "friend's" cures for acne.
- If acne rash is unresponsive to initial antibiotic, consider culture of pustule.
- If acne rash is located on legs, consider possibility of shaving folliculitis; treat with antibiotic and instruct to change razor or blades routinely.
- Sunscreens ≥30 SPF and moisturizers are required daily.
- Topical products
  - Topical antibiotics increase drug resistance more than oral antibiotics.
  - Tea tree oil may reduce the number of papules and comedones.
  - Topical gels seem to work better in females; topical solutions (roll-ons) are better tolerated by males; if the skin is dry, use creams; if the skin is oily, use gels.
  - Retinoids decrease follicular plugging but cause erythema of the skin; encourage use of moisturizers over retinoids at night.
  - Topical retinoids may decrease active acne and slow scar formation.
- Discourage picking at papules or squeezing bumps.
- Makeup brands that do not normally irritate acne are Almay, Neutrogena, Clinique, or any that are accurately labeled as hypoallergenic/noncomedogenic.
- Suggest a low-glycemic diet and avoidance of junk foods. This does not worsen or have any effect on acne per se, but most teenagers with significant acne are usually obese to some extent and eat as a comfort measure.
- Wash after sweating because perspiration makes acne worse.
- Shampoo hair more often with oily hair.
- Avoid tanning beds because UV light damages skin and increases sensitivity to medications.
- Azelaic acid may decrease post-inflammatory hyperpigmentation.

ATOPIC DERMATITIS (ECZEMA)

   I. Description
      A. Cases usually stem from familial predisposition to eczema or seasonal allergies.
      B. Increased prevalence of flare-ups with food allergies; smoke exposure, change in climate, perfumes, and cosmetics.
      C. Patients may have acute exacerbations with periods of remission.

● = *non-urgent referral*

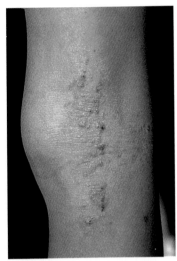

Fig. 5.1 Flexural atopic dermatitis with lichenification. (From White, G. M., & Cox, N. H. (2002). *Diseases of the skin: A color atlas and text.* St. Louis: Mosby.)

    D. Lesions can be diffuse erythematous macules, papules, or scaly plaques that may have grouped vesicles

        1. Lesions associated with itch-scratch cycle and paroxysmal itching are usually worse at night.

        2. May produce exudation with wet crusts and fissures; this increases the risk of secondary bacterial infections and molluscum.

    E. Distribution of lesions is common on the face, antecubital and popliteal spaces, joints, and other areas of friction; distribution of lesions may be symmetrical but may be isolated and/or discrete (see Fig. 5.1); usually spares groin and axilla.

II. Treatment

    A. Primary goal: to relieve itching and improve hydration of skin, with prevention and maintenance of symptoms to minimize use of steroids

        1. Increase oral hydration and also ambient moisture with a humidifier.

        2. Wear all-cotton clothing and use cotton bed linens.

        3. Avoid triggers that may worsen itching

           (a) Do not over heat skin.

           (b) Do not use harsh soaps and detergents.

           (c) Use dust mite covers on bed pillows and linens.

        4. Topical therapy, when used consistently, may decrease exacerbations

           (a) Decrease time to 10 min daily and use only tepid water and mild unscented soap (Dial, Dove, Aveeno, Basis).

           (b) Apply emollient moisturizers (Eucerin, Aquaphor, mineral, or baby oil) on the skin immediately after bathing and 3–4 times daily.

           (c) Ointments are better moisturizers in dry environments or for very young children or infants.

           (d) Apply moisturizers, when not using steroid ointments, to prevent flare-ups.

           (e) For acute itching, soak in tepid bath and then use emollient with a soft, cotton wrap over the area, and do not let the cloth become dry.

    5. Apply sunscreen to all exposed areas whenever outdoors.

    6. Vitamin E: 400–800 International Units daily >12 yr of age

    7. Apply calamine lotion or spray (not for open, weeping areas).

B. Prompt identification and treatment of flare-ups or infections will improve overall outcomes.

C. Pharmacological therapy

    1. First-line therapy is topical steroids (see Table 5.3; and PRACTICE PEARLS FOR STEROIDS, see later in chapter)

        (a) Initial therapy with low-potency steroids (e.g., hydrocortisone 0.5%–1% OTC) bid on the face or skin folds; for moderate eczema, can use mid-potency steroids bid on the trunk until symptoms resolve.

        (b) Use steroids for the shortest amount of time.

        (c) High-potency steroids would be reserved for the most severe flare-ups and for the shortest amount of time (e.g., less than 2 wk). *Do not use on face and genital.*

    2. Second-line therapy for frequent, hard-to-control flare-ups with moderate-to-severe symptoms is topical immunomodulators

        (a) Tacrolimus (Protopic) ointment; apply to lesions bid

            (i) For patients 2–15 yr of age: use 0.03%.

            (ii) For patients >15 yr of age: use 0.03%–0.1%.

        (b) Pimecrolimus 1% (Elidel): >2 yr of age; apply bid to lesions; can be used in sensitive areas where steroids may cause serious or systemic reactions

        (c) Crisaborole 2% ointment (Eucrisa): >3 mo of age; apply thin layer bid; not for eyes, oral, or intravaginal use

    3. Oral steroids in "burst" therapy can be used short-term for severe, refractory cases in adults; must be closely monitored for side effects (see Table 5.4 and PRACTICE PEARLS FOR STEROIDS, see later in chapter).

    4. Oral antihistamines for sedative effect as needed to break the itch-scratch cycle; dose based on age

        (a) Diphenhydramine (Benadryl) 12.5–50 mg q6h

        (b) Hydroxyzine (Atarax) 10–100 mg q6–8h

        (c) Cetirizine 1 mg/mL daily

            (i) Patients 2–5 yr of age: give 2.5–5 mL

            (ii) Patients >6 yr of age: give 5–10 mL

        (d) Cyproheptadine (Periactin) 2 mg/5 mL syrup or 4 mg tab tid; dose dependent on age

    5. Topical antihistamines have an increased potential to cause contact dermatitis to already inflamed skin

        (a) Topical diphenhydramine cream or spray

        (b) Calamine spray

        (c) Doxepin 5% cream (adults only) qid as needed

    6. Emollients can be used for maintenance therapy and are safe for any age

        (a) Nonprescription creams decrease water loss in skin (e.g., EpiCeram, CeraVe, Cetaphil).

        (b) Should be applied directly after bathing.

        (c) Plain petrolatum is well tolerated for flares.

        (d) Using emollient about 10–15 min before using topical steroid may enhance steroid absorption and shorten the length of time for steroid use.

    7. Consider using mupirocin ointment for localized infection bid for 1–2 wk; using it nasally for 3 days prior to any invasive procedures can decrease risk of post procedure infections.

8. Suggested antibiotic therapy given for 5–10 days for *secondary* infections

Drug	Pediatric Dose	Adult Dose
Dicloxacillin	<40 kg: 12.5–25 mg/kg/day ÷ q6h >40 kg: 125–250 mg q6h	125–500 mg q6h
Cephalexin	25–50 mg/kg/day ÷ q6–8h	250–500 mg q8–12h
Erythromycin	30–50 mg/kg/day ÷ q6–12h	250–400 mg qid

●   **III.** *Referral to dermatologist if atopic dermatitis is severe or unresponsive to treatment; start therapy while awaiting appointment.*

CONTACT DERMATITIS

I. Description
  A. Inflammation of the epidermis and dermis caused by irritative agents or allergens
    1. Latex dermatitis affects health care providers primarily, but can affect the general population.
    2. Latex is found in multiple places; there are some foods that cross-react with latex IgE
      (a) In any health care setting: ambu bags, gloves, BP cuffs; IV tubing, and urinary catheter and tubing; medical office: cervical dilators, rubber stoppers, pillow covers, dental dams, elastic bandages, elastic support hose, electrode pads, surgical implants, endotracheal tubes, tourniquets
      (b) Common foods that might cross-react: avocado, banana, chestnut, cantaloupe, kiwi, potato, tomato; reported foods that might cross-react: apple, mango, peach, spinach, celery, melon, pear, turnip, cherry, papaya, pineapple, wheat
    3. Poison ivy, oak, and sumac are common causes with a typical pattern of distribution; the symptoms can occur in sites unrelated to the contact exposure (see Fig. 5.2).
  B. Characteristics are itching, burning, redness, and swelling, with well-demarcated areas where the irritant/allergen has touched the skin; scaly, vesicular, or maculopapular lesions appear in scattered, linear lines (rhus lines), or clustered groupings in the area of direct contact (see Fig. 5.2).
  C. Uncontrolled scratching can cause secondary skin infections and scarring.
  D. Scarring can be caused by actual direct contact and any secondary infections.
II. Treatment
  A. Remove irritant and cleanse skin thoroughly with soap and water.
  B. Control itching with oral antihistamines (e.g., diphenhydramine, hydroxyzine, cyproheptadine—see ATOPIC DERMATITIS, C for dosing); may cause drowsiness.
  C. Topical treatment for relief of itching with moderate-to-severe contact dermatitis
    1. Aluminum acetate (Domeboro)
    2. Oatmeal baths
    3. Calamine lotion/spray
    4. Vinegar in water 50:50 solution
  D. Topical steroids, mid-potency applied 2–3 times daily (see Table 5.3; and PRACTICE PEARLS FOR STEROIDS, and see later in chapter)

● *= non-urgent referral*

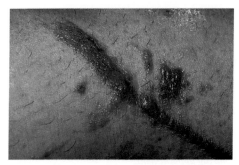

Fig. 5.2 Allergic contact dermatitis to Rhus. The classic appearance of allergic contact dermatitis is illustrated in this patient who came into contact with poison oak. The lesions are linear but not following Blaschko's lines. The eruption is microvesicular and extremely pruritic. (From White, G. M., & Cox, N. H. (2002). *Diseases of the skin: A color atlas and text*. St. Louis: Mosby.)

TABLE 5.3 ■ **Selected Topical Steroid Potencies**

Potency	Product	Vehicle	Sizes
Very high potency	Augmented betamethasone dipropionate (Diprolene) 0.05%	Cream, ointment	15 and 45 g
	Clobetasol propionate (Temovate) 0.05%	Cream, ointment	15, 30, 45, and 60 g
	Halobetasol 0.05%	Ointment, cream	50 g
High potency	Desoximetasone (Topicort) 0.25%	Cream, ointment	15 and 60 g
	Fluocinonide (Lidex) 0.05%	Gel, ointment, cream	15, 30, 60, and 120 g
	Halcinonide (Halog) 0.1%	Cream, ointment	15, 30, 60, and 240 g
	Triamcinolone acetonide (Aristocort) 0.5%	Ointment	15 and 60 g
	Diflorasone topical (Psorcon E) 0.05%	Ointment/cream	15, 30, and 60 g
Medium potency	Triamcinolone topical (Kenalog) 0.1%	Spray	63 and 100 g
	Fluocinolone acetonide (Synalar) 0.025%	Cream, ointment	15, 30, and 60 g
	Mometasone furoate (Elocon) 0.1%	Cream	15 and 50 g
	Betamethasone valerate (Luxiq) 0.1%; foam 0.12%	Cream, lotion, foam, ointment	15, 45, and 60 g
	Hydrocortisone valerate (Westcort) 0.2%	Ointment, cream	15, 45, and 60 g
Low potency	Desonide (DesOwen) 0.05%	Cream, lotion, foam	15, 60, and 90 g; 60 and 120 mL
	Fluocinolone acetonide (Synalar) 0.025%–0.01%	Cream, ointment, solution	120 g; 60–90 mL
	Triamcinolone topical 0.025%	Lotion	15 and 80 g
	Hydrocortisone (OTC brands) 1%	Cream	15 and 45 g

1. With more severe reactions, oral prednisone may be needed in "burst" therapy (see PRACTICE PEARLS FOR STEROIDS, see later in chapter), especially if the reaction involves the face.
2. Do not use topical steroids in the diaper areas or on the face of infants/children because of the risk of systemic or local reactions.
3. Taper for poison ivy with oral steroids over 1–3 wk to prevent recurrence. Methylprednisolone dose pack is too short.

DIAPER DERMATITIS

I. Description
   A. Inflammation occurs in the diaper area of infants or elderly people who wear incontinence diapers/pads (see Fig. 5.3).
   B. Usual cause is irritation from urine/stool in close contact with the skin for long periods of time or highly acidic urine/stool.
      1. Causes skin breakdown and secondary bacterial infection.
      2. *Candida* is the most common agent (see Fig. 5.4).

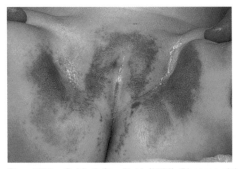

Fig. 5.3 Diaper dermatitis. (From White, G. M., & Cox, N. H. (2002). *Diseases of the skin: A color atlas and text*. St. Louis: Mosby.)

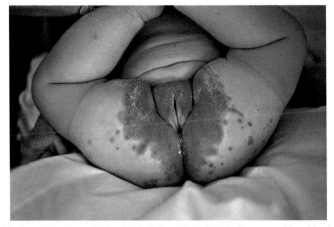

Fig. 5.4 Candida dermatitis. (From White, G. M., & Cox, N. H. (2002). *Diseases of the skin: A color atlas and text*. St. Louis: Mosby.)

     C. Lesions are bright red and beefy in the diaper area, with papular and sometimes pustular lesions; satellite lesions can occur; *lesions may spare inguinal folds.*

     D. More common with history of atopic dermatitis/eczema.

  II. Treatment (for any patient using protective undergarments for incontinence)

     A. Frequent diaper changes.

     B. Discourage use of commercial diaper wipes; if infant, bathe in tepid bath after stooling/urinating and use dabbing technique or use a spray bottle to cleanse the area instead of wiping.

     C. After performing skin care, leave the diaper area open to air or use a blow dryer on low setting at arm's length from the baby/adult after each diaper change.

     D. Encourage use of a barrier cream/ointment with each diaper change (e.g., zinc oxide, white petroleum, or Aquaphor).

     E. Encourage using super-absorbent diapers if frequent diaper changes are not an option, and avoid rubber pants.

     F. Discourage intake of highly acidic foods/juices when dermatitis is present.

 III. Mimics of Diaper Dermatitis

     A. Candida does not spare skin folds and satellite pustules/papules are common (see Fig. 5.4)

       1. Use topical antifungals if *Candida* infection is suspected (nystatin cream, clotrimazole, miconazole); apply 2–3 times daily to the diaper area; use barrier cream over this. Consider oral fluconazole (Diflucan) therapy for incontinent *adults* for recurrent or refractory *Candida.*

       2. With worsening inflammation, use a combination steroid and antifungal (nystatin/triamcinolone topical [Mycolog II ointment]) preparation applied 2 times daily for a short period of time to the diaper area until improvement (e.g., 1 wk).

       3. If the mother is breastfeeding, consider the possibility of thrush in the infant's mouth and treat both simultaneously.

     B. If no improvement with Candida treatment, consider secondary infection with *Streptococcus pyogenes* or *Staphylococcus aureus* (see IMPETIGO, this chapter)

       1. Consider wound culture for confirmation.

       2. Avoid neosporin or bacitracin, these may cause allergic reaction.

       3. Anogenital area may have small pustules to bullous blisters or bright red erythema with maceration that involves skin folds.

       4. May have household contact with streptococcal pharyngitis.

       5. Treat with oral antibiotics (see ATOPIC DERMATITIS, C, Treatment).

  IV. *Referral to dermatologist if symptoms cannot be controlled.*

HYPERHIDROSIS

  I. Description

     A. Excessive sweating, which can be localized or generalized, predominantly noted in the axilla, groin, or palms of hands and soles of feet, sometimes with resultant skin sloughing.

     B. Can disrupt lifestyle and cause embarrassment in social settings.

     C. Symptoms do not occur at night.

● = *non-urgent referral*

D. Begins in childhood or adolescence; if adult onset, look for a secondary cause; condition will decrease as the person ages.

E. Usually has a positive family history.

II. Treatment

A. Start treatment with an OTC *antiperspirant* (not deodorant) to block sweat production (e.g., Certain Dri, Secret clinical strength, Sweatblock, and Hydrosal), and use at night.

B. Pharmacological treatment

1. Apply aluminum chloride 20% (Drysol) for 7–10 nights initially, then 1–2 times a week; wash off every morning.

2. Aluminum chloride 6.25% (Xerac AC) at night to the axilla and palms, and wash off in the morning.

3. Oxybutynin 5–10 mg po bid (off label) to decrease pedal sweating symptoms; caution with geriatric patients; do not use in patients with glaucoma, urinary retention, or gastrointestinal (GI) disorders.

4. Glycopyrrolate 1–2 mg po 1–2 times daily (max dose 8 mg/daily) or glycopyrrolate Tosylate 2.4% (Qbrexza) topically daily to axilla area; for >9 yr of age.

5. Can try Botox injections for axillary sweating (off-label use approved by FDA).

C. Sweating and tachycardia associated with social phobia and/or public speaking may be relieved with propranolol 10–20 mg prior to event.

⬤ **III.** *Referral to a dermatologist if uncontrolled or if the condition is affecting life.*

PSORIASIS

I. Description

A. Lesions are inflamed, thickened, pruritic, violaceous plaques with powdery white or silver scales (see Fig. 5.5).

B. Familial tendency which usually occurs before age 35 and is accompanied by relapses and remissions

1. Lesions vary in size and distribution; most common over extensor aspects of elbows and knees, presacral area, ears, and scalp, but can occur anywhere.

2. Pustular type: most common on palms and soles

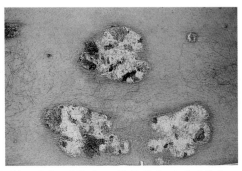

Fig. 5.5 Psoriasis vulgaris. (From Callen, J. P., Greer, K. E., Paller, A. S., & Swinyer, L. J. (2000). *Color atlas of dermatology* (2nd ed.). Philadelphia: W.B. Saunders.)

⬤ = *non-urgent referral*

    3. Guttate psoriasis: involves skin over most of the torso/extremities and appears as small red macular/papular lesions.

    4. Pitting and dystrophy of nails, which can increase risk for onychomycosis.

II. Treatment

    A. Topical treatment (see PRACTICE PEARLS FOR STEROIDS, see later in chapter)

      1. Emollients to maintain skin hydration and minimize itching.

      2. Mid- or high-potency topical steroids (see Table 5.3) for up to 5 days on the skin for acute exacerbations; use low- to mid-potency steroids in intertriginous areas.

      3. Small, mild, hyperkeratotic lesions respond to low-potency topical steroids (hydrocortisone 1%) with tar preparations (e.g., phototar or anthralin) 1–2 times daily.

      4. Scalp lesions often require tar shampoo, salicylic acid, and/or steroids (under an occlusive shower cap for the first or second treatment, to increase contact time).

      5. Calcipotriene topical 0.005% (Dovonex) applied bid; avoid face, mucous membranes, and eyes; wash hands after application

      6. Can use combined calcipotriene and betamethasone dipropionate (Taclonex) ointment daily up to 4 wk for decreased side effect profile.

      7. Calcitriol (Vectical) apply bid to psoriasis plaques up to 4 wk.

      8. Tazarotene topical cream/gel 0.05%, 0.1% (Tazorac) applied qhs; if the patient is of child-bearing age, perform pregnancy test before starting treatment

        (a) Effective in decreasing scales and can be used as monotherapy for chronic plaques; can be used on face and in intertriginous areas.

        (b) Most common side effect is local irritation; irritation is decreased when tazarotene is combined with topical steroids.

    B. Discourage scratching and rubbing of lesions.

    C. Discourage oral steroids.

    D. Consider tanning bed phototherapy for maintenance.

III. *Referral to a dermatologist if unresponsive to treatment.*

ROSACEA

I. Description

    A. Rosacea is a cutaneous vascular disorder that develops later in life, usually between 30 and 50 yr of age, and is most common in fair-skinned people; women are affected 3 times more often than men, but men have more severe symptoms, including rhinophyma (see Fig. 5.6).

    B. Distribution of lesions occurs on the center of the face (cheeks, chin, nose, or forehead), with inflammatory papules and pustules on an erythematous base.

    C. Many have flushing and blushing reactions to emotional or environmental triggers (before actual lesions occur)

      1. Alcohol ingestion

      2. Irritating cosmetics

      3. Excessive washing of face

      4. Emotional stress

      5. Spicy foods, smoking, caffeine, or sun exposure

II. Signs and symptoms

    A. Occurs bilaterally without comedones; there is very little to no scarring

    B. Central facial flushing (transient)

    • = *non-urgent referral*

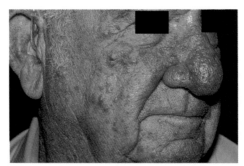

Fig. 5.6 The classic appearance of rosacea. Multiple papules and a few pustules are scattered on the nose and cheeks. The nose shows almost confluent erythema. (From White, G. M., & Cox, N. H. (2002). *Diseases of the skin: A color atlas and text*. St. Louis: Mosby.)

C. Nontransient erythema or persistent redness of the face
D. Papules and pustules in clusters
E. Telangiectasia
F. Burning or stinging, which can occur with the use of sunscreens or moisturizers
G. Plaques and dryness with itchy, scaly skin (resembles xerosis)
H. Edema after prolonged flushing
I. Rhinophyma (usually in men)
J. Ocular manifestations
   1. Watery, bloodshot eyes; dryness with photophobia
   2. Conjunctivitis and blepharitis

III. Treatment
  A. Topical pharmacological treatment
    1. For flushing/blushing—apply daily to entire face, avoiding contact with eyes
      (a) Brimonidine 0.33% (Mirvaso) gel
      (b) Oxymetazoline 1% (Rhofade) cream
    2. For pustules and/or papules with mild to moderate disease, apply to affected area
      (a) Metronidazole 1% cream daily or metronidazole 0.75% gel bid
        (i) If severe, may need to add an oral antibiotic (tetracycline) until remission.
        (ii) May take several weeks for the effects to be seen and the usual course of treatment is up to 2 wk.
      (b) Azelaic acid 15%–20% (Azelac) cream/lotion or gel apply 1–2 times daily up to 3 mo; may combine with ivermectin (Soolantra) if unresponsive to single therapy.
      (c) Ivermectin 1% cream (Soolantra) apply daily.
      (d) Clindamycin 1% lotion or erythromycin 2% solution bid; treatment course may take up to 2–3 mo.
      (e) Minocycline 1.5% FOAM apply daily to affected areas.
      (f) Sulfacetamide-sulfur 10%/15%; apply 1–2 times daily.
    3. Antibiotics (either oral or topical) are not curative; may need to repeat dosing with flare-ups.
  B. Systemic therapy is used to treat hard-to-control rosacea with or without ocular manifestations; once improved, return to topical treatment
    1. Tetracycline 250–500 mg q12h; then decrease to daily dosing

2. Doxycycline 50–100 mg bid or 40 mg DR daily.
3. Minocycline 50–100 mg bid; then may need daily dosing
4. Metronidazole 250 mg daily for 4–6 wk
   C. Avoid using steroids on the face.
   D. Daily facial moisturizers, sunscreens, and mild cleansers.
   E. For flushing, consider clonidine 0.5 mg bid.
   IV. Referral to a dermatologist if symptoms are unresponsive or disfiguring.

SEBORRHEIC DERMATITIS

I. Description
   A. Inflammatory papulosquamous dermatitis that affects sebaceous areas.
   B. Occurs in infants, adolescents, and adults; triggers can be stress, and cold dry winters.
   C. May be associated with vitamin B deficiencies, such as B2, B6, and niacin. Start vitamin B therapy, such as B-complex and niacin (B3) daily.
   D. Characterized by mild-to-severe red, dry, flaky, patchy lesions on the face, ears, scalp, and trunk (see Fig. 5.7)
      1. Patches are poorly defined and appear greasy over inflamed skin with mild itching or burning sensation.
      2. Lesions typically appear on nasolabial folds, ears, eyebrows, or hairline; can occur in the groin, axilla, and mid-chest areas.
   E. It is usually a chronic condition with a bothersome appearance but can manifest as infection in intertriginous areas and eyelids.
II. Treatment
   A. Scalp: treat twice weekly until improved then maintenance with medicated shampoo weekly
      1. Selenium sulfide 2.5% shampoo (can also be used on face)

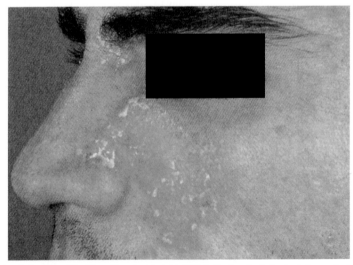

Fig. 5.7 Seborrheic dermatitis. (From Swartz, Mark H. (2014). *Textbook of physical diagnosis*. Philadelphia: Saunders.)

● = non-urgent referral

    2. Zinc pyrithione or salicylic acid shampoo (can also be used on face)

    3. Ketoconazole 2% shampoo

    4. Ciclopirox 1% shampoo

  B. Face: treat 1–2 times a day until improved, steroids should not be used for >5 days; maintenance therapy once weekly with antifungals

    1. Low potency steroids (see Table 5.3)

    2. Antifungals (e.g., ketoconazole cream)

    3. Ciclopirox 1% cream

    4. Tacrolimus (off label) or pimecrolimus (off label); check pregnancy status if child-bearing age

  C. Torso and intertriginous areas: topical steroid treatment 1–2 times daily *until* improvement seen then continue treatment with antifungals

    1. Low potency topical steroids (see Table 5.3) to intertriginous areas

    2. Medium potency steroids (see Table 5.3) to chest or upper trunk

    3. Antifungal cream (e.g., ketoconazole) or ciclopirox 1–2 times daily until resolution

  D. Gentle cleansing with a soft toothbrush to remove patches/plaques will improve treatment; for blepharitis, use baby shampoo and Q-tips to remove crust.

III. *Referral: to a dermatologist if unresponsive to treatment.*

URTICARIA (HIVES)

  I. Description

    A. Transient eruptions of well-defined papular lesions or wheals anywhere on the body, with severe pruritus (see Fig. 5.8)

      1. Any size from mm to inches or greater; complete blanching with pressure

      2. Lesions are transient in nature; can last for <1 hr up to weeks and usually are self-limiting

    B. Associated with

      1. Stinging insects (e.g., hymenoptera [bees] or triatoma [kissing bugs])

      2. Latex exposure

      3. Ingestion of foods such as fish, berries, nuts, eggs, and wheat

      4. Medications such as antibiotics, NSAIDs

      5. Occasionally associated with infection, stress, and temperature changes

    C. Evaluate for angioedema and respiratory distress.

    D. Evaluate psychosocial stressors for cause of urticaria.

    E. If chronic urticaria (>6 wk) is present, check CBC, CMP, A1c, ESR, ANA, and TSH to rule out systemic diseases (e.g., infection, DM, hypothyroidism, cancer).

  II. Treatment

    A. Avoid triggers

    B. Pharmacological treatment

      1. *Urgent treatment for angioedema or respiratory distress to ED per ambulance, initiate treatment while waiting for ambulance*

        (a) Epinephrine 0.1–0.3 mL SQ; may repeat in 15–30 min

        (b) Diphenhydramine 25–50 mg PO, IM or IV

        (c) O$_2$ therapy

      2. OTC medications for less severe urticaria (i.e., no angioedema or respiratory distress)

        (a) H1 nonsedating antihistamines are now first-line therapy; give daily for ≥2 wk (fexofenadine, cetirizine, loratadine, levocetirizine).

▲ = *urgent referral*

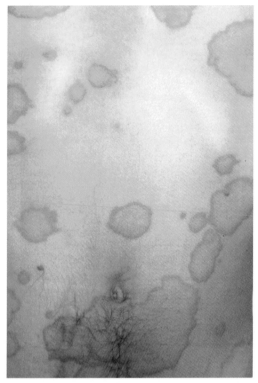

Fig. 5.8   Urticarial hive. (From Marks, J., Miller, J. (2018). *Lookingbill and Marks' Principles of Dermatology* (6th ed.). London: Elsevier.)

   (b) H1 blockers: sedating antihistamines are best given at hs (e.g., hydroxyzine, diphenhydramine, cyproheptadine).
   (c) H2 blockers may decrease reaction on a daily basis and can be used for up to 1 mo (e.g., nizatidine, famotidine).
   (d) Cyproheptadine (H1 blocker)
       (i) Children: 2 mg/5 mL, 0.25 mg/kg/day divided q8–12h
       (ii) Adults: 4 mg qid
 3. Prescription treatment
   (a) May need to give oral steroids for 5–7 days (children 0.5–1 mg/kg/day or adults 30–60 mg/day) or single steroid injection
   (b) Montelukast may be recommended for cold urticaria.
       (i) Children: 4–5 mg daily, based on age
       (ii) Adults: 10 mg daily
   (c) Doxepin (H1 and H2 blocker) 10 mg orally bid-qid (adults only)
 4. Chronic urticaria
   (a) Patient may need daily oral antihistamines and/or H1 and/or H2 blockers for maintenance therapy.
   (b) If chronic itching is not relieved at night with oral antihistamines, try switching to tricyclic antidepressants such as doxepin 10–50 mg at hs (adults only).
 III. *Referral to a dermatologist if there is no improvement in symptoms.*

 ⬤ = *non-urgent referral*

XEROSIS (XERODERMA)

I. Description
   A. Moderate-to-severe dry, scaly, rough skin with fissuring that is pruritic
      1. Appears on the extremities and "high use" skin areas (outer thighs, buttocks, midback, extremities, feet/hands)
      2. Usually spares the face, scalp, groin, and axilla areas
   B. Occurs predominantly in winter and with lower humidity and can occur in any age group.
   C. May have pruritus with no obvious rash.
II. Treatment involves conservation of skin moisture from evaporation and exposure; prevention and maintenance of symptoms is essential to decrease use of steroids
   A. Increase ambient moisture with a humidifier.
   B. Limit bathing, use tepid water and mild soap to decrease moisture loss; proper nail care hygiene.
   C. Topical therapy
      1. Lubricants/emollients (petrolatum, mineral oil, baby oil, Eucerin, Lubriderm, Aquaphor) 3–4 times daily and after bathing
      2. Lotions with menthol or camphor (Sarna); pramoxine (Pramisone OTC) 3–4 times daily to help control itching
      3. Liquid vegetable shortening can be used and is cost-effective
      4. Apply lubricant to feet or hands at bedtime and wear white cotton socks and/or gloves to bed. Wear the same socks or gloves every night if there are no excoriations (could lead to secondary infection), as this can decrease the amount of lubricant needed. This will soften callused areas, especially on feet
      5. Ammonium lactate topical (Lac-Hydrin): bid and rub in thoroughly
      6. Lactic acid creams (Eucerin Plus, Lacticare 5%): apply 3–4 times daily; can alternate ammonium lactate and lactic acid creams if the skin is sensitive
      7. Can use low- to mid-potency topical steroids 1–2 times daily (see Table 5.3)
   D. Consider wet wrap therapy (or wet-to-dry wrap) if poor result with other therapies
      1. First layer is "wet" with low-potency steroid or moisturizer (or both).
      2. Cover with dry gauze layer and over-wrap of area with dry gauze roll.
      3. Can leave on for several hours to 24 hr but can be longer. This increases penetration of topical agent and decreases itch-scratch cycle.
   E. Treat any underlying infection (usually *Staphylococcus aureus*).
III. *Referral to dermatologist if not improving.*

PRACTICE PEARLS FOR STEROIDS

- Topical steroids are antiinflammatory agents that control inflammation and pruritic conditions of the skin. Remember to consider the potency, location, and desired duration of action when prescribing a topical steroid preparation. (See Table 5.3 for selected topical steroid potencies; this list is not all-inclusive.)
- Twice-a-day application is most useful and economical; more frequent applications do not hasten improvement because topical steroids have a repository effect; start with bid applications and decrease as improvement occurs.
- Areas of use for less than 2 wk:
  High potency for palms and soles
  Medium-low potency on groin, axilla, face
  Low potency around eyes

Continued

= *non-urgent referral*

PRACTICE PEARLS FOR STEROIDS—CONT'D

- Adverse reactions such as skin thinning, striae, rebound lesion flares, and HPA axis suppression can occur (especially with higher potency and/or longer use).
- High-potency steroids
  - *Do not use "very-high-potency" steroids on the face or groin area or with occlusive dressings.*
  - If using topical high or very high steroids, limit use to 2 wk.
  - Topical steroids, especially at higher concentrations and in children, can affect the hypothalamic–pituitary–adrenal (HPA) axis; beware of the dosage and slowly withdraw the drug if it has been used for a long time.
  - When a high- or very-high-potency steroid is ordered, indicate on the prescription "not for use on the face."
  - Use of oral steroid pulse therapy (i.e., using moderate-to-high doses of steroids daily for <5 days) will decrease the chance of tachyphylaxis; there should be an interval of at least 1 mo between pulse therapies.
    - Children: 0.5–1 mg/kg/day
    - Adult: 30–60 mg/day
- Pediatric use
  - Do not use topical steroids for diaper rash; children have a greater body surface area; therefore, absorption will be greater.
  - For an infant <6 mo of age, low-potency steroids (e.g., hydrocortisone 1% OTC cream) can be used for <7 days.
  - For a child 6 mo to 12 yr of age, low-mid-potency steroids can be used for short periods of time (e.g., 7–10 days).
  - Use after bathing to enhance absorption.
- Vehicles for administration: steroids come in various vehicles to maximize effects
  - *Ointments* are more occlusive; use for dry, cracked, scaly lesions; more potent than creams or lotions in the same group; may cause maceration and folliculitis; do not use on open, draining wounds.
  - *Creams* are less occlusive and more drying; used for oozing lesions and in intertriginous areas; increase anesthetic action; rub in well; these are good for treating dermatitis in hot, humid climates.
  - *Gels, lotions, foams, and aerosols*: gels have some occlusive properties; gels and foams are used on hairy areas; urea-containing creams increase skin hydration, facilitate cortisone penetration, and may be cooling to the skin; lotions are better for use on the face.
- Occlusive dressings (wet wrap therapy)
  - Can be used in areas where increased uptake of topical steroids is required.
  - Should not be used for >12 hr daily because of enhanced penetration and concomitant systemic effects.
  - Patient instructions regarding occlusive dressings:
    - Soak the area in warm water or wash well with warm water.
    - While the skin is still slightly wet, rub the topical steroid into the affected area (increased moisture increases penetration).
    - Cover the area with a plastic wrap, such as Saran Wrap, and seal the edges with tape or a cloth bandage; ensure a good seal between the steroid and the skin; gloves may be worn on the hands; sandwich bags for the feet and shower caps for the scalp may also be used.
    - Leave the dressing in place overnight or approximately 6 hr; *do not use an occlusive dressing with very-high-potency steroids.*
    - Patients should report signs of infection such as pain, increased warmth, exudate, and worsening redness to the practitioner; discontinue occlusive dressing immediately.
- Some conditions may require oral steroid therapy (Table 5.4).

▨ = *not to be missed*

TABLE 5.4 ■ Oral Steroid Equivalency

Name	5 mg	10 mg	15 mg	20 mg	25 mg	30 mg	35 mg	40 mg
Prednisone or prednisolone 5 mg tablets	1 tab	2 tab	3 tab	4 tab	5 tab	6 tab	7 tab	8 tab
Prednisone 5 mg/5 mL (liquid Pred syrup)	1 tsp	2 tsp	3 tsp	4 tsp	5 tsp	6 tsp	7 tsp	8 tsp
Prednisolone 15 mg/5 mL (Prelone syrup)	$1/3$ tsp	$2/3$ tsp	1 tsp	1.3 tsp	1.6 tsp	2 tsp	2.3 tsp	2.6 tsp
Prednisolone sodium phosphate 5 mg/ 5 mL (Pediapred)	1 tsp	2 tsp	3 tsp	4 tsp	5 tsp	6 tsp	7 tsp	8 tsp
*Methylprednisolone 4 mg tablets (Medrol)	1 tab	2 tab	3 tab	4 tab	5 tab	6 tab	7 tab	8 tab
*Triamcinolone 4 mg tablets (Aristocort)	1 tab	2 tab	3 tab	4 tab	5 tab	6 tab	7 tab	8 tab

* Drugs marked with an asterisk (*) are equivalent to 5 mg of prednisone.

Disorders Caused by Bacterial Infections

CELLULITIS/ERYSIPELAS

I. Description

   A. Cellulitis: deeper dermis and subcutaneous skin infection without purulent discharge, usually caused by *Streptococcus pyogenes (most common)* or *Staphylococcus aureus*
      1. Painful and warm erythema with poorly defined margins and usually with red "streaking" in lymphatic channels.
      2. May have constitutional symptoms of fever, tachycardia, malaise, leukocytosis.
      3. Most commonly occurs in head and neck in children and lower extremities in adults, but can occur anywhere.
      4. Suspect methicillin-resistant *Staphylococcus aureus* (MRSA) if abscess is present and infection does not improve with treatment; may need to culture site.

   B. Erysipelas: superficial form of cellulitis with lymphatic involvement, usually caused by β-*hemolytic Streptococcus* bacteria
      1. Sudden onset redness with well demarcated, elevated border that is advancing with swelling and pain (see Fig. 5.9).
      2. Aggressive infection leading to bullae, ulcers, and necrosis.
      3. Often associated with pruritus, burning, tenderness, and constitutional symptoms of fever, chills, malaise, leukocytosis, tachycardia.
      4. Most common sites are face and hands; and lower legs, especially in the elderly; but can occur anywhere; not usually associated with abscesses.

II. Treatment

   A. Identify bacteria with wound cultures.
   B. Cold compresses for erysipelas and warm moist compresses for cellulitis.
   C. Rest and elevate extremity.
   D. If caused by penetrating injury, inquire about tetanus prophylaxis (see Table 5.5).
   E. If on lower extremity, check between toes for sites of infection or tinea.
   F. Should reassess patient in 24 hr, and ***if no improvement, refer to hospital.***

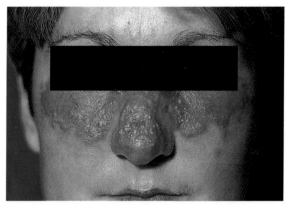

Fig. 5.9   Erysipelas. (From Walker, B. R., Colledge, N. R., Ralston, S. H., Penman, I. D. (2014). *Davidson's Principles and Practice of Medicine* (22nd ed.). Elsevier.)

● = *non-urgent referral*

TABLE 5.5 ■ Postexposure Tetanus Prophylaxis for People Who Previously Received Tetanus Toxoid Doses

	Significant Wounds*		Minor Wounds	
	Vaccine[†]	Tetanus Immune Globulin	Vaccine[†]	Tetanus Immune Globulin
Unsure of the tetanus status or <3 doses	Yes	Yes (do not mix vaccines and do not give in the same extremity)	Yes	No
Has had at least 3 doses	Yes, if the last dose was >5 yr ago	No	Yes, if the last dose was >10 yr ago	No

Note: Tdap (Adacel: ages 11–64 yr; Boostrix: ≥10 yr) to boost tetanus, diphtheria, and pertussis immunity can be given once any time and then return to q10yr schedule with Td.
* Including contaminated wounds, those related to necrotizing infections, or those from crush injury, burns, frostbite, bullets, or shrapnel.
[†] Patients ≥7 yr of age receive adult Td vaccine; patients <7 yr of age receive pediatric DT vaccine.

G. Can use topical mupirocin or retapamulin bid to lesions for both children and adults if few lesions are seen.

H. Outpatient oral antibiotic treatment
1. Should be active against *Streptococci pyogenes* and *Staphylococcus aureus*.
2. If there are no constitutional signs (e.g., fever, malaise, confusion, necrosis), start antibiotic treatment for 5 days; if symptoms continue (but not worsen), may extend treatment up to 14 days.

Condition	Drug	Pediatric dose	Adult
Cellulitis	Dicloxacillin	<40 kg: 12.5–25 mg/kg/day ÷ q6h >40 kg:125–500 mg q6h	125–500 mg q6h
	Clindamycin	10–25 mg/kg/day ÷ q8h	300 mg qid
	Cefadroxil	30 mg/kg/day ÷ q12h	1 g ÷ q12h
	Cephalexin	25–50 mg/kg/day ÷ q6–8h	500 mg qid
Erysipelas	TMP-SMZ	≥2 mo of age: TMP 6–12 mg/kg ÷ bid	≤120 kg: DS 1 q12h >120 kg: DS 2 q12h
	Pen VK	25–50 mg/kg/day ÷ q6h	500 mg qid
	Amoxicillin/clavulanate	≥3 mo of age: 25–50 mg/kg/dose ÷ q8h	875 mg bid
	Cephalexin	25–50 mg/kg/day ÷ q6–12h	500 mg qid
	Clindamycin	10–25 mg/kg/day ÷ q8h	300 mg q6h
PCN allergy or MRSA	Doxycycline	<45 kg: 2 mg/kg/dose q12h >45 kg: 4.4 mg/kg/d ÷ q12h (or adult dose)	100 mg bid

Continued

Condition	Drug	Pediatric dose	Adult
	Delafloxacin (Baxdela)	Not recommended	450 mg q12h for 5–14 days
	Minocycline	>8 yr of age: 4 mg once then 2 mg/kg/ dose ÷ q12h	200 mg once then 100 mg bid
	Clindamycin	10–25 mg/kg/day ÷ q8h	300 mg q6h
	TMP-SMZ	≥2 mo of age: TMP 8–12 mg/kg ÷ bid	≤120 kg: DS 1 q12h >120 kg: DS 2 q12h

▲   **III.** *Referral to ED/hospital*
    A. *Person appears ill (e.g., fever >100.4°F, tachycardic, chills) and will need IV antibiotics*
    B. *Infection located over prosthetic joint or other medical device(s)*
    C. *Poorly controlled diabetes*
    D. *Immunocompromised person*
    E. *Worsening constitutional symptoms to include change in mental status or hypotension*
    F. *Patient noncompliant with therapy*
    G. *Wound appears to be necrotizing*
        1. *Bullae formation or crepitus and any skin anesthesia*
        2. *Discoloration affecting the limb or edema beyond the area of erythema*

FOLLICULITIS

  I. Description
    A. Superficial inflammation of hair follicles, usually due to *Staphylococcus aureus*; usually heals without scarring; rarely seen in infants/children
    B. Scattered discrete papules/pustules are seen at the base of hair follicles in hairy areas (e.g., buttocks, axilla, groin, scalp, beard)
    C. Hot tub folliculitis occurs after sitting in a hot tub; usually seen on the buttocks, thighs, and lower trunk, and is commonly caused by *Pseudomonas aeruginosa*; usually *self-limited with good personal hygiene and chlorination of pool/hot tub*
  II. Treatment
    A. Hot moist compresses, antiseptic washes, and antibacterial soaps with good hand washing
    B. Hygiene measures
        1. Stop shaving until lesions are resolved.
        2. Change razors or other personal hygiene items.
        3. If induced by a hot tub, clean and disinfect the tub thoroughly.
        4. Clean/disinfect any type of exercise mat that is used by multiple people.
    C. Improve glycemic control
    D. Topical antibiotics until lesions are healed in mild-to-moderate cases of non-MRSA
        1. Mupirocin ointment tid
        2. Retapamulin ointment bid

▲ = *urgent referral*

E. If infection persists, start oral antibiotics for 10 days (*Staphylococcus aureus* may be penicillin resistant)

Drug	Pediatric Doses	Adult Doses
Dicloxacillin	<40 kg: 12.5–25 mg/kg/day ÷ q6h >40 kg: 125–250 mg q6h	250–500 mg q6h
Cephalexin	25–50 mg/kg/day ÷ q6–8h	250–500 mg qid
Clindamycin*	25–30 mg/kg/day ÷ q6h	450 mg tid
Ciprofloxacin	Not for children	250–750 mg bid (severe hot tub folliculitis)
Doxycycline*	<45 kg: 2 mg/kg/dose q12h >45 kg: 100 mg bid	100 mg bid

* Can be used for MRSA infection.

III. *Referral to a dermatologist if unresponsive to treatment in 2–3 wk.*
IV. Prevention: good personal hygiene, avoid sharing personal skin care items, keep exposure to sources of contamination at a minimum (i.e., exercise mats, showers)

FURUNCLE/CARBUNCLE

I. Description
   A. A furuncle (abscess) is an acute, red, hot, very tender fluctuant nodule with well-defined borders that can evolve from folliculitis and can occur anywhere on the body (see Fig. 5.10).
   B. A carbuncle is a collection of multiple coalescing furuncles that can occur anywhere on the body.

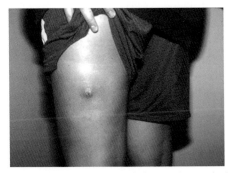

Fig. 5.10   Abcess. (From Cohen, P. R., Kurzrock, R. (2004). Community-acquired methicillin-resistant *Staphylococcus aureus* skin infection: An emerging clinical problem. *Journal of the American Academy of Dermatology* by the American Academy of Dermatology, Inc, Elsevier.)

___

 = *non-urgent referral*

C. Patient may have fever, malaise, and mild-to-moderate pain with or without purulent discharge from abscess.

D. Because of the increase in MRSA infections, treat as MRSA until wound culture results are obtained; suspect MRSA in case of the following
   1. Exposure at home or school
   2. Recent hospitalizations or daycare
   3. History of past MRSA infection
   4. Abscessed wound can occur from other bacteria also (e.g., *Staphylococcus aureus* or *Streptococci pyogenes*)

II. Treatment
   A. Most abscesses resolve with warm moist compresses; may consider use of OTC products, such as Prid or Crest toothpaste (Cavity Protection Regular Paste) apply daily until resolution.
   B. If no resolution, then incision and drainage (I&D) is required and antibiotics may or may not be needed
      1. If an abscess enlarges or starts to drain but has inadequate core opening, then I&D will be required.
      2. An abscess is "ready" to be incised with good results if the central portion of the abscess is "soft" to touch (e.g., feels like the tip of your nose), but the surrounding skin may stay firm.
      3. The area is usually "under pressure," so beware of injecting local anesthesia and during the first incision—either of these procedures may produce an eruption of purulent material that could "spew" up to one foot!
      4. Post wound abscess care
         (a) Can continue warm packs over dressing tid.
         (b) Change packing q2–4d but change the outer dressing more often, depending on the amount of drainage from the abscessed wound.
         (c) The amount of packing needed should gradually decrease with each packing change; monitor for decrease in the redness and size of the wound.
         (d) If the wound continues to drain and apparent infection is noted, start oral antibiotics.
         (e) ***Referral to surgeon if unresponsive to antibiotic therapy after 3 days.***
         (f) Recurrence of an abscess in the same location is usually due to inadequate incision depth, premature wound closure or tunneling.
   C. Culture the area if it is a first-time abscess.
   D. Improve hygiene by washing with antibacterial soaps, keep fingernails clean and short, do not share towels or personal items
   E. Change all razors and do not shave affected areas until the abscess has healed.
   F. Antibiotic therapy: 5–7 days for non-MRSA and 14 days for MRSA infections if
      1. Temperature >38°C (100.4°F).
      2. WBC >12,000 or <400 cells/μL.
      3. Unable to I&D abscess.
      4. Lack of response to initial treatment.
      5. Rapid progression of disease.

● = *non-urgent referral*

Pathogen	Drug	Pediatric Doses	Adult Doses
Non-MRSA			
	Dicloxacillin	<40 kg: 12.5–25 mg/kg/day ÷ q6h	125–500 mg q6h
	Cephalexin	25–50 mg/kg/day ÷ q8h	250–500 mg q6h
MRSA			
	Doxycycline	<45 kg: 2 mg/kg/dose q12h >45 kg: adult dose	100 mg q12h
	Minocycline	>8 yr of age: 4 mg/kg once then 2 mg/kg bid	200 mg once then 100 mg bid
	Clindamycin	30–40 mg/kg/day ÷ q6–8h	≤120 kg: 450 mg tid >120 kg: 600 mg tid

G. **Referral to surgeon if unresponsive to therapy or if the symptoms worsen.**
H. No sports until healed, but can return to school if the wounds are covered.
I. Suggested *decolonization* protocol for MRSA (with recurrent skin infections, even with adequate wound care and hygiene measures)
  1. All members of the household should complete the protocol simultaneously.
  2. Mupirocin intranasally bid for 5–10 days monthly for up to 6 mo with
    (a) Chlorhexidine baths daily for 5–14 days monthly for up to 6 mo (check the protocol with your institution) OR
    (b) Dilute bleach baths for 15 min, twice a week for up to 3 mo (add $^{1}/_{4}$ cup bleach to ¼ bath tub of water).
  3. Wash clothes in bleach and use a hot dryer.
  4. Clean surfaces at home with a disinfectant (1 Tbsp bleach in 1 qt water).
  5. Improve overall hygiene of the person and the family, with focus on hand washing and linen management.

IMPETIGO

I. Description
  A. Highly contagious infection of the skin; usually seen in children (but can occur at any age), with incubation period of 1–10 days and can be spread from direct contact or inanimate objects.
  B. Caused by *Staphylococcus aureus* or *group A β-hemolytic streptococci*
    1. Bullous impetigo (neonates or older infants) is usually caused by *Staphylococcus aureus; can occur in the diaper area.*
    2. Nonbullous impetigo (most common type) is seen in all ages of children, usually caused by *group A β-hemolytic streptococci.*
  C. Initial lesion is a vesicle that ruptures and becomes encrusted with thick, honey-colored fluid, followed by the crust; usually found on exposed skin such as face or extremities (see Fig. 5.11).

● = *non-urgent referral*

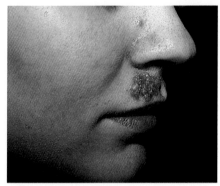

Fig. 5.11   Impetigo. Honey-colored, moist crust just above the upper lip. (From Weston, W. L., Lane, A. T., & Morelli, J. G. (2002). *Color textbook of pediatric dermatology* (3rd ed.). St. Louis: Mosby.)

     D. Can be itchy and painful and is quite contagious, but does not have associated constitutional symptoms.

  II. Treatment

     A. Improve overall hygiene and keep fingernails short.

     B. May need oral antihistamines (e.g., diphenhydramine) at night to prevent scratching; can have the child wear gloves at night.

     C. Gently soak and remove the crust with an antibacterial soap.

     D. Topical treatment can be used if few lesions are present

        1. Mupirocin tid for 5–7 days and cover with bandage

        2. Retapamulin (Altabax) bid for 5 days and cover with bandage

     E. Systemic oral antibiotic treatment for 7 days

Drug	Pediatric Dose	Adult Dose
Amoxicillin/ clavulanate	<3 mo of age: 30 mg/kg/day ÷ q12h >3 mo of age, <40 kg: 25 mg/kg/ day ÷ q12h	500–875 mg q8–12h
TMP-SMX	TMP 8–12 mg/kg/day q12h	≤120 kg: DS 1 tab bid >120 kg: DS 2 tab bid
Clindamycin	10–20 mg/kg/day ÷ tid	300 mg qid–450 mg tid
Cephalexin	25–50 mg/kg/day ÷ qid	250–500 mq qid
Dicloxacillin	<40 kg: 12.5–25 mg/kg/day ÷ q6h >40 kg: 125–250 mg q6h	250 mg qid

     F. No daycare or school for 24 hr after antibiotics started.

     G. Culture the lesion if there is no response to treatment. This condition usually resolves within 7 days of starting treatment.

  ● **III.** *Referral to infectious disease specialist if not improving.*

● *= non-urgent referral*

Disorders Caused by Viral Infections

ERYTHEMA INFECTIOSUM (FIFTH DISEASE)

I. Description
   A. Caused by parvovirus B19; lesions usually seen in clusters.
   B. Incubation period 4–14 days; the virus spreads via respiratory droplets.
   C. Patients are contagious 1 wk prior to the rash but *not* once the rash appears.
   D. More common in children than adults.
II. Signs and symptoms (see Figs. 5.12 and 5.13)
   A. Initially fever, rhinorrhea, H/A; nausea, diarrhea, and malaise occur within 2–5 days.
   B. This is followed by a red, macular blush that looks like a "slapped cheek" and then migrates to abdomen and then extensor surfaces of the extremities with a characteristic lacy, reticular pattern.
   C. The rash finally resolves but can recur intermittently over 3–4 wk, especially with exposure to sunlight, heat/cold, or exercise.
   D. May have painful and swollen joints of hands, feet, or knees; more common in adults.
III. Treatment
   A. No treatment but conservative care.
   B. Increase fluids to prevent dehydration.
   C. Use antipyretics and analgesics (see Appendices C and D) routinely while fever/pain is present.
   ▲ D. *Referral for pregnant women to OB immediately if exposed because the virus is fatal to the fetus.*

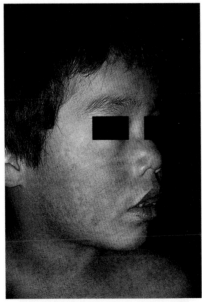

Fig. 5.12 Slapped-cheek appearance of a child with parvovirus B19 infection (erythema infectiosum). (From Weston, W. L., Lane, A. T., & Morelli, J. G. (2002). *Color textbook of pediatric dermatology* (3rd ed.). St. Louis: Mosby.)

▲ = *urgent referral*

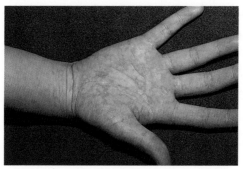

Fig. 5.13 Lacy pink eruption over the palms in erythema infectiosum. (From Weston, W. L., Lane, A. T., & Morelli, J. G. (2002). *Color textbook of pediatric dermatology* (3rd ed.). St. Louis: Mosby.)

HAND, FOOT, AND MOUTH DISEASE (HFMD)

I. Description
  A. Caused by either enterovirus or coxsackievirus A16; most contagious for the first 7 days of illness but can be infective for several weeks after symptoms resolve.
  B. Transmission is by direct contact with blisters, droplets, and fecal content (diaper changes); both adults and children can be infected.

II. Signs and symptoms
  A. Mouth and throat pain with oral lesions most commonly found on buccal mucosa and tongue may be the primary cause for refusal to eat (see Figs. 5.14 and 5.15).
  B. Abrupt onset of scattered macular, maculopapular, papular, and vesicular lesions found on palms, between fingers, and on the soles of feet, buttocks, legs, and arms.
  C. Constitutional symptoms: fever, malaise, joint aches, and cervical adenopathy

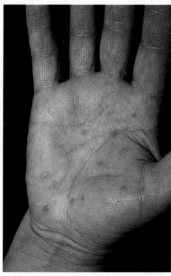

Fig. 5.14 Hand-foot-and-mouth disease. (From Callen, J. P., Greer, K. E., Paller, A. S., & Swinyer, L. J. (2000). *Color atlas of dermatology* (2nd ed.). Philadelphia: W.B. Saunders.)

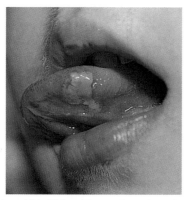

Fig. 5.15 Erosion of the tongue in a child with hand-foot-and-mouth syndrome. (From Weston, W. L., Lane, A. T., & Morelli, J. G. (2002). *Color textbook of pediatric dermatology* (3rd ed.). St. Louis: Mosby.)

III. Treatment
  A. Self-limiting illness; usually resolves in ~ 10 days; however darker skin types may have post-inflammatory pigmentation for longer periods of time.
  B. May have occasional itching.
  C. Use antipyretics for fever (no ASA in children).
  D. Increase fluid intake; cold liquids may soothe the pain.
  E. Treatment for mouth lesions in older children and adults
    1. OTC numbing mouthwashes or lozenges (e.g., Cepacol, Sucrets); do not use more than 10 lozenges/day.
    2. May try diphenhydramine liquid 5 mL PRN swish and spit, to decrease pain.
    3. Magic mouthwash mixture: mix equal parts of one of the following; swish and spit out 1–2 tsp, 3–4 times daily (each component can also be used individually)
      (a) Diphenhydramine + viscous Xylocaine 2%
      (b) Viscous Xylocaine 2% + Maalox + diphenhydramine
      (c) Viscous Xylocaine 2% + Maalox + prednisone liquid (can substitute nystatin suspension) + diphenhydramine
  IV. *Referral to hospital if child/adult is unable to maintain hydration.*

HERPES SIMPLEX (FEVER BLISTERS)

  I. Description
    A. Usually caused by herpes simplex virus type 1.
    B. Infection occurs about 2–12 days after exposure and can last 2–3 wk.
    C. Transmitted by skin-to-skin contact with mucous membranes, through open or abraded skin, or through contact with contaminated objects.
  II. Signs and symptoms
    A. Initial outbreak may be preceded by fever, malaise, H/A, and adenopathy.
    B. Lesions appear as grouped vesicles, followed by erosions and ulcerations, and may appear on the lips, oral mucosa, epidermal areas, and genitalia (see Fig. 5.16).
    C. Subsequent outbreaks may start as a "tingling sensation," which indicates active infection; subsequent outbreaks have few constitutional symptoms.
    D. Recurrent episodes are common, especially after stress, fever, and sun exposure.

⬤ = *non-urgent referral*

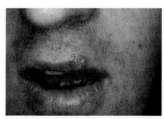

Fig. 5.16 Herpes simplex labialis-recurrent lesions. (From Callen, J. P., Greer, K. E., Paller, A. S., & Swinyer, L. J. (2000). *Color atlas of dermatology* (2nd ed.). Philadelphia: W.B. Saunders.)

III. Treatment
 A. Diagnosis is usually based on symptoms and appearance of lesions; provide education on transmission and treatments.
 B. May consider viral cultures (unroof vesicle and swab fluid for best results), but diagnosis is usually based on appearance of lesions.
 C. Keep lesions moist at all times with OTC products such as Carmex or lip balm.
 D. Lysine (OTC herbal product) orally or as a topical ointment; may shorten the illness duration or lessen the intensity of symptoms.
 E. Topical therapy: less effective and has to be applied frequently for best results; apply at first sign of infection
   1. Zilactin OTC or Zilactin-B OTC (>2 yr of age) for pain relief; use up to qid
   2. Abreva OTC (>12 yr of age); apply 5 times daily; apply with a finger cot or rubber glove; use until healed
   3. Viscous Xylocaine 2% mouth rinse for short-term pain relief; 1–2 tsp q8h; rinse and spit out
   4. Penciclovir (Denavir) cream (>12 yr of age), apply q2h while awake for 4 days; apply with rubber gloves
   5. Acyclovir 5%/hydrocortisone 1% (Xerese) cream (>6 yr of age), applied 5 times daily for 5 days
 F. Pharmacological therapy for *initial outbreaks*
   1. Acyclovir for 5 days
     (a) Children: 20 mg/kg/dose qid; max single dose 200 mg
     (b) Adults: 200 mg 5 times daily
   2. Acyclovir 400 mg tid (>12 yr of age) for 7–10 days
   3. Famciclovir 250 mg q8h or 500 mg bid for 7–10 days (adults only)
   4. Valacyclovir 1000 mg q12h for 7 days or 2 gm bid for 1 day (adults only)
 G. Pharmacological therapy for *recurrence* (adults only) started at earliest sign of infection
   1. Acyclovir for 5 days: 400 mg tid or 800 mg q12h
   2. Acyclovir oropharyngeal MBT 50 mg (Sitavig) applied as a single dose to the upper gum line on the same side of symptoms within 1 hr of onset of symptoms
   3. Valacyclovir 2000 mg bid for 1 day
   4. Famciclovir 750 mg bid 1 day or 1500 mg as single dose
 H. Pharmacological therapy for *suppression* (adults only); reassess the need for continued therapy annually
   1. Acyclovir 400 mg bid
   2. Valacyclovir 500 mg daily if breakthrough symptoms occur

HERPES ZOSTER (SHINGLES)

I. Description
   A. Discrete, vesiculopustular, grouped lesions (see Fig. 5.17); follows dermatomal line (see Fig. 13.1).
   B. Lesions do not normally cross the midline, but zoster multiplex involves multiple dermatomes and possibly bilateral distribution.
   C. Very painful, occasional itching that may precede actual eruption.
   D. Postherpetic neuralgia (PHN): residual burning pain that occurs at the site of lesions after the rash is resolved; can occur after the initial episode of zoster and may disrupt life activities because of nerve pain.
   E. Transmitted from person to person via contact with lesion.
      1. Highest risk with elderly and under-immunized children.
      2. Keep lesions covered until appearance of crust.

II. Treatment
   A. *Initiate treatment within 72 hr of outbreak; if patient is immunocompromised, can start treatment >72 hr.*
   B. Nonpharmacological therapy
      1. Wet-to-dry dressings with sterile saline or Domeboro solution qid
      2. Calamine lotion 4–5 times daily
      3. Zinc oxide, which will help decrease itching and can decrease infection; also helps dry lesions
   C. Pharmacological therapy for acute episodes (adults)
      1. Acyclovir 800 mg 5 times daily for 7 days *or*
      2. Famciclovir 500 mg tid for 7 days *or*
      3. Valacyclovir 1000 mg tid for 7 days
      4. Steroids alone or in combination with antiviral have not been proven to aid in the resolution of herpes zoster and may increase risk of infection.
      5. Pain management with Tramadol 50 mg tid, opioids, acetaminophen, and/or NSAIDs (unless contraindicated) (see Chapter 14, PHARMACOLOGICAL THERAPIES)
      6. Amitriptyline 10–25 mg at hs
   D. Until all lesions are crusted, avoid contact with immunocompromised people, pregnant women, and people with no history of chicken pox infection/immunization.
   ▲ E. *Referral to an ophthalmologist as soon as possible if around the eyes (because this can permanently affect vision).*

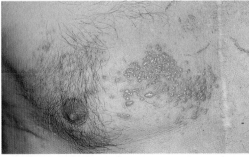

Fig. 5.17 Herpes zoster. (From Callen, J. P., Greer, K. E., Paller, A. S., & Swinyer, L. J. (2000). *Color atlas of dermatology* (2nd ed.). Philadelphia: W.B. Saunders.)

▨ = *not to be missed;* ▲ = *urgent referral*

F. Therapy for PHN: the goal is to prevent PHN with early treatment, but if unsuccessful, use one or more of the following
   1. Amitriptyline 10–25 mg or nortriptyline 25 mg (off-label) at hs (better tolerated at lower doses)
   2. Gabapentin 300 mg for 1 day, then 300 mg bid for 1 day, then tid
   3. Gabapentin ER (Gralise) start with 300 mg and slowly increase to a maximum of 1800 mg daily
   4. Pregabalin (Lyrica) 150–300 mg bid
   5. Venlafaxine 150–300 mg/day (off label)
   6. Topical capsaicin cream applied 5 times daily (use gloves and wash hands well after use)
   7. Topical lidocaine transdermal patches 5% (Lidoderm); patches may be applied for up to 12 hr a day in a 24 hr period; may be cut to size; no more than three patches at a time; never reuse a patch and do not place on open skin
   8. Consider TENS unit
   9. Acupuncture
III. *Consider referral to a pain management specialist.*
IV. Prevention
   A. Varicella-zoster virus vaccine (Zostavax) is no longer available in U.S.
   B. Zoster vaccine recombinant (Shingrix) for adults >50 yr of age (recommended)
      1. Two dose series, first dose followed by second dose at 2–6 mo.
      2. If >6 mo after first shot, give one dose, but do not restart series.
      3. Can be given if history of shingles and/or has previously had Zostavax (persons receiving Zostavax are encouraged to revaccinate with Shingrix).
      4. For use in immunocompetent adults; it can be given to immunocompromised adults on low-dose suppressive therapy but vaccine effectiveness may be reduced.
      5. Do not give during an acute outbreak of shingles or while still on antiviral medications.
      6. Do not give if the person is undergoing moderate to high-dose "biologic therapy" for other illnesses.
   C. Give varicella-zoster immune globulin (VZIG) for patients that are high risk; can give up to 96 hr after exposure and protection lasts about 3 wk.

MOLLUSCUM CONTAGIOSUM

I. Description
   A. A viral lesion that is a smooth, flesh- to pink-colored, raised, umbilicated papule; may have redness or scaling around lesions (see Fig. 5.18).
   B. Lesions are considered contagious and are transmitted by skin-to-skin contact or skin to fomite (e.g., towels, clothing, gym mats); found anywhere on the body (although rarely on palms or soles)
      1. Face and torso are common areas in children.
      2. Genitals, anal area, groin, and lower abdomen are common areas in adults.
   C. In general, lesions resolve without treatment in about 12–18 mo if the person has a competent immune system; if immunocompromised, lesions generally will not resolve without treatment and may be a marker for HIV.
   D. Even with treatment, lesions may recur.

● = *non-urgent referral*

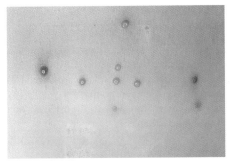

Fig. 5.18 Molluscum contagiosum. Small papules with a central umbilication. (From Callen, J. P., Greer, K. E., Paller, A. S., & Swinyer, L. J. (2000). *Color atlas of dermatology* (2nd ed.). Philadelphia: W.B. Saunders.)

II. Treatment
   A. If inflammation is noted surrounding individual molluscum, do not treat; this is indicative of resolution.
   B. Surgical: curettage, cryosurgery with liquid nitrogen, electrodessication, and laser
   C. Suggested nonsurgical therapies (apply to lesions)
      1. Cantharidin 0.7% topical application (painful)
      2. Imiquimod 5% cream 3 times a week for 12 wk (can be self-applied)
      3. Potassium hydroxide (KOH) 10% applied bid until lesions disappear (can be applied at home)
   D. Many sports require clearance before play
      1. No play for 48 hr after curettage.
      2. Cover small lesions with occlusive dressing while playing.

ROSEOLA

I. Description
   A. Common in children 3 mo to 4 yr of age
   B. Caused by human herpesvirus 6
   C. Presumed transmission is via saliva
   D. Incubation period may be 5–15 days
II. Signs and symptoms
   A. Starts with high fever (up to 105°F), may have mild irritability, rhinorrhea, and sore throat; as fever decreases in 2–4 days, a rose-pink maculopapular rash appears.
   B. The rash first appears on the trunk and may spread to the face, neck, and extremities.
   C. The child does not appear ill; symptoms last for about 7 days.
III. Treatment
   A. No treatment but conservative care.
   B. Increase fluids to prevent dehydration.
   C. Use antipyretics (e.g., acetaminophen [not aspirin due to potential for Reye syndrome]) routinely while fever is present; may use cool sponge baths.
   D. Caution parents that the maximum height of a fever, instead of the rapid rise, may cause febrile seizures. Fever, usually >100.4°F sustained, may be the stimulus required for some pediatric patient to exhibit seizure activity.

VARICELLA (CHICKEN POX)

I. Description
   A. Highly contagious viral illness with transmission through respiratory droplets and direct contact with vesicles; incubation period 10–21 days.
   B. Multistaged papular, vesicular, pustular lesions on a red base that crust (see Fig. 5.19)
   C. Lesions begin on the trunk and are scattered.
   D. Pruritus, fever, H/A, coryza, cough, anorexia, malaise, and sore throat are common.
   E. Usually seen in young children.

II. Treatment
   A. Nonpharmacological therapy in healthy children
      1. Control pruritus
         (a) Calamine lotion or pramoxine gel
         (b) Oatmeal baths
         (c) Oral antihistamines (e.g., diphenhydramine, hydroxyzine)
      2. Fever and pain (see Appendices C and D)
   B. Adults, elderly, or immunocompromised people who never had varicella need to be treated to prevent complications
      1. VZIG administered as soon as possible after presumed exposure; may be effective within 6 hr after initial exposure.
      2. Protection with VZIG lasts for approximately 3 wk; may be repeated once if re-exposed >3 wk after prior dose.
   C. Monitor and treat secondary bacterial infections.
   D. Pharmacological treatment, if given, should be started within 24 hr after the rash starts and continued for 5 days
      1. Acyclovir
         (a) Children >2 yr of age: acyclovir 20 mg/kg/dose qid (not over 800 mg/dose)
         (b) Adults: 800 mg 5 times daily

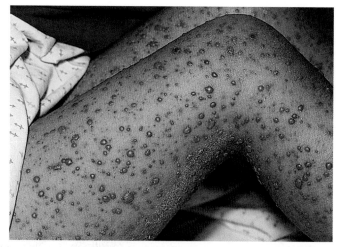

Fig. 5.19 Chicken pox. (From Swartz, Mark H. (2014). *Textbook of physical diagnosis: History and examination* (7th ed.). Philadelphia: Saunders.)

2. Valacyclovir (off label)
   (a) Children >2yr of age: 20 mg/kg/dose tid
   (b) Adults: 1000 mg tid

VERRUCA VULGARIS (WARTS)

I. Description: a viral lesion caused by HPV and transmitted by direct contact
   A. Clinical presentation
      1. Common warts are firm, small, skin-colored papules anywhere on the body, especially on hands and feet (see Fig. 5.20)
      2. Plantar warts are thickened, rough, skin-colored plaques found on the plantar surface of feet.
   B. Lesions do not itch but may be painful if in high-stress area such as the sole of feet.
II. Treatment: lesions may spontaneously resolve without any treatment
   A. Surgical option with excision
   B. Cryotherapy
      1. Liquid nitrogen can be used for all warts; may require several treatments before resolution.
      2. When using liquid nitrogen, let the lesion thaw between treatments; watch for a ring around the lesion to ensure adequate freezing.
      3. Do not use liquid nitrogen on the skin for >15 sec at a time; if using in children, have them count or recite letters to distract them or sing songs during treatment.
   C. Flat warts may respond to tretinoin acid 0.05% cream (Retin-A) daily with or without occlusion; can use benzoyl peroxide 5% or salicylic acid 5% cream with Retin-A until healed.
   D. Plantar warts may respond to occlusive salicylic acid 40%; keep in place for 2–3 days, then pare down the wart(s), and may repeat again.
   E. Anogenital warts may respond to imiquimod 5% cream applied at home 3 times a week for 16 wk (see Chapter 10, Gynecological Infections, SEXUALLY TRANSMITTED DISEASES, II, D).
   F. Hand warts may respond to cryotherapy weekly for 3 wk.
   G. Subungual or periungual warts may respond to salicylic acid followed by imiquimod.
   H. Duct tape can be tried for wart(s)
      1. Apply tape and leave on for several days; then remove the tape, pare down the wart, leave open for at least 12 hr, and reapply the tape.

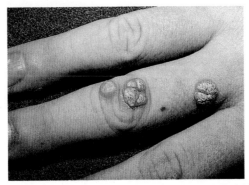

Fig. 5.20 Common warts on a child's fingers. (From Weston, W. L., Lane, A. T., & Morelli, J. G. (2002). *Color textbook of pediatric dermatology* (3rd ed.). St. Louis: Mosby.)

2. May take several months, but this procedure is relatively painless.
3. Another technique is to put a salt compress on the wart and then apply duct tape.
   I. When athletes return to play, they should cover the warts when the sport involves skin-to-skin contact.
III. Referral to a podiatrist if no resolution of plantar warts and/or dermatologist for other warts and advanced therapies.

Disorders Caused by Fungal Infection

ONYCHOGRYPHOSIS

I. Description
   A. Nails are very thickened, yellow, and usually curving, and can resemble a claw or horn, especially the great toenails (see Fig. 5.21B).
      1. Very large overgrowth of the nail plate can override the toe and rest on the plantar aspect of the toe.
      2. Has no relationship to fungal infection but may be confused with tinea.
      3. Nail may loosen at the base or along the body of the nail.
   B. Caused by repeated trauma (e.g., too short shoes, trauma to nail matrix) or poor hygiene; usually seen in the elderly.
   C. Treatment
      1. This is a chronic problem and cannot be solved with removing the nail or occasional trimming; ablation of the nail plate may correct the problem.
      2. Use strong nail clippers or motorized tool (e.g., dremel) to cut or grind the surface of the nail in order for the shoe to fit without pain.
      3. Evaluate the type of shoe and size and recommend larger toe box on shoe.
      4. Usually need to perform nail care q3mo after nail ablation.
   D. Referral to a podiatrist if unable to reduce the size of the nail sufficiently to get shoes on comfortably and is affecting QOL.

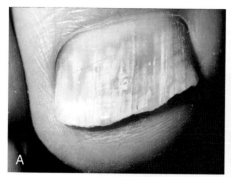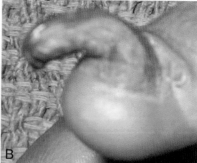

Fig. 5.21 A: Onychomycosis. B: Onychogryphosis. (Panel A: From Rai, Ashish, et al. (2014). An algorithmic approach to posttraumatic nail deformities based on anatomical classification. *Journal of Plastic, Reconstructive & Aesthetic Surgery, 67*, 540–547, Elsevier. Panel B: From Coleman, N. W., Fleckman, P., & Huang, J .I. (2014). Fungal Nail Infections. *Journal of Hand Surgery, 39*(5). American Society for Surgery of the Hand. Elsevier.)

⬤ = *non-urgent referral*

ONYCHOMYCOSIS

I. Description (see Fig. 5.21A)
  A. Fungal infection of nail bed or nail plate.
  B. Can affect finger nails but is more common in toenails.
  C. Can limit quality of life due to pain and disrupted gait.
  D. Immunocompromised people (e.g., DM with neuropathy) are at higher risk for more serious complications.
  E. Most common dermatophyte is *Trichophyton rubrum* and least common is *Candida.*
II. History and appearance
  A. Usually asymptomatic and presents to office for cosmetic reasons.
  B. History of environmental (e.g., work in damp, humid conditions, poor hygiene facilities, inability to keep feet dry) and occupational exposures (e.g., constant hand washing, frequent travel, and use of communal bathing facilities).
  C. Hyperkeratotic nails with
    1. Yellow-white color, either solid or with streaking at the junction of the nail and the bed.
    2. Milky white discoloration of nail plate that moves distally with nail growth.
    3. Small, white, speckled powdery patches with easy nail crumbling.
  D. Toenail(s) are usually slightly thickened and can be separated at nail bed, which can cause pain with poorly fitting shoes; can lead to undetectable injury/infection if neuropathy exists.
  E. May interfere with walking, balance, and exercise.
III. Diagnostics
  A. Should confirm diagnosis of onychomycosis prior to treatment, although a negative result does not rule out disease.
  B. Direct microscopy using a special preparation of KOH 20% in dimethyl sulfoxide (DMSO) preparation is useful to rule out presence of fungi.
  C. Fungal culture may be beneficial to identify the species of organism prior to treatment.
IV. Treatment
  A. This infection is not life-threatening, and many insurance companies will not pay for treatment because it is considered cosmetic. If immunosuppressed, treatment should be available because of potential for systemic spreading and worsening of disease.
  B. Keep nails trimmed and smooth to decrease potential to tear nail.
  C. Topical treatments generally do not cure because of poor penetration through nail plate, especially toenails.
    1. Ciclopirox 8% solution nail lacquer (Penlac): apply to either toenails or fingernails daily for 48 wk and then re-evaluate; good option for persons with hands in water frequently (adults only)
    2. Efinaconazole 10% (Jublia) topical solution: apply to toenails daily for 48 wk (adults only)
    3. Tavaborole 5% solution (Kerydin): apply to toenails daily for 48 wk; ≥6 yr of age.
    4. Apply Mentholatum (popular home remedy) to toenails every night until fungal infection is resolved or stabilized; this may take months
    5. Have person fill a pan with warm water and add 1 capful of bleach to 1 qt of water; soak feet in this solution for 10–15 min bid for 2 wk (wash feet after each treatment); toenails will turn white; new nails should regrow in 2–3 mo
  D. Systemic treatments
    1. Terbinafine (Lamisil)

   (a) Pulse therapy
     (i) Fingernails: 250 mg daily for 1 wk each mo for 6–9 mo
     (ii) Toenails: 250 mg daily for 1 wk each mo for 9–12 mo
     (iii) No need to monitor lab work
   (b) Daily continuous therapy
     (i) Fingernails: 250 mg daily for 6 wk
     (ii) Toenails: 250 mg daily for 12 wk
     (iii) Monitor CBC, AST/ALT every 4 wk for 2 mo.
  2. Itraconazole (Sporanox) (do not use in patients with HF)
   (a) Pulse therapy
     (i) Fingernails: 200 mg q12h for 7 days then off 21 days; may repeat once
     (ii) Toenails: 200 mg q12h for 7 days then off 21 days; may repeat twice
     (iii) No need to monitor lab work
   (b) Daily continuous therapy
     (i) Fingernails: 200 mg daily for 6 wk
     (ii) Toenails: 200 mg daily for 12 wk
     (iii) Monitor CBC, AST/ALT every 4 wk for 2 mo.
 E. Surgical removal has not been shown to promote a cure.
 F. Lifestyle changes to prevent recurrence
  1. Avoid communal showers.
  2. Wear properly fitting shoes.
  3. Wear water proof shoes (e.g., flip flops, lake shoes) when showering in communal facilities.
  4. Treat comorbidity (e.g., DM).
  5. Prevent nail damage with routine nail care.
● **V. Referral to a podiatrist if unresponsive to treatment and/or effects QOL.**

TINEA

 I. Description
  A. Highly contagious, superficial, mildly pruritic infection caused by dermatophytes.
  B. Well-demarcated plaques with or without pustules or papules; usually have scaling at the edges with central clearing.
  C. Predisposes the person to bacterial infections or dyshidrotic eczema.
  D. Treatment is usually started before identification of particular fungal species, if treatment is ineffective: scrape multiple areas on the leading edge of a lesion with a scalpel and place the scrapings on a slide; add one drop of KOH and then heat the slide; examine under a microscope for hyphae and spores or send specimen for fungal culture.
 II. Types
  A. Tinea capitis
   1. Poorly defined, scattered areas of white scales on the head where hair is present (e.g., scalp, eyebrows, or eyelashes), with varying degrees of hair loss, more common in children.
   2. Scalp lesions can be large, with an exudate under scales that mats hair.
   3. Culture should be done to determine species for effective treatment; most common species involved with tinea capitis is *Trichophyton* or *Microsporum*.

● = *non-urgent referral*

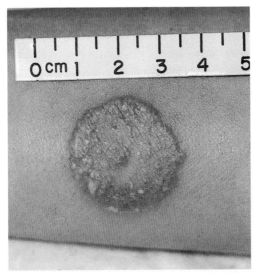

Fig. 5.22 Tinea corporis. (From Schwartz, M. H. (2014). *Textbook of Physical Diagnosis* (7th ed.). Philadelphia: W.B. Saunders.)

    4. ***Referral to dermatologist (systemic treatment is recommended because topical treatment is ineffective).***

B. Tinea corporis (ringworm)

    1. Asymmetrically distributed, erythematous scaly patch with central clearing; usually found on skin areas other than scalp, groin, palms, or soles of feet (see Fig. 5.22).

    2. Scales are prominent on the edges of patches and are usually associated with itching.

    3. Usually spread from infected animals (e.g., cats and dogs), people (e.g., especially wrestlers) and fomites.

    4. Topical treatment should be applied at least 2 in. beyond infected ring

      (a) Tolnaftate (OTC) apply bid for 1–4 wk

      (b) Butenafine 1% (Mentax) gel/solution, apply daily for 1–4 wk

      (c) Ciclopirox 0.77% (Loprox) cream/gel/suspension bid up to 4 wk

      (d) Terbinafine (Lamisil) cream, apply daily for 7 days up to 4 wk

      (e) Naftifine 1%–2% (Naftin) cream/gel apply 1–2 times daily for 2–4 wk

      (f) Oxiconazole 1% (Oxistat) cream/lotion 1–2 times daily for 2 wk

    5. Can also prescribe terbinafine 250 mg po daily for 1–2 wk

C. Tinea cruris (jock itch)

    1. Pruritic, well-demarcated patches with central clearing, centered over inguinal creases and extending down the medial thighs and may involve buttocks; in males, scrotum is usually spared (see Fig. 5.23)

    2. Scales are seen at the periphery and may be moist and exudative or dry with barely perceptible scale

    3. Can have corresponding tinea pedis

    4. Associated with wearing tight-fitting clothing and wearing wet underclothing for extended periods of time; may worsen with DM or other immunocompromised illnesses

_____

● = *non-urgent referral*

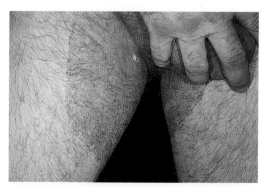

Fig. 5.23 Tinea cruris. (From Callen, J. P., Greer, K. E., Paller, A. S., & Swinyer, L. J. (2000). *Color atlas of dermatology* (2nd ed.). Philadelphia: W.B. Saunders.)

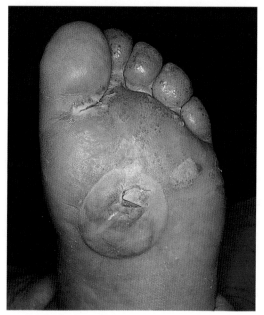

Fig. 5.24 Tinea pedis. (From Swartz, Mark H. (2014). *Textbook of physical diagnosis*. Philadelphia: Saunders.)

5. Topical treatment is recommended along with weight loss and control of DM
  (a) Tolnaftate OTC (Tinactin) apply bid for 2–3 wk
  (b) Butenafine 1% (Mentax) apply daily for 4 wk
  (c) Ciclopirox 0.77% (Loprox) apply bid for 2–4 wk
  (d) Terbinafine (Lamisil AT) apply bid for 1–4 wk
  (e) Econazole 1% (Ecoza) apply daily for 2 wk

D. Tinea pedis (athlete's foot)
1. Redness with maceration, fissuring, itching, and scaling; usually between the fourth and fifth toes, sparing the dorsum of the foot, but may have hyperkeratotic eruptions on dorsum and sides of feet (see Fig. 5.24).
2. Occasional painful vesicular or ulcerative lesions; often, peeling of the skin on feet and between toes and can lead to bacterial infections.
3. Can use Burrow's solution as a wet to dry compress or as a soak for maceration between toes or plantar aspect of foot; soak for ~20 min 2–3 times a day.
4. Treatment with topical agents for approximately 2–6 wk; treatment should last until symptoms are resolved. Re-evaluate progress at end of treatment
   (a) Terbinafine 1% (Lamisil) apply bid
   (b) Butenafine 1% (Mentax) gel/solution apply bid
   (c) Naftifine 2% (Naftin) gel apply daily (>12 yr of age)
   (d) Ciclopirox 0.77% (Loprox) apply bid
   (e) Clotrimazole 1% (Lotrimin) apply q12h
   (f) Econazole 1% (Ecoza) cream or foam apply daily
   (g) Ketoconazole 2% (Nizoral) apply daily
   (h) Oxiconazole 1% (Oxistat) apply 1–2 times daily
   (i) Sertaconazole 2% (Ertaczo) cream apply bid
   (j) Luliconazole 1% (Luzu) cream apply daily
5. If severe, may require oral treatment
   (a) Terbinafine 250 mg daily for 2 wk
   (b) Fluconazole 150 mg once weekly for 2–6 wk
6. Prophylaxis
   (a) Desiccating foot powder daily to feet, socks and shoes (e.g., Dr Scholl's foot powder, Gold Bond medicated foot powder or corn starch).
   (b) Keep feet dry, especially in the summer; consider open sandals.
E. Tinea versicolor (Pityriasis versicolor)
1. A cosmetic condition caused by yeast infection; usually asymptomatic and does not itch.
2. Patches or spots of hypopigmentation or hyperpigmentation with mild erythema on the trunk, neck, and upper arms; are more apparent in the warmer months and can be recurrent.
3. Topical treatment applied to rash area
   (a) Selenium sulfide 2.5% shampoo (Selsun) applied daily for 1 wk; should remain on skin for at least 10 min before washing off; can use weekly or monthly to prevent recurrence
   (b) Zinc pyrithione 1% or 2% shampoo daily for 2 wk
   (c) Ketoconazole 2% (Nizoral) shampoo or cream applied daily for 2–6 wk (wash off after 10 min) and then as needed for recurrence
   (d) Terbinafine (Lamisil) applied bid daily for 1 wk
   (e) Miconazole cream (Monistat) applied 1–2 times daily until resolved
   (f) Ciclopirox 0.77% cream bid for 2 wk
4. Systemic treatment for adults
   (a) Fluconazole 300 mg (Diflucan) once weekly for 2 wk
   (b) Itraconazole 200 mg (Sporanox) daily for 5 days (do not use with HF)

Disorders of Pigmentation

ACANTHOSIS NIGRICANS

I. Description
   A. Symmetrical, thickened, darkened areas of skin that feel "velvety" and are located predominantly in axilla, neck, and groin; also may be seen on face, elbows, knees, dorsum of hands, breasts, and genitalia (see Figs. 15.1 and 15.2)
   B. Commonly associated clinical conditions are obesity, DM, insulin resistance, hyperandrogenic and hypogonadal states
   C. Associated with malignancy (e.g., stomach, colon, liver and lung)
   D. Can be familial and seen at birth
   E. Can be caused by certain medications such as steroids, OCP, insulin and niacin
II. Treatment
   A. Treat the cause
      1. Control endocrine disorder.
      2. Lose weight.
      3. Medication consideration: metformin (see Chapter 8, METABOLIC SYNDROME), topical retinoic acid or salicylic acid (see Table 5.1), and fish oil.
   B. Laser treatments may correct discoloration.
III. *Referral to dermatologist or endocrinologist if unresponsive to treatment.*

LICHEN SCLEROSIS

I. Description
   A. Hypopigmentation disorder resulting in loss of color, tissue thinning, and scarring appearance; most commonly seen in the vulvar area and often causes severe pruritus.
   B. Dry, papery thin skin starting above the clitoral arch and going down the labia majora to the perianal area (often in the shape of an "hourglass"); does not involve the vaginal tissue (see Fig. 5.25).
   C. Can result in introital stenosis with scarring, and fusion of the labia, which causes discomfort with sexual intercourse and can cause bleeding.
   D. Common in prepubertal girls and older women.
II. Diagnostics: biopsy is indicated because it can progress to squamous cell carcinoma (SCC) in 5% cases
III. Treatment
   A. Avoid harsh soaps.
   B. Wear ventilated cotton clothes and avoid panty liners.
   C. Use Cetaphil as a cleanser and moisturizer.
   D. Use mild vaginal lubricants daily and with intercourse.
   E. For severe pruritus, try Domeboro solution in cool water as a sitz bath.
   F. High to very high potency steroids in ointment (see Table 5.3) are given to relieve severe symptoms; start with nightly treatments for 6–12 wk, and then follow-up
      1. Treatment can be PRN for flare-ups.
      2. Maintenance therapy, if needed, with steroids 2–3 times a week.
      3. Continue daily emollients (e.g., petrolatum, lanolin, olive oil) indefinitely.
   G. Estrogen creams may relieve symptoms (see Chapter 10, Table 10.4).
IV. *Referral to a dermatologist or gynecologist for persistent symptoms.*

● = *non-urgent referral*

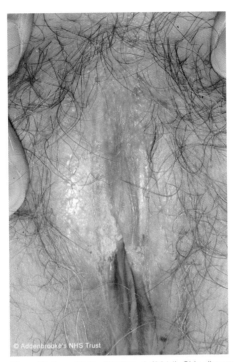

Fig. 5.25 Lichen sclerosus. (From Shaheen H. H., Sterling, J. (2014). Skin diseases affecting the vulva, *Obstetrics, Gynecology, and Reproductive Medicine, 24*(5). Philadelphia: Elsevier.)

MELASMA

I. Description: considered a chronic disease
  A. Mostly symmetrical distribution of macular hyperpigmentation (bronzing) in sun-exposed areas, predominantly over the cheeks, forehead, nose, chin, jaw angle, and above the upper lip but can appear in other sun-exposed areas.
  B. Seen most often in women of reproductive age with a darker complexion; can appear with pregnancy (e.g., chloasma) or use of oral contraceptives.
  C. Triggers
     1. Sun (common in summer and improves in winter)
     2. Initiation of OCs or HRT
     3. Some antiseizure and anticancer medications
     4. Scented cosmetics, toiletries, and soaps
     5. Hypothyroidism
II. Treatment
  A. Cosmetic treatment involves camouflaging with facial tones to hide the darkening.
  B. Sun protection and sunscreens containing broad spectrum UV-A and -B with SPF >50 are beneficial and *must* be used for any sun exposure, even on cloudy days.
  C. Wear wide-brimmed hats and sunglasses.
III. Pharmacological therapy (not to be used with pregnancy)
  A. Hydroquinone 4% cream: apply bid (apply a small amount on the arms to test for hypersensitivity first); contraindicated with breast feeding or pregnancy.
  B. Azelaic acid 20% (Azelex [off-label]): apply bid for up to 8 mo

    C. Fluocinolone/hydroquinone/tretinoin (Tri-Luma): apply at hs up to 24 wk for severe symptoms

    D. Kojic acid 2% or niacinamide 4% cream daily may lighten some dark spots.

    E. Steroids alone result in initial clearing, but subsequently lead to rapid recurrence and poor overall response.

IV. Referral to dermatologist for enhanced skin lightening therapies.

VITILIGO

I. Description

    A. Discrete areas of the skin and mucus membranes are depigmented; the most commonly affected sites are as follows

      1. Dorsal hands and arms

      2. Body creases and genitalia

      3. Buccal mucosa, face, neck, scalp, anus, and nose

    B. Tends to occur between 10 and 30 yr of age and can be progressive.

    C. May be associated with the following conditions

      1. Alopecia

      2. Thyroiditis, Graves' disease

      3. Pernicious anemia

      4. Irritable bowel syndrome (IBS), psoriasis, type 1 DM

II. Treatment: no permanent cure, and resolution with treatment is less than optimal; suggest

    A. Camouflage with cosmetics

    B. Mild symptoms (<10% body surface area [BSA])

      1. Mid-to-high potency topical steroids daily for 2 mo

      2. Tacrolimus (off label) or pimecrolimus (off label) bid for 2 mo

      3. Tattooing is contraindicated.

III. Referral to a dermatologist.

Skin Lesions

ACTINIC KERATOSIS

I. Description

    A. Premalignant lesion(s) usually caused by sun exposure, with an increased risk for SCC.

    B. Lesion is symmetrical and has a scaly appearance (see Fig. 5.26); it is common to see multiple lesions.

    C. Lesion has usually been present for a long time as a chronic scale that can be scratched off but will always come back without treatment.

II. Treatment

    A. Cryotherapy

    B. Curette excision

    C. Topical products for multiple lesions

      1. Imiquimod 5% cream (Aldara) bid at hs for 16 wk

      2. Diclofenac sodium 3% gel (Solaraze) bid for 60–90 days

---

● = non-urgent referral

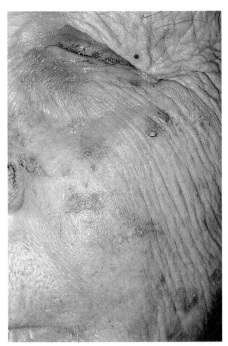

Fig. 5.26   Multiple actinic keratosis. (From Callen, J. P., Greer, K. E., Paller, A. S., & Swinyer, L. J. (2000). *Color atlas of dermatology* (2nd ed.). Philadelphia: W.B. Saunders.)

   3. Fluorouracil 0.5% cream (Carac); daily for 4 wk; better tolerated, least systemic absorption
   4. Fluorouracil 5% cream (Efudex); bid hs for ~16 wk; better outcomes, but more irritation
   5. Tirbanibulin 1% ointment (Klisyri) daily for 5 day; *remove* ointment after 8 hr
  III. *Referral to a dermatologist if lesions do not respond to treatment, large area of the skin is involved, if the lesion returns after therapy, or if there are concerns for cancerous changes.*

EPIDERMOID CYST (ALSO CALLED SEBACEOUS, KERATIN, OR EPITHELIAL CYST)

 I. Description
  A. A stable or slow-growing firm subcutaneous nodule that is flesh-colored, smooth and usually nontender; does not require treatment unless inflamed or bothersome to patient.
  B. There may be a history of intermittent drainage with discharge
   1. Has a small central punctum (core) that differentiates it from lipoma.
   2. Cyst contents, when present, are usually cream-colored with a cottage cheese-like consistency and foul odor.
  C. Can be small (0.5 cm) to large (>2.5 cm); usually a solitary nodule.
  D. Can become inflamed with persistent irritation or infected from bacteria on skin.

⬤ = *non-urgent referral*

II. Treatment is excision, drainage, and removal of the cyst and cyst wall
  A. For the best results, wait until cyst inflammation/infection is resolved
    1. Remove contents by either squeezing or flushing it out with saline or hydrogen peroxide.
    2. Cyst wall can be removed easier if contents have been removed.
  B. Excision techniques
    1. Punch biopsy for smaller, singular cyst (see PUNCH BIOPSY, later in this chapter)
    2. Superficial incision with #11 blade

KERATOACANTHOMA

  I. Description
    A. Lesion is symmetrical and dome shaped, with a central plug and crust; borders are smooth, well demarcated; nodule is firm and not painful.
    B. The lesion grows rapidly and may double within a 2-wk period up to 2 cm in size; in contrast, basal cell carcinoma (BCC) or squamous cell carcinoma (SCC) is typically slower growing and may take months to years to double in size.
    C. Found primarily on sun-exposed areas such as the face and extremities.
  II. Treatment
    A. Cryotherapy for smaller lesions.
    B. Deep shave or conventional excision with free margins; send to pathology.
    C. Can recur; monitor the area after treatment every month for at least 3 mo.
  III. *Referral to dermatologist or surgeon if resistant to treatment.*

SKIN CANCER

  I. Basal cell carcinoma (BCC)
    A. Description
      1. Lesion is usually round with small central ulcerated depressions on a pearly raised base. Borders are smooth with increased vascularity around the rim (see Fig. 5.27)
      2. Can be nonhealing or recurrent, irregularly shaped, and bleeds easily
      3. Color variation: from pale white to pink, flesh-colored to red, but can be darker in color

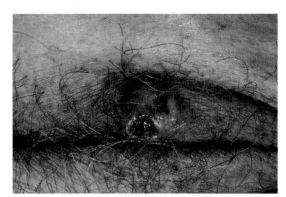

Fig. 5.27 Basal cell carcinoma of nodular type with ulceration affecting the vulva. (From White, G. M., & Cox, N. H. (2002). *Diseases of the skin: A color atlas and text*. St. Louis: Mosby.)

● = *non-urgent referral*

4. Usually develops on sun-exposed skin in middle-aged, fair-skinned people with significant outdoor exposure

5. Does not usually metastasize, but has an increased rate of recurrence, especially in nasolabial folds and preauricular areas

B. Treatment

1. Any nonhealing lesion should be biopsied.

2. Remove superficial lesions with

   (a) Cryotherapy or shave excision

   (b) Imiquimod 5% and apply once daily 5 days/wk; leave on for 8 hr, then wash off; maximum use up to 16 wk; apply 1 cm outside margin of lesion

C. *Referral to dermatologist*

   1. *The lesion appears deep with poorly defined edges.*

   2. *Facial lesions of any significant size.*

   3. *Located in an area of high recurrence (mask area of face, genitalia, hands, and feet).*

   4. *Recurrent after treatment/removal.*

II. Melanoma

A. Description: not all lesions appear the same; lesions may be found in obscure areas (thorax) or hard to see areas (posterior arms, legs or buttocks) (see Fig. 5.28). Use the following mnemonic for identifying abnormal skin lesions:

A = Asymmetry, such as a lumpy, bump-on-bump appearance

B = Border irregularity, such as a scalloped, cauliflower, or spreading pattern

C = Color variation, such as two or more colors present in the lesion (e.g., red, white, blue, brown, or black)

D = Diameter ≥6 mm (approximately the size of a pencil eraser)

E = Evolving/elevating lesion that was previously flat, change in texture, dimpling, or itching; growth either vertically (indicated by puckering of the surrounding skin [poor prognosis]) or horizontally

B. Risk factors

1. Family history of numerous nevi, prominent, irregular moles, or past melanomas

2. Recurrent personal history of melanoma with or without treatment

3. Previous sun exposure

4. Changes noted in moles

5. Family history of pancreatic cancer or astrocytomas

▲ C. *Treatment is urgent referral to a dermatologist or surgeon.*

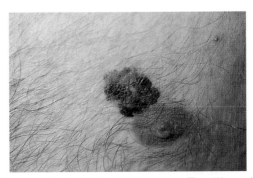

Fig. 5.28 Malignant melanoma on the chest of an adolescent male. (From Weston, W. L., Lane, A. T., & Morelli, J. G. (2002). *Color textbook of pediatric dermatology* (3rd ed.). St. Louis: Mosby.)

● = *non-urgent referral;* ▲ = *urgent referral*

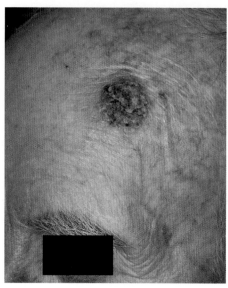

Fig. 5.29 Squamous cell carcinoma. Malignant degeneration occurred in an actinic keratosis that had been present for years. (From Habif, T. P. (1996). *Clinical dermatology: A color guide to diagnosis and therapy* (3rd ed.). St. Louis: Mosby.)

   III. Squamous cell carcinoma (SCC)
     A. Description
       1. Nonhealing lesions that are slightly raised with scaling, having irregularly shaped, sharply demarcated raised borders (see Fig. 5.29)
         (a) May be ulcerated, with a crust in the center on a firm, moveable base
         (b) Usually found at the base of actinic keratosis
         (c) Diameter varies
       2. Found mainly on sun-exposed areas such as head, neck, forearms and back of hand.
       3. More aggressive than BCC and can metastasize into surrounding areas.
     B. ***Referral to a dermatologist or surgeon for biopsy and treatment.***

SKIN TAGS

   I. Description
     A. Flesh-colored, soft, and pliable papilloma with a stalk; occurs anywhere on the body, but mostly in intertriginous areas.
     B. Varying sizes; small at the base (<1 mm up to 10 mm).
     C. Causes cosmetic disfigurement and discomfort at the site because of friction; is not usually malignant.
   II. Treatment
     A. Remove by snipping off with a sharp scalpel or scissors, cryotherapy, or punch biopsy; if excising, use a pressure dressing for 24 hr (if possible); these lesions are quite vascular.
     B. Send to pathology if indicated.

● = *non-urgent referral*

Wound Care

ABRASIONS, SCRATCHES, SKIN TEARS

   I. Clean the area thoroughly with soap and water.
   II. Keep covered with a clean, dry bandage during the day and while working; may remove at night.
   III. Consider using OTC or prescription antibiotic ointments or petroleum jelly to prevent sticking; do not use triple antibiotic ointment (Neosporin) ointments, as this can oftentimes cause tissue irritation.
   IV. May need to use a butterfly dressing for a small, superficial laceration to hold the edges together.
   V. May use Dermabond with a simple, clean laceration that is easily approximated.
   VI. Skin tears usually occur in the elderly and are found on extremities
      A. After injury, control bleeding with pressure; clean the area gently with soap and water.
      B. Approximate the flap edge with the outer edge of wound by using moistened Q-tip or gloved finger
         1. If appropriate, can use Steri-strips or butterfly closure to help maintain wound flap edges.
         2. If unable to approximate edges, use nonstick dressing and bandage.
      C. Outer dressing cover can be either gauze dressing or stockinette to cover extremity.
      D. Dressing should be left in place for 2–4 days and monitored closely for infection.
      E. ***Caution should be used in removing dressing to ensure the wound edge is not peeled away from outer edge (i.e., remove dressing in the direction the tear occurred; this could be noted by marking with an arrow on dressing).***
      F. Follow-up should be based on size of wound and patient's risk of infection.
      G. Flap may deteriorate at the outer edges and may darken in color, debride if necessary.
   VII. Ask about tetanus prophylaxis (see Table 5.5).

BITES

   I. Domestic Animal
      A. Guidelines
         1. Bites are usually related to cats or dogs.
         2. ***Referral to ED any child with facial or scalp wounds.***
         3. Infection risk is highest on hands or with puncture wounds and crush injuries.
      B. Treatment
         1. Tetanus prophylaxis (see Table 5.5).
         2. Anesthetize the wound and cleanse thoroughly with copious amounts of antibacterial soap (e.g., dilute 1:10 solution of betadine:saline), ***except for facial wounds; refer to ED or plastic surgeon for cleansing and repair.***
         3. If the wound is >8 hr old, consider culture of the wound site.
         4. Debride the devitalized or necrotic tissue—***except on the face.***
         5. Use mupirocin ointment and bandage with a clean dressing daily; wound closure is not recommended for puncture wounds, simple lacerations can be closed if <12 hr old.
         6. Splinting of the extremity may aid in healing.

■ = *not to be missed;* ▲ = *urgent referral*

Drug	Pediatric Dose	Adult Dose
Amoxicillin/Clavulanate *This is drug of choice.*	22.5 mg/kg/dose bid (maximum 875 mg)	875/125 mg q12h
Penicillin V	12.5 mg/kg/dose qid (maximum 500 mg)	500 mg qid
Cefuroxime *preferred if PCN allergic*	10–15 mg/kg/dose bid (maximum 500 mg)	500 mg bid
Clindamycin	10 mg/kg/dose ÷ q8h (maximum 450 mg)	450 mg tid
TMP-SMX *preferred if PCN allergic*	4–6 mg/kg/dose bid (maximum 160 mg TMP dose)	160/800 mg bid
Ciprofloxacin	Not recommended	500–750 mg bid
Levofloxacin	Not recommended	750 mg daily
Doxycycline	<45 kg: 1–2 mg/kg bid (maximum 100 mg/dose) >45 kg: adult dose	100 mg bid

     7. Systemic antibiotics for 3–5 days prophylactically; 5–14 days for infection.
     8. Follow the state laws for reporting animal bites.
     9. Follow up in the office in 24 hr to evaluate the wound and refer if needed.
   C. **Referral to ED**
     1. *If infection in wound is present or wound not healing*
     2. *If there is no record of rabies vaccination for the offending animal or if the animal cannot be quarantined and the risk is high, rabies immune globulin (RIG) and vaccine may be needed.*
 II. Feral or Wild Animal Bites
   A. Primary concern is possible rabies
     1. Principal carriers of rabies: bats, foxes, ferrets, raccoons, skunks, coyote, cats/dogs
     2. Rarely carry rabies: squirrels, mice, rats, rabbits
   B. Signs and symptoms of rabies may not appear for up to 10 days; bat bites may go undetected because of the size of the bite area and the painless act of biting
     1. Initial symptoms include the following
       (a) H/A, jaw pain
       (b) Photophobia; dizziness
       (c) Numbness
       (d) Fever, nausea and vomiting (N/V)
     2. As the disease progresses, symptoms include changes in cognition and gait disturbances.
     3. Final stage of the disease is cardiovascular collapse.
   C. Treatment
     1. Tetanus prophylaxis (see Table 5.5).
     2. Individuals who have been attacked by wild animals carrying an increased risk of rabies should have postexposure prophylaxis; the animal should be tested, if possible.
     3. Wound care
       (a) *If wound is on face, refer to ED or plastic surgeon.*

● = *non-urgent referral;* ▲ = *urgent referral*

      (b) After anesthetizing the wound, thoroughly cleanse with gentle irrigation using copious amounts of sterile saline or dilute 1:10 betadine/saline solution (can prevent up to 90% of rabies transmission).

      (c) Debride the necrotic tissue—*except on the face.*

      (d) Wound closure is discouraged.

    4. Prophylactic antibiotics, the same as with dog bites (see previous section).

  D. Follow the state laws for reporting animal bites.

  E. ***Referral to ED for rabies treatment.***

III. Human Bites

  A. Clean thoroughly with soap and water, followed by gentle irrigation with normal saline or dilute 1:10 solution betadine/saline.

  B. Ask about tetanus prophylaxis (see Table 5.5).

  C. Oral antibiotics are given for 10 days:

Drug	*Pediatric Dose*	*Adult Dose*
Amoxicillin/ Clavulanate	<3 mo of age: 30 mg/kg/day ÷ q12h >3 mo of age: <40 kg: 25–45 mg/kg/ day ÷ q12h >3 mo of age: >40 kg: use adult dosing	500–875 mg q8–12h
Doxycycline	Not recommended	100 mg bid
Clindamycin	30–40 mg/kg/day ÷ q6h	300–450 mg q6h
Levaquin	Not recommended for children	750 mg daily for 3–5 days

  D. Use hot moist soaks or hot packs minimum of qid.

  E. Monitor for cellulitis; recheck in the office at least once within the first 24 hr regardless of the size of the bite.

  F. Do not suture human bites.

BURN CARE

  I. Superficial burns should be gently cleaned with cool water and plain soap

    A. Apply cool compress; should heal in 3–7 days.

    B. May try aloe gel (plain), aloe gel with Xylocaine, or aloe gel spray for pain relief.

  II. Second-degree burns usually blister; keep covered with a nonstick dressing and possibly silver sulfadiazine (Silvadene) and do not attempt to break open the blisters; change the dressing twice daily.

  III. Minor burns are painful; adult dose for acetaminophen 500–1000 mg tid or ibuprofen 400–800 mg tid

    A. Weight-directed dosing for acetaminophen

      1. Infants >3 mo of age up to adolescence: 10–15 mg/kg q4–6h as needed

      2. Do not exceed 5 doses or 75 mg/kg in 24 hr

    B. Weight-directed dosing for ibuprofen

      1. Infants >6 mo of age up to age 12 yr of age: 10 mg/kg/dose q6–8h as needed

      2. Maximum single dose 400 mg; maximum daily dose 40 mg/kg

  IV. Tar burns can cause deep tissue injuries because of continued burning until removal.

    A. Can try using mayonnaise or mineral oil to remove tar prior to treatment/transfer.

■ = *not to be missed;* ● = *non-urgent referral*

    B. These injuries are very painful and will require pain medications, (e.g., opioid, see Chapter 14, PHARMACOLOGICAL THERAPIES).

  V. Consider tetanus prophylaxis (Table 5.5)

▲ VI. *Referral the following burns to the burn center or ED:*

    A. *Circumferential burns; burns involving the face, chest, or neck; or burns in children with a poor and concerning history of injury or burn pattern*

    B. *Burns of a severity greater than second degree and/or involving the fascia and tendons, ligaments, or muscle*

    C. *Electrical or tar burns*

LACERATIONS (INCLUDING CLOSURE TECHNIQUES)

  I. Description

    A. Methods for primary closure of wounds within 8–12 hr of injury (except on the face and scalp) include sutures, Steri-Strips, staples, and Dermabond.

    B. Secondary closure/healing involves allowing the wound to close on its own; the wound must be cleansed *very well* and debrided if necessary; assess "dirty" wounds more frequently during the healing process; a Penrose drain can be placed to facilitate drainage.

  II. Use of anesthesia

    A. Before using a local anesthetic on the wound, drizzle/spray a small amount into the laceration to decrease some of the pain when infiltrating.

    B. No need to shave area, use lubricant or tape to hold hair away from laceration (shaving increases risk of infection); may need to trim hair in laceration area.

    C. Anesthetize the wound using the smallest needle possible (e.g., 27–30 gauge); inject slowly along the wound edges, not into the intact skin; inject each side of laceration with as few punctures as possible.

    D. Simple digital blocks work well for providing anesthesia in finger and toe wounds; advanced blocks can be used for larger extremity wounds and for facial wounds.

    E. *Never use an anesthetic with epinephrine in or on fingers, toes, ears, nose, penis, or any area with poor vascular supply.*

  III. Suture points to consider when repairing wounds (see Table 5.6)

    A. Before suturing lacerations that involve the extremities, assess for sensation, strength, and movement distal to injury.

    B. Assess the degree of wound tension by observing the wound edges; if the edges are close with minimal tension, a good cosmetic closure will result.

    C. If the edges are >5 mm apart, there is increased tension and the wound should be repaired in layers for best results.

    D. When removing a lesion, make the incision parallel to the skin tension lines (Langer lines); this will decrease scarring (gently pull the intact skin in different directions to see which way the natural line of the skin moves).

    E. To check wound thickness, use the stick end of the applicator and set into the injury; if it will not drop through the skin, consider partial thickness.

    F. After the wound is anesthetized, clean vigorously and irrigate profusely with saline or dilute betadine: saline solution 1:10 (the cleaner the wound, the less likely that infection will occur). *Do not suture highly contaminated wounds, human or animal bites, wounds older than 24 hr, or puncture wounds.*

■ = *not to be missed;* ▲ = *urgent referral*

TABLE 5.6 ■ Suture Points

Location	Suggested Suture Size		Suture Removal (Days)	
	Skin	Deep Absorbent	Adult	Child
Scalp	4–0, 5–0	4–0	6–7	5–6
Face or forehead	6–0	5–0	4–5	3–4
Eyebrow	5–0, 6–0	5–0	4–5	3–4
Lip, nose, or ear	6–0	5–0 (n/a for ear)	4–5	3–4
Trunk	4–0, 5–0	3–0	7–10	5–9

Arm or leg	4–0, 5–0	3–0	Joint spared: 7–10
			Joint (extensor
			  surface): 8–14
			Joint (flexor surface):
			  8–10
				Joint spared: 5–9
				Joint (extensor surface):
				  7–12
				Joint (flexor surface): 6–8

Hand	5–0	5–0	Dorsal: 7–9 Palm: 7–12	Dorsal: 5–7 Palm: 7–10
Plantar foot	3–0, 4–0	4–0	7–12	7–10

    IV. Alternate closures (e.g., Dermabond)

        A. Tissue adhesive

            1. Comparable with suture healing, cosmetic appearance, and infection rates.

            2. No local anesthesia or follow-up needed because adhesive peels off in about 10 days.

            3. Can only be used in low-tension skin areas (e.g., scalp) with good approximation of skin edges and clean wounds.

            4. Not to be used on jagged or contaminated wounds and in high-tension skin areas (e.g., over joints); not to be used in mouth, groin, or axilla.

        B. Skin staples

            1. Used to close linear wounds in non-cosmetic areas (e.g., posterior thorax, scalp) with good wound edge approximation.

            2. Easy to perform, quick to apply, but patient will need to return for removal.

            3. Can be removed on same time frame as sutures (see Table 5.6).

            4. Will need to keep wound line clean, dry, and covered (can use antibiotic ointment on wound line) until removed.

        C. Skin closure strips

            1. Easy to apply but will need adhesive (e.g., tincture of benzoin) to help secure strips.

            2. May be difficult to keep in place in high-tension areas.

            3. Will need to keep skin and tape clean, dry, and covered.

            4. Skin strips should come off on their own in about 5–7 days.

            5. Can place skin strips over laceration and then secure with tissue adhesive; will peel off in ~1wk or can be peeled off gently after wound healed.

    V. Post-wound care

        A. Wound care re-checks should be done in 24 hr for contaminated wounds, in 5–7 days for "clean" wounds, and before removing sutures.

        B. Instruct the patient to keep the wound dry and clean; if the dressing accidentally becomes wet, change the dressing immediately.

        C. Have the patient (or caregiver) gently clean the edges of the wound daily with a cotton swab saturated with peroxide to remove crusts (this will decrease scarring by facilitating the healing of wound edges).

    D. To decrease scarring, apply thin layer of antibiotic ointment (without Neosporin) or Vaseline daily to suture line.

    E. Caution the patient to return immediately if signs of infection occur, or in cases of the following
       1. Redness or red streaks progressing up an extremity
       2. Increasing pain or swelling
       3. Recurrent bleeding, skin line comes open, or change in color to the skin line or surrounding area
       4. Fever
       5. Trouble moving extremity

    F. For the following lacerations, use broad-spectrum oral antibiotics (see CELLULITIS/ERYSIPELAS earlier in this chapter)
       1. Traumatic injury and contamination
       2. Contaminated wounds with inadequate debridement
       3. Joint wounds
       4. Wounds >6–12 hr old
       5. Animal and human bites
       6. Compromised host

VI. Ask about tetanus prophylaxis (see Table 5.5).

PUNCH BIOPSY

    I. Can easily remove small skin lesions/tags and embedded ticks; can facilitate obtaining a sample for pathologic examination.

    II. After anesthetizing and prepping the skin, stretch the skin around the lesion 90 degrees to the proposed direction of the linear closure.

    III. Lightly depress the instrument over the lesion while turning it; remove the instrument and release skin tension.

    IV. Excise the cored-out lesion from the punch; the resulting incision should be an ellipse that can be easily sutured, if needed.

    V. Suture with respect to skin lines to decrease scar formation.

Things That Bite and Sting

MOSQUITO-BORNE DISEASES

    I. Malaria
      A. Description
        1. The disease is a major problem for world travelers.
        2. Symptoms usually occur 7–9 days after exposure.
      B. Signs and symptoms
        1. Cyclic fever and shaking chills after exposure
        2. H/A, cough, malaise, fatigue
        3. N/V/D, abdominal pain, splenomegaly, bloody diarrhea
        4. Muscle aches, back pain
        5. Jaundice, dark urine
        6. Tachycardia, tachypnea
      C. Diagnosis
        1. Diagnosis can be made from a history of recent visit to an endemic tropical area.

▲

    2. *Blood smear for Plasmodium species is confirmative; if positive, refer to an infectious disease specialist.*

  D. Prevention/prophylaxis

    1. Consult the CDC website (www.cdc.gov) for information on prevention according to the country of travel and any prophylactic treatment before traveling.

    2. Preventive treatment depends on the destination; medication should be started before traveling to endemic countries (may be 2 days to 2 wk prior to departure, depending on the medication).

    3. Use an insect repellant on all exposed skin areas whenever outdoors; use mosquito netting and avoid going outdoors between dusk and dawn.

II. West Nile virus (WNV)

  A. Description

    1. The disease is spreading throughout United States.

    2. The illness can be very mild, similar to "cold" symptoms lasting about 3–6 days, or can be very severe (lasting weeks), leading to death; incubation period is 3–14 days.

    3. Infection usually provides immunity from WNV.

  B. Signs and symptoms

    1. May include acute febrile illness followed by the following

      (a) Malaise, myalgia, anorexia with N/V

      (b) Headache, eye pain, conjunctivitis

      (c) Nonpruritic, papular rash on trunk, arms, and legs; lymphadenopathy

    2. May progress to severe neurological disease with encephalitis, ataxia, seizures, flaccid paralysis and neuritis.

  C. Treatment

    1. Diagnosis is based on positive IgM antibody to WNV in the serum or spinal fluid.

    2. Supportive treatment with antipyretics, analgesics, rest, and hydration.

    3. This is a reportable illness; notify the local health department.

  D. Prophylaxis

    1. Mosquito control by draining all standing water, cleaning out drains, and removing all items that might hold water.

    2. Wear long sleeves and long trousers with sleeve and cuff tucked into shoes.

    3. If going outdoors at night, use mosquito repellant with DEET for adults and children >2 yr of age or wear permethrin-impregnated clothing.

▲

  E. *Referral to ED with unresolving respiratory infection or no response to treatment in 24 hr.*

III. Zika virus

  A. Description

    1. Mosquito-borne disease similar to dengue virus, yellow fever virus, and WNV, found worldwide and in the United States.

    2. Associated with birth deformity and neurological complications.

    3. Transmission occurs through

      (a) Bite of infected mosquito (primary route), during the day or at dusk

      (b) Maternal-fetal transmission

      (c) Sex (vaginal, oral, and anal)

      (d) Blood product transfusion

      (e) Organ transplants

      (f) Laboratory exposure

▲ = *urgent referral*

      4. Onset of symptoms occurs between 2 and 14 days, and symptoms usually resolve after about 2–7 days; immunity is conferred after initial infection.

      5. Of importance is the possibility of intrauterine infection through vertical transmission during pregnancy. Infection is highest during the first and early second trimester.

  B. Signs and symptoms

    1. Low-grade fever, H/A, and eye pain

    2. Pruritic rash with erythematous macules and papules noted on face, palms, soles, extremities, and trunk

    3. Pain in smaller joints of hands and feet

    4. Nonpurulent conjunctivitis

    5. Significant life-threatening signs include

      (a) Guillain-Barré syndrome

      (b) Encephalitis

      (c) Changes in mental status

      (d) Transverse myelitis

      (e) With intrauterine infection, testing should include microcephaly for the fetus (i.e., microcephaly may not be present at birth and may occur up to the first year)

  C. Diagnosis

    1. Zika virus IgM blood testing, but will need to do secondary testing if positive to determine if this is recent infection or false-positive result.

    2. All pregnant women who have been to high-risk areas or with clinical symptoms should be tested for Zika, and the unborn baby should be tested with U/S for microcephaly.

  D. Treatment

    1. There is no treatment for Zika.

    2. Manage symptoms with rest, increase in fluid intake, and acetaminophen for fever or pain.

  E. Prevention

    1. Protection from mosquito bites with insect repellants.

    2. Full clothing coverage when outdoors.

    3. Decrease areas where free water stands (e.g., cans, old tires, buckets).

    4. To prevent transmission to partners, abstain from unprotected sexual intercourse

      (a) Men should wait at least 3 mo after symptoms resolve.

      (b) Women should wait for at least 8 wk after symptoms resolve.

      (c) If partner is pregnant, the couple should abstain from intercourse for entire pregnancy.

  F. *Referral to OB if pregnant.*

PARASITIC INFESTATION

  I. Bed bugs

  A. Description

    1. Number one urban pest; incidence has increased since the banning of DDT.

    2. Transmission occurs when bed bugs attach to personal belongings (e.g., luggage, clothing, furnishings) and travel to home or the next destination.

● = *non-urgent referral*

3. Bed bugs present a distinct odor of sweetness or musty/stale odor, and there may be small, dark blood stains on bedding (especially seams), pillows, and other furniture in the room.
4. Bed bugs are small, blood-sucking insects that hide during the day and come out at night. It is the saliva that causes the allergic response and may vary from person to person.
5. Bed bugs feed on humans but do not live on the skin, and at this time, there has been no known transmission of disease to humans.
6. Superficial skin infections may occur due to scratching of bites.

B. Signs and symptoms
1. The chief complaint is intense itching and mild skin inflammation with clustered lesions, which are usually found on the head, neck, and upper body, especially around the elastic portions of clothing.
2. Mild reactions include small, maculopapular erythematous lesions that appear in a curve or line at the feeding site and may appear up to 11 days after exposure; if not scratched, will resolve after ~1 wk.
3. Moderate-to-severe reaction includes wheals, diffuse urticaria, blood blisters; reaction continues as long as exposure remains; can have occasional systemic reaction with angioedema.
4. Insomnia (from itching)
5. Emotional distress secondary to thought of infestation

C. Treatment
1. Remove/destroy any infested items that cannot be properly cleaned.
2. Wash everything with soap and hot water (sustained temperature >49°C [120°F]); if items cannot be washed, place them in plastic bags and leave them outside in the sun or in a closed car during the day (the heat will kill the bugs).
3. For itching
   (a) Topical application of low-mid potency topical steroids (see Table 5.3), pramoxine liquid (OTC) or doxepin cream.
   (b) Oral antihistamines (e.g., hydroxyzine or diphenhydramine) can be used at night to decrease the "itch-scratch" cycle and help with sleeping.
4. If infection occurs (usually from scratching), use mupirocin ointment.
5. Whenever traveling
   (a) Examine your room furnishings and bed/mattress for any unusual stains along the mattress seams and pillow.
   (b) Do not put luggage on the floor or near the bed; put used clothing in sealed plastic bag for transport home.
   (c) When you get home, put all clothing in a hot dryer for at least 15 min.

II. Head lice (Pediculosis capitis)
A. Description
1. Common infestation by a small parasite called *Pediculus humanus capitis*.
2. Found worldwide; is most common in children 3–12 yr of age.
3. Transmission occurs when hats, combs, hairbrushes, and caps are shared; lice are spread through direct contact.
4. Resistance has been developing to standard medications used in the US; however most treatment failures are due to poor adherence to therapy or continued exposure to source.

B. Signs and symptoms
1. The adult louse is small, grayish in color, and very agile; it is approximately 3 mm long with six legs.

2. The scalp is the most commonly affected area, but can be found on eyelashes, eyebrows, and beard.
3. Louse eggs (nits) are most commonly found behind the ears, on the nape of the neck, and on the crown of the head; nits are usually located near the hair shaft and are usually of dark color; as the eggs hatch, the casing turns white and is easier to see.

C. Treatment
   1. Should always involve removing the nits; this can be time-consuming, and many caregivers will not take the time to remove all nits
     (a) Use bright light and several hair clips, and section off the hair for easier identification of nits.
     (b) Nit combs may miss nits but will remove actual lice—use q2–3d to decrease reinfestation.
     (c) Shaving the head is an easy treatment for boys, but not for girls.
   2. Head lice preparations should be applied based on the package instructions with recommendations
     (a) Do not use hair conditioner before using lice medications.
     (b) Rinse with warm water over sink to limit exposure to lice shampoo.
   3. Topical head lice preparations should be left on for 10 min
     (a) Permethrin 1% OTC cream rinse (e.g., Nix); can retreat in 9 days; approved for children ≥2 mo of age; least allergenic
     (b) Pyrethrin 0.3%/piperonyl butoxide 3%–4% OTC liquid, gel, or shampoo (e.g., Rid); can retreat in 9 days; approved for children ≥2 yr of age
     (c) Benzyl alcohol 5% (Ulesfia) lotion; can retreat in 7 days; approved for infants ≥6 mo of age
     (d) Spinosad topical suspension 0.9% (Natroba); can retreat in 7 days if live lice; approved for children ≥6 mo of age
     (e) Ivermectin lotion 0.5% (Sklice) *single application only*; approved for infants ≥6 mo of age
     (f) Malathion 0.5% lotion (e.g., Ovide); DO NOT use hair dryer, *allow hair to dry naturally (malathion is flammable) for 8 hr then wash out*; avoid getting in eyes; can retreat in 7–9 days; approved for children ≥6 yr of age
   4. Oral head lice medications for *resistant* head lice
     (a) TMP/SMX 10 mg/kg/day (based on TMP) bid for 10 days; works best if used with Nix shampoo; not FDA approved for lice
     (b) Ivermectin 200 mcg/kg (Stromectol) (off label) once and may be repeated in 10 days if needed; not approved for pregnancy
       (i) Children: 200 mcg/kg once and repeat in 10 days; approved for children weighing >15 kg
       (ii) Adult: 400 mcg/kg/day once and repeat in 7 days
   5. If there are still numerous live active lice after 8–12 hr, you may need to retreat with a different product; if there are a few live lice seen but they are more sluggish, do not retreat; comb out the live lice and all nits.
   6. Tea tree oil can be used daily and may eliminate live head lice; nits still have to be removed manually.
   7. Environmental cleaning must be started with other treatments
     (a) Wash/soak all head gear, combs, and bedding worn or slept on over the last 24–48 hr in hot water (130°F) and dry for 20 min on hot cycle in a dryer.
     (b) Store nonwashable items in a closed plastic bag for 2 wk.
     (c) Vacuum the floor and furniture where the person sat or lay; lice only survive about 48 hr off the scalp.

   (d) Avoid sharing head gear (e.g., hats, head bands, helmets).
   (e) Store hats and coats separately at home and school.
III. Scabies (*Sarcoptes scabiei*)
   A. Description: scabies is a skin infestation caused by a mite and is spread by close contact
   B. Signs and symptoms (can take up to 6 wk to develop reaction if person is naive to scabies)
      1. Intense nocturnal itching is the presenting symptom.
      2. Primary lesions are linear groupings of papules with burrows, but vesicular lesions without burrows may be present.
      3. In adults, mites are rarely found above the neck; in infants, these areas are not spared, and lesions also may be found on palms and soles.
      4. Burrows are common between the fingers, flexor areas of the wrist, penis, vulva, nipples, axilla, and buttocks; vesicles can be found on the sides of fingers.
   C. Pharmacological therapies for scabies control
      1. Permethrin 5% cream (Elimite)
         (a) For adults and pregnant women apply to the skin from the neck down, including soles of feet.
         (b) For infants ≥2 mo of age and the elderly, also apply to hairline, neck, scalp, and forehead.
         (c) Leave on for 8–14 hr, and then wash off.
         (d) May repeat once in 14 days.
      2. Ivermectin (off label)
         (a) Children 2 mo of age or ≥15 kg: 200 mcg/kg/dose once and repeat in 14 days
         (b) Adults: 200 mcg/kg/dose once and repeat in 14 days
         (c) ***Not approved for pregnant women.***
      3. Avoid direct physical contact with others for 8 hr after treatment.
   D. Pharmacological therapies for pruritus (which may continue even after treatment because of increased sensitivity to dead mites and mite byproducts)
      1. Oral antihistamines (e.g., diphenhydramine, hydroxyzine)
      2. Pramoxine (OTC) lotion
      3. Medium to high potency topical steroid (see Table 5.3)
      4. Topical menthol base creams (e.g., Sarna)
   E. Oral or topical antibiotic if any infections occur (e.g., cephalexin, TMP-SXZ, mupirocin).
   F. Treat all close contacts and try to treat everyone at the same time; wash all linens and clothes in hot water (130°F) and dry on hot cycle in a dryer; for nonwashable items, store in a tightly closed plastic bag for 2 wk.
   G. If the skin has not healed and itching continues, consider retreatment.

SPIDER BITES

   I. Black widow
   A. Description: slightly aggressive spider; lives in dark, secluded places such as wood piles and barns (close, dark areas); majority of the bites occur in summer.
   B. Symptoms may not occur immediately after the bite, but the patient will complain of severe pain, burning, redness, and swelling at the site with muscle pain and spasm near bite, possibly followed by more severe symptoms within 1–12 hr
      1. H/A, dizziness

▨ = *not to be missed*

    2. Itching with rash that can be localized to the bite location or spread into the region of the bite

    3. Restlessness, anxiety, and sweating or tachycardia

    4. Dysautonomia symptoms (i.e., eyelid edema, ptosis, HTN, salivation, weakness, N/V)

    5. Intractable pain with rigid muscles in the abdomen, back, and chest

    6. Muscle tremor, fasciculations, and cramping in major muscle groups

    7. Symptoms can last from a few hours to a few days from the time of the bite

C. Treatment

    1. Treatment is usually supportive with local wound care.

    2. Tetanus prophylaxis if indicated (see Table 5.5).

    3. Application of ice to the bite area.

    4. Significant analgesia along with benzodiazepines and muscle relaxants may be needed to relieve anxiety and control pain with moderate-to-severe symptoms.

▲   D. ***Referral to ED with life-threatening symptoms or with intractable pain.***

II. Brown recluse

A. Description: not an aggressive spider; likes dark, little-used areas; bites usually occur when the spider is caught in clothing or bed linens

B. Signs and symptoms

    1. Within 1–24 hr after the bite, which is usually painless, the patient complains of "pin-pricking" sensation followed by irritation, itching, redness, and a small white blister.

    2. After 24 hr, the site of bite turns deep blue-purple, surrounded by a white ring and a large outer ring; may be raised or bullous; will be painful.

    3. After 48–72 hr, the site will develop ulceration in the center, which often gradually enlarges and sloughs.

    4. May experience H/A, body aches, rash, fever, and N/V.

    5. Wounds are commonly found on upper arms, thorax, or inner thighs and are usually worse if they occur in highly adipose tissue.

C. Treatment

    1. Cleanse the area thoroughly.

    2. Apply ice packs.

    3. Use NSAIDs or acetaminophen for pain.

    4. Tetanus prophylaxis if indicated (see Table 5.5).

    5. Antihistamine for any itching.

    6. Wound care

       (a) Conservative wound care; there is no specific treatment for bite wound; not all bites progress to tissue sloughing.

       (b) ***Referral to a surgeon or wound care provider if the lesion is enlarging, sloughing, and necrotic.***

       (c) Antibiotics, either systemic and/or topical, may be needed if secondary infection occurs.

    7. Ineffective therapies (no proven benefits)

       (a) Dapsone has been tried to slow the sloughing process.

       (b) Nitroglycerin patch has been tried to increase circulation to the ulcer by applying over the wound.

       (c) Steroid injections into the site have been tried with little success.

● = *non-urgent referral;* ▲ = *urgent referral*

STINGING INJURIES

I. Bee stings (hymenoptera)
  A. Description
  1. Non-Africanized bees sting only once and never in swarms.
  2. Africanized bees can sting multiple times and in swarms.
  3. Venom is protein-based and has a high risk for causing allergic reactions that can be lethal in sensitive people.
  B. Signs and symptoms (there is no correlation between the number of stings and allergic reaction)
  1. Local reactions: pain at the site with redness, edema, and pruritus
  2. Systemic reactions: pain at the site with N/V, syncope, wheezing, H/A, seizures, hypotension, muscle spasms, cardiopulmonary arrest
  3. Can have delayed serum sickness 10 days after being stung
  C. Treatment
  1. Local treatment involves removing the stinger, if possible, by scraping with a card or similar object.
  2. Apply ice to the area.
  3. Use OTC antihistamines (e.g., diphenhydramine) and NSAIDs routinely q6h for the first 24 hr.
  4. Try low-to-medium potency topical steroids to area for pruritus and pain (see Table 5.3).
  5. If the patient has a more severe reaction, consider using epinephrine 1:1000 solution, 0.1–0.5 mL SQ (or EpiPen); consider corticosteroid IM (e.g., dexamethasone 8 mg).
  ▲ 6. *Transfer to ED if the symptoms are not resolving quickly or if respiratory distress has occurred.*
  D. Prophylaxis: prescribe EpiPen and encourage the patient to obtain a Medic Alert bracelet
II. Fire ant stings
  A. Description
  1. An aggressive ant that resides in southern states, lives in underground burrows, and will swarm victims if the anthill is threatened; each ant can sting numerous times.
  2. The site of sting is immediately painful with a burning sensation, followed by development of a vesicle that will progress to a pustule and can cause tissue necrosis and superficial scarring.
  3. Extreme pruritus follows.
  4. Generally localized symptoms with multiple stings; systemic reactions may be seen; stings are more severe in young children.
  B. Treatment
  ▲ 1. *Monitor for severe systemic allergic reactions and transfer to ED if present (may need EpiPen treatment before transfer) or if patient is a child.*
  2. Immediate application of a moistened meat tenderizer to the bite may decrease local reaction.
  3. Supportive treatment with ice and elevation of the extremity
  4. Pharmacological therapy may be needed to decrease pruritus and pain
    (a) Topical antihistamine (e.g., pramoxine OTC) and low to medium potency topical steroids (see Table 5.3).
    (b) Oral antihistamines (e.g., diphenhydramine, cetirizine) with doxepin cream or high potency topical steroids (see Table 5.3) for more severe stings.

▲ = *urgent referral*

(c) May need a brief course of high dose oral prednisone (see PRACTICE PEARLS FOR STEROIDS).

5. Monitor for infection at the site(s) and treat with oral antibiotics.

C. Prevention

1. Wear shoes and avoid anthills or regions where ants are commonly found; monitor young children closely.
2. To keep anthills away from the house, use approved chemicals to dispense on lawns or in fire ant hills.

TICK-BORNE DISEASES

I. Alpha-gal (Galactose-alpha-1,3 galactose) allergy
  A. Description
    1. IgE allergy (delayed reactions) acquired from tick bite by Lone Star tick.
    2. Delayed anaphylaxis, of varying intensity can occur after
      (a) Eating mammalian meats or meat products, including milk and milk products; rarely occurs after ingestion of poultry or fish
      (b) Intake of gelatins in foods, candies, OTC supplements
      (c) Exposure to some medical products (e.g., vaccines, heart valves)
  B. Signs and symptoms
    1. Sneezing, rhinorrhea, H/A.
    2. Reactions involve hives, angioedema, N/V/D, and asthma-like symptoms.
    3. Reactions can be delayed up to 6 hr after ingestion.
  C. Diagnostic testing: can request IgE test (i.e., IgE anti-alpha-gal antibody) or can send for skin testing
  D. Treatment
    1. *If true anaphylaxis, emergent referral to ED; use EpiPen at first sign of allergic reaction.*
    2. Avoid mammalian meats or milk or other triggering products.
    3. Reaction may go away with time (especially if original reaction was mild) but may recur with repeated exposure.
II. Ehrlichiosis
  A. Description
    1. Caused by the Lone Star tick found mainly in the Southeastern and South-Central United States.
    2. Tick bites frequently occur from May to August, and transmission occurs immediately after the bite.
    3. Signs and symptoms occur within 7–14 days of exposure
      (a) At onset, the symptoms include fever, chills, H/A, myalgia, and malaise.
      (b) Later, N/V, anorexia, and weight loss occur.
      (c) Petechial, maculopapular rash (not pruritic) and edema in the hands and feet are more common in children.
      (d) Adults are more likely to have cough, confusion, and lymphadenopathy.
    4. Can progress to renal failure, meningoencephalitis, coagulopathy, GI hemorrhage, and pulmonary complications.
  B. Laboratory values
    1. Thrombocytopenia (50,000/µL to 140,000/µL, but can be <20,000/µL)
    2. Mild-to-moderate leukopenia (neutropenia and lymphopenia)

▲ = *urgent referral*

3. Elevated liver enzymes, alkaline phosphatase
4. Peripheral blood smear for *Ehrlichia* serial immunofluorescent antibody (IFA) IgG taken initially and then 2–4 wk later

C. Treatment
1. Diagnosis is based on suspicion of the disease, history of tick bites, fever and leukopenia; antibiotics should not be delayed for blood smear or antibody results.
2. *Ehrlichia* organisms are resistant to most antibiotics, and therapy is limited to doxycycline bid for 7–14 days
(a) Children: 2.2 mg/kg/day ÷ q12h; maximum 100 mg/dose
(b) Adult: 100 mg bid
3. Supportive treatment for other symptoms.

▲ **D. Referral to ED with significant symptoms.**

III. Lyme disease
A. Description
1. Caused by *Borrelia burgdorferi* carried by black legged ticks (*Ixodes scapularis* and *pacificus*).
2. Occurs more often in late spring and summer months primarily in the Northeastern, upper Midwestern, and along the Pacific coast of the United States.
3. There is increased risk of transmission if the tick is attached for >24 hr.

B. Signs and symptoms (may not appear for 30 days)
1. *Early localized symptoms*
(a) Erythema migrans (rash may appear 3–30 days later, at bite site)
(b) Fever, malaise, myalgia
(c) Lymphadenopathy and H/A
2. *Early disseminated*
(a) Multiple erythema migrans
(b) Bell palsy (common cause of facial palsy in children)
(c) Asymptomatic first-degree atrioventricular (AV) block
(d) Meningitis
3. *Late symptoms* are the same as those for early localized symptoms plus the following
(a) Acrodermatitis chronica atrophicans on distal extremities (e.g., dorsum hand and heels, knees, and elbows)
(b) Severe fatigue, sleep disorders, and confusion
(c) Paralysis and cranial nerve defects
(d) Short-term memory disruption
(e) Migratory arthritis (e.g., knee and TMJ)

C. Diagnostic testing (diagnosis is difficult because of unreliable testing)
1. Recommended two-step testing
(a) Enzyme-linked immunosorbent assay (ELISA)
(b) If positive or equivocal and symptoms <30 days, then Western immunoblot test IgM and IgG; if symptoms >30 days, IgG only for confirmation
2. CBC (for leukopenia or thrombocytopenia, which indicates coinfection)
3. Liver function test (AST may be elevated)
4. ESR/CRP (may be elevated)
5. Urinalysis for microscopic hematuria or proteinuria
6. Electrocardiogram (ECG) to check for heart block

D. Treatment
1. Supportive care with rest, hydration, and NSAIDs for pain.
2. Early intervention with oral antibiotics for prophylaxis or treatment when erythema migrans is present, may prevent later adverse effects.

▲ = *urgent referral*

Drug	Pediatric Dose	Adult Dose
Doxycycline	Prophylaxis: 4.4 mg/kg once Treatment: 2.2 mg/kg/ dose ÷ q12h × 10 days	Prophylaxis: 200 mg once Treatment: 100 mg bid 10 days
Amoxicillin	50 mg/kg/day ÷ q8h × 14 days	500 mg tid 14 days
Cefuroxime	30 mg/kg/dose ÷ q12h × 14 days	500 mg bid 14 days
Azithromycin (not first line therapy)	10 mg/kg/day × 5–10 days	500 mg daily × 5–10 days

3. Can use macrolides if allergic to amoxicillin, doxycycline, or cefuroxime, but they are less effective, and patients should be closely monitored for resolution of symptoms.
4. ***Referral to an infectious disease specialist for more severe symptoms.***

IV. Rocky Mountain spotted fever (RMSF)
  A. Description
    1. Caused by *Rickettsia* bacteria from Rocky Mountain wood tick and the American dog tick.
    2. Infection found predominantly in Southeast and Midwest United States and commonly occurs from April to September.
    3. Transmission occurs within hours of the bite, and symptoms occur within 2–14 days
      (a) Symptoms occur suddenly with fever, H/A, and rash (classic triad); may also have N/V, abdominal pain, and myalgia.
      (b) Initially, a blanching pink macular rash appears on the ankles, wrists, and forearms; the rash then becomes maculopapular and spreads to the trunk; rash may occur 2–4 days after fever.
      (c) Later symptoms include: altered mental status, respiratory distress, renal failure
  B. Diagnostic testing
    1. Always ask about travel history and tick exposure.
    2. Diagnosis relies on heightened suspicion, predominance of endemic area, and season of the year.
    3. CBC may show a normal or low leukocyte count with a left shift, decreased RBCs, decreased platelets; CMP may show hyponatremia and elevated liver enzymes.
▲   C. ***Referral to ED if RMSF is suspected.***

● = *non-urgent referral;* ▲ = *urgent referral*

CHAPTER 6

Eye, Ear, Nose, and Throat Conditions

For details regarding complete history and physical examination, see Chapters 1 and 2.

Common Eye Conditions

- General eye examination
  - Record visual acuity in the right and left eyes and both eyes together, and ask the patient if vision has been affected (see Chapter 1, **EYES**, III).
  - Determine the amount of inflammation: look at the eyes. Where is the redness in relation to the pupil? Is it localized or diffuse? Is it symmetrical or asymmetrical in one or both eyes? Are the eyelids swollen?
  - Check pupils' responses for equality and reactivity to light and accommodation (PERRLA) and assess peripheral vision; failure of the pupils to react appropriately or loss of peripheral vision indicates a more serious problem (see Tables 1.1 and 1.2).
- Recommended preventative eye examinations
  - Children at risk: annual exam
    - Premature or low birth weight with known O_2 supplementation
    - Strabismus, nystagmus
    - Known developmental delay, CP, hydrocephalus, seizures, etc.
  - Children without risk
    - Birth to 24 mo of age: at 6 mo of age or as recommended
    - 2–5 yr of age: average 3 yr of age
    - 6–18 yr of age: every 2 yr if indicated
  - Adults at high risk: annual exam
    - DM with/without known retinopathy (examinations may be more frequent with progressing disease)
    - Any patient receiving chronic steroids, chemotherapy, or biologic agent treatments
    - Use of any medications with ocular side effects (e.g., quetiapine)
    - Working in occupations that are visually hazardous
  - Adults without risk
    - 18–60 yr of age: approximately q3–5yr
    - >61 yr of age: approximately q1–2yr
- When instilling eye drops, place drop(s) into the inner canthus while eye is closed and head slightly tilted to outside, then have patient "open" eye(s) and drop(s) will automatically "run" into eye. This is an easy and "nonscary" way to instill drop(s).
  - Ointment is preferred over drops for children.
  - Drops are preferred for adults, unless only hs instillation.
  - Fluoroquinolone drops are preferred when treating abrasions in contact users.
- Fluorescein staining is used to detect injuries to the surface of the cornea (e.g., abrasion, foreign body). This is done easily with minimal discomfort and is a good tool for determining further care and/or referral for care.
  - Make sure patient is not wearing contact lens.

Continued

PRACTICE PEARLS FOR EYES—CONT'D

- Instill 1–2 gtts of local anesthetic. *Do not let patient touch eyes for the next 60 min*: this can injure the cornea because the corneal reflex is now absent. If anesthetic eye drops give immediate relief, the problem is most likely caused by surface pain; if pain remains, the pain is most likely deep in the eye itself (more serious).
- Put a drop of saline on a fluorescein paper and touch the paper to the inner, lower eyelid. The conjunctiva will turn orange immediately (if it does not, remoisten the fluorescein strip). Have the patient open and close the eye(s) a few times.
- Using a cobalt blue pen light, inspect the cornea and under the eyelids (see Fig. 1.1, Eyelid Eversion Technique); if there is an injury or foreign object (FO), the dye will enhance the area. Possible findings:
    - "Ice rink sign": scratches on the cornea from blinking due to FO in the upper eyelid
    - Dendrite appearance: possibly herpes zoster or other virus
    - Abrasions seen at the 3 and 9 o'clock positions on the cornea are common with contact lens wearers.
    - Isolated dots across the cornea from poorly fitted contact lenses or dry eyes
    - Lesion located in the central vision (over the pupil) will decrease visual acuity and depth perception (may not be seen with dye but patient will report this during exam).
- After examination, irrigate the eye(s) with saline solution until clear and reevaluate in same manner; injury or FO will be seen.
- If abrasion is noted, refer to section on corneal abrasion in this chapter.
- Remind patient not to touch eye if anesthetic drop(s) are used and may need to place an eye patch for *short-term* use if concern for touching is present.
    - Explain to patient that orange drainage may be present after "blowing nose" for the next hour. This is due to dye running down tear ducts.
    - Anesthetic eye drops are for examination purposes only and not for continued pain relief; *do not* send home with patient.
- Eversion of upper eyelid (see Fig. 1.1) is an important tool for inspecting under the upper lids for injury, FO, or swelling.
- *Retinal artery occlusion*
    - Sudden, painless, total (or near total) loss of vision in one eye
    - Retina is pale and edematous with a central macular cherry-red spot.
    - Have the patient breathe into a paper bag (CO_2 retention causes vasodilation) and **refer immediately to ED or ophthalmologist.**
- *Ophthalmologist referral*
    - **Urgent with acute onset eye pain, diminished visual acuity, and photophobia**
    - **Nonurgent referral with chronic conditions such as red eyes and scratchy feelings that are not controlled with current medications**

CATARACTS

   I. Description

      A. Caused from clouding of the lens secondary to DM, age, or chronic prednisone use

      B. Signs and symptoms

         1. Subtle progressive changes in visual acuity and dimming of color spectrum

         2. Increasing nearsightedness

         3. No pain or discharge, no redness to eye

         4. May have some dryness and increased tearing

■ = *not to be missed;* ▲ = *urgent referral;* ● = *non-urgent referral*

5. Halos noted around lights at night
6. Decreased ability to see internal structures of eye with ophthalmoscope and background of eye has a "spider web" appearance
C. Treatment is *referral to ophthalmologist for further evaluation and surgical options*

CONJUNCTIVITIS

I. Allergic conjunctivitis
  A. Signs and symptoms (bilateral; if unilateral investigate for another cause)
    1. Itching, grittiness, redness, and watery discharge
    2. Varying levels of conjunctival edema (chemosis), eyelid swelling
    3. May have sneezing, rhinorrhea, "throat itching"
    4. May have history of eczema, atopic dermatitis, or seasonal allergies
  B. Nonpharmacological treatment
    1. Avoid allergens (triggers)
    2. Cold or warm compresses
    3. Artificial tears to decrease irritation
    4. Decrease contact use
  C. Pharmacological treatment
    1. OTC drops to relieve symptoms; avoid OTC allergy drops containing tetrahydrozoline, which may cause rebound injection
      (a) Ketoprofen (Zaditor): ≥3 yr of age: 1 gtt q8–12hr prn
      (b) Olopatadine ophthalmic 0.2% (Pataday): ≥2 yr of age: 1 gtt in eye(s) daily or 0.1% Patanol; ≥2 yr of age: 1 gtt in eye(s) bid
      (c) Naphazoline 0.25%–pheniramine 0.3% (Naphcon-A): ≥6 yr of age: 1–2 gtts up to 4 times a day
    2. Prescription drops
      (a) Nedocromil ophthalmic 2% (Alocril) solution: ≥3 yr of age: 1–2 gtts in eye(s) bid
      (b) Azelastine ophthalmic 0.05% (Optivar) solution: ≥3 yr of age: 1 gtt in eye(s) bid
      (c) Ketorolac ophthalmic 0.5% (Acular) solution: ≥2 yr of age: 1 gtt in eye(s) qid
      (d) Cetirizine 0.24% (Zerviate) solution: ≥2 yr of age: 1 gtt eye(s) bid
  D. *Referral to ophthalmologist if not improving in 5–7 days*
II. Bacterial conjunctivitis
  A. Signs and symptoms (usually start unilateral and may progress to both eyes)
    1. Tearing, and redness, with a "gritty" or FO sensation; very little itching.
    2. No pain to eyeball and no vision loss, but may have blurring to vision that can be "blinked" away.
    3. Yellow-green *mucopurulent discharge* from the inner canthus that usually lasts all day; limbus is spared and conjunctiva is injected.
    4. If profuse purulent discharge with preauricular adenopathy, ask about sexual partners, as this could be a gonococcal infection and can progress to vision loss.
    5. Cornea is clear with mild eyelid swelling.
  B. Nonpharmacological treatment
    1. Cold compresses over eyes during the day; may need warm compresses in the morning to loosen the exudate.
    2. Artificial tears prn.

● = *non-urgent referral*

  3. Remove contacts (if wearing), until infection resolved then use new contact lens.

  4. This is quite contagious—recommend handwashing, separate towels, and avoid handshaking.

  5. Children attending daycare or school can return after 24 hr of treatment.

 C. Antibiotic treatment for 5–7 days

  1. Erythromycin 5 mg/g ophthalmic ointment: one-half inch in eye(s) qid

  2. Trimethoprim-polymyxin B 10,000 u/mL (Polytrim) ophthalmic drops: 1 gtt in eye(s) q3hr while awake

  3. Ofloxacin (Ocuflox) ophthalmic solution: 1–2 gtts in eye(s) qid (recommended for contact wearers)

  4. Ciprofloxacin (Ciloxan) ophthalmic drops: 1–2 gtts in eye(s) qid (recommended for contact wearers)

  5. Azithromycin 1% solution: 1 gtt bid for 2 days; then 1 gtt daily for 5 days

 D. ***Referral to ophthalmologist if considered herpetic infection or if not markedly better in 4 days, can cause permanent damage***

III. Viral conjunctivitis

 A. Signs and symptoms (unilateral and/or bilateral infection)

  1. Burning, itching, tearing (may cause some blurred vision, but resolves with blinking)

  2. Conjunctival injection (limbus *not* spared), "gritty" or "scratchy" feeling

  3. Watery, mucoid discharge with matting on eyelids/lashes usually in the morning

  4. May have preauricular lymph node enlargement

  5. Recent history of URI with fever

 B. Treatment

  1. Cold or warm compresses to eyes.

  2. Gently cleanse with water.

  3. Artificial tears to decrease irritation 1–2 times daily.

  4. Remove contacts immediately and when infection is resolved, use new contact lens.

  5. This is very contagious, recommend frequent handwashing, separate towels, and avoid handshaking; symptoms may last up to 2 wk.

  6. Children attending daycare or school cannot return until 24 hr after treatment, and child may not be allowed back in school until antibiotic eye drops are started (even though drops not indicated).

  7. Do not use vasoconstrictor eye drops (e.g., Visine), as this may cause rebound injection.

 C. ***Referral to ophthalmologist if suspected herpetic infection, or if symptoms worsen within 24 hr or continue past 7 days.***

CORNEAL INJURIES/ABNORMALITIES

 I. Corneal abrasion

  A. Commonly caused by trauma, foreign objects, or improper contact lens use

  B. Signs and symptoms

   1. Unilateral severe eye pain; patient may have a foreign object sensation.

   2. Photophobia and inability to easily open eye.

   3. Vision may be normal, decreased, or have "halo" effect.

   4. Contact lens wearers will commonly wear contacts to bed and awaken with pain when opening eye(s).

● = *non-urgent referral*

C. Examination
   1. Exam for FO and if no penetrating eye injury, instill 1–2 gtts of preferred anesthetic eye drops; relief should be immediate; if not, consider other diagnosis.
   2. Test for visual acuity and document.
   3. Fluorescein staining (see **PRACTICE PEARLS FOR EYES** earlier in this chapter) to detect abrasion, foreign object, or pus in the anterior chamber.
D. Treatment (uncomplicated abrasion, small, <4 mm abrasion)
   1. General recommendations
      (a) Ointments are preferred.
      (b) No steroid eye drops.
      (c) Avoid eye patches.
      (d) Continue medications for 24 hr after symptom resolution.
      (e) Do not resume wearing contacts until eye is completely healed.
   2. *Noncontact lens wearers* for 3–5 days; follow-up in 24 hr if symptoms continue
      (a) Erythromycin 0.5% (Ilotycin) ointment: one-half inch in eye(s) qid
      (b) Sulfacetamide 10% (Bleph-10) ointment: one-half inch in eye(s) qid
      (c) Sodium sulfacetamide (Bleph-10) solution: 1–3 gtts in eye(s) qid
   3. *Contact lens wearers* for 3–5 days; follow-up should be in 24 h
      (a) Ciprofloxacin 0.3% (Ciloxan) ointment: one-half inch in eye(s) qid
      (b) Ofloxacin 0.3% (Ocuflox) solution: 1 to 2 gtts in eye(s) qid
      (c) Tobramycin 0.3% ointment: one-half inch in eye(s) 2–3 times daily
   4. Oral NSAIDs (e.g., ibuprofen) or topical NSAIDs for 2–3 days as needed
      (a) Ketorolac 0.4% or 0.5% solution: 1 gtt 4 times a day
      (b) Diclofenac 0.1% solution: 1 gtt 4 times a day
E. *Urgent referral to ophthalmologist, or ED if unable to be seen that day if*
   1. *Corneal infiltrate or large abrasion*
   2. *Purulent discharge that is persistent*
   3. *Unable to open eye(s)*
   4. *Foreign body that cannot be removed or any type of globe puncture wound*
   5. *Decreased vision or no vision*
   6. *Corneal abrasion that does not heal within 3 days*

II. Pinguecula
   A. Caused by sun exposure/damage or chronic dry eyes and with advancing age
   B. Small yellowish growth/elevation seen near the inner or outer margins of the cornea on the nasal side
   C. Treated with topical ophthalmic NSAIDs (e.g., ketorolac) and artificial tears
   D. *Referral to ophthalmologist if vision is affected*

III. Pterygium
   A. Signs and symptoms
      1. Clear to flesh-colored, thin tissue growth that can extend over the cornea and impair vision
      2. Commonly seen at the inner side of eyeball
      3. Can cause irritation (sensation of foreign object in eye) and can be swollen and red
   B. Treatment
      1. Treat with natural tears frequently
      2. If inflamed, can use ketorolac ophthalmic (Acular) 1 gtt qid for 5 days
   C. *Referral to ophthalmologist if vision is impaired*

■ = *not to be missed;* ● = *non-urgent referral;* ▲ = *urgent referral*

IV. Subconjunctival hemorrhage (collection of blood occurring under the conjunctiva but not into iris/pupil)

  A. Caused by trauma, excessive straining (Valsalva) with vomiting or coughing, HTN, or rubbing of eyes; can also be seen with asphyxiation

  B. Signs and symptoms
   1. May have felt a mild "stinging" sensation when it occurred
   2. No change in visual acuity and no foreign sensation
   3. No photophobia

  C. Treatment
   1. Rule out HTN, trauma, or bleeding disorders, and treat if needed.
   2. No treatment needed, reassure that it should resolve in approximately 2 wk.
   3. Use artificial tears frequently.
   4. No rubbing
   5. Treat presumed cause, if cough or vomiting.
   6. Limit use of ASA or NSAIDs until resolution.

  D. *Referral to ophthalmologist if no resolution in 2 wk or if there is a vision disturbance.*

EYELID ABNORMALITIES

  I. Blepharitis: inflammation of the inner portion of eyelid margin or base of eyelashes, which can be acute or chronic

  A. Causes
   1. Inflammatory skin disorders
    (a) Eczema, psoriasis
    (b) Rosacea, seborrheic dermatitis
   2. Infection
    (a) *Staphylococcus aureus*
    (b) Parasitic (e.g., *Demodex* species)
   3. Irritants or allergens
    (a) Contact lens wearer
    (b) Smoke exposure
    (c) Contact dermatitis
   4. Medications
    (a) Retinoids (e.g., isotretinoin)
    (b) Chemotherapeutics (e.g., 5-FU)

  B. Signs and symptoms
   1. Redness, itching, and irritation to eyelids which cause gritty feeling to eye
   2. Pink eyes with excessive tearing
   3. Crusting or matting of eyelashes in the morning (does not recur during day)
   4. Blurred vision (can be blinked away) with minimal light sensitivity
   5. Oily white plugs at Meibomian gland openings
   6. "Sleeves" on eyelashes that resemble dandruff; this may be mites

  C. Nonpharmacological treatment for mild symptoms
   1. Warm moist compresses 1–2 times daily.
   2. Daily lid massage followed by washing with baby shampoo; include the bases of lashes, and rinse off after a few min.
   3. Artificial tears prn.

● = *non-urgent referral*

4. Tea tree oil eyelid scrubs or tea tree shampoo used to cleanse eyelids/lashes if suspect parasitic infection.
5. Eliminate allergic triggers (e.g., cigarette smoke, contact lens, cosmetics).
6. *Daily* eyelid hygiene even after treatment.
D. Pharmacological treatment if nonpharmacological treatment fails
   1. Mild to moderate infection (topical)
      (a) Erythromycin ointment (Ilotycin) one-half inch to eyelid(s) hs for 1–2 wk
      (b) Bacitracin ointment one-half inch to eyelid(s) at hs for 1–2 wk
      (c) Azithromycin ophthalmic (AzaSite) 1 gtt eye(s) bid for 10–14 days
   2. Moderate to severe blepharitis infection, if unresponsive to topical therapy
      (a) Doxycycline 100 mg bid for ~ 2–4 wk
      (b) Azithromycin 500 mg daily for 3 days or 500 mg day 1, then 250 mg daily for 4 days
      (c) Ivermectin 200 mcg/kg once and repeat in 7 days (if suspect parasitic infection)
E. *Referral criteria for ophthalmologist*
   1. *Severe eye redness and pain*
   2. *Light sensitivity and/or impaired vision*
   3. *Poor response to treatment*

II. Hordeolum (Stye)
A. Types
   1. Acute inflammation/abscess of Meibomian gland (*internal inflammation*)
   2. Acute inflammation/abscess on eyelash follicle or tear gland at eyelid (*external infection*)
B. Signs and symptoms (unilateral)
   1. Localized area of redness that is raised and painful on conjunctival side of eyelid below the lash line (abscess) or noted as a plug on outer lower lid (not abscess).
   2. Usually self-limited and resolves in 5–7 days.
C. Treatment
   1. Warm, moist compresses followed by gentle compression on hordeolum qid.
   2. Gently remove any eyelid debris.
   3. Topical antibiotics may not improve outcomes.
D. Chronic hordeolum (aka Chalazion)
   1. Chronic inflammatory lesion from Meibomian tear gland obstruction that can result in cancerous lesion.
   2. Lesion evolves into painless, rubbery nodule on inside of eyelid margin (e.g., usually lower lid) with continued mild erythema and eyelid swelling.
   3. Treatment is same as hordeolum and antibiotics are not required because this is not an infection.
E. *Referral to ophthalmologist if*
   1. *Poor response to treatment and affects QOL*
   2. *Frequent hordeola*
   3. *History or presence of rosacea*
   4. *Hordeola hardens and becomes chalazion or suspect cancerous lesion*

III. Xanthelasma
A. Cause
   1. Lipoprotein abnormalities
   2. Primary biliary cholangitis
   3. Possible association with atherosclerosis

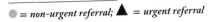

● *= non-urgent referral;* ▲ *= urgent referral*

   B. Signs and symptoms
1. Benign soft, yellow plaques that are cholesterol-filled
2. Appear on the medial aspects of the eyelids bilaterally
3. Seen mainly in elderly, but can occur in younger population

   C. Treatment
1. No treatment except for cosmetic reasons
2. Treat underlying lipid abnormality
3. Encourage healthy lifestyle

GLAUCOMA (ACUTE ANGLE-CLOSURE)

I. Due to narrowing or closure of anterior chamber angle that can lead to vision loss and increased intraocular pressure (IOP)
II. Predisposing factors
   A. Female, age >60 and FH of glaucoma
   B. Hyperopia
   C. Pseudoexfoliation
   D. Medications
      1. Stimulants, both oral and ophthalmic
      2. Anticonvulsants, antihistamines
      3. Diuretics
      4. TCAs, SSRIs, SNRIs
III. Signs and symptoms
   A. *Severe eye pain*
   B. *Decreased or loss of peripheral vision and visual acuity; halos around lights with photophobia*
   C. *Headache, N/V*
   D. *As intraocular pressure (IOP) ↑ may see conjunctival redness, pupil in fixed, midposition*
IV. Treatment is *immediate referral to ED or ophthalmologist*

IRITIS (UVEITIS)

I. Caused by inflammation of anterior uveal tract and ciliary body often involved
II. Signs and symptoms
   A. Ciliary flush (red ring around the iris) (see Fig. 6.1)
   B. Photophobia with aversion to penlight in both eyes
   C. *No sensation of foreign body*, no discharge and minimal tearing
III. Treatment is *immediate referral to ED or ophthalmologist*

PERIORBITAL CELLULITIS

I. Types
   A. Periorbital (AKA pre-septal): involves soft tissues in anterior portion of orbital septum, not involving other ocular structures
   B. Orbital: involves ocular muscle and fat in the orbit (more severe infection)
II. Signs and symptoms (usually unilateral)
   A. Periorbital
      1. Eyelid swelling with redness

■ = *not to be missed;* ▲ = *urgent referral*

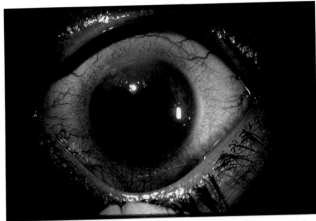

Fig. 6.1 Color, external photograph of left eye shows severe ciliary flush. (From Harpal, S., & Kaplan, H. (2019). *Clinical case in uveitis*. Philadelphia: Elsevier.)

    2. May have eye pain or tenderness

    3. May have fever and ↑ WBCs

  B. Orbital

    1. Eyelid swelling with or without redness

    2. Eye pain/tenderness with movement

    3. Proptosis, chemosis

    4. Vision impairment, ophthalmoplegia with diplopia

    5. Fever with increased WBCs

▲ C. *If patient has pain with eye movements, proptosis, vision impairment, and loss of eye muscle movement, this indicates possible orbital involvement; immediate referral to ED or ophthalmologist.*

III. Testing if there is a concern for orbital cellulitis

  A. Confirm with contrast enhanced CT of orbits and sinus areas

  B. CBC

IV. Treatment as O/P (if no systemic signs) for 5–7 days

  A. *Give one of the following* (also, see B below)

    1. Clindamycin

      (a) Children: 30–40 mg/kg/day ÷ tid

      (b) Adult: 300 mg q8hr

    2. TMP-SMX

      (a) Children: 8–12 mg/kg/day (trimethoprim) ÷ q12hr

      (b) Adults: DS 1–2 tab q12hr

  B. *Plus one of the following*

    1. Amoxicillin or amoxicillin/clavulanate

      (a) Children: 45 mg/kg/day ÷ q12hr

      (b) Adults: 875 mg q12hr

    2. Cefpodoxime

      (a) Children <12 yr of age: 10 mg/kg/day ÷ q12hr; >12 yr of age: use adult dose

      (b) Adults: 400 mg q12hr

▲ = *urgent referral*

   3. Cefdinir
     (a) Children: 14 mg/kg/d ÷ q12hr
     (b) Adults: 300 mg bid
  V. *Referral to ophthalmologist if not improving in 24–48 hr.*

TEAR DUCT ABNORMALITIES

I. Dacryostenosis: nasolacrimal duct obstruction in infants
  A. Signs and symptoms
    1. Persistent tearing (most common complaint)
    2. Debris on eye lashes
    3. No conjunctival redness, unless from rubbing
    4. May see enlargement of tear duct opening
    5. Gentle palpation may elicit tears or mucus into inner canthus.
  B. Treatment
    1. Gentle massage to inner canthus 2–3 times daily.
    2. Warm moist compresses.
  C. *Referral*
    1. *Usually resolves spontaneously within 2–3 mo; if not, referral to a pediatric ophthalmologist*
    2. *If any signs of infection (e.g., redness to conjunctiva or surrounding facial skin or fever), urgent referral to ED*
II. Dry eye syndrome
  A. Causes
    1. Allergens (e.g., smoke, dust, fans); cold and dry environments
    2. Disorders of tear ducts/glands
    3. Contact lens use
    4. Medications (e.g., antihistamines, diuretics, anti-Parkinson drugs, anticholinergics, some antiarrhythmics)
    5. Vitamin A deficiency
    6. Older adults
    7. Systemic diseases (e.g., DM, Parkinson, Sjögren)
  B. Signs and symptoms
    1. Symmetrical irritation, with redness and dryness
    2. Burning and foreign object sensation or gritty feeling
    3. Blurred vision that resolves with blinking
    4. Excessive tearing and blinking
    5. Light sensitivity
  C. Treatment
    1. Artificial tears (preservative free) 1 gtt qid
    2. Humidifier all year
    3. Warm moist compresses daily
    4. Elimination of allergens and treatment of known causes
    5. Consider oral flaxseed or omega-3 fatty acids daily
  D. *Referral to ophthalmologist if condition is not controlled and affecting quality of life (QOL)*

● = *non-urgent referral;* ▲ = *urgent referral*

Common ENT Conditions

PRACTICE PEARLS FOR ENT

- Aphthous ulcer treatments
  - Buccal: Kenalog in Orabase or compounded clobetasol propionate 0.05% oral paste 2–3 times daily.
  - Suggested "magic mouthwash" formulas: 1–2 tsp swish, gargle and spit out qid prn; for all formulas, each component in equal portions.
    - Prednisolone 5 mg/mL + nystatin susp 100,000 u/mL + lidocaine viscous 2% + diphenhydramine + Maalox or Mylanta susp + water
    - Lidocaine viscous 2% + diphenhydramine + Kaopectate
    - Prednisolone 5 mg/mL + lidocaine viscous 2% + diphenhydramine + Maalox or Mylanta susp
  - Chlorhexidine gluconate (i.e., Peridex) mouth rinses 1–2 times daily may reduce pain.
  - PPI for 5–7 days
  - Consider B12 1000 mcg po daily for prophylaxis
  - ▲ *Usually lasts about 7–10 days; if the lesions worsen or ulcerative gingivitis is noted, refer to ENT or ED emergently.*
- Gingivitis treatment bid for 10 days for adults
  - Antibiotic treatment: cefadroxil 500 mg or clindamycin 300 mg
  - Encourage the patient to perform good dental hygiene
  - Chlorhexidine (i.e., Peridex) rinse (swish and spit out)
  - May need pain medicine short term
  - *Referral to dentist or oral surgeon if unresponsive to treatment*
- Herbal preparations for various URI disorders (not exclusive)
  - Echinacea: for prophylaxis and treatment of respiratory and flu symptoms; 1 cap bid for 10 days; DO NOT use for >8 wk or at all in patient with an autoimmune disease; 2–4 cups of tea with echinacea daily may lessen cold symptoms.
  - Hyssop: for coughs, colds, and as expectorant; can use as tea, as gargle, and to rub on the skin prn, but DO NOT take if pregnant.
  - Slippery elm: for cough and sore throat pour 2 cups boiling water over 2 tbsp powdered bark and steep for 3–5 min and drink 1 cup tid *or* take 400–500 mg cap 3–4 times daily
  - Honey alone or mixed with lemon will decrease cough; can be used for patients >1 yr of age.
- Nose bleed (epistaxis)
  - Have patient sit forward and pinch the nose shut for 10–15 min *by the clock* and not to release pressure for that amount of time.
  - If unrelieved in 15 min, try oxymetazoline (e.g., Afrin) 2–3 sprays in nostril that is bleeding and continue pressure; apply cold compress over nasal area.
  - *Referral to ED if bleeding continues for >30 min.*
  - Ask patients *not* to "pack" nose with tissues, tampons, or other linens. This may restart bleeding when removed.
  - Question patient about BP control, discourage "nose picking" (this is number one cause in children)
  - Encourage humidifier in house and in bedroom, use saline nasal spray or gel to keep nasal mucosa moist
- Hypertonic saline nasal spray
  - Acts to clean mucus crusts, decongests nose by shrinking membranes to open passages, and improves nasal drainage.
  - Mix ½ tsp sea, pickling, or kosher salt (table salt has too many preservatives) to 6 oz boiled or distilled water; allow to cool, and pour into a nasal spray bottle or can purchase already prepared OTC solution (i.e., AYR-hypertonic).

Continued

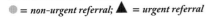

● = *non-urgent referral;* ▲ = *urgent referral*

PRACTICE PEARLS FOR ENT—CONT'D

- Use frequently; keep the "homemade" saline in the refrigerator when not using and discard any remaining liquid after 3 days and make new solution.
- Normotonic saline nasal spray
  - Acts as a cleansing solution to remove mucus and keep nasal passages open and moist; this improves cilia function to remove debris and reduces postnasal drip.
  - Saline nasal spray: mix ¼ tsp sea salt in 6 oz of boiled water; allow to cool; and pour into a nasal spray bottle or can purchase OTC.
  - Use numerous times a day; keep the "homemade" saline in the refrigerator when not using and throw away any remaining liquid after 3 days and make new solution.
- CPT code to bill for removing ear cerumen: 69210 with curette, 69209 with irrigation
- To soften ear wax
  - Use Debrox, peroxide, olive oil, or liquid Colace and put 5–10 gtts in ear canal(s) and leave in for 15 min.
  - Use bulb syringe and warm water to remove wax with flushing.
- Ear candles are not recommended due to lack of evidence and possible burns to ears.

ALLERGIC RHINITIS

I. Signs and symptoms
   A. Pruritus of the nose, eyes, palate, and oropharynx
   B. Excessive tearing, allergic shiners, puffiness around eyes and eyelids, and conjunctival injection
   C. Cough and nasal congestion with sneezing, clear rhinorrhea, and anosmia
   D. Nasal mucosa is pale, swollen, and has bluish tint with cobble-stoning to posterior pharynx
   E. Transverse nasal crease with "allergic salute"

II. General treatment
   A. Limit exposure to allergens (see Chapter 7, ASTHMA, VII, Allergen Control Measures)
   B. Air purifiers and dust filters
   C. Air conditioner in house, especially where sleeping
   D. Remove pets from house
   E. Consider first generation antihistamines (e.g., diphenhydramine) for children
      1. Caution in children, may cause excitation
      2. Caution in elderly, may cause dizziness and falls

III. Pharmacological treatment
   A. Steroid nasal spray, 1–2 sprays each nostril
      1. Beclomethasone dipropionate (Beconase) bid
      2. Ciclesonide (Omnaris) daily
      3. Mometasone (Nasonex) daily
      4. Fluticasone propionate (Flonase Allergy Relief) OTC or fluticasone furoate (Flonase Sensimist) OTC daily
      5. Triamcinolone nasal (Nasacort Allergy 24 HR) OTC daily
      6. Budesonide nasal (Rhinocort) OTC daily
   B. Antihistamine nasal sprays each nostril bid
      1. Azelastine (Astelin) nasal spray: 2 sprays
      2. Azelastine/fluticasone propionate (Dymista): 1 spray
      3. Olopatadine nasal (Patanase): 2 sprays bid
   C. Ipratropium bromide nasal spray (Atrovent): 2 sprays bid-tid
   D. Antihistamine daily (may be given in addition to or instead of nasal steroids)
      1. Loratadine 10 mg
      2. Cetirizine 10 mg

3. Fexofenadine 180 mg
4. Levocetirizine (Xyzal) 5 mg
5. Desloratadine (Clarinex) 5 mg
E. Montelukast (Singulair) 10 mg hs
IV. *Referral to allergist if symptoms worsen and/or affect QOL*

BACTERIAL SINUSITIS
(ALSO SEE CHAPTER 16, UPPER RESPIRATORY TRACT DISORDERS, BACTERIAL SINUSITIS, ACUTE)

I. Acute inflammation/infection of nasal cavity and paranasal sinuses; symptoms present for >10 days or recur after an initial period of improvement ("double sickening")
II. Signs and symptoms
  A. Pressure/pain
    1. In face: increases with bending forward or down; often has maxillary dental pain
    2. In ethmoid, frontal, and sphenoid sinuses: greater in the supine position
  B. Persistent cough (worse when lying down), purulent nasal and postnasal drainage; often lymphoid hyperplasia of pharynx; halitosis
  C. Nasal mucosa inflamed and boggy; TMs retracted with effusion and are hypomobile
  D. Fever >102°F, nausea, fatigue, anosmia/hyposmia, decreased hearing, and fullness in ears
  E. Sore throat, frequent clearing of throat; nasal voice; H/A
III. Treatment
  A. Initial illness; antibiotics for 5–7 days initially
    1. Amoxicillin or amoxicillin/clavulanate 875 mg bid
    2. Doxycycline 100 mg bid or 200 mg daily
    3. Cefpodoxime 200 mg q12hr
    4. Cefixime 400 mg daily
    5. Clindamycin 150–300 mg qid
    6. Moxifloxacin 400 mg or levofloxacin 500–750 mg daily for high-risk patients
  B. Complicated infection (e.g., worsening symptoms or no improvement in 7 days); antibiotics for 10 days
    1. Amoxicillin/clavulanate ER 2000 mg/125 mg q12hr
    2. Levofloxacin 500 mg daily
    3. Moxifloxacin 400 mg daily
    4. Doxycycline 100 mg bid
  C. Chronic rhinosinusitis (CRS)
    1. Nasal steroids (e.g., fluticasone, mometasone, beclomethasone) daily
    2. Nasal saline flushes 1–3 times daily
    3. May consider antibiotics for 7–10 days with broad-spectrum coverage if exacerbation occurs (e.g., anterior/posterior nasal mucopurulent drainage, nasal blockage, facial pain/pressure, anosmia/hyposmia)
      (a) Amoxicillin/clavulanate 875 mg bid or 1000 mg bid
      (b) Clindamycin 300 mg qid
      (c) Moxifloxacin 400 mg daily
  D. If patient initially responds to second-line therapy but again relapses, extend antibiotics again for another 10 days; if little or no response, then *referral to ENT* and order noncontrast CT sinuses.

● = *non-urgent referral*

IV. Adjunct therapy
  A. Acetaminophen or ibuprofen as needed for pain
  B. Nasal decongestants (e.g., oxymetazoline nasal spray) 1–2 times daily for up to 5 days
  C. Nasal steroid, 2 sprays each nostril daily for 1 mo (e.g., fluticasone or mometasone)
  D. Atrovent nasal spray: 2 sprays 2–3 times a day to decrease rhinorrhea
  E. Use a humidifier in the bedroom, warm compresses on the face, and steam inhalation and steamy showers
  F. Hypertonic saline nasal spray frequently (e.g., 8–10 times daily) or Neti pot/sinus rinse 2–3 times daily
  G. Increase oral fluids
  H. Lifestyle changes: stop smoking and wear a mask around environmental allergens
  I. Probiotics 1–2 times daily during the antibiotic course and for the next 2–3 mo
  J. Vitamin D 4000 International Unit daily for 1 mo or turmeric 1/2 tsp daily for 1 mo to decrease inflammation
  ● K. *Referral to ENT if the symptoms do not resolve after 3–4 wk of treatment*

COVID-19—ACUTE RESPIRATORY SYNDROME CORONAVIRUS 2 (SARS-COV-2)

I. Unique viral illness that is highly contagious with varying degrees of symptoms and severity
  A. General information
    1. *Acute COVID* illness: occurring up to 4 wk of symptoms
    2. *Post-COVID* illness ("long haulers"): symptoms continue >4 wk after infection and can last for several months without identifiable reason
  B. Incubation period: up to 14 days after exposure (average 3–5 days)
  C. High-risk populations
    1. Immunocompromised, >65 yr of age, very young with underlying medical conditions
    2. Asthma, COPD or other respiratory illness
    3. Cardiac, DM, cancer, CKD, CVA
    4. Lower socioeconomic populations (e.g., homeless), HIV
    5. Pregnancy, obesity, smoking
    6. Use of chronic corticosteroids or immunosuppressive therapies
II. Signs and symptoms of *acute* COVID-19
  A. Adults
    1. Cough, H/A, fever, and myalgia (most common)
    2. Sore throat, N/V/D, smell/taste abnormality (may not occur with all strains)
    3. Mild upper respiratory symptoms (e.g., nasal congestion, rhinorrhea, sneezing)
    4. Confusion, falls, delirium (most common in elderly)
    5. Pneumonia, chills, dyspnea
    6. Decreased cognitive skills ("brain fog"), postural tachycardia
  B. Children (usually have milder symptoms)
    1. Asymptomatic infection is common
    2. Fever, cough, shortness of breath (most common)
    3. Myalgia, rhinorrhea, sore throat, H/A, N/V
    4. N/V/D may occur without respiratory symptoms
    5. Less than 12 mo of age symptoms may be minimal but can include
      (a) Feeding difficulty
      (b) Fever without cause

● = *non-urgent referral*

   (c) Intussusception
   (d) Bronchiolitis, apnea
   6. Usual recovery is 1–2 wk
   C. *Post-COVID* symptoms lasting more than 4 wk.
   1. Tachycardia with minimal exertion, fatigue, poor endurance
   2. Joint pain without swelling
   3. Dyspnea, cough, chest pain
   4. Insomnia, sweating
   5. Depression, PTSD, anxiety
   6. Decreased cognition with poor concentration and impaired memory
III. Laboratory and radiological testing
   A. Acute testing
   1. Antigen testing within 5–7 days of symptom onset; nasopharyngeal or nasal swab; results usually within the hour
   2. NAATs (RT-PCR) preferred test; nasopharyngeal or nasal swab; may take up to 3 days for results to return
   3. Single positive test is confirmatory; if symptoms continue and initial test was negative, recommend second test using NAATs
   B. Post-COVID testing
   1. It is not necessary to retest after recovery (antibodies can be present for months)
   2. For continued symptoms (either acute or post-COVID), consider
   (a) CBC, CMP, liver enzymes
   (b) TSH (continued fatigue), BNP (chest pain, edema)
   (c) D-dimer (unexplained new dyspnea)
   (d) ANA and CK (arthralgias, myalgias)
IV. Nonpharmacological treatment (as of current CDC guidelines at the time of publication)
   A. Primarily supportive care with rest, fluids and proper nutrition
   ▲ B. ***Referral or transfer to ED if patient is having acute respiratory distress, chest pain or inability to care for self at home; acute symptoms can occur rapidly.***
   C. Isolation at home during acute phase
   1. Separate patient from others in home and limit number of visitors.
   2. Wear face covering when in same room with others.
   3. No sharing of personal items or eating utensils, private bathroom and dining room, if available.
   4. Consistent, same caregiver.
   D. Discontinuation of isolation is individually based on symptoms and may be stopped:
   1. Asymptomatic illness
   (a) 5 days after positive test
   (b) No symptoms during illness
   (c) Should wear mask in public setting for another 5 days
   2. Mild to moderate symptomatic illness
   (a) 5 days after illness started
   (b) Afebrile for 24 hr
   (c) Wear mask in public setting for another 5 days
   (d) If rebound symptomatic COVID, restart 5 days of isolation and consider pharmacological treatment

▲ = *urgent referral*

  V. Pharmacological treatment for out-patients based on risk and symptoms

    A. If patient is hypoxemic with O2 sat <90%, consider home oxygen to maintain pulse ox at or >90%

    B. If history of asthma/COPD, continue current regimen but may need to change steroid inhalers to oral steroids and inhaled medication to nebulized (caution with nebulizers around others due to aerosolization of virus)

    C. Ibuprofen (monitor for GI effects) or acetaminophen routinely for at least 5 days or longer

    D. Cough: dextromethorphan (caution with elderly) or benzonatate 100–200 mg tid

    E. Refer to CDC guidelines for other pharmacological outpatient treatments, such as:

      1. Nirmatrelivir-ritonavir (Paxlovid)

      2. Remdesivir

      3. Molnupiravir

      4. Bebtelovimab

  VI. Follow up in office or by telehealth for mild out-patient illness

    A. Follow up within first 24 hr of diagnosis, either in person or by telephone, as symptoms may progress rapidly and hospitalization may be required.

    B. For high-risk individuals, if stable after 24–48 hr, consider visit in 1–2 wk.

    C. With persistent mild symptoms after 1–3 mo, and consider screening for

      1. Depression, PTSD or anxiety

      2. Respiratory evaluation with: CXR, PFT, pulse ox at rest and with exertion

      3. Cardiac evaluation with ECG and possible referral to cardiologist

  VII. Vaccine recommendations

    A. mRNA vaccine (Pfizer and Moderna) for everyone >6 mo of age should get vaccine at earliest opportunity to help prevent spread of virus

    B. mRNA booster

      1. Pfizer: first >5 yr of age; second >12 yr of age

      2. Moderna: first booster >18 yr of age

    C. Novavax and J&J vaccine indicated for >18 yr of age (no authorized booster); CDC recommends mRNA booster after initial J&J vaccine

    D. Can give other vaccines at same time as COVID vaccine/booster

    E. If tested positive COVID infection, can have vaccination or booster when symptoms resolve

    F. If tested positive for covid and had monoclonal antibodies or convalescent plasma, *wait 90 days.*

    G. Do not take NSAIDs, acetaminophen, ginger, or turmeric prior to vaccine but can take *after* vaccine.

    H. Defer mammograms for 90 days if any lymph node enlargement noted after injection.

    I. Side effects of vaccines

      1. Local site reactions with itching, swelling, pain; may see redness at site up to 3 wk later.

      2. Axillary lymph node swelling and pain, could be on opposite side of injection.

      3. Fever, fatigue, H/A.

      4. Anaphylaxis rarely occurs; monitor patient for at least 15 min after injection.

    J. Contraindications

      1. Prior anaphylaxis (immediate response)

      2. Wheezing or hives (within 4 hr of last vaccine)

      3. Clotting disorders

VIII. Post-COVID syndrome

    A. Occurs more frequently after severe illness and hospitalization; may persist up to 6 mo for all COVID positive patients

    B. Most common post-COVID symptoms

        1. Fatigue: pace self in regards to daily activities, frequent rest breaks and slowly increase endurance

        2. Cough: suggest humidifier, benzonatate, dextromethorphan, bronchodilators

        3. Dyspnea: breathing exercises (e.g., deep breathing or purse-lip breathing, home oxygen as needed

        4. Chest pain/tightness: warm packs, NSAIDs or acetaminophen as needed

        5. Decreased mental cognition (more frequent after hospitalization): simple video games, crossword puzzles, word search, etc.

    IX. *Referral based on continued symptoms to appropriate specialist (e.g., cardiologist, pulminologist, OT/PT, nutritionist, neurologist)*

INFLUENZA (ALSO SEE CHAPTER 16, UPPER RESPIRATORY TRACT DISORDERS, INFLUENZA)

    I. Signs and symptoms

    A. Sudden onset of fever (usually >102°F and may last up to 3 days), malaise, myalgia, and H/A (most common)

    B. Coryza, nonproductive cough, and sore throat

    C. Vomiting and diarrhea (occasionally in children)

    D. Elderly and immunocompromised may exhibit lower grade fever (if any), lassitude, confusion, and pulmonary complications

    II. Diagnostic testing: antigen detection tests for flu A and B

    III. Treatment

    A. Supportive therapy: increase fluids, prevent dehydration, antipyretics (no ASA in children), and analgesics

    B. STAY HOME and rest; if going out, wear mask. Perform good hand washing and cleaning surfaces with bleach-based disinfectant.

    C. Acute antiviral therapy should be started within 48 hr of symptoms for best results and given for 5 days.

        1. Oseltamivir (Tamiflu) adult 75 mg bid (may need to extend dose if severely ill or immunocompromised)

        2. Zanamivir adult (Relenza) 10 mg (2 inhalations) bid; not recommended for patients with lung disease

        3. Baloxavir (Xofluza) *as a single dose*

            (a) <80 kg: 40 mg

            (b) ≥80 kg: 80 mg

        4. Prophylaxis after household exposure should be started within 48 hr

            (a) Oseltamivir po 75 mg daily for 7 days after last exposure

            (b) Zanamivir (Relenza) inhaled 2 inhalations (10 mg) daily for 7 days (not recommended in persons with lung disease)

            (c) Baloxavir (Xofluza) *as a single dose*

                (i) <80 kg: 40 mg

                (ii) ≥80 kg: 80 mg

    D. Encourage seasonal flu immunizations to all ages

  ● = *non-urgent referral*

OTITIS EXTERNA (SWIMMER'S EAR)
(ALSO SEE CHAPTER 16, UPPER RESPIRATORY TRACT DISORDERS, OTITIS EXTERNA)

I. Causes
   A. Swimming (too much water in ears)
   B. Excessive cleaning (irritates canal)
   C. Hearing aids, ear phones/buds
   D. Chemical in cosmetics or shampoos
   E. Psoriasis and allergic dermatitis
   F. Anatomical variations of canal (e.g., small, curved canal)

II. Signs and symptoms
   A. Otalgia (worse with movement of pinna and tragus) and otorrhea
   B. The external auditory canal (EAC) swollen, red, and painful, with an exudate present
   C. TM can be normal or red; frequent complaint of fullness and loss of hearing is usually due to swollen canal and debris
   D. With repeated infection, consider seborrhea, eczema, fungal, and undiagnosed DM

III. Treatment
   A. Cleaning EAC with irrigation can be done if TM is visualized
      1. If possible, the *provider* can clean the EAC gently with a dry Q-tip or loop curette through an otoscope, or try placing an ear wick to "soak up" the debris; ***do not curette out the debris or flush ear unless you can fully visualize the TM.***
      2. Irrigation solution can be either warm water, hydrogen peroxide, or saline or combination.
      3. Use manual irrigation system for better control with less pain.
   B. After the EAC has been cleaned, use topical agents for 7–10 days; if available may use same ophthalmic drops, which can be less expensive than otic drops.
      1. Ofloxacin otic 10 gtts daily (bacterial or fungal); *can be used with TM perforation.*
      2. Ciprofloxacin/dexamethasone (Ciprodex) otic 4 gtts bid (bacterial or fungal); do not use if suspected TM rupture.
      3. Ciprofloxacin/hydrocortisone otic 3 gtts bid (bacterial or fungal); do not use if suspected TM rupture.
      4. Neomycin/polymixin B/hydrocortisone otic suspension (Cortisporin otic) 3 gtts 3 to 4 times daily (bacterial); do not use if suspected TM rupture.
      5. 2% acetic acid otic sol (VoSol) *or* hydrocortisone/acetic acid 1%/2% otic sol (VoSol HC; if suspected fungal) 4 gtts q8hr; do not use if suspected TM rupture.
   C. Pain management with acetaminophen or ibuprofen
   D. Monitor immunocompromised patients or those with DM closely for worsening disease.
   E. For 2 wk, gently place cotton balls impregnated with petroleum jelly into the outer EAC to keep water out; discourage ear buds.

IV. Prevention
   A. Keep the ears dry; the *patient* should not use anything to clean or scratch in the ears
   B. After water exposure, use a blow dryer on low setting at least 12 inches from EAC opening to dry the EAC
   C. To alleviate itching and prevent OE after swimming, instill a few drops of vinegar, rubbing alcohol, or peroxide in the ears and immediately let it drain out
   D. May use ear plugs after infection has resolved and if wearing hearing aids, take the aids out at night and clean

───────────────

■ = *not to be missed*

ACUTE OTITIS MEDIA (AOM) (ALSO SEE CHAPTER 16, UPPER RESPIRATORY TRACT DISORDERS, ACUTE OTITIS MEDIA)

I. Cause can be either bacterial, viral, or associated with allergic rhinitis.

II. Signs and symptoms have acute onset and are usually seen after URI.
   A. Significant otalgia; if TM perforates, pain will diminish immediately.
   B. TM
      1. Cloudy, bulging, and impaired mobility
      2. Bright red or hemorrhagic appearance
      3. May have bullae or perforations with or without purulent fluid
   C. Loss of appetite, N/V, fever, purulent otorrhea
   D. Tinnitus, vertigo, and decreased hearing or ear stuffiness due to fluid
   E. H/A, irritability, and confusion in the elderly

III. Treatment
   A. Pain management: acetaminophen or ibuprofen; may need stronger pain meds
   B. Antibiotics (5–7 days if mild illness)
      1. Amoxicillin/clavulanate 500 mg tid or 875 mg bid
      2. PCN allergy
         (a) Cefuroxime: 500 mg q12hr
         (b) Cefdinir 300 mg q12hr or 600 mg daily
         (c) Cefpodoxime 200 mg bid
      3. PCN and cephalosporin allergy
         (a) Doxycycline 100 mg bid
         (b) Azithromycin: 500 mg daily for 3 days or clarithromycin 500 mg bid
   C. For more severe disease or high-risk patient (e.g., >65 yr of age, immunocompromised, recent hospitalization or recent course of antibiotics); amoxicillin/clavulanate 1000 tid or 2000 mg bid for 10 days.
   D. If PCN allergy, or failure after first PCN course; use cephalosporin (as above) for 10 days

IV. *Referral to ENT if the symptoms do not improve*

OTITIS MEDIA WITH EFFUSION (ALSO SEE CHAPTER 16, UPPER RESPIRATORY TRACT DISORDERS, OTITIS MEDIA WITH EFFUSION, IV)

I. Causes: high-altitude activity, URI, allergies, orthodontic malocclusion with mouth breathing, or eustachian tube dysfunction

II. Signs and symptoms (do not have acute onset)
   A. Decreased hearing
   B. Feeling of fullness or pressure in the ear(s)
   C. "Popping" sensation with yawning, swallowing, or nose blowing
   D. TM retracted with clear to yellowish or bluish colored fluid; decreased mobility and poor visibility of landmarks

III. Treatment if no infection noted
   A. With mild symptoms, the condition often spontaneously resolves in 2–3 wk but can take up to 12 wk
   B. Medications to consider
      1. Pseudoephedrine 30 mg tid
      2. Oxymetazoline (Afrin) 1–2 sprays q12hr (Note: this should be used only for 3 to 5 days because of nasal rebound congestion); can restart again after 7 days off

---

● = *non-urgent referral*

3. Loratadine 10 mg or cetirizine 10 mg or fexofenadine 180 mg daily
4. Azelastine (Astelin) nasal spray 2 sprays each nostril bid
5. Azelastine/fluticasone propionate (Dymista) 1 spray each nostril bid
6. Consider nasal steroids (e.g., fluticasone, mometasone) 1–2 sprays each nostril daily

C. Consider chewing gum or frequent auto-insufflation (trying to gently "pop ears," pinch nose closed and swallow or blow out with lips closed, or blow-up balloons).
D. Use hypertonic saline nasal spray often (e.g., 8–10 times daily) or Neti-pot or nasal rinse 2–3 times daily (see **PRACTICE PEARLS FOR ENT**, earlier in this chapter).
E. Follow up in 3 wk and consider hearing testing if still symptomatic after 8–12 wk.
F. *Referral to ENT or allergist if symptoms continue and/or hearing loss*

PHARYNGITIS (ALSO SEE CHAPTER 16, UPPER RESPIRATORY TRACT DISORDERS, PHARYNGITIS)

I. Cause: usually viral but can be bacterial or allergic; need to identify any treatable causes and prevent complications
II. Signs and symptoms
   A. Common presentation of bacterial pharyngitis
      1. Acute-onset sore throat with erythema and tonsillar exudates bilaterally (one tonsil may be affected more than other)
      2. Fever, H/A, and tender/enlarged bilateral cervical nodes
      3. May have sandpaper rash on torso and petechiae of soft palate
      4. Children may present with N/V and stomach pain
      5. Absence of cough and stuffy nose
   B. Common presentation of viral pharyngitis
      1. Sore throat
      2. Coryza
      3. Conjunctivitis
      4. Cough and hoarseness
   C. May also have malaise, myalgia, anorexia, and difficulty swallowing
III. Diagnostic testing
   A. Rapid strep test (testing not indicated if <3yr of age unless other family members positive); throat culture if indicated
   B. CBC and mono spot (if concerned about other diagnoses)
IV. Treatment (see Chapter 16, Upper respiratory Tract Disorders, PHARYNGITIS, for pediatric dosing)
   A. *If unilateral enlarged tonsil with exudate and fullness in palatal area, consider peritonsillar abscess, referral immediately to ED*
   B. Supportive therapy
      1. Antipyretics and analgesics (e.g., acetaminophen or ibuprofen) routinely for 2 to 3 days
      2. Throat lozenges (e.g., with benzocaine, dyclonine, and menthol)
      3. Throat sprays (e.g., with phenol, benzocaine, or chlorhexidine)
      4. Saltwater gargles and can add ½ to 1 tsp liquid diphenhydramine
      5. Encourage soft, cold foods, and ice chips
      6. Increase humidity in house
      7. If severe pain, consider swish/swallow with topical steroid + diphenhydramine (see **PRACTICE PEARLS FOR ENT**, earlier in this chapter).

___

● = *non-urgent referral;* ▲ = *urgent referral*

    C. If bacterial pharyngitis or history of rheumatic fever, start antibiotics
      1. Penicillin VK 500 mg bid for *10 days*
      2. Amoxicillin/clavulanate 500 mg tid or 875 mg bid for *10 days*
      3. Penicillin G benzathine (Bicillin LA) 1.2 million units IM *once*
      4. With PCN allergy; treat for *10 days*
        (a) Cefdinir 300 mg bid or 600 mg daily
        (b) Cephalexin 500 mg q12hr
        (c) Cefixime 400 mg daily
      5. PCN or cephalosporin allergy
        (a) Azithromycin (Z-Pak) for *5 days*
        (b) Clarithromycin 250 mg bid for *10 days*
    D. If viral pharyngitis, supportive therapy measures only
    E. If the tonsils and pharynx are severely swollen, consider prednisone; start with 30–50 mg daily and taper over 10–14 days
    F. Follow-up
      1. Visit in 1 to 3 days; monitor closely for peritonsillar abscess.
      2. May return to school after 24 hr on antibiotics and fever resolution.
      3. Throw away current toothbrush and start using a new brush after 48 hr.
      4. Do not put toothbrush in communal holder at home.
   ● **V. *Referral to ENT if the symptoms are recurrent or do not resolve***

TINNITUS

   I. Description: perception of sound heard by the patient that is not attributable to an external sound (e.g., hissing, ringing, whining, buzzing)
    A. May be unilateral or bilateral, consistent or intermittent
    B. Usually perceived as louder at night (because there are fewer distractions and extraneous sounds)
  II. Possible causes
    A. Aging and history of high noise levels for long periods of time
    B. Cerumen impaction, acute and chronic otitis media (OM), eustachian tube dysfunction
    C. Head and neck injuries, TMJ, acoustic neuroma, DM, thyroid disorders, Meniere disease, and vascular diseases
    D. Allergies and eustachian tube dysfunction
    E. Medications
      1. ASA, NSAIDs, loop diuretics, SSRIs, and caffeine
      2. Some antihypertensives (e.g., beta blockers, especially metoprolol)
 III. Diagnostic testing
    A. Otoscopy with a pneumatic otoscope and insufflation
    B. Rinne and Weber tests (see Fig. 1.3)
    C. Cranial nerve testing (see Table 1.5)
    D. CBC, ESR, ANA titer, Lyme disease titer (if suspected), rheumatic factor, RPR (if syphilis is suspected), TSH, and FBG
    E. Audiology testing
    F. MRI/MRA if suspect a mass or vascular causes

● = *non-urgent referral*

IV. Treatment
- A. Stop any ototoxic medications
- B. Hearing aids (if hearing loss is the cause) or tinnitus maskers (resemble hearing aids but produce soft background noises)
- C. Cognitive behavioral therapy (e.g., relaxation techniques, biofeedback); patient can experience depression or insomnia
- D. Decrease salt intake
- E. Medications that might help but are not proven
  - 1. Antianxiety drugs to help manage stress/anxiety
  - 2. Melatonin (if having insomnia because of the noise) or other medication to help induce sleep

V. Treatment is *referral to ENT (or other specialty based on diagnosis)*

● = *non-urgent referral*

CHAPTER 7

Respiratory Conditions

For details regarding complete history and physical examination, see Chapters 1 and 2.

ASSESSING PULMONARY FUNCTION

I. Pulse oximetry
  A. A noninvasive method of estimating and monitoring oxygen saturation in the blood
  B. Normal is >92%
II. Peak expiratory flow rate (PEF) (see Appendix B for the PEF chart)
  A. Reflects large airway flow; it is decreased in obstructive diseases and with age.
  B. Normal is >80% predicted.
  C. May be used in office or at home to monitor the effects of treatment and the status of the disease process, but results may be misleading and do not always reflect the severity of symptoms.
III. Pulmonary function testing (PFT)/office spirometry
  A. A noninvasive test used to detect obstructive and/or restrictive lung diseases; all results are based on standardized charts of predicted values by age and percentage.
    1. Obstructive
      (a) Seen with decreased outflow of air from lungs due to resistance of lung tissue.
      (b) Conditions include COPD (i.e., emphysema and chronic bronchitis), asthma, cystic fibrosis; also bronchiectasis or bronchiolitis in children.
    2. Restrictive
      (a) May be related to lung pathology or extrinsic factors (i.e., outside the lungs) related to inability of chest muscles to fully expand or reduction in lung volume.
      (b) Conditions include pneumonia, sarcoidosis, tuberculosis (TB), tumors, pulmonary edema, pulmonary fibrosis, scoliosis, obesity, and ascites.
    3. Mixed or neuromuscular: conditions include amyotrophic lateral sclerosis (ALS), diaphragmatic paralysis, myasthenia gravis, muscular dystrophy, polio
  B. May be used to
    1. Evaluate patients with SOB, dyspnea on exertion (DOE), or restrictive diseases
    2. Monitor chronic lung disease
    3. Evaluate chronic cough
    4. Evaluate lung function prior to general anesthesia for patient with current lung disease
    5. Physical exams, including DOT exams, for anyone over 40–45 yr of age who smokes
    6. Evaluate effectiveness with medication changes in respiratory conditions
  C. Do not test the patient
    1. During an acute illness/exacerbation—wait for at least 6 wk after the illness has resolved
    2. Within 6 wk of COVID illness (i.e., bronchodilators will increase cough and may be responsible spread of occult infection)

D. Relative contraindications to PFT/office spirometry
   1. Hemoptysis
   2. Pneumothorax
   3. Unstable cardiac status, recent MI or PE
   4. Aneurysms
   5. Recent eye, ear, thorax, or abdominal surgery
   6. Acute illness (would give false readings and may increase droplet spread of illness)
E. PFT/office spirometry values used for interpretation (see Table 7.1)
   1. Values for interpretation: always assess flow volume loops for accuracy and patient effort
   2. Always perform pre- and post-bronchodilator testing, if possible

TABLE 7.1 ■ How to Read Pulmonary Function Test/Spirometry Quickly

Measure	Normal	Obstructive	Restrictive	Mixed
FEV₁*	>80% predicted	Decreased Used to stage COPD (Post bronchodilator reading): Mild: ≥70% Moderate: 50%–69% Mod-severe: 50%–59% Severe: 30%–49% Very severe: <30%	Decreased to normal	Decreased
FVC*	>80% predicted	Normal or decreased	Decreased: Mild: 70%–79% Moderate: 50%–69% Severe: <50%	Decreased
FEV₁/FVC ratio	>70% predicted	Normal early on, then decreases <70% post bronchodilator	Increased to normal (>80%)	Increased to normal
TLC		Increased to normal (>100%)	Decreased: Mild: 65%–80% Moderate: 50%–65% Severe: <50%	Decreased
FEF 25%–75%	>80%	Decreased Mild: 60%–79% Moderate: 40%–59% Severe: <40%	Increased, decreased or normal	
Examples		Limitation of expiratory airflow-airways cannot empty due to: COPD, asthma, cystic fibrosis	Reduced lung volumes/ compliance due to: Muscle weakness Obesity, scoliosis Pregnancy Chest wall deformity Pleural effusion Interstitial fibrosis Neuromuscular disease	Cystic fibrosis Bronchiectasis HF Sarcoidosis Guillain-Barre syndrome

* Most useful tests.

Note: FEV₁ represents FEV_1 and FEV₁/FVC represents FEV_1/FVC.

3. Forced vital capacity (FVC)
    (a) Total volume of air forcefully exhaled after a full inspiration
    (b) Measures the severity of restriction and should be followed up with a complete PFT
4. Forced expiratory volume in 1 sec (FEV_1)
    (a) Volume of air forcefully expired in the first second during maximal expiratory effort; detects airway obstruction in early stages
    (b) Measures large airway flow and can be used to monitor asthma/COPD and severity of airway obstruction
    (c) Normal is >80% predicted
    (d) Greater than 12% improvement in FEV_1 after bronchodilator treatment shows reversibility (i.e., asthma)
5. FEV_1/FVC ratio (normal 70%)
    (a) Used to determine the degree of airflow limitations (e.g., asthma/COPD)
    (b) Normal values are age-based.
        (i) <20 yr of age: ≥85%
        (ii) 20–39 yr of age: ≥80%
        (iii) 40–59 yr of age: ≥75%
        (iv) 60–80 yr of age: ≥70%
    (c) Restrictive disorders may have near normal to above normal values.
6. Total lung capacity (TLC): air volume in lungs after maximum inspiration; used to determine difference between obstructive and restrictive diseases
7. FEF 25%–5% (normal >65%): reflects small airway function
F. Steps for interpretation of spirometry (see Table 7.1)
1. If FEV_1/FVC <70% (this shows obstruction), then look at FEV_1 to determine grade of severity.
2. If FEV_1/FVC >70% (shows possible restriction), then look at FVC, and if this is <80%, you can determine the grade of restriction.
3. If FVC >80%, this could indicate mixed disease; look at FEF 25%–75%; if this is >50%, this would be considered normal, and if >50%, this could indicate a mixed disease.

COUGH

I. Acute cough lasts <3 wk and has sudden onset
    A. Common causes with associated signs and symptoms
        1. ACE inhibitors (for treatment see Chapter 8, **PRACTICE PEARLS FOR HTN**)
            (a) Daily nonproductive cough; can occur anytime during treatment
            (b) "Tickling" or "scratchy" sensation in throat
        2. Acute bronchitis
            (a) Usually presents after URI and cough starts within 3 days of onset of symptoms and may last up to 10 days
            (b) Cough often occurs in spasms; may have clear sputum production
            (c) No consolidation on chest exam
            (d) Absence of high fever
        3. Asthma (see later in this chapter)
            (a) First episode of asthma may be hard to distinguish between asthma and bronchitis
            (b) History of or current episodic wheezing, cough (especially at night), SOB
            (c) Usually caused by allergen, exercise, or irritant
            (d) No constitutional symptoms

    4. Common cold (also called URI)
- (a) May have low-grade fever and myalgia; sputum production is usually clear to white (may become mucopurulent)
- (b) Rhinorrhea, sneezing, scratchy throat
- (c) Malaise and headache

    5. GERD (see Chapter 9, Upper Abdominal Conditions, GASTROESOPHAGEAL REFLUX DISEASE (GERD))
- (a) Cough may be only presenting symptom
- (b) Cough mainly after meals
- (c) May have heartburn, regurgitation, dysphagia
- (d) May have silent aspiration

    6. HF (for treatment see Chapter 8, HEART FAILURE)
- (a) Cough can be first sign of sudden onset HF
- (b) SOB with exertion or lying flat, peripheral edema, gallop rhythm

    7. Flu/COVID (for treatment see Chapter 6, Common ENT Conditions, INFLUENZA, COVID-19)
- (a) Acute fever, myalgia
- (b) Clear rhinorrhea, H/A
- (c) Deep, nonproductive "barky" cough with clear sputum

    8. Pneumonia (for treatment see later in this chapter)
- (a) Fever, tachypnea, tachycardia
- (b) Change in mental status, especially in the elderly
- (c) Signs of consolidation on chest exam
- (d) Initial chest X-ray may or may not show evidence of pneumonia; repeat in 2–5 days

    9. Postnasal drip (PND; also known as upper airway cough syndrome [UACS])
- (a) Frequent clearing of throat
- (b) Clear rhinorrhea

  10. Pulmonary embolism
- (a) Dyspnea, pleuritic chest pain, hemoptysis
- (b) Tachypnea, tachycardia
- (c) Symptoms can be mild or dramatic

B. Generalized treatment that may be beneficial for short-term symptoms caused by acute illness

    1. Throat lozenges (do not exceed 10–12 daily), hot tea, cold beverages, honey 1–2 tsp (use for >12 mo of age), encourage smoking cessation and avoiding second-hand smoke, and minimizing exposure to irritants

    2. Intranasal sprays for common cold and PND until symptoms subside
- (a) Anticholinergic: Ipratropium (Atrovent nasal): 2 sprays 3–4 times a day
- (b) Antihistamine: Azelastine (Astepro): 2 sprays daily
- (c) Steroid nasal spray
  - (i) Fluticasone (Flonase Allergy Relief, OTC): 1–2 sprays daily
  - (ii) Triamcinolone (Nasacort Allergy 24HR, OTC): 1–2 sprays daily
  - (iii) Mometasone (Nasonex, Rx): 2 sprays daily

    3. Consider albuterol or albuterol/ipratropium (Duoneb) nebulized (for bronchospastic cough due to bronchitis or COPD, whether person is smoker or nonsmoker)

    4. Antihistamine/decongestants may be more beneficial together than given individually (e.g., brompheniramine/pseudoephedrine)

    5. Naproxen; may not be beneficial for cough, but will help with myalgia if present

    6. Consider Vicks VapoRub to soles of feet at hs, with socks overnight (can be used for any age; unclear benefits)

7. Hypertonic nasal saline spray 8–10 times daily; increase humidification in home
8. Antitussive agents (for acute bronchitis, pneumonia) such as benzonatate, codeine sulfate, dextromethorphan (avoid with SSRIs and tramadol), menthol, and guaifenesin
9. Antibiotics not recommended unless bacterial causes or symptoms present >14 days

II. Subacute cough lasts 3–8 wk
  A. Common causes
    1. Allergic rhinitis (see Chapter 6, Common ENT Conditions, ALLERGIC RHINITIS)
    2. Asthma (see later in this chapter)
    3. GERD (see Chapter 9, Upper Abdominal Conditions, GASTROESOPHAGEAL REFLUX DISEASE (GERD))
    4. Medication-induced (e.g., ACE inhibitor therapy)
      (a) Stop therapy and choose alternate HTN medication (see Table 8.16).
      (b) Consider inhaled or nasal corticosteroid for 3–4 wk.
    5. Pertussis should be considered if cough is getting progressively worse over 2 wk *and* preceded by URI *and*
      (a) Cough is paroxysmal with post-cough vomiting or whooping sound; testing for pertussis is recommended but results may take several wk.
      (b) Treat with azithromycin (or TMP-SMX if allergic to macrolide) if in the first 3 wk of illness.
    6. Postinfectious cough usually starts with or shortly after acute viral/bacterial illness and continues past 3 wk
      (a) Nonproductive cough
      (b) Persistent inflammation of nose/sinuses seen with upper airway cough syndrome
      (c) Affects daily routine and nighttime sleep
    7. Bacterial sinusitis (see Chapter 6, Common ENT Conditions, BACTERIAL SINUSITIS)
    8. Current smoker or exposure to second hand smoke
  B. Generalized treatment for subacute cough is aimed at relief of symptoms
    1. Smoking cessation and avoidance of second-hand smoke or environmental irritants
    2. No antibiotics, unless bacterial infection present or positive for pertussis
    3. Usually resolves without treatment but may need antitussive medications to help with sleep
    4. Consider intranasal ipratropium (Atrovent), antihistamine (azelastine) or inhaled or intranasal corticosteroids
    5. Antitussive
      (a) Benzonatate
      (b) Dextromethorphan (avoid with SSRIs and tramadol)
      (c) Codeine 30–60 mg q4–6 h (use when cough is most bothersome; will cause drowsiness; use only for short period of time)
    6. Cough may mean loss of or poor control of asthma; monitor asthma action plan
    7. First- or second-generation oral antihistamines
      (a) Brompheniramine, chlorpheniramine, and/or in combination with pseudoephedrine (avoid 1st generation in the elderly, due to drowsiness and fall risk)
      (b) Cetirizine, loratadine, and fexofenadine (nonsedating), and/or in combination with pseudoephedrine
    8. Mucolytics: guaifenesin
    9. Consider gabapentin (off-label) if all other options have failed

III. Chronic cough lasts >8 wk in adults and >4 wk in children; it is usually an annoying cough that interrupts sleep or daily activity; may be productive or nonproductive

    A. Common causes (*most common causes of chronic cough)

        1. Airway disease (see later in this chapter)

           (a) Asthma*

           (b) COPD

           (c) TB

        2. Airway irritants

           (a) Smoking: productive cough in the morning and dry cough the rest of the day

           (b) Non-eosinophilic airway disease (NEAD)

        3. Allergic rhinitis (see Chapter 6, Common ENT Conditions, ALLERGIC RHINITIS)

        4. Chronic sinusitis (see Chapter 6, Common ENT Conditions, BACTERIAL SINUSITIS))

        5. Congenital anomalies

        6. GERD* (see Chapter 9, Upper Abdominal Conditions, GASTRO-ESOPHAGEAL REFLUX DISEASE (GERD))

        7. Habit or idiopathic cough

        8. Mass (benign or malignant) of the upper or lower airways

        9. Medications (e.g., ACE inhibitor, beta-blockers)

      10. Nonallergic rhinitis

      11. PND*

      12. Silent aspiration caused by disruption of swallowing mechanism after CVA

    B. History related to chronic cough

        1. Present or past smoking

        2. Taking ACE inhibitor for HTN

        3. Exposure to TB, fungal agents, or other irritants in the environment

        4. History of cancer, TB, AIDS

        5. History of CVA/TIA (possible silent aspiration)

    C. *Not to be missed regarding chronic cough*

        1. *Smoker with >20 pack year history*

        2. *Smoker >45 yr of age with new or changed cough*

        3. *Hemoptysis*

        4. *Unintended weight loss*

        5. *Worsening dyspnea, especially at night*

        6. *Hoarseness, dysphagia, pain with swallowing*

        7. *Recurrent pneumonia*

        8. *Anemia, unexplained fatigue, or weight loss*

        9. *Increased sputum production (without exacerbation of COPD)*

    D. Diagnostic testing for chronic cough

        1. Chest X-ray and if abnormal, consider CT chest

        2. PFT/office spirometry

        3. Speech pathology evaluation (if suspect silent aspiration)

        4. *Helicobacter pylori* test (if suspect infection)

        5. CBC, metabolic panel; ESR or CRP

        6. TB skin testing

        7. Consider sinus CT

    E. Treatment is based on the cause

        1. Stop smoking or decrease exposure to irritants both at home and at work; wear mask at work, if needed

---

■ = *not to be missed*

    2. Increase humidification in home

    3. Antihistamines

       (a) First-generation (e.g., brompheniramine, chlorpheniramine) are stronger than second-generation but have more sedating effects.

       (b) Second-generation (e.g., cetirizine, loratadine, fexofenadine).

    4. Inhaled ipratropium, azelastine, intranasal or inhaled steroids

    5. Antitussive

       (a) Dextromethorphan (avoid with SSRIs and tramadol) with guaifenesin

       (b) Codeine 30–60 mg q4–6 hr (use when cough is most bothersome; will cause drowsiness; use only for short period of time)

       (c) Benzonatate

    6. Mucolytic: guaifenesin

    7. Consider montelukast (Singulair) 10 mg daily

  IV. *Referral to pulmonologist for further evaluation if cough continues.*

ASTHMA (REACTIVE AIRWAY DISEASE)

  I. Description

    A. Chronic inflammatory condition of the airways

      1. Associated with widespread bronchospasm and variable airflow obstruction that is reversible either spontaneously or with treatment

       (a) Children may have a cough (e.g., nocturnal, with exercise, or seasonal allergies), fatigue, and decreased exercise tolerance but less wheezing.

       (b) Adults typically have widespread high-pitched expiratory wheezes that do not resolve with cough and also nocturnal cough.

       (c) Elderly may have intermittent wheeze, cough, chest tightness, but no dyspnea.

    B. Signs and symptoms

      1. Nonproductive cough (at rest, with exercise, at night), bronchospasm

      2. Wheeze at rest or at night (may not have any wheezing unless patient is active)

      3. Shortness of breath with activity and decreased pulse ox

      4. Exercise intolerance (any age) or child may exhibit inability to keep up with others

    C. Symptoms may be triggered by the following:

      1. Environmental allergens (e.g., smoking, dust mites, pets) or occupational irritants (e.g., chemical irritants or pollutants)

      2. Exercise-induced asthma (EIA)

      3. Drug (e.g., ASA, NSAIDs, nonselective beta blockers, ACEI)

      4. Structural defects (e.g., nasal polyps)

      5. Exposure to extreme temperatures and cold foods

      6. Emotional stressors (e.g., crying and laughing, which can cause bronchospasm)

      7. Food and drinks (e.g., peanuts and other nuts; food additives [for taste or color and preservation])

      8. Acute illness (e.g., acute viral and/or bacterial infections)

  II. General guidelines

    A. Early diagnosis and treatment are essential for maintaining normalcy.

      1. Recognizing triggers of symptoms, treatment, and control of allergens/irritants (see **VII**, below)

      2. Minimizing the severity of attacks with early treatment

      3. Monitoring frequency of nocturnal symptoms which indicate worsening of the disease

---

● = *non-urgent referral*

4. PFT or office spirometry
   (a) At initial diagnosis for baseline
   (b) Every 1–2 yr recommended to monitor progress of disease; may need to do this more often during medication changes
   (c) When stable after acute illness
   (d) Anytime there is an increase of SABA use >2 days a wk for symptom control, this may indicate poor control and possible need to change treatment

B. Treatment goals
   1. Reduce impairment caused by asthma.
   2. Allow the patient to lead a normal life.
   3. Decrease number of exacerbations requiring ED visits or hospitalization.

C. Instruct patient to perform PEFR daily or weekly, depending on control, to establish a base line "personal best" and to be able to identify any changes in actual symptoms.

D. There should be an "asthma action plan" (refer to *https://lung.org/search.jsp?query= asthma+action+plan*) in place to allow the patient to start rescue therapy immediately when exacerbations occur, and this plan should be reviewed at each visit related to asthma or respiratory illness.

E. Monitor for other triggers (e.g., GERD) and treat promptly.

F. Routine follow-up in office with or without spirometry, every 3–12 mo, depending on severity of illness and need for inhalers.

III. Treatment of asthma by type (also see **IV**, Treatment for Exacerbations)

A. *Intermittent asthma* (which includes EIA and incidental occurrences)
   1. Symptoms
      (a) Persistent cough (may be only sign) occurring at night or with exercise, especially in cold and dry air
      (b) Episodic, mild diffuse wheezing, chest tightness with mild dyspnea, tachypnea and/or SOB, usually for short periods of time, which resolves with or without treatment
      (c) May wake up during nighttime ≤ 2 nights/mo; no reportable fatigue in the mornings
      (d) Episodes are infrequent or with activity and do not interfere with overall ADLs
      (e) During an episode, the patient can speak in short sentences with minor difficulty
   2. Spirometry
      (a) FEV_1 >80% predicted and is normal between episodes; FEV_1 increases by 12% after use of bronchodilator
      (b) FEV_1/FVC ratio normal (70% predicted) between exacerbations
   3. Medications (see Table 7.2) should be reevaluated every 6–12 mo, depending on disease progression
      (a) Long-term control requires no routine medications, only rescue as needed.
      (b) Use SABA prn for symptom control with good relief of symptoms (if having to use ≥ 2 days/wk, then should consider cause and/or increase therapy).
      (c) Can consider using LTRA for EIA; must take 2 hr prior to any activity, effects may last up to 12 hr; recommend having rescue inhaler available.
   4. Exacerbations are usually predictable with activity, weather or seasonal allergies and there should be no hospitalization or use of oral glucocorticoids (OGC) within the past yr.
   5. Patient education should include an asthma educator (if available) and should occur at each visit for asthma.
      (a) Review proper use of inhalers and when to use inhaler or other medications.
      (b) Allergen avoidance (see Review "asthma action plan," see **II. D**, above).

B. *Mild persistent asthma*
1. Symptoms similar to intermittent but occur more than 2 days/wk (not daily) consistently
    (a) Awaken at night with symptoms not more than 3–4 times/mo; awakens without fatigue.
    (b) Symptoms cause a minor limitation to ADLs; patient is able to keep up with peers but may need rescue inhaler.
2. Spirometry
    (a) $FEV_1 \geq 80\%$ predicted
    (b) FEV_1/FVC ratio > 70% predicted
3. Medications (see Table 7.2) should be reevaluated every 3–6 mo, depending on disease progression
    (a) Use daily low-dose range inhaled corticosteroid (ICS).
    (b) Rescue inhaler (SABA) used > 2 days/wk to control symptoms, but not more than once a day.
    (c) Can consider leukotriene receptor antagonist (LTRA), instead of daily ICS, if symptoms are controlled.
4. Exacerbations (also see **IV**, Treatment for Exacerbations)
    (a) May experience exacerbations ≥ 2/yr that require OGC.
    (b) For children with *intermittent exacerbations*: can use dexamethasone 0.3–0.6 mg/kg orally daily (up to 16 mg/dose) for 1–2 days (instead of 3–5 days with prednisone or prednisolone).
    (c) If any hospitalization for asthma during any 1 yr period; this may be indication of poor control and need to increase therapy.
5. Patient education should include an asthma educator (if available) and should occur at each visit for asthma
    (a) Monitor daily PEFR logs and actual symptoms that may accompany exacerbations.
    (b) Monitor frequency of SABA rescue inhaler use, if increasing, need to investigate reasons for use.
    (c) Review "asthma action plan" (see **II.D**, above) at each visit for asthma; also see allergen control (see **VII**, below).
    (d) Consider *referral to allergist if symptoms poorly controlled or < 12 yr of age.*
C. *Moderate persistent asthma*
1. Symptoms
    (a) Wheezing and shortness of breath occur daily with nighttime cough > 1×/wk that awakens patient.
    (b) Fatigue, cough, wheeze causing some limitation in ADLs.
    (c) Unable to keep up with peers without using SABA.
2. Spirometry
    (a) FEV_1 between > 60% and < 80% predicted
    (b) FEV_1/FVC below normal by about 5% (> 70% predicted is normal)
3. Medications (see Table 7.2) should be reevaluated every 3–6 mo, depending on disease progression
    (a) Continues with SABA to control symptoms and ICS + LABA
    (b) Daily ICS (low dose) with daily LABA; use combined inhaler ICS + LABA to enhance compliance and safety *or*
    (c) Daily medium dose ICS *or* low-dose ICS + LTRA
    (d) Consider *short course* (3–7 days) of oral steroids, if indicated with exacerbation

---

● = *non-urgent referral*

   (e) Do not use LABA as *monotherapy*
   (f) Can consider theophylline as an alternative to ICS or LABA if poor control or physical limitations for person using inhalers; side effects and drug levels MUST be monitored monthly to prevent toxicity
  4. Exacerbations: >2/yr that require OGC and/or hospitalization (also see **IV**, Treatment for Exacerbation)
  5. Patient education should include an asthma educator (if available) and should occur at each visit for asthma
   (a) Monitor daily PEFR logs and consider adjustments based on PEFR and symptoms.
   (b) Monitor frequency of SABA rescue inhaler and if usage is increasing, investigate reasons why.
   (c) Review "asthma action plan" (see **II. D**, above) at each visit for asthma; also review allergen control (see **VII**, below).
   (d) Consider adding LTRA (montelukast or zileuton) if control not adequate.
   (e) Consider *referral to pulmonologist or allergist.*
 D. *Severe persistent asthma*
  1. Symptoms
   (a) Occur throughout the whole day with nighttime symptoms up to 7 days/wk causing poor sleep and fatigue in the mornings
   (b) Extreme limitations in ADLs due to cough and wheezing
   (c) Unable to keep up with peers
  2. Spirometry
   (a) FEV_1 <60% predicted
   (b) FEV_1/FVC reduced >5% (>70% predicted is normal)
  3. Medications (see Table 7.2) should be reevaluated every 3 mo, depending on disease progression.
   (a) SABA multiple times daily to control symptoms
   (b) Medium dose ICS + LABA (*do not use LABA as monotherapy*)
   (c) Medium dose ICS + LTRA (montelukast or zileuton)
   (d) High dose ICS + LABA
  4. *Referral*
   (a) *To ED with an acute exacerbation*
   (b) **To pulmonologist or allergist** *if generally uncontrolled with above regimen*
 IV. Treatment for exacerbations
  A. Assess severity of symptoms with goal to reverse airflow obstruction and minimize hospitalization
  1. Symptoms of exacerbation
   (a) Worsening of SOB/dyspnea, cough, wheezing or chest tightness, and nocturnal cough/wheeze, marked breathlessness.
   (b) Patient can only speak in short sentences.
   (c) If home or office pulse ox < 90%, use supplemental oxygen with inhaler therapy.
  2. *Emergent transfer to ED recommended if patient is showing signs of deterioration (see C below)*
  B. *Immediate treatment with inhaled or nebulized SABA 2–8 puffs q20min up to 4 times, then q1–4 h or until symptoms improve*

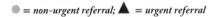 = *non-urgent referral;* ▲ = *urgent referral*

1. *Improvement* in symptoms (i.e., resolution of wheezing, dyspnea and PEFR ≥80% predicted, oxygen saturation >90% on room air; decreased tachypnea in young children)
   (a) Continue inhaled or nebulized SABA q3–4h for the next 24–48 hr.
   (b) Consider short course of OGC (e.g., prednisone 40–60 mg daily for 3–7 days).
   (c) Discuss triggers for exacerbation.
   (d) Reevaluate "asthma action plan" (see **II.D**, above) and consider severity of asthma; if poor control with current plan, consider changing maintenance medications.
2. *Continued* symptoms after initial treatment (i.e., persistent wheezing/dyspnea and tachypnea and PEFR 50%–79% predicted)
   (a) Continue with inhaled or nebulized SABAs q3–4h. Consider albuterol/ipratropium nebulized, especially if patient is a current/past smoker.
   (b) OGC 60 mg initially in office and then prednisone 40–60 mg daily for 3–7 days.
   (c) Remove any allergens/irritants that were causing symptoms.
   (d) Continue to measure PEFR every hour (if possible).
   (e) Oxygen by mask to keep pulse ox >90%. Home oxygen if needed.

C. *Deteriorating symptoms (i.e., PEFR <50% plus any of the following)*
   1. *Worsening wheeze, dyspnea, tachypnea*
   2. *Tachycardia*
   3. *Unable to speak except in short, gasping sentences*
   4. *Unable to lie flat and assumes a "tripod" position*
   5. *Using accessory muscles to breathe or has retractions*
   6. *Distant breath sounds, hyperresonance, "silent chest" (inaudible breath sounds)*
   7. *Fatigue, drowsiness, or confusion*
   8. *Cyanosis of lips and diaphoresis*

V. Diagnostic testing during exacerbations (if indicated)
   A. *Do not attempt diagnostic testing if patient is in dire distress*
   B. WBC may be elevated indicating infective process
   C. Pulse ox continuously to evaluate hypoxia (if available)
   D. CXR to evaluate for pneumonia or mass
   E. Complete metabolic profile to evaluate electrolytes, kidney/liver function
   F. PEFR/Spirometry to monitor improvement in treatment process

VI. *When to refer for consultation or co-management to pulmonologist, allergist, or ENT specialist*
   A. *Any patient ≤12 yr of age requiring ICS + LABA*
   B. *Has been in hospital >2 times or had >2 bursts of OGC in the last year*
   C. *Poor control or unresponsiveness to current treatment*
   D. *There is a question as to correct diagnosis of asthma*
   E. *Other physical anatomical restrictions causing poor control of asthma (e.g., nasal polyps, chronic URI, COPD, vocal cord dysfunction)*
   F. *Unknown severe environmental/occupational allergy triggers (referral to allergist for testing and management of medications)*

VII. Allergen control measures
   A. Because environmental stimuli exacerbate asthma, allergen control is important. These measures can be beneficial for any allergy-induced symptoms; they must be used daily at home and other places where the person spends a lot of time.
   B. Outdoor allergens
      1. Determine if there is a particular aggravating season.

■ = *not to be missed;* ● = *non-urgent referral;* ▲ = *urgent referral*

  2. Keep windows closed; use air conditioning with ultrasensitive filters.
  3. When in a car, keep windows up and use air conditioning.
  4. Limit outdoor activity to late evening; wear a mask if doing yard work.
  5. Have patient leave shoes outside when coming inside and wash hands after putting shoes on or taking shoes off.
C. Indoor allergens
  1. Wear a mask when vacuuming or cleaning draperies.
  2. Limit the number of houseplants at home.
  3. Dust mite control includes the following:
     (a) Covering or encasing mattresses and pillows with plastic dust proof covers
     (b) Using filter over air ducts, especially in bedroom
     (c) Washing bedding weekly in hot water (e.g., temperature >130°)
     (d) Replacing bedroom carpets with hardwood floors or linoleum
     (e) Vacuuming house and bedroom carpets frequently using HEPA ultra-sensitive filters to remove pet dander and dust; consider having ducts cleaned and changing air intake filters quarterly.
     (f) Removing any upholstered pieces of furniture and other dust collectors.
  4. Decreasing humidity in the house, especially in the bedroom.
  5. Limiting exposure to cockroaches and their feces using the following measures:
     (a) Promptly cleaning up after meals and sealing all food sources and dishes tightly
     (b) Sealing gaps around the kitchen and bathroom pipes
     (c) Using either OTC roach bait stations or professional extermination
     (d) If using "insect spray," stay out of room until odor has resolved
  6. Cat and dog allergens are other possible causes.
     (a) If possible, remove cats and/or dogs from the environment; if not possible, keep pets out of the bedroom and off frequently used furniture.
     (b) Minimize contact with animals whenever possible.
     (c) Wash pets weekly in water to decrease dander and loose hair, and check for fleas or ticks.
  7. Stop smoking and avoid second-hand smoke; do not allow smoking in the house.
  8. Clean any moldy surfaces and food preparation areas with bleach solution.

PRACTICE PEARLS FOR ASTHMA

- Inhaled corticosteroids DO NOT affect long-term growth in children.
- Inhaled low-dose corticosteroids are the best treatment for adults who have to use SABAs >2 times a wk for symptom control.
- *Always taper to lowest effective dose* of inhaled corticosteroids, but do not be afraid to increase dose if needed. You can always taper later.
- The use of systemic prednisone (40–60 mg daily for 3–5 days) will generally improve symptoms of acute asthma and reduce the risk of relapse.
- SABA use
  - Nebulized or inhaled albuterol is preferred over the liquid oral form (which causes severe irritability).
  - Nebulized SABA may be more beneficial than inhaled during an exacerbation.
  - If more than two SABA inhaler canisters are used a month, asthma control is in question.
  - Use albuterol inhaler 15 min before activity to control the symptoms of exercise-induced asthma (EIA).
- Patients should not trust the "float" test to determine fullness of the inhalers (not accurate); most new inhalers have counters on the canister.
- Always use a spacer device with inhalers (especially with children). This delivers about 30% more medication into the lungs. This is a separate prescription.

TABLE 7.2 ■ **Drugs for Asthma**

Drug	Adult Dose	Child Dose (Use of Spacer Will Improve Delivery of Drug)
Drugs for Asthma		
Inhaled SABA Rescue or Maintenance		
Albuterol MDI 90 mcg	2 inhalations q4–6h prn	>4 yr of age:
	2 inhalations 15–30 min before exercise	1–2 inhalations q4–6h prn
	2–8 puffs q 20 min initially for exacerbations	2 inhalations 15–30 min before exercise
Albuterol nebulized solution 0.083%: 2.5–5 mg/3 mL	2.5–5 mg/3 mL q4–6h prn (rescue) 2.5–5 mg/3 mL q20 min x3 doses, then q3–4h until symptoms resolve with exacerbations	>5 yr of age: 2.5 mg/3 mL q4–6h prn (rescue) >12 yr of age: use adult dose
Levalbuterol (Xopenex) nebulized solution 1.25 mg/3 mL, 0.63 mg/3 mL	0.63–1.25 mg/3 mL tid prn	6–11 yr of age: 0.31–0.63 mg/3 mL tid prn >12 yr of age: use adult dose
Levalbuterol (Xopenex HFA) 45 mcg	2 inhalations q4–6h prn	>4 yr of age: 2 inhalations q4–6h prn
ICS[†] (Asthma Maintenance) start with lowest effective dose and increase or decrease as needed		
Beclomethasone MDI (Qvar RediHaler) 40 mcg/inhalation 80 mcg/inhalation	1–4 inhalations bid	4–11 yr of age: 1 inhalation q12h and increase as needed >12 yr of age: use adult dose
Budesonide DPI (Pulmicort Flexhaler) 90 mcg/inhalation 180 mcg/inhalation	2 inhalations bid	≥6 yr of age: use adult dose
Budesonide respules (nebulized) 0.25 mg/2 mL 0.5 mg/2 mL ***Do not mix in nebulizer with other nebulized medications***	0.5 mg/2 mL q6h	>6 yr of age: 0.25 mg/2 mL daily to bid
Ciclesonide HFA (Alvesco) 80 mcg/inhalation 160 mcg/inhalation	1 inhalation bid	>12 yr of age: use adult dose
Fluticasone propionate[†] HFA (Flovent) 44 mcg/inhalation 110 mcg/inhalation 220 mcg/inhalation	2–4 inhalations bid	4–11 yr of age: 2 inhalation bid (start with 44 mcg) >12 yr of age: use adult dose
Fluticasone propionate DPI (Flovent diskus) 50 mcg/inhalation 100 mcg/inhalation 250 mcg/inhalation	1–2 inhalations bid	4–11 yr of age: 1 inhalation bid (start with 50mcg) >12 yr of age: use adult dose
Fluticasone propionate (ArmonAir RespiClick) 55 mcg/inhalation 113 mcg/inhalation 232 mcg/inhalation	1 inhalation q12h	>12 yr of age: use adult dose

Continued

■ = *not to be missed*

TABLE 7.2 ■ Drugs for Asthma—cont'd

Drug	Adult Dose	Child Dose (Use of Spacer Will Improve Delivery of Drug)
Fluticasone furoate (Arnuity Ellipta) 50 mcg/inhalation 100 mcg/inhalation 200 mcg/inhalation	1 inhalations daily	5–11 yr of age: 1 inhalation daily (start with 50 mcg) >12 yr of age: use adult dose
Mometasone HFA (Asmanex) 50 mcg/inhalation (HFA) 100 mcg/inhalation (HFA) 200 mcg/inhalation (HFA) 220 mcg/inhalation (Twisthaler)	2 inhalations q12h	5–11 yr of age: 2 inhalation q12h (start with 50 mcg) >12 yr of age: use adult dose
Combination of LABA and ICS† (Maintenance Asthma Only) ***Do not use LABA as monotherapy***		
Fluticasone/salmeterol* (Advair Diskus) 100/50 mcg 250/50 mcg 500/50 mcg	1 inhalation q12h Start with lowest effective dose and increase as needed	4–11 yr of age: 1 inhalation q12h, start with 100/50 mcg ≥12 yr of age: use adult dose
Mometasone/formoterol (Dulera) MDI 50/5 mcg 100/5 mcg 200/5 mcg	2 inhalations bid Start at lowest effective dose; if already requiring two maintenance medications, start with higher dose	5–11 yr of age: 2 inhalations bid, start with 50/5 mcg >12 yr of age: 2 inhalations, start with adult dose
Budesonide/formoterol (Symbicort) MDI 80/4.5 mcg 160/4.5 mcg	2 inhalations bid Start with lowest effective dose and then increase if needed after 2 wk	6–11 yr of age: 2 inhalations bid, start with 80/4.5 mcg >12 yr of age: use adult dose
Fluticasone furoate/vilanterol (Breo Ellipta) 100/25 mcg 200/25 mcg	1 inhalation daily	Not available
LTRA (Asthma Maintenance)		
Montelukast (Singulair) 4 and 5 mg chewable 10 mg tablet	10 mg at hs	2–5 yr of age: 4 mg hs 6–14 yr of age: 5 mg hs >15 yr of age: 10 mg hs *EIA*: 6–14 yr of age: start 5 mg ~2 hr before exercise >15 yr of age: EIA, start 10 mg ~2 hr before exercise
Zafirlukast (Accolate) 10 mg tab 20 mg tab	20 mg bid Take 1 hr before or 2 hr after meals	5–11 yr of age: 10 mg bid, 1 hr before or 2 hr after meals >12 yr of age: use adult dose
Zileuton (Zyflo) (Zyflo CR) 600 mg tablet	600 mg qid 600 mg CR 2 tabs bid; give <1 hr after am and pm meals	>12 yr of age: use adult dose
Other Medications to Consider for Asthma		
Theophylline	Dosing individualized; refer to pharmacology reference of choice Monitor drug and liver enzymes	Dosing individualized; refer to pharmacology reference of choice Monitor drug and liver enzymes
Systemic oral steroids	5–60 mg/day Usually given as "burst" therapy; start with a high dose and taper down over 5–7 or 10–14 days depending on symptoms	1–2 mg/kg/day Usually given as "burst" therapy for 5 days; start with a high dose and taper down over 10–14 days

■ = *not to be missed*

TABLE 7.3 ■ Drugs for Chronic Obstructive Pulmonary Disease

Drug	Adult dose	Considerations
Drugs for COPD (Adults only)		
SABA (Rescue or Maintenance Therapy)		
Albuterol MDI 90 mcg/inhalation	Maintenance: 2 inhalations qid and/or prn Exacerbation: 2–8 inhalations q20min initially	Side effects are nervousness, anxiety, and tachypnea If using routinely, should consider daily LABA or LAMA
Albuterol nebulized solution 0.083%: 2.5–5 mg/3 mL	Rescue: 2.5–5 mg/3 mL q4–6h prn Acute exacerbation: 2.5–5 mg/3 mL q20minx3 doses, then q3–4h prn	Side effects are nervousness, anxiety, and tachypnea
Levalbuterol (Xopenex) nebulized solution 1.25 mg/3 mL, 0.63 mg/3 mL	0.63–1.25 mg/3 mL tid prn	Fewer and less intense side effects than albuterol
Levalbuterol (Xopenex HFA) 45 mcg/inhalation	2 inhalations q4–6h prn	Fewer side effects and less intense than albuterol
SAMA		
Ipratropium (Atrovent HFA) 17 mcg/inhalation	2 inhalations qid	Combining with SABA will improve symptom control
Ipratropium nebulized 0.5 mg/2.5 mL	0.2 mg/mL q6–8h	Can mix with albuterol neb solution May cause paradoxical bronchospasm
SABA+SAMA		
Ipratropium bromide/albuterol (Combivent respimat) 20 mcg/100 mcg/inhalation	1 inhalation qid	Routine use is acceptable as long as symptoms are controlled Can use the meds in separate inhalers with same dose schedule (depends on cost)
Ipratropium/albuterol nebulized 0.5 mg/2.5 mg/3 mL	3 mL qid	Depending on cost, can mix individual albuterol and ipratropium tubules with same results
LABA		
Salmeterol* (Serevent) 50 mcg	1 inhalation q12h	Use as initial treatment for mild COPD
Formoterol* (Perforomist) 20 mcg/2 mL nebulizer	2 mL q12h	Use as initial treatment for mild or moderate COPD
Arformoterol (Brovana) 15 mcg/2 mL nebulizer	2 mL q12h	
Olodaterol (Striverdi respimat) 2.5 mcg/inhalation	2 inhalations daily	
LAMA*		
Tiotropium Spiriva respimat: 2.5 mcg/ inhalation Spiriva handihaler: 18.6 mcg/cap	Respimat: 2 inhalation daily Handihaler: 2 inhalations (1 cap) daily	LAMAs alone may prevent more exacerbations
Aclidinium (Tudorza pressair) 400 mcg/inhalation	1 inhalation q12h	Improves QOL and reduces exacerbations
Umeclidinium (Incruse Ellipta) DPI 62.5 mcg/inhalation	1 inhalation daily	Can be used for long-term maintenance
Glycopyrrolate (Lonhala Magnair) nebulized 25 mcg/1 mL	25 mcg nebulized bid	Do not use with other SAMA/LAMAs

Continued

TABLE 7.3 ■ Drugs for Chronic Obstructive Pulmonary Disease—cont'd

Drug	Adult dose	Considerations
Combination LABA+LAMA		
Glycopyrrolate/formoterol (Bevespi Aerosphere) 9/4.8 mcg/inhalation	2 inhalations bid	Can be used for moderate to severe COPD
Tiotropium/olodaterol (Stiolto Respimat) 2.5/2.5 mcg/inhalation	2 inhalations daily	
Umeclidinium/vilanterol (Anoro Ellipta) 62.5/25 mcg/inhalation	1 inhalation daily	
Combination LABA+LAMA+ICS[†]		
Fluticasone/umeclidinium/vilanterol (Trelegy Ellipta) 100/62.5/25 mcg/dose	1 inhalation daily	Can be used for long term maintenance control for moderate to very severe COPD
Budesonide/glycopyrrolate/ formoterol (Breztri Aerosphere) MDI 160 mcg/9 mcg/4.8 mcg per inhalation	2 inhalations bid	Can be used for long term maintenance control for moderate to very severe COPD
Combination LABA/ICS[†]		
Formoterol/budesonide (Symbicort) 160/4.5 mcg/inhalation	2 inhalations bid	Can be used for severe or very severe COPD with exacerbations
Fluticasone/salmeterol* Advair diskus 250/50 mcg, 500/50 mcg/inhalation	1 inhalation bid Start at 250/50 mcg/spray and increase as needed	Can be used with LAMA (triple therapy) for frequent exacerbations and/or poor control of symptoms
Fluticasone furoate/vilanterol (Breo Ellipta) DPI 100/25 mcg/inhalation	1 inhalation daily	
Other Medications for Worsening COPD		
Roflumilast (Daliresp)	Start with 250 mcg daily×4 wk then ↑ to 500 mcg daily	Phosphodiesterase-4 inhibitor Used for very severe COPD with exacerbations
Azithromycin 250 mg daily	With acute exacerbations use azithromycin (5-day ZPAK)	For severe to very severe COPD, can also be given 1 tab daily for maintenance
Oral prednisone	Can be given in "burst" of 40 mg daily × 5 days for acute exacerbations or 2.5–10 daily routinely (when all other treatments have failed)	Burst therapy useful with onset of exacerbations Continuous therapy for very severe and uncontrolled COPD (may or may not help to control symptoms) Attempt to wean down frequently
Theophylline 100–600 mg	Dosing individualized; refer to pharmacology reference of choice	Side effects based on dose Recommend routine monthly evaluation of drug levels Only used with stable COPD Not recommended unless other long-term bronchodilators have been ineffective or not available due to cost
Oxygen therapy	As needed to maintain pulse ox >90%	Used for resting hypoxemia either continuous or minimum 15 hr/day

* Contraindicated with soy, milk, or peanut allergy.
[†] Rinse mouth after use.

CHRONIC OBSTRUCTIVE PULMONARY DISEASE

I. Description

    A. It is an obstructive airway disease that is not fully reversible and is progressive.

    B. Goals for treatment are to decrease symptoms (e.g., dyspnea, increase exercise tolerance), decrease exacerbations with fewer hospitalizations, and improve health status and mortality.

    C. Common findings of chronic bronchitis and emphysema:

        1. Chronic bronchitis is seen with obstruction of small airways and productive cough >3 mo at a time over a 2 yr period.

            (a) Skin has a bluish tinge from hypoxemia and hypercapnia (blue bloater)

            (b) Peripheral edema secondary to HF

            (c) Chronic cough with large amounts of sputum produced

        2. Emphysema is characterized by loss of lung elasticity and enlargement of air spaces.

            (a) Patient appears more cachectic

            (b) Pink skin color due to more normal oxygenation (pink puffer)

            (c) SOB, tripod posturing, and pursed-lip breathing

    D. *There is no cure*—only management of disease processes with lifestyle changes and medications.

II. Causative factors

    A. Chronic exposures to tobacco smoke, air pollution, airway infections, and dust and chemical exposures from environmental sources

    B. Familial factors or hereditary factors (i.e., alpha-1-antitrypsin glycoprotein)

    C. Allergy predisposition and hyperresponsiveness

III. Signs and symptoms usually occur in midlife with slow progression

    A. Most common symptoms associated with COPD

        1. Chronic cough, usually worse in the mornings; may have rhonchi, hyper-resonant breath sounds or wheezes

        2. Chronic sputum production: excessive clear to white amount

        3. Progressive, persistent dyspnea with any activity or at rest

        4. May also have wheezing and chest tightness in later stages

        5. Spirometry shows $FEV_1/FVC < 70\%$ predicted and it is not significantly reversible with bronchodilator (see Table 7.1).

    B. As the disease progresses, the patient will often experience

        1. Weight gain or loss (weight loss usually seen in advanced disease)

        2. Progressive limitation of daily activity and loss of exercise tolerance

        3. Depression/anxiety

        4. "Cough syncope"

        5. Frequent viral or bacterial URIs

        6. Tripod positioning when sitting upright

    C. In the end stages of COPD, symptoms are severe with

        1. Feelings of anxiousness, impending doom

        2. Complete dependence on oxygen therapy

        3. Unable to hold a conversation

        4. Barrel chest appearance with clubbing of fingers and toes

        5. Central cyanosis and cachexia (later signs)

        6. Cor pulmonale

IV. Diagnostic tests

    A. PFT is the gold standard for diagnosing COPD (see Table 7.1)

1. PFT/office spirometry (using pre- and post-bronchodilator administration) should be done annually to monitor progression of disease.
2. After any increase in symptoms.
3. Any time there is decrease in exercise tolerance.

B. Can use COPD Assessment Test (CAT) and/or Modified MRC dyspnea scale (mMRC) at each visit to assess for quality of life and for progression of dyspnea (both found at GOLD guideline at *www.goldcopd.org*). These tests are not diagnostic for COPD but help to guide treatment and determine the severity of the limitations.
   1. CAT is used to assess the perceived effects/impact of COPD on daily life and health status.
   2. mMRC is used to assess the perceived effect of dyspnea during ADLs.
C. Obtain baseline pulse ox, which may be <88%–90%; goal is to maintain pulse ox above 90%. If considering oxygen therapy, pulse ox at rest must be <88% and improve to >88% with oxygen therapy for insurance/Medicare reimbursement.
D. Chest X-ray: has poor sensitivity for finding COPD but could show hyperinflation and air trapping with flattening of diaphragm and bullae.
E. Offer low-dose CT to all current asymptomatic (italics for asymptomatic) smokers between 55–77 yr of age and those having quit within past 15 yr.
F. CBC may show
   1. Elevated HCT, which increases risk for PE/DVT.
   2. If eosinophils are elevated ≥300 cells/µL, ICS may be beneficial in decreasing exacerbations.
G. 6-min walk test

V. Lifestyle changes to improve survival rates
   A. Smoking cessation can reduce the rate of decline in lung function; to help with smoking cessation
      1. Smoking cessation classes
      2. Long-acting nicotine patches + prn nicotine gum or lozenges
      3. Can consider bupropion for the anxiety related to smoking cessation
      4. Strong recommendation for smoking cessation for all in close proximity to patient
   B. Encourage patient to wear a mask when working with irritants, fumes, or particulate matter (e.g., painting, lawn mowing).
   C. Avoid temperature extremes: if not possible, wear protective cover over the mouth and nose in cold temperatures.
   D. Increase humidification at home, especially in the winter.
   E. Bronchial hygiene with pursed-lip breathing and deep breathing exercises before coughing and at bedtime.
   F. Increase fluids if not contraindicated because of HF.
   G. Participate in pulmonary rehab program when first diagnosed and 4 wk after any exacerbations.
   H. Use oxygen daily and at night, if needed to maintain oxygen level >90%.
   I. Encourage COVID vaccine, annual flu shot and the pneumonia shot(s) (see Chapter 3, PRACTICE PEARLS FOR RESPIRATORY SYSTEM for current recommendations).
   J. Encourage exercise as tolerated.

VI. At each visit, discuss
   A. Smoking status.
   B. Dyspnea (at rest, with exertion), cough (normal or worsening), sputum production (color and amount) and sleep quality.

   C. Use of oxygen, what liter flow rate, how often used (e.g., is it continuous or intermittent, with activity or at rest), and the delivery system (continuous or on demand).
   D. Review CAT or mMRC results and document.
   E. Discuss any hospitalizations and/or exacerbations of COPD.
   F. Were there any treatment changes? What were they?
   G. Have there been any medication changes and what were they? Can the patient afford their medications?
   H. Review last spirometry results.
   I. Review cost of medications; also how to use inhaler or nebulizer based on patient's physical and mental ability.
   J. Develop, discuss, and review COPD "action plan" (refer to *www.lung.org/assets/documents/copd/copd-action-plan.pdf*).

VII. Treatment of COPD based on levels of COPD (see Table 7.1 for Spirometry and Table 7.3 for Medications)
   A. See Fig. 7.1 for Quick Reference for COPD staging/treatment.
   B. *Mild COPD*: based on spirometry (see Table 7.1) with no exacerbation and no COPD hospitalizations, with CAT score <10 or mMRC 0–1 within last year
      1. Having only mild intermittent symptoms (e.g., dyspnea with strenuous exercise; fair exercise tolerance).
      2. SABA, SAMA, or SABA/SAMA combination inhaler (see Table 7.3) to control intermittent dyspnea and for rescue use.
      3. If dyspnea not controlled, consider LABA routinely.
      4. Overnight pulse ox, and if indicated, consider nocturnal O_2 if ≤88% predicted for more than 5 min in 2 hr time period.
      5. Consider sleep study for apnea.
   C. *Moderate COPD*: based on spirometry (see Table 7.1) with ≤1 exacerbation and no COPD hospitalizations, with CAT score ≥10 or mMRC ≥2 within last year
      1. Dyspneic symptoms with walking slowly and must stop frequently to "catch breath" on level ground; symptoms are worse with walking on incline.
      2. Start with either a LAMA (LAMA may decrease number of exacerbations) *or* LABA routinely based on symptoms (see Table 7.3).
      3. Use SABA, SAMA, or SABA/SAMA inhaler for rescue (see Table 7.3).
      4. If poor control (e.g., SOB/dyspnea) with single LABA or LAMA, can use combination inhaler with LABA + LAMA (see Table 7.3).
      5. Recommend oxygen with activity (if needed) and continuous oxygen at bedtime to maintain pulse ox >90%.
      6. Consider pulmonary rehabilitation program.
   D. *Severe COPD*: based on spirometry (see Table 7.1) with ≥2 exacerbations and/or ≥1 COPD hospitalization, with CAT score ≤10 or mMRC ≤1 within last year
      1. Continuous oxygen with activity and at bedtime; may not need when resting.
      2. Dyspnea worsens when exercising on level ground or walking up slight incline.
      3. Regular treatment with LAMA, and if continued poor control (e.g., SOB/dyspnea or exacerbations), add LABA (see Table 7.3).
      4. Consider blood eosinophils to see ICS will be beneficial.
      5. Consider adding ICS if LABA + LAMA (see Table 7.3) not controlling symptoms and/or with frequent exacerbations, history of asthma, or ↑ risk of pneumonia; *discontinue* ICS at earliest opportunity and monitor symptoms.
      6. Continue SABA/SAMA for control of exacerbations even when using LABA + LAMA routinely.

7. Consider noninvasive positive pressure respiratory assist devices (NiPPRA), such as BiPAP or HMV; must have documented criteria for Medicare/insurance to cover:
   (a) Hypercapnia ($PaCO_2 \geq 52$ mmHg) with oxygen ≥ 2 L/min
   (b) Hypoxia ($PaO_2 \leq 60$ mmHg) on oxygen ≥ 2 L/min
   (c) $FEV_1 < 50\%$ predicted
   (d) Nocturnal desaturation of $\leq 88\%$ for at least 5 min while on oxygen ≥ 2 L/min
   (e) Positive use of NiPPRA while in hospital during exacerbation of COPD

Quick Reference COPD treatment chart

MILD	MODERATE
Mild, infrequent dyspnea, worsens with strenuous activity or walking fast FEV_1 >80% predicted CAT score* <10 mMRC score* 0–1 Exacerbations ≤1 OR No COPD hospitalizations	Has to stop and "catch breath" while walking on level ground and walks slower due to dyspnea, mild exercise intolerance FEV_1 50–79% predicted CAT score* ≥10 mMRC score* ≥2 Exacerbations ≤1 AND No COPD hospitalizations
No need for supplemental oxygen Start with SABA inhaler (Proventil HFA) intermittently or routinely as needed to control symptoms	May need oxygen at bedtime Daily treatment with either LAMA or LABA Continue with SABA inhaler or consider SAMA inhaler or combination SABA/SAMA inhaler
SEVERE	**VERY SEVERE**
Has breathlessness with strenuous exercise and mild dyspnea at rest; moderate decrease in exercise tolerance FEV_1 30–49% predicted CAT score* ≤10 mMRC score* 0–1 Exacerbations ≥2/yr AND/OR COPD hospitalization ≥1/yr	Worsening dyspnea with walking any speed or on level ground, severe exercise intolerance FEV_1 <30% predicted CAT score* ≥10 mMRC score* ≥2 Exacerbations ≥2/yr AND/OR COPD hospitalizations ≥1
Oxygen at rest and at bedtime Daily treatment LAMA and based on symptoms, add LABA for control Continue SABA, SAMA or combination inhaler and may need to consider nebulized medications	Continuous oxygen Daily treatment with LAMA or LAMA/LABA combination If symptoms poorly controlled, consider ICS/LABA/LAMA combination or single ICS with above daily treatment Continue SABA/SAMA inhaler or switch to nebulized medications If exacerbations and hospitalizations continue, consider daily roflumilast (Daliresp) and/or daily antibiotic May need short course(s) of oral prednisone

*See CHRONIC OBSTRUCTIVE PULMONARY DISEASE, IV, B.

■ **Fig. 7.1** Quick reference for COPD staging/treatment *(see also* Table 7.2 *and CHRONIC OBSTRUCTIVE PULMONARY DISEASE).*

■ = *not to be missed*

    E. *Very severe COPD*: based on spirometry (see Table 7.1) with ≥2 exacerbations and/
       or ≥1 COPD hospitalization, with CAT score ≥10 or mMRC ≥2 within last year
       1. Symptoms of dyspnea limiting QOL with very poor exercise tolerance.
       2. Regular treatment with LAMA/LABA (see Table 7.3) for better control of
          persistent symptoms, considering adding ICS.
       3. Use LABA + ICS if positive for asthma.
       4. Can still use SABA/SAMA (see Table 7.3) for control of exacerbations even
          when using LABA + LAMA routinely.
       5. *Discontinue* ICS at earliest opportunity unless this is controlling symptoms.
       6. Continuous oxygen.
       7. Consider roflumilast (Daliresp) if FEV_1 <50% predicted with chronic bronchitis
          and continued exacerbations and hospitalizations.
       8. Consider daily macrolide (especially with smokers) to prevent hospitalizations
          and decrease exacerbations.
       9. Consider nebulized medications if person cannot physically use inhaler, or has
          low inspiratory flow rate or cannot afford inhalers.
      10. Consider NiPPV (BiPAP or HMV) at home (see D. 7., above).

VIII. Control comorbidities
    A. Smoking: encourage and educate that smoking cessation is critical to patient's health
       and will *slow* progression of disease
    B. Anxiety: consider antidepressant or antianxiety medications at hs (see Tables 17.1
       and 17.2)
    C. Malnourished or underweight (based on BMI)
       1. Encourage high-protein foods and small frequent meals.
       2. Monitor weight monthly as the disease progresses.
       3. Nighttime dose of mirtazapine 7.5 mg can stimulate appetite.
    D. End-of-life care and palliative care
       1. This should be approached as early as possible, especially when patient is classified
          as having severe to very severe COPD.
       2. Advanced directives and Personal Will should be completed with or without
          family involvement in decision-making.
    E. Asthma: make sure patient is taking/using correct medications
    F. Diabetes
       1. Monitor A_{1c} routinely.
       2. Discuss diet and activity.
       3. As patient loses weight or becomes more debilitated, may need to reduce doses of
          medications.
    G. GERD is associated with increased risk for exacerbations.
       1. Symptoms can simulate chest tightness and cause cough; control reflux symptoms
          to decrease cough reflex.
       2. Start with H_2 blockers (see Chapter 9, Upper Abdominal Conditions,
          GASTROESOPHAGEAL REFLUX DISEASE (GERD)) daily or bid, and
          if still uncontrolled with medication and diet adjustment, consider PPIs daily or
          alternate with H_2 blocker daily.
    H. Osteoarthritis
       1. There is a direct correlation between fractures and COPD due to smoking, non-
          weight-bearing activity, low BMI, and steroid use.
       2. Encourage diet high in calcium (see Appendix A) and calcium/vitamin D
          supplements 1 bid.
       3. BMD every 2 yr and patient may need bisphosphonates.

IX. Management of exacerbations
- **A.** Acute worsening of CARDINAL SYMPTOMS (*worsening dyspnea, increased sputum volume, sputum purulence*), not controlled with current medications, indicates impending exacerbation
  1. Mild exacerbation: one of the above cardinal symptoms
  2. Moderate to severe exacerbation: 2 out of 3 cardinal symptoms
- **B.** Other symptoms related to acute exacerbation
  1. Chest tightness
  2. Fluid retention and HF
  3. Wheeze
  4. Fatigue and "doesn't feel well"
  5. Inability to hold a conversation due to SOB
- **C.** Evaluate risk factors leading to poor outpatient outcomes with treatment
  1. Antibiotic use within last 3 mo
  2. >2 exacerbations leading to hospitalization within the last yr
  3. FEV_1 <50% predicted
  4. Continued smoking
  5. Nonadherence to oxygen therapy at home
  6. >60 yr of age
  7. Co-morbidity (e.g., DM, CVD, HTN)
- ▲ **D.** *Indications for hospitalization (recommend urgent transfer to ED)*
  1. *Sudden, severe worsening of symptoms with resting dyspnea, ↑ respiratory rate, ↓ oxygen level (pulse ox <90%), confusion*
  2. *Changing or worsening in peripheral edema, cyanosis*
  3. *Failure to respond to treatments*
  4. *History of comorbidities under poor control (e.g., HF, arrhythmias, DM)*
  5. *Lack of home support*
- **E.** Pharmacological treatment for exacerbations (see Table 7.3)
  1. Initiate oxygen therapy with targeted pulse ox 88%–92%.
  2. Increase the frequency of SABA and may add SAMA (nebulizer may work better than inhaler based on severity of symptoms).
     - (a) SABA works even with LABA.
     - (b) If already using tiotropium, consider using SABA, instead of SAMA.
     - (c) Dose SABA 6–8 puffs (with spacer) or nebulizer every 30 min to 2 hr.
     - (d) Dose SAMA (ipratropium) 6–8 puffs (with spacer) q3–4h or use nebulizer every 30 min to 2 hr.
  3. If no response or poor response, add OGC for 5 days (e.g., oral prednisone 40 mg daily).
  4. If all three of the CARDINAL SYMPTOMS (see A, above) are present or if two are present with one being sputum purulence, will likely need antibiotic for 5–7 days (evaluate local resistance patterns for choice in antibiotic); for mild to moderate outpatient exacerbation
     - (a) No risk factors (see C, above) and no pseudomonas suspected
       - (i) Azithromycin 500 mg day one then 250 mg days 2–4 days
       - (ii) Clarithromycin 500 mg q12h
       - (iii) Cefuroxime 500 mg bid
       - (iv) Cefdinir 300 mg daily
     - (b) Positive risk factors (see C above) but no pseudomonas suspected
       - (i) Amoxicillin/clavulanic acid 875/125 mg bid
       - (ii) Moxifloxacin 400 mg daily

■ = *not to be missed;* ▲ = *urgent referral*

        (iii) Levofloxacin 500 mg daily (based on kidney function)

    (c) Positive risk factors (see above) and probable pseudomonas

        (i) Ciprofloxacin 750 mg q12h

        (ii) Levofloxacin 500 mg daily (based on kidney function)

F. Outpatient management after numerous exacerbations/hospitalizations

  1. Consider roflumilast (Daliresp) 500 mcg daily

    (a) May cause gastrointestinal (GI) upset

    (b) Start with ½ tab 2× wk and gradually increase to once daily in the evening over about 3 mo

  2. Azithromycin 250 mg daily may be needed to decrease number of exacerbations, especially if past or current smoker, on maximum LAMA + LABA + ICS regimen and supplemental oxygen.

  3. Start mucolytic agents daily to try to decrease exacerbations by increasing mucus mobility

    (a) Guaifenesin (Mucinex OTC) 600 mg bid

    (b) Guaifenesin + dextromethorphan (Mucinex DM OTC) 2 tsp q4h

  4. Consider BiPAP or HMV (NiPPV) (see above criteria Section VII, C, 7).

X. *Refer to pulmonologist if poorly controlled and/or treatment failure*

PRACTICE PEARLS FOR COPD

- COPD is not curable only manageable; treatment guidelines are just that. Keep the patient comfortable with lifestyle changes and medications. You may have to increase and decrease medications to maintain control.
- Smoking is the number one factor that contributes to COPD and many of your patients will continue to smoke! This is their choice and you need to try encourage them to stop smoking, but they still need medical attention. It is very frustrating for the provider.
- ICS + LABA are more effective together than individually.
- LABA or LAMA are preferred over SABA, SAMA, or SABA/SAMA for daily use, unless patient symptoms are very mild and only need rescue treatment.
- You can use SABA for rescue even when on LABA.
- Triple therapy (ICS + LABA + LAMA) has been shown to improve lung function, improve overall health status and decrease exacerbations.
- Long-term OGC show no true benefits and have long-term side effects; short courses of OGC (3–7 days) have been shown to decrease exacerbations.
- Daily long-term use of azithromycin (e.g., 250 mg daily or 500 mg 3 times a wk) has been shown to decrease number of exacerbations but can increase bacterial resistance, decrease hearing and prolong QT.
- Blood eosinophils >300 cells/µL can help to identify patient with greatest benefit profile for continuous ICS use.
- NiPPV (BiPAP, HMV) has been shown to decrease mortality and morbidity and prolong need for readmission with exacerbation.

COMMUNITY-ACQUIRED PNEUMONIA (CAP)

I. Definition: acute pulmonary infection in a person not recently hospitalized

  A. Bacterial causes: *Streptococcus pneumoniae* (most common bacteria and is common after influenza), *Haemophilus influenzae* (typically seen in smokers and in children of smokers), or *Moraxella catarrhalis* (may resolve without treatment, if person is healthy)

  B. Atypical causes: *Mycoplasma pneumoniae*, *Legionella*, and respiratory viruses

---

● = *non-urgent referral*

II. Signs and symptoms
   A. Specific signs and symptoms
      1. Bacterial (typically): sudden onset and rapid progression of fever, rigors, cough with purulent sputum production, pleuritic chest pain, and lobar consolidation on imaging
      2. Atypical: signs usually present with scant or watery sputum and may show interstitial infiltrates on chest X-ray
   B. General symptoms of CAP
      1. Tachypnea (most sensitive sign with the elderly) with RR >24, tachycardia, cyanosis
      2. Fever (may not be present in the elderly), malaise, myalgia
      3. Exertional dyspnea, pain in posterior thorax with inspiration, hypoxia
      4. Anorexia; possible abdominal pain, N/V/D, or weight loss
      5. Decreased breath sounds, wheezing, rhonchi, crackles that do not clear with cough
      6. Egophony ("e" to "a" sound) on auscultation, pleural friction rub, dullness to percussion
      7. Decline in functional and mental status commonly seen in the elderly as presenting symptoms

III. Diagnostic testing
   A. Pulse ox (normally, should be >95% on room air and should not drop with exertion)
   B. Consider CBC (i.e., if the patient is >65 yr of age, comorbidity exists, or possible hospital admission)
      1. Leukocytosis with left shift may indicate bacterial infection; elderly people may not have a competent immune system to generate this response.
      2. Leukopenia (leukocytes <5000 mm^3) may indicate impending sepsis.
      3. Hgb <9 mg/dL and/or Hct <30% is indicative of higher mortality.
   C. Complete metabolic profile to evaluate BUN/creatinine/GFR for kidney function; liver enzymes may be elevated with sepsis and glucose may be elevated if DM poorly controlled.
   D. CRP (if >40 mg/L could be bacterial infection).
   E. Consider test for influenza/COVID.
   F. Chest X-ray (AP and lateral) should show frank consolidation in the area of pneumonia and possible pleural effusion, or may show interstitial infiltrates if atypical pneumonia.
      1. Chest X-ray is indicated in all symptomatic patients >40 yr of age, current smokers, or past smokers; repeat chest X-ray should be obtained in 12 wk.
      2. False-negative results can occur with dehydration or within 3 days of onset of pneumonia.
      3. If the patient has positive clinical signs and symptoms with elevated suspicion of pneumonia but CXR is negative, treat the patient for pneumonia or obtain chest CT.
   G. Consider CT scan chest with atypical presentation or immunocompromised person to help differentiate causes.
   H. Sputum culture is recommended if failure to respond to treatment.

IV. Decisions on whether to admit or treat in the community are based on patient symptoms, ability to care for self at home, and accessibility of health care
   A. CURB-65 is an algorithmic tool that can be used as a good predictor of both severity of illness and possible complications that could result in death.
   B. CURB-65 criteria, 1 point each:
      1. Confusion

    2. BUN >20 (if unable to get BUN: check urine and if dark or specific gravity is elevated; add 1 point)

    3. Respiratory rate >30/min

    4. SBP <90; DBP <60

    5. Age ≥65

  C. Scoring

    1. Score of 0–1 indicates low severity of illness and could be treated as an O/P, especially if score of 1 is related to age ≥65 yr with no comorbidity.

    2. Score of 2 indicates moderate severity of illness and should be sent to hospital or close observation at home.

    3. Score of 3–4 indicates high severity of illness and admission is usually required to ICU.

V. Treatment (see Chapter 16, Lower Respiratory Tract Disorders, COMMUNITY ACQUIRED PNEUMONIA, I, II, III)

  A. No comorbidity, has been healthy, <65 yr of age and no antibiotics within the last 3 mo: give antibiotics for 5 days.

    1. Amoxicillin 1000 mg tid PLUS

    2. Azithromycin 500 mg on day one, then 250 mg daily for 4 days OR

    3. Clarithromycin 500 mg q12h

    4. If PCN allergy:

      (a) Cefuroxime 500 mg bid or cefpodoxime 200 mg daily PLUS

      (b) Doxycycline 100 mg bid or azithromycin or clarithromycin

    5. If unable to take PCN, cephalosporin, or doxycycline, use monotherapy with fluoroquinolone (see **B. 3**, below)

  B. Persons with comorbid conditions such as DM, COPD, renal or liver disease, immunosuppression, asplenia, or cancer; >65 yr of age, or have had antibiotics within the last 3 mo: give antibiotics for 5 days.

    1. Amoxicillin/clavulanate 2000 mg bid PLUS one of the following:

      (a) Azithromycin 500 mg on day one, 250 mg daily for 4 days

      (b) Clarithromycin 500 mg q12h

      (c) Doxycycline 100 mg bid

    2. If PCN allergy: cefpodoxime 200 mg daily or cefuroxime bid PLUS one of the above

    3. If unable to tolerate above medications, can use fluoroquinolone as monotherapy daily.

      (a) Moxifloxacin 400 mg

      (b) Gemifloxacin 320 mg

      (c) Levofloxacin 750 mg

  C. Antibiotics may be needed longer depending on comorbid conditions and health status, such as

    1. Age >65 yr of age, alcoholism, or multiple medical comorbidities: at risk for drug-resistant pneumococcal infection

    2. Living in a long-term care facility or with multiple medical comorbidities: at risk for infection with an enteric gram-negative organism

    3. Structural lung disease and recent broad-spectrum antibiotic use for >7 days in the last month: at risk for *Pseudomonas* infection

    4. Current exposure to daycare situations increases the risk for viral and streptococcal infections

VI. Other pharmacologic therapies

  A. Consider O_2 therapy for the duration of illness if pulse ox drops <88% at rest or with activity.

    B. NSAIDs or Tylenol for discomfort.

    C. Consider a nebulized bronchodilator (SABA), muscarinic antagonist (SAMA) and budesonide (Pulmicort) if patient is a smoker.

    D. Antitussives with nocturnal cough; consider benzonatate (Tessalon Perles) for cough during the day and possible narcotic cough suppressant at night.

    E. Because of the increased risk of recurrent pneumonia, consider stopping PPI, or switch to an H_2 blocker, for 1 mo after the illness subsides, if possible.

VII. Nonpharmacological

    A. Maintain adequate hydration, use a humidifier at home, rest as much as possible.

▲   B. Follow-up in the office in 24–48 hr, and if not improving, ***refer to ED.***

VIII. After the illness has resolved, consider annual flu vaccine and pneumococcal vaccines (if applicable) and COVID vaccine

OBSTRUCTIVE SLEEP APNEA (OSA)

I. Description

    A. Chronic airway obstruction occurring while sleeping, which disrupts normal sleep patterns and causes symptoms of chronic sleep deprivation

    B. Decreases O_2 to vital organs

    C. Can be a contributing factor for HTN, obesity, depression, and RLS

II. Risk factors

    A. Obesity (e.g., BMI >30 kg/m^2) is the primary factor

    B. Traumatic craniofacial injuries and tonsillar hypertrophy

    C. Male gender, age >40 yr of age, and smoking

    D. Type 2 DM, COPD, HF, CVA, hypothyroidism

III. Signs and symptoms

    A. Snoring and apnea periods and nocturnal restlessness are commonly noted by sleeping partner

    B. Daytime sleepiness; napping/dozing off during the day at inappropriate times (e.g., while talking, driving, eating)

    C. Poor concentration, cognitive deficits, and inattentiveness at work, school, or home

    D. Does not feel rested upon awaking and frequently has morning headaches

    E. Poor control of weight, HTN, and depression with mood swings

    F. Neck circumference >16 in. in women and >17 in. in men, and waist circumference greater than hip circumference

    G. Vivid and strange dreams, GERD, moodiness and irritability, nocturnal gasping and choking

    H. Decreased libido and impotence, nocturia

    I. Epworth Sleepiness Scale can be used to quantify patient's perception of sleepiness and is considered normal if score is ≤10/24

IV. Diagnostic testing should be considered for anyone with excessive daytime sleepiness, snoring, and especially if they work in an area that requires alertness and quick reactions (e.g., truck driver, airline pilots, bus drivers)

    A. Overnight pulse ox to determine nocturnal hypoxia; if positive, prescribe oxygen to improve alertness and QOL

    B. Home sleep apnea testing

▲ = *urgent referral*

    C. Polysomnography (gold standard for diagnosis) performed in a sleep lab; test is positive if the apnea-hypopnea index (AHI: number of apnea and hypopnea events/hr) is >5 events/hr with symptoms
      1. Mild OSA: 5–14 events/hr
      2. Moderate OSA: 15–29 events/hr
      3. Severe OSA: >30 events/hr
    D. CBC, CMP, TSH may be obtained to rule out other causes for symptoms.
  V. Treatment: ***referral to a pulmonologist or ENT depending on the cause***
  VI. Follow-up (in addition to above referral)
    A. For changes in sleep habits and feeling of refreshed sleep
    B. Monitor use of equipment that was ordered (CPAP machine); if the patient is not using their CPAP, ask why and have them contact the supplier for alternative equipment
    C. Encourage weight loss and exercise and monitor progress; send to dietician, if available
    D. BP control
    E. Decrease alcohol intake and any medications that might cause CNS depression
    F. Sleep in lateral position if possible

TUBERCULOSIS

  I. Description
    A. Primary lung infection acquired via droplets from contaminated people. Usually the TB bacterium is inhaled, the normal defense system is activated, and the bacterium is walled off without further incident; 90%–95% of TB bacteria are dormant.
    B. TB can become active when the patient's immune defenses undergo periods of stress or are fighting off current infections, with corticosteroid therapy, or with aging of the immune system.
    C. Common sites are apices of the lungs, but disseminated TB can affect any body system.
    D. The risk of TB increases with chronic disease, drug abuse, and living in a nursing home, shelter, or a crowded home with poor hygienic conditions.
    E. Early and latent TB can be asymptomatic and are best diagnosed with a TB skin test and CXR.
  II. Signs and symptoms
    A. Fatigue; unintentional weight loss, anorexia
    B. Fever (usually low grade) that peaks in late afternoon and early evening
    C. Night sweats lasting longer than 1–3 wk (no associated fever)
    D. Productive cough (initially dry, progresses to purulent; may see blood)
    E. Can have mouth/tongue ulcers, some extending into larynx and GI tract
  III. Diagnostic testing
    A. Tuberculosis skin test (TST) is a screening test only; interpret in 48–72 hr and measure *induration*, not redness. Obtain CXR with any positive TST.
      1. Induration ≥5 mm is most likely positive in a patient with any of the following:
        (a) HIV (also considered positive if ≤5 mm *and* positive for HIV)
        (b) Recent close contact with someone who has known TB
        (c) Immunosuppression therapy or immunocompromised
        (d) Chest X-ray showing old TB lesions
        (e) Fibrosis of lung or organ transplant recipient

● = *non-urgent referral*

2. Induration ≥10 mm is positive if the patient
   (a) Is a recent immigrant from a high-prevalence country (within the last 5 yr)
   (b) Is an IV drug user
   (c) Is a resident or staff of a high-risk facility (e.g., nursing home, correctional facility, hospital, homeless shelter, or works in laboratory setting)
   (d) Has a comorbid illness (e.g., DM, chronic renal or liver disease, malnourished) or is <4 yr of age exposed to adults at high risk
3. Induration ≥15 mm is usually positive; however, healthy people with no risk factors can still have positive results without having TB

B. People who have been vaccinated with BCG may have false-positive TST. Suggest using QuantiFERON-TB Gold (QFT-Plus) blood test or T-SPOT-TB (T-Spot) blood test.
1. Preferred for persons who have received BCG (TB vaccine) or person at increased risk who may fail to follow-up.
2. Positive test indicates person has been infected and will need further testing to determine if active or latent disease.

C. Chest X-ray

D. Sputum culture for acid-fast bacilli is time-consuming and difficult to obtain in a clinical setting.

IV. Treatment: identification and *referral to the health department and pulmonologist*

● = *non-urgent referral*

CHAPTER 8

Cardiovascular Conditions

For detailed history and physical examination, see Chapter 1, CARDIOVASCULAR.

Cardiac Conditions

AMBULATORY DYSRHYTHMIAS

As a general rule, significant dysrhythmias require oxygen therapy.
I. Fast rhythms
  A. Atrial fibrillation
    1. Description: irregular ventricular rhythm with absence of P waves
    2. May be paroxysmal (intermittent or lasting < 7 days), persistent (lasting > 7 days to 1 yr), or permanent (lasting > 1 yr)
    3. Increased risk with CHD, COPD, AMI, hypoxia, holiday heart syndrome (associated with excessive alcohol bingeing), hyperthyroidism, hypomagnesemia, OSA
    4. Treatment

▲   (a) *Emergency transfer to ED if the patient is hemodynamically unstable.*
      (b) Depends on the ventricular rate and how long the rhythm has been present; controlling symptoms is important, but reducing the risk of CVA is critical.
      (c) With a rapid rate, may try: a beta blocker or diltiazem; digoxin may be used, primarily in a sedentary patient > 80 yr of age.
      (d) Anticoagulation therapy should be started as soon as possible after diagnosis with high-risk patients, as documented by a CHA_2DS_2-VASc score (see Table 8.1).
        (i) Female, 3 or higher and male, 2 or higher
        (ii) Treatment choices include warfarin or direct oral anticoagulant (DOAC) (see Tables 8.20 and 8.22); DOAC is preferred over warfarin except with concomitant moderate or severe mitral stenosis or a presence of mechanical valve.

▲   5. *Referral: Patient with any new-onset (or newly diagnosed) atrial fib should be urgently referred to a cardiologist or electrophysiologist for evaluation.*
  B. Paroxysmal supraventricular tachycardia (PSVT)
    1. Description: sudden onset of regular rhythm with narrow QRS complexes and a rate usually > 150/min.
    2. Causes include CHD, medications, mitral valve prolapse, hyperthyroidism, digoxin toxicity, excessive stimulants (e.g., caffeine, ETOH, nicotine, drugs such as cocaine), Wolff-Parkinson-White (WPW) syndrome.

▲ = *urgent referral*

TABLE 8.1 ■ CHA$_2$DS$_2$-VASc Score*

Clinical Finding	Points
Diagnosed heart failure (any type)	1
HTN, treated or untreated	1
Age 65–74 yr	1
Diabetes	1
Vascular disease (e.g., MI, PAD, aortic plaque)	1
Female sex	1
Previous CVA or TIA	2
Age ≥ 75 yr	2

* For a score of ≥ 2, anticoagulation therapy should be started as soon as possible. Consider anticoagulation with a score of 1.

    3. Treatment: rhythm may terminate spontaneously or require therapy to stop.
      (a) Simple measures to try include Valsalva maneuver and cough.
      (b) Possible medications include adenosine, verapamil, diltiazem, propranolol.
      (c) ***Referral of a stable patient with newly diagnosed PSVT to cardiologist (consider an electrophysiologist, if available) as soon as possible for evaluation and treatment plan.***
      (d) Consider 48–72 hr Holter monitor or an event monitor to try to "catch" the rhythm while awaiting appointment with specialist.
    4. ***Emergency transfer to ED if the patient shows signs of hemodynamic instability.***
  C. Sinus tachycardia
    1. Description: normal components with a rate of > 100/min
    2. May be normal in children but never found in adults without a cause (e.g., fear, pain, anxiety, fever, HF, hypoxia, hyperthyroidism, hypotension, AMI, volume depletion, shock)
    3. Treatment
      (a) Treat the cause
      (b) Requires appropriate diagnostic workup after analysis of the history and possible causes
    4. ***Referral: to cardiologist if unable to detect and treat the cause***
 II. Premature ventricular complexes
  A. Description: wide QRS complexes interspersed in normal rhythm; may be occasional to frequent; also, may look similar (uniform) or different from each other (multiform).
  B. Causes include AMI, CHD, electrolyte imbalance, hypoxia, and medications
  C. Treatment
    1. Often do not require treatment, but development of ventricular tachycardia may be a concern (three or more PVCs in a row at a rate of > 100/min)
    2. PVCs should not be treated unless determined significant by a physician.
    3. Verify normal serum potassium and magnesium levels.

● = *non-urgent referral;* ▲ = *urgent referral*

      D. *Emergent transfer to ED if ventricular tachycardia develops (even in brief runs).*

III. Slow rhythms (sinus bradycardia or AV blocks)

    A. Description: ventricular rate < 60/min; if < 40/min, consider the presence of an AV block.

    B. Causes include medications, hypothyroidism, vagal response, AMI, HF, electrolyte abnormality, and athletic heart (i.e., patient in a very good physical shape).

    C. Treatment

       1. Attempt to treat the cause if possible (e.g., decrease beta blocker dose; check CMP and TSH).

       2. *If the patient is symptomatic (e.g., hypotensive, altered mentation, SOB, chest pain) or if the ventricular rate is < 40/min, consider giving atropine 0.5 mg rapidly IV (if available), while awaiting emergency transport.*

    D. *Referral: to a cardiologist if the patient is stable and the cause is not known.*

BACTERIAL ENDOCARDITIS ANTIBIOTIC PROPHYLAXIS* GUIDELINES

    I. High risk (always pretreat prior to any invasive procedure)

      A. Prosthetic heart valve (including transcatheter implanted valve) or prosthetic material used for heart valve repair

      B. History of endocarditis

      C. Unrepaired cyanotic congenital heart disease

      D. Repaired congenital heart disease with residual defects at the site of or adjacent to the site of the prosthetic device

      E. Heart transplant that develops problems in a heart valve

    II. Negligible risk (*do not need* to pretreat prior to any invasive procedure)

      A. Surgically repaired congenital heart defects

      B. History of CABG surgery

      C. Calcified aortic stenosis

      D. Mitral valve regurgitation and mitral valve prolapse

      E. Rheumatic heart disease

      F. Bicuspid valve disease

      G. Physiologic, functional, or innocent murmurs

      H. Previous rheumatic fever without valve damage

      I. Pacemakers or implanted defibrillators

      J. Before an EGD, colonoscopy, or GU procedure

      K. After joint replacements *unless* patient has severe immunosuppression or prior joint infection

    III. See Table 8.2 for antibiotic prophylaxis regimens

---

* For dental procedures (*not* including routine dental cleaning) or respiratory tract procedures involving incision or biopsy of the respiratory tract mucosa.

■ = *not to be missed;* ● = *non-urgent referral;* ▲ = *urgent referral*

TABLE 8.2 ■ Antibiotic Prophylaxis Regimens for Bacterial Endocarditis

Patient Status	Agent	Regimen*
Not allergic to penicillin; is *able* to take oral medication	Amoxicillin	*Adult:* 2 g 1 hr before procedure *Child:* 50 mg/kg 1 hr before procedure
Not allergic to penicillin; is *unable* to take oral medication	Ampicillin	*Adult:* 2 g IM or IV within 30 min of procedure *Child:* 50 mg/kg IM or IV within 30 min of procedure
	OR	
	Cefazolin *or* ceftriaxone	*Adult:* 1 g IM or IV 30–60 min before procedure *Child:* 50 mg/kg IM or IV 30–60 min before procedure
Allergic to penicillin; is *able* to take oral medication	Cephalexin	*Adult:* 2 g 1 hr before procedure *Child:* 50 mg/kg 1 hr before procedure
	OR	
	Clindamycin	*Adult:* 600 mg 1 hr before procedure *Child:* 20 mg/kg 1 hr before procedure
	OR	
	Azithromycin	*Adult:* 500 mg 1 hr before procedure *Child:* 15 mg/kg 1 hr before procedure
Allergic to penicillin; is *unable* to take oral medication	Clindamycin	*Adult:* 600 mg IV within 30 min of procedure *Child:* 20 mg/kg IV within 30 min of procedure
	OR	
	Vancomycin	*Adult:* 15–20 mg/kg, not to exceed 2 g dose, IV 2 hr before procedure *Child:* 15 mg/kg, not to exceed 1 g dose, IV 2 hr before procedure

* Maximal dose in children should not exceed recommended adult dose.

CORONARY HEART DISEASE (CHD)

I. Risk factors
  A. CHD risk equivalents: these conditions have been associated with a risk of a cardiovascular event (e.g., MI, CVA) equivalent to that of a patient with known CHD; patients with these risks should be treated as aggressively as those with known disease.
    1. Any noncoronary atherosclerotic disease (e.g., carotid artery disease, PAD, AAA)
    2. DM (which is also associated with other risk factors such as obesity and dyslipidemia)
    3. Chronic kidney disease (CKD), even in mild-to-moderate stages
  B. Nonmodifiable risk factors
    1. Age: prevalence of any vascular disease increases significantly with each decade of life
    2. Gender
    3. Family history of CHD: increased risk for a younger person with an FH of premature CHD (MI or death from CHD in a parent or sibling before 50 [males] or 60 [females] yr of age)
  C. Modifiable risk factors
    1. Smoking: increases total cholesterol, LDL cholesterol, triglycerides, and non-HDL cholesterol; lowers HDL cholesterol
    2. Dyslipidemia (see DYSLIPIDEMIA, IV. A)
    3. Hypertension: see Table 8.13
    4. Abdominal obesity: waist at umbilicus > 40 inches (males) or > 35 inches (females)
    5. Psychosocial factors (e.g., stress, depression, anger)

6. Diet: specifically *low* in fruits, vegetables, or foods with fiber and *high* in foods with higher glycemic indices (i.e., sugary foods, simple carbs) and saturated and/or trans fats
7. Lack of or more than moderate alcohol consumption in patients ≥ 65 yr of age
   (a) "Moderate" means more than two drinks a day (males) and more than one a day (females)
   (b) One drink: 12 oz beer, 5 oz wine, or 1.5 oz 80-proof liquor
8. Lack of regular physical activity: even moderate exercise protects against CHD and all-cause mortality

D. Other risk factors
1. Androgen deficiency in men
2. Collagen vascular diseases (e.g., RA, SLE)
3. Obstructive sleep apnea (OSA)
4. Nonalcoholic fatty liver disease (NAFLD)
5. Postmenopausal state, hormone replacement therapy

E. Tools to assess risk factors for CHD (all available online)
1. Framingham risk score (*www.framinghamheartstudy.org/risk/coronary.html* or *www.framinghamheartstudy.org/risk/gencardio.html*)
2. Reynolds risk score (*www.reynoldsriskscore.org*)

II. Risk stratification for significant disease
A. High likelihood
1. History of CHD or one or more risk equivalents
2. Men > 60 yr of age; women > 70 yr of age
3. Changes in hemodynamics
4. ECG changes: ST-segment elevation or depression of more than 1 mm, marked symmetric T-wave inversion in multiple precordial leads (V_1–V_6) or bipolar T waves in leads II, III, and aVF (see **12-LEAD ECG**, Figs. 8.2 and 8.3 for examples)

B. Moderate likelihood
1. Two or more CHD risk factors (especially HTN, dyslipidemia, and smoking)
2. ECG changes: ST-segment depression of 0.5–1 mm or T-wave inversion of more than 1 mm in leads with dominant R waves

C. Low likelihood
1. One risk factor
2. No changes on ECG (Note: one-half to one-third of patients with angina have normal ECG readings; see **12-LEAD ECG**, Fig. 8.1 for example.)

III. Classification of angina
A. Stable angina occurs at predictable times (e.g., with exercise or at stressful times) (see Table 8.3).

TABLE 8.3 ■ **Classification of Angina**

Class	Activity/Onset	Limits to Normal Activity
I	Prolonged exertion	None
II*	Walking 2 blocks	Slight
III*	Walking <2 blocks	Marked
IV	Minimal or rest	Severe

* A practical differentiation between class II and III is the ability to walk 2 blocks or climb a flight of stairs.

B. Unstable angina
   1. In most patients, this diagnosis has changed to non-ST elevation MI (NSTEMI) because of widespread use of the troponin test (see **D**, Acute Coronary Syndrome, below).
   2. Consider with
      (a) New-onset angina that markedly limits physical activity
      (b) Angina that is more frequent, lasts longer, or occurs with less exertion than previously
      (c) Rest angina lasting > 20 min
C. Vasospastic angina (previously called Prinzmetal's or variant angina): angina at rest, promptly relieved with short-acting NTG; caused by coronary artery vasospasm
D. ***Emergency transfer to ED if suspecting Acute Coronary Syndrome (ACS)***
   1. *Non-ST-elevation MI (NSTEMI)—see B, Unstable angina, above*
   2. *ST-elevation MI (STEMI)* (see **12-LEAD ECG**, Figs. 8.2 and 8.3 for examples)
IV. Diagnostics for CHD
   A. Initial
      1. ECG (keep in mind that the initial ECG may be normal, even with acute MI)
      2. Chemistry profile (be sure it includes serum magnesium)
      3. Fasting lipid profile
      4. Consider high-sensitivity C-reactive protein (hs-CRP) if no known CHD; it can help with risk stratification.
      5. Stress testing
         (a) Exercise treadmill testing is best for patients who can exercise
         (b) Nuclear single-photon emission computed tomography (SPECT) myocardial perfusion study (Lexiscan without treadmill) if patient cannot exercise satisfactorily or has a pacemaker, LBBB, left ventricular hypertrophy, or abnormal ST segments
         (c) Dobutamine SPECT myocardial perfusion study or dobutamine stress echocardiogram if patient cannot exercise satisfactorily and has asthma or bronchospastic disease
      6. Echocardiogram
   B. Definitive workup
      1. Cardiac catheterization
      2. Thallium studies or chemical (e.g., dipyridamole or dobutamine) stress test
V. Outpatient treatment for CHD, with the goal to reduce the risk of MI or CVA/TIA
   A. ***Consult a cardiologist if angina is new onset or has changing characteristics.***
   B. Medications (see Table 8.4)
      1. Nitrates (short-acting, usually sublingual) are used for acute treatment.
      2. For "prevention" (i.e., reducing angina episodes and improving exercise tolerance)
         (a) Beta blockers are the first-line choice (effective for exertional angina and also can prevent reinfarction and improve survival post-MI). Do not use with vasospastic angina.
         (b) Calcium channel blockers (CCB) can be used alone, instead of beta blockers (BB), or in combination with them. The preferred CCB are diltiazem, verapamil or amlodipine (long-acting medications).
         (c) Long-acting nitrates are an alternative to BB or CCB; isosorbide mononitrate is the first choice.

■ = *not to be missed;* ▲ = *urgent referral*

TABLE 8.4 ■ **Medications for Angina**

Medication	Advantages and Disadvantages	Examples
Nitrates*	Reduce angina and improve exercise tolerance with stable angina Decrease the risk of AMI in unstable angina Extended-, sustained-, and controlled-release forms are for prevention; they are *not* used to treat an acute anginal episode Most require a 6–8-h period of abstinence to prevent tachyphylaxis Disadvantages include tolerance, H/A, hypotension, and need to regularly space doses	Nitroglycerin sublingual 0.4 mg (range 0.3–0.6 mg) q5min, up to 3 tabs or 3 sprays; *transfer to ED for further evaluation if angina persists* Nitroglycerin extended-release capsule 2.5–18 mg tid-qid Nitroglycerin transdermal patch 0.2–0.8 mg worn for 12 hr daily Isosorbide dinitrate sustained-release cap/tab 40–80 mg 1–2 times daily Isosorbide mononitrate (Monoket 10–20 mg *or* ISMO 20 mg given bid, 7 hr apart *or* Imdur 60–120 mg given once daily)
Beta blockers	Improve exercise tolerance and reduce angina with stable angina Reduce angina and the risk of AMI in unstable angina Particularly helpful if the patient has exercise-associated tachycardia with angina Disadvantages include bronchoconstriction, AV block, reduced contractility (may induce HF), and changes in blood lipids	***Noncardioselective* agents** Propranolol immediate-release 20–80 mg tid-qid *or* extended-release (Inderal-LA) 80–320 mg daily Nadolol 40–240 mg daily ***Cardioselective* agents** Atenolol 50–100 mg daily Metoprolol tartrate (Lopressor) 50 mg bid *or* extended release (Toprol XL) 100 mg daily; maximum dose for both is 400 mg daily
Calcium channel blockers	Given if contraindications to or adverse reactions with beta blockers *or* added to treatment if beta blockers alone are not successful Improve exercise tolerance and reduce angina in chronic angina Reduce angina in unstable angina (especially nicardipine) Disadvantages include hypotension, AV block, reduced contractility (verapamil, diltiazem, nifedipine may induce HF), constipation, edema, and tachycardia with some agents	Nifedipine (Procardia XL) 30–90 mg daily Diltiazem extended-release cap 120–480 mg daily *or* tab 180–360 mg daily Nicardipine 20–40 mg tid Verapamil immediate-release 80–120 mg tid Amlodipine 5–10 mg daily
Sodium channel blocker	Exact mechanism of action unknown Caution in patients with HF or recent MI, ≥75 yr of age, or if eGFR <60 mL/min	Ranolazine (Ranexa) ER tab start with 500 mg bid; maximum 1000 mg bid

* If given more than once a day, leave a 12–14-hr nitrate free interval to decrease risk of tolerance.

C. Dietary therapy: after a review of the lipid profile, suggest an appropriate diet (see DYSLIPIDEMIA, **IV**, A); consider calorie reduction for overweight or obese patients.
D. Exercise: after clearance by a physician, exercise 65%–75% of the maximum heart rate for the age.

▲ = *urgent referral*

E. Smoking cessation (the risk of recurrent MI decreases 50% within 1 yr of cessation and normalizes to that of a nonsmoker within 2 yr)
F. Consider a moderate- or high-intensity statin (see Table 8.8), even if cholesterol levels are not elevated.
G. Manage comorbid conditions
1. HTN: consider goal of < 130/80 mmHg if tolerated, < 140/90 mmHg if lower goal is not tolerated; start with an ACE or ARB.
2. DM: start with metformin; if A1c goal not met, consider adding empagliflozin (Jardiance) or liraglutide (Victoza) to reduce CV risk.

PRACTICE PEARLS FOR ANGINA

- Do not obtain a stress test with unstable angina (ACS).
- "Chest pain"
  - Women often have atypical angina: vague, but descriptive; unexplained SOB; exhaustion; "full" feeling or discomfort; indigestion; profound fatigue; disturbances in sleep or thinking; often occurs with arm activities.
  - A BP cuff left on and inflated too long may mimic the left arm pain of a patient with a cardiac disorder.
- Noncardiac chest pain
  - Constant aching pain that may occur in the substernal area and persist all day
  - Pain that is present in only one position and not in others
  - Pain over the apex of the heart or over the right anterior chest region
  - Fleeting, momentary pain (lasting only 1–2 sec) described as a needle jab or stick
  - If the patient is able to localize the pain with a finger or two to a small region, it is usually not cardiac in nature; cardiac pain tends to be diffuse.
- Patients with AMI frequently complain of feeling unusually tired for months or weeks preceding MI.
- Have the patient keep a diary of symptoms and precipitating events; *referral to cardiologist if the patient continues to have symptoms, even with a normal treadmill test*.
- Medications
  - Do not give isosorbide mononitrate (Imdur, ISMO, or Monoket) as q12h dosing (see Table 8.4); it is designed with an abstinence period to prevent tachyphylaxis.
  - *Primary prevention* with ASA 81 mg is no longer recommended because it has not been shown to reduce risk of CV events. It is often prescribed as antiplatelet therapy for *secondary* prevention.
  - Nitroglycerin (NTG) sublingual tablets are good until the expiration date on the bottle as long as they are kept in the original bottle, tightly capped, and at room temperature.
  - Omega-3 fatty acids can decrease triglycerides, inhibit blood clotting, and may decrease dysrhythmias associated with sudden cardiac death; encourage two servings of fish weekly (primarily salmon, tuna, mackerel, herring, or sardines); *fish oil supplements* (Rx or OTC fish oil caps) *do not* improve CV outcomes in high-risk patients.
  - NSAIDs (except ASA)
    - Limit use in cardiac patients; use the lowest dose for the shortest time.
    - Naproxen has the least CV risk; avoid selective COX-2 medications (e.g., celecoxib) and diclofenac.
- Education
  - Encourage family CPR training.
  - Teach the patient and family when to call 911 or the emergency medical system.
  - Teach the patient and/or family how to read labels and calculate fat and sodium intake.
- For chest pain differential diagnoses, see Table 8.5.

● = *non-urgent referral*

TABLE 8.5 ■ Chest Pain Differential Diagnosis

Description	Confirm by	Exclude by
Acute MI or Acute Coronary Artery Insufficiency		
Severe, oppressive, constricting retrosternal discomfort; often radiates to the left shoulder and down the left arm (on the inside of the arm) Women are more likely to have unexplained fatigue, nausea and/or SOB Onset is usually at rest Lasts >30 min Often accompanied by anxiety, restlessness, diaphoresis, or dyspnea Prior history of angina or MI Levine sign (holding fist to chest) Possible dysrhythmias or HF	ECG changes Serial cardiac enzymes	Usually by normal serial ECGs or observation in the hospital Normal serial cardiac enzymes (if no MI)
Aortic Dissection		
Very abrupt, tearing pain in the anterior or posterior chest, frequently between the shoulders; often migrates to the arms, abdomen, and legs Pulse deficits Shocky but hypertensive Possible neurologic changes (especially in the legs) Diastolic HTN with aortic diastolic murmur	May be found on an echocardiogram or abdominal U/S Usually found with angiography, CT scan, or MRI	Normal mediastinum on CXR
Biliary Colic		
Constant epigastric or right upper quadrant pain; may extend to the back Often positive Murphy sign Lasts 15 min to 6 hr Associated with N/V; possible fever	Clinical history Abdominal U/S or HIDA scan	Absence of gallstones and/or normal HIDA scan
Esophageal Spasm		
Substernal constricting pain, often at the time of swallowing History of dysphagia Pain related to cold and carbonated drinks or food	Barium swallow Endoscopy Esophageal manometry	Normal esophageal manometry
Esophagitis		
Heartburn and acid brash Worse when bending over or supine Better with antacids	Endoscopy Biopsy UGI series	Normal endoscopy and biopsy or UGI series
Musculoskeletal Chest Wall Pain/Costochondritis		
Sharp pain, usually worse with deep breath or certain movements (e.g., twisting) Often associated with back pain, which is worse in the supine position Often associated with a history of lifting or moving a heavy object	Reproducible pain with pressure along the costosternal and/or paravertebral junctions (often T_{8-10}; T_7 level is at the low end of scapulae)	Pain not reproducible with pressure to the painful area
Pancreatitis (Acute)		
Severe epigastric or periumbilical pain radiating to the back Clinically looks very sick Associated with N/V History of alcohol use or gallstones; may be associated with high triglycerides and DM Current use of HCTZ	Elevated serum amylase and lipase CT abdomen	Normal amylase and lipase Normal CT scan

Continued

TABLE 8.5 ■ Chest Pain Differential Diagnosis—cont'd

Description	Confirm by	Exclude by
Peptic Ulcer Disease		
Epigastric postprandial discomfort Often relieved with antacids or food May respond to antacid or H_2 antagonist trial	Upper GI series or endoscopy	Normal GI series or endoscopy
Pericarditis		
Pleuritic chest pain, often worse in the supine position, better when sitting up; referred to the trapezius ridge Pericardial friction rub Often associated with disease (e.g., viral infection, recent MI, connective tissue disease)	Typical ECG: concave ST-segment elevation in all leads except aVR and V_1 Pericardial friction rub Echocardiography	Normal ECG Normal echocardiogram Absence of friction rub
Pneumonia		
Usually pleuritic chest pain with cough and fever Dull to percussion (affected area) A–E changes (affected area)	CXR	Normal CXR (> 24 hr after symptom onset)
Pneumothorax or Pneumomediastinum		
Sudden dyspnea or retrosternal pain, cough, and lateral chest pain Diminished breath sounds with possible mediastinal shift Possible history of asthma, COPD, or chest trauma Possible subcutaneous emphysema (skin "crackles" on touch)	CXR	Normal CXR (including lateral view)
Pulmonary Embolism		
Pleuritic chest pain or sudden dyspnea, apprehension, and palpitations Occasionally, acute nonpleuritic chest "pressure" with hemoptysis Clinical signs of DVT Factors predisposing to venous thrombosis (e.g., postpartum, use of OCs, prolonged bed rest, HF)	V/Q scan or CT pulmonary angiography (CTPA) or both ECG changes typical of PE (right ventricular strain)	Normal V/Q scan or CTPA Observation in hospital

12-LEAD ECG

I. Description
   A. See Fig. 8.1 for a normal 12-lead ECG.
   B. Ischemia, injury, and infarction of the ventricle are reflected in the 12-lead ECG; each area of the ventricle is reflected in certain leads. With MI, there is a strong correlation between the leads showing changes and the location of actual disease. (See Tables 8.6 and 8.7 for acute changes and Figs. 8.2 and 8.3 for examples.)
   C. Generally progressive changes on ECG tracing indicate an ST elevation MI (STEMI).
      1. T waves initially heighten and become peaked
      2. ST segments elevate
      3. T waves become inverted
      4. Q waves form and R waves lose some of their height (NSTEMI do not develop Q waves)

Text continued on page 220

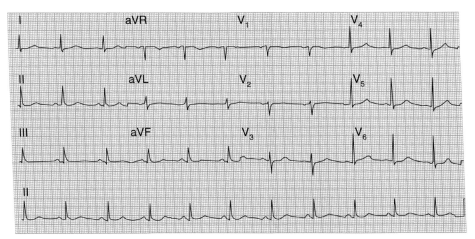

Fig. 8.1 12-Lead electrocardiogram

Because 12-lead ECG tracings do not look alike, it is important to know the criteria for "normal":

- Sinus rhythm
- Normal measurements (i.e., PR: 0.12–0.2 sec, QRS: 0.04–0.1 sec, and QT: 0.32–0.44 sec)
- All ST segments level with baseline (i.e., no depression or elevation)
- All T waves usually upright except aVR; may be inverted in lead III or V_1
- QRS complex in leads I, II, and aVF upright
- Normal R-wave progression: in looking at leads V_1 through V_6, the QRS complex becomes more positive than negative in either V_3 or V_4

Any deviation from these criteria will create an abnormal ECG, which is not necessarily life threatening.

TABLE 8.6 ■ Acute Changes on 12-Lead ECG

Acute Changes	ECG Findings
Ischemia	ST-segment depression > 1 mm and T-wave inversion (if the inversion is deeply symmetric, it is more significant); consider ischemia with just T-wave inversion (normal ST segments)
Injury	ST-segment elevation > 1 mm is generally significant
Necrosis	Q waves are signs of necrosis; to be diagnostic of MI, the Q wave must be ≥ 0.04 sec wide *or* greater than one-quarter the total height of the QRS complex

TABLE 8.7 ■ Location of Changes on 12-Lead Electrocardiogram

	Leads	Artery Involved
Left Ventricle		
Anterior	V_1, V_2, V_3, V_4	LAD coronary artery
Inferior	II, III, aVF	Usually RCA but may be left circumflex
Lateral	I, aVL, V_5, V_6	Left circumflex
Posterior	V_1, V_2 (acute changes include tall R wave and ST-segment depression)	RCA
Right Ventricle		
Right ventricular MI (associated with inferior MI)	V_4 on the right side of the chest (V_4R) (acute change is ST-segment elevation > 1 mm)	RCA

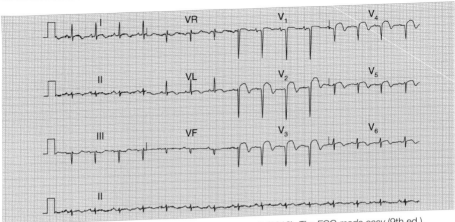

Fig. 8.2 Anterior MI, acute. (From Hampton, J., & Hampton, J. (2019). *The ECG made easy* (9th ed.). Elsevier.)

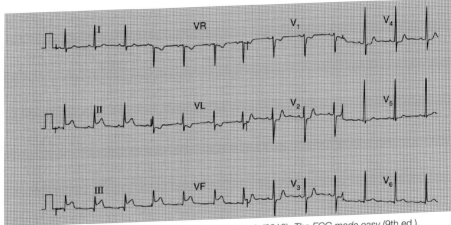

Fig. 8.3 Inferior MI, acute. (From Hampton, J., & Hampton, J. (2019). *The ECG made easy* (9th ed.). Elsevier.)

      D. *It is important to treat the patient and not the ECG. Refer for clinical symptoms. Do not wait for ECG changes.*

    ▲ **II.** *Emergency treatment of suspected AMI* (see Figs. 8.2 and 8.3)

      A. Administer oxygen and start intravenous line (if equipment is available).

      B. Have the patient chew 325 mg of ASA (rule out aortic dissection or peptic ulcer disease).

      C. Transport patient to the hospital by Advanced Life Support means immediately.

DYSLIPIDEMIA

  I. Screening recommendations (based on 2018 ACC/AHA guidelines)

    A. Adults

      1. 20 yr of age or older: obtain either a fasting or nonfasting lipid profile (total cholesterol, HDL, LDL, and triglycerides). While fasting is not required for lipids, there

---

■ = *not to be missed;* ▲ = *urgent referral*

is a possibility of elevated triglycerides (> 400 mg/dL) in a nonfasting test, which would require the patient to have a fasting lipid profile drawn at a later date.

2. Repeat lipid screening and risk factor assessment every 4–6 yr for patients > 20 yr of age, not on medications and with low risk; repeat every 3 yr for those close to a threshold, to consider treatment (e.g., LDL value or calculated CVD risk).
3. There is no consensus on when to stop lipid screening; Up-to-Date suggests
   (a) In good health without known CVD: stop at 79 yr of age
   (b) With at least one prior normal lipid panel: stop at 65 yr of age

B. Pediatrics
   1. Normal lipid values vary by age and sex; research has not conclusively shown overall benefit vs possible harms for screening.
   2. Considerations
      (a) FH of either early ASCVD or significant hypercholesterolemia: fasting or nonfasting lipid panel, starting as early as 2 yr of age
      (b) No FH as listed above: once between 9 and 11 yr of age and again between 17 and 21 yr of age
      (c) If the patient is obese or has other metabolic risk factors, obtain fasting lipid profile.

II. Risk factors
   A. Major risk factors
      1. Elevated LDL; possible causes are
         (a) Diet: saturated or trans fats, weight gain, anorexia
         (b) Drugs: diuretics, cyclosporine, glucocorticoids, amiodarone
         (c) Diseases: biliary obstruction, nephrosis, hypothyroidism, obesity
      2. Cigarette smoking
      3. HTN
      4. Blood glucose abnormalities (e.g., pre-DM, DM)
      5. Age
      6. Calculated 10-yr ASCVD risk (based on the pooled cohort equation [PCE], see **IV**, B, below)
   B. Risk-enhancing factors *supplement the PCE*, to aid in patient discussion (i.e., if these factors are present, they help to confirm higher CV risk)
      1. FH of premature ASCVD (males < 55 yr of age, females < 65 yr of age)
      2. Persistently elevated LDL ≥ 160 mg/dL
      3. Metabolic syndrome (see METABOLIC SYNDROME, later in this chapter)
      4. CKD (eGFR 15–59 mL/min, with or without albuminuria), not treated with dialysis or kidney transplant
      5. History of preeclampsia or premature menopause (< 40 yr of age)
      6. Chronic inflammatory disorder (e.g., RA, psoriasis, or chronic HIV)
      7. High-risk ethnic group (e.g., South Asian)
      8. Persistently elevated triglycerides ≥ 175 mg/dL
      9. Additional tests, if ordered: high-sensitivity CRP ≥ 2 mg/L; ABI < 0.9; lipoprotein (a) ≥ 50 mg/dL or 125 nmol/L or apolipoprotein B ≥ 130 mg/dL

III. Treatment goals (adult)
   A. LDL: based on patient age, presence/absence of clinical arteriosclerotic cardiovascular disease (ASCVD), and LDL levels (see Treatment, **IV**, B and C, below)
   B. HDL: > 40 mg/dL (males) or > 50 mg/dL (females)
   C. Triglycerides: < 150 mg/dL
      1. If triglycerides are elevated, LDL is small and dense regardless of its value.
      2. Trigs ÷ HDL value > 3 indicates the presence of insulin resistance.

IV. Treatment

    A. Therapeutic lifestyle changes should be emphasized for every patient regardless of other treatments

        1. Diet therapy should be tried for 3 mo before medications are started (unless CHD exists or the patient has diabetes).

            (a) Diets should emphasize vegetables, fruits, whole grains, legumes, healthy proteins (i.e., low-fat dairy, low-fat poultry, fish/seafood, nuts), and nontropical vegetable oils. Sweets, sugar-sweetened beverages, and red meat should be limited.

            (b) Mediterranean diet decreases the relative risk of CV events by 30% in 5 yr (similar to some statins).

            (c) People who eat a diet rich in plant-based foods lower their risk of CVD by > 50%, in a research study published in the *Journal of the AHA* (8/4/2021).

            (d) With elevated triglycerides, the patient should avoid all refined carbohydrates (the "whites"—flour, sugar, white rice or potatoes), alcohol, and fried foods.

        2. Regular exercise (e.g., moderate to vigorous activity 3–4 times a week, for average of 40 min)

        3. Weight loss, if applicable

    B. LDL (from 2018 ACC/AHA Cholesterol Guideline)

        1. The focus is on treatment of cholesterol to decrease ASCVD risk using the appropriate intensity of statin therapy in those most likely to benefit (no improved ASCVD outcomes by simply meeting a specific LDL goal). The primary principle when treating LDL is "lower is better." Generally, lowering the LDL by 1% lowers the ASCVD risk by 1%.

        2. The Pooled Cohort Equations are recommended to estimate 10-yr ASCVD risks for CHD and CVA in patients 20–75 yr of age who *do not have clinical ASCVD* (e.g., acute coronary syndrome; history of MI, stable/unstable angina, CABG or other arterial revascularization surgery, CVA, TIA, or PAD). See *http://my.americanheart.org/cvriskcalculator*

           Low risk   < 5%

           Borderline risk   5% to < 7.5%

           Intermediate risk   ≥ 7.5% to < 20%

           High risk   ≥ 20%

            (a) If the patient is already on a statin, use pretreatment cholesterol values (if known).

            (b) Consider statins if the 10-yr risk is ≥ 7.5%; see below for specific patient variable(s).

        3. Nonstatin therapies (except ezetimibe and PCSK9 inhibitors) do not acceptably decrease ASCVD risk compared with the potential for adverse outcomes.

    C. Statin benefit groups (see Table 8.8 for high-, moderate-, and low-intensity statin therapy)

        1. Patients up to 75 yr of age *with clinical ASCVD:* high-intensity statin therapy should be initiated/continued to achieve ≥ 50% reduction; moderate-intensity therapy is the second option. If the patient has very high-risk ASCVD, consider adding a nonstatin if the LDL is not < 70 mg/dL.

        2. Patients ≥ 21 yr of age *with no clinical ASCVD*

            (a) LDL ≥ 190 mg/dL: high-intensity statin therapy; often a nonstatin cholesterol-lowering medication is needed as well (Table 8.9).

            (b) If the patient is > 75 yr of age, without preexisting cardiovascular disease, statins are not indicated.

        3. Patients 40–75 yr of age *with DM and LDL ≥ 70 mg/dL:* moderate-intensity statin therapy; in patients < 40 or > 75 yr of age, individualize statin therapy according to the benefits of ASCVD risk reduction vs possible side effects or drug interactions.

Text continued on page 224

TABLE 8.8 ■ High-, Moderate-, and Low-Intensity Statin Therapy

Therapy	Effectiveness	Statins
High-intensity therapy	Lowers LDL, on average, approximately ≥50% when taken daily	Atorvastatin 80 mg* Rosuvastatin 20 (40) mg
Moderate-intensity therapy	Lowers LDL, on average, approximately 30%–49% when taken daily	Atorvastatin 10 (20) mg Rosuvastatin (5) 10 mg Simvastatin 20–40 mg Pravastatin 40 (80) mg Lovastatin 40 mg Fluvastatin 40 mg bid
Low-intensity therapy	Lowers LDL, on average, by <30% when taken daily	Pravastatin 10–20 mg Lovastatin 20 mg

Dosages in italics are approved by the US Food and Drug Administration but were not tested in the trial reviewed for the guidelines.
* Decrease dose to 40 mg daily if 80 mg is not tolerated.

TABLE 8.9 ■ Nonstatin Therapy

Medication	Initial Dose	Monitoring
Bile Acid Sequestrants		
Cholestyramine (Questran, Cholybar)	4 g tid-qid	Obtain fasting lipid profile before starting, in 3 mo, and q6–12 mo thereafter Discontinue if triglycerides exceed 400 mg/dL
Colestipol (Colestid)	6 g daily	
Colesevelam (Welchol)	3 tablets bid or 6 tablets daily with food	
Fibric Acid Derivatives (Fibrates)		
Gemfibrozil (Lopid)	600 mg bid ac	Monitor LFTs and lipids at the start of therapy, at 12 wk, and periodically thereafter; stop if ALT >100 U/L. Gemfibrozil: avoid if creatinine >2 mg/dL and use cautiously with hepatic impairment* Should not be used with statins (increased risk of rhabdomyolysis)
Fenofibrate	67–200 mg daily	Monitor renal status (serum creatinine and eGFR) before starting, in 3 mo, and q6 mo thereafter. Do not use if eGFR <30 mL/min; do not exceed 54 mg/day if eGFR 30–59 mL/min May use with low- or moderate-intensity statin *only* if the benefits exceed the potential risk for side effects or if triglycerides >1000 mg/dL
Niacin (Do Not Use With Statins; Increased Risks and No Benefit)		
Niacin (nicotinic acid)	1–3 g tid with or after meals	Obtain baseline ALT/AST, FBG or hemoglobin A1c, and uric acid before starting, during dose increases, and q6mo thereafter Do not use if ALT/AST >2–3 times the normal or with gout or persistent hyperglycemia Use cautiously with renal impairment and do not use with active liver disease
Niacin, extended release (Niaspan)	500 mg hs, adjust dose by 500 mg daily at 4-wk intervals	
Miscellaneous Medications		
Ezetimibe (Zetia)	10 mg daily	Monitor lipids periodically Do not use with moderate-to-severe hepatic impairment*

Continued

TABLE 8.9 ■ **Nonstatin Therapy—cont'd**

Medication	Initial Dose	Monitoring
Omega-3 capsules (Lovaza, Vascepa)	4 caps daily	Monitor lipids periodically Used when triglycerides ≥ 1000 mg/dL
PCSK9 Inhibitors		
Alirocumab (Praluent)	75 mg SQ q2wk; may increase to 150 mg q2wk after 4–8 wk **OR** 300 mg SQ q4wk	No routine lab monitoring recommended No dosage adjustment for renal or hepatic conditions
Evolocumab (Repatha)	140 mg SQ q2wk **OR** 420 mg SQ qmo	No routine lab monitoring recommended No dosage adjustment for renal or hepatic conditions Caution with latex sensitivity

* Includes history of liver disease, consuming substantial quantities of ETOH, and/or unexplained elevations in ALT and AST.

4. Patients 40–75 yr of age *with no DM and*
   (a) LDL ≥ 70 mg/dL and 10-yr ASCVD risk of ≥ 7.5%: moderate-intensity statin, if discussion of treatment options favors statin therapy
   (b) 10-yr ASCVD risk of 7.5%–19.9%: begin a statin if risk-enhancing factors favor it
   (c) LDL 70–189 mg/dL and 10-yr ASCVD risk of ≥ 7.5%–19.9%: if decision about statin therapy is not certain, consider measuring coronary artery calcium
5. *For patients with NYHA class II–IV HF* (see HEART FAILURE, **V**) *or undergoing hemodialysis: consult with or referral to a cardiologist regarding statin therapy.*

D. Monitoring statin therapy
   1. Obtain fasting lipid profile before starting, in 4–12 wk (determines patient adherence), and then every 3–12 mo as clinically indicated and patient continues the medication.
   2. Obtain baseline ALT/AST before starting therapy; if normal, further hepatic monitoring is not needed unless hepatotoxicity signs/symptoms occur (e.g., unusual fatigue, abdominal pain, dark urine). Asymptomatic increases in ALT/AST (i.e., > 3 times ULN) are often resolved with a dose reduction.
   3. Measure CK only with complaints of severe muscle symptoms and/or *objective* muscle weakness. With rhabdomyolysis (rare condition), the CK levels are > 10 times ULN with evidence of acute kidney injury.
   4. If also using nonstatin cholesterol-lowering medications, more intensive monitoring may be indicated.
   5. New-onset DM may occur with statin use, in patients at high risk for developing DM. The statin should be continued because of the benefit of taking the statin with DM.
   6. Discontinue the statin in an elderly patient with physical and/or cognitive decline, a limited life expectancy from whatever cause, or multiple comorbid conditions.
   7. Female patients of child-bearing age taking a statin, who are sexually active
      (a) Should use reliable contraception; if she gets pregnant while taking the statin, stop it as soon as she discovers the pregnancy.
      (b) If planning a pregnancy, stop the statin 1–2 months in advance.
E. For muscle pain associated with statins, consider the following:
   1. Stop statin if CK level is > 10 times the normal or if the symptoms are intolerable.

● = *non-urgent referral*

     2. Try lowering the dose or give less frequently (e.g., rosuvastatin or atorvastatin q2–3d).

     3. Change to pravastatin or low-dose rosuvastatin.

     4. Correct low vitamin D or hypothyroidism (both can cause myalgias).

  F. Statin administration

     1. If insomnia occurs, split the tablet in half and take twice daily.

     2. Atorvastatin and rosuvastatin may be given any time of the day; others work better if given in the evening.

     3. Do not give simvastatin > 40 mg daily or > 20 mg daily if the patient is taking a CCB.

  G. Use statins cautiously with fibrates because rhabdomyolysis may occur (consider this with myalgias, dark urine, and CK level ≥ 10 times the upper limit of normal).

  H. Reassure patient that the CV benefits of statins outweigh any small risk of DM; associated liver disease is rare; and these drugs do not cause dementia or cancer.

  V. *Referral*

    A. *To cardiologist if unable to reach lipid goals*

    B. *To pediatric cardiologist for patients < 18 yr of age with dyslipidemia*

PRACTICE PEARLS (FOR NONSTATIN THERAPY)

- Prescription omega-3 capsules (e.g., Lovaza) are recommended only for *secondary* prevention of CHD and sudden cardiac death in patients with prevalent CHD or *secondary* prevention of outcomes in patients with HF.
- Niacin (see Table 8.9): to decrease the frequency and severity of skin side effects
  - Take with food or take ASA 325 mg 30 min before niacin.
  - With extended-release niacin, increase the dose by 500 mg q1–2wk to a maximum of 2000 mg daily.
  - With immediate-release niacin, start with 100 mg tid and titrate up to 3000 mg daily divided in two to three doses. Do *not* use with statins; there are increased risks and no benefits.
- Bile acid sequestrants (BAS) (see Table 8.9)
  - Do not use BAS or statins for the treatment of isolated elevations of VLDL because both may increase VLDL levels.
  - Can elevate triglycerides; do not use with fasting triglycerides ≥ 300 mg/dL.
  - Constipation resulting from BAS can be reduced by increasing the dose slowly and by concomitant administration of psyllium (Metamucil) or methylcellulose (Citrucel).
- PCSK9 inhibitors (i.e., Praluent [alirocumab], Repatha [evolocumab]) are potent nonstatin therapies, given by SQ injection q2–4wk.
  - They are added on to statin and ezetimibe therapy and can lower LDL by an additional 43%–64%.
  - However, they are very expensive.
- OTC supplements
  - Omega-3 fatty acids can lower lipids; encourage two servings of fish per week (salmon, tuna, mackerel, herring, or sardines); OTC fish oil capsules may lower values but *have not* been shown to decrease mortality.
  - Flaxseed supplement (2 tbsp oil daily) may cause a minor reduction in triglycerides but has no effect on LDL.
  - Garlic extract: no significant long-term change in lipids.
  - Guggul or guggulipid: overwhelming evidence showed it to be *ineffective* for lipids.
  - CoQ10: no solid evidence whether it helps limit muscle pain with statins, but it is not likely to harm.
  - Consider ezetimibe (Zetia) if patient needs an add-on to statin (e.g., has CV disease but does not reach the LDL goal or cannot tolerate a high-intensity statin). It lowers LDL by 13%–20%.

= non-urgent referral

HEART FAILURE

I. Description
   A. Heart failure (HF) is a chronic illness characterized by progressive deterioration and punctuated by periodic symptomatic exacerbations.
   B. Causes result in failure of the heart to keep up with the metabolic demands of tissues; possible etiologies include the following
      1. Cardiovascular
         (a) Ischemia (i.e., CHD), HTN and hypertensive heart disease
         (b) Valvular: aortic stenosis or regurgitation, mitral regurgitation
         (c) Cardiomyopathy (dilated, hypertrophic, or viral [inflammatory])
         (d) Atrial fibrillation
      2. Respiratory: severe lung disease (e.g., COPD), OSA
      3. Toxins: alcohol, tobacco use, chemotherapy
      4. Metabolic: DM, obesity, hyperthyroidism
      5. Kidney disease, volume overload
      6. Anemia
II. Clinical manifestations
   A. HF with reduced ejection fraction (HFrEF) (previously called systolic HF) occurs when the heart muscle is dilated and thin-walled.
      1. Low EF (e.g., <40%) occurs because of reduced contractility of the weakened muscle.
      2. It often results from CHD or MI.
   B. HF with preserved EF (HFpEF) (previously called diastolic dysfunction) is associated with a hypertrophied myocardium with elevated filling pressures.
      1. The EF is >50%.
      2. Diastolic dysfunction is often the result of HTN; it is also found with ischemic heart disease, hypertrophic obstructive cardiomyopathy, DM, and CKD.
   C. Left ventricular vs right ventricular failure
      1. Left ventricular (LV) failure is associated with reduced cardiac output systemically.
         (a) There is associated pulmonary congestion.
         (b) It is often the result of CHD, MI, valvular heart disease, cardiomyopathy, and/or HTN.
      2. Right ventricular failure is associated with systemic congestion (e.g., hepatic congestion and peripheral edema).
         (a) Right ventricular failure is usually the result of LV failure (in which case, there may also be pulmonary congestion) and also occasionally pulmonary HTN, right ventricular MI, or COPD.
         (b) HF caused by COPD is called *cor pulmonale*.
   D. Acute vs chronic
      1. Acute (days to weeks): mainly SOB at rest and/or with exertion; also orthopnea
      2. Chronic: paroxysmal nocturnal dyspnea (PND); fatigue, anorexia, abdominal distention, and peripheral edema may be more pronounced than dyspnea
III. Signs and symptoms
   A. Signs
      1. Crackles (specific but not a very sensitive finding; clear lung fields tell very little about the fluid status of the heart)
      2. Increased JVD (best physical finding for determining fluid status) (see Chapter 1, CARDIOVASCULAR, IV and V)

      3. Laterally displaced PMI

      4. Peripheral edema

      5. Hepatomegaly and ascites

      6. May have an S_3 heart sound (especially with HFrEF)

  B. Symptoms.

      1. Exertional dyspnea

      2. Exercise intolerance

      3. Cough, worse in the recumbent position

      4. Nocturnal symptoms

        (a) Orthopnea: difficulty breathing beginning < 1 min after lying down

        (b) PND: occurs 2–4 hr into sleep

      5. Abdominal discomfort

      6. Fatigue or altered mental status

IV. Diagnostics

  A. Not all patients will have evidence of fluid retention.

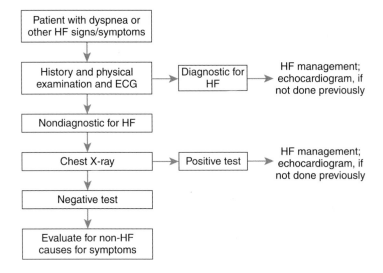

  B. There is no single diagnostic test for HF. Tests (e.g., labs, ECG) are done to determine the degree and type of HF and if there is a reversible cause; for recommended testing, see Table 8.10.

V. Classification

  A. New York Heart Association (NYHA) classification describes the severity of symptoms; EF does not correlate with the class.

I	No limitations to physical activity
II	Symptoms with usual activities
III	Symptoms with minimal activities; correlates to Stage C (see B, below)
IV	Inability to carry out physical activity without discomfort; symptoms at rest; correlates to Stage D (see B, below)

TABLE 8.10 ■ Additional Recommended Testing for Signs and Symptoms of Heart Failure

Test	Finding	Possible Diagnosis
ECG	Acute ST-T changes	Ischemia
	Atrial fibrillation	Thyroid disease, result of acute MI
	Bradycardia	HF due to slow rate
	Previous MI	Depressed LV function
	LVH	Diastolic dysfunction
Troponin T or I	Elevated	Myocardial ischemia/injury
CBC	Anemia	Decreased O_2 carrying capacity
UA	Proteinuria	Nephrotic syndrome
	Casts	Glomerulonephritis
Serum BUN/creatinine	Elevated	Renal failure or CKD
Serum albumin	Decreased	Increased extravascular volume or poor nutrition
TSH	Abnormal	Hypothyroidism or hyperthyroidism
Echocardiogram	Abnormal	Systolic or diastolic dysfunction Valvular heart disease Pulmonary HTN Coronary heart disease
BNP	Increased > 400*	HF (not all patients with symptomatic HF have elevated BNP levels and not all asymptomatic patients have low ones; elevated in some patients with acute decompensated HF) Often elevated with CKD with or without HF

* Result below 100 is not HF; 100–400 is not sensitive or specific enough for diagnosis of HF.

B. American College of Cardiology (ACC)/American Heart Association (AHA) guidelines classify patients, in stages, at risk for having HF.

Stage		Patient Description
A	High risk for developing HF	HTN CAD DM FH of cardiomyopathy
B	Asymptomatic HF	Previous MI Left ventricular systolic dysfunction Asymptomatic valvular disease
C	Symptomatic HF	Known structural heart disease SOB and fatigue Reduced exercise tolerance
D	Refractory end-stage HF	Marked symptoms at rest despite maximal medical therapy

VI. Treatment

    A. ***HF should be managed in collaboration with a physician.***

    B. Risk reduction (all stages)

        1. Weight reduction if the patient is obese

        2. Control lipids, HTN, and DM

        3. Maintain fluid balance: sodium restriction and daily weights

           (a) Stages A & B: < 2–3 g sodium daily

■ = *not to be missed*

  (b) Stages C & D: <2 g sodium daily
  (c) Fluid restriction
    (i) With Stage D HF or hyponatremia (i.e., sodium <130 mEq/L)
    (ii) With chronic fluid retention despite diuretics and sodium restriction: restrict fluids to no more than 2000 mL a day
C. Stop smoking and ETOH consumption.
D. Encourage regular exercise (e.g., walking) to tolerance.
E. Consider evaluation for OSA (patients rarely report excessive daytime sleepiness).
F. Emphasize the importance of taking the prescribed medications (according to the ACC/AHA guidelines) (see Table 8.11); multiple medications are given to treat

TABLE 8.11 ■ Medications for the Treatment of Heart Failure

Stage	Suggested Medical Therapy
A	Risk reduction measures
B	ACE* (ARB,* if intolerant to ACE) • Patients with recent or remote MI or acute coronary syndrome and EF <40% • All patients with decreased EF (<40%)
	Beta blocker • Patients with recent or remote MI or acute coronary syndrome and EF <40% • All patients with decreased EF (<40%) • Carvedilol (Coreg) 3.125 mg bid, doubling q2wk to 25 mg bid if tolerated *or* carvedilol CR 10 mg daily, titrate to 80 mg daily if tolerated • Metoprolol succinate extended release (Toprol XL) 12.5–25 mg daily, doubling q2wk to 200 mg daily if tolerated
	Statin • All patients with recent or remote MI or acute coronary syndrome
C	ACE* (or ARB,* if intolerant to ACE): all patients
	Beta blocker: all patients • Carvedilol (Coreg) 3.125 mg bid, doubling q2wk to 25 mg bid if tolerated *or* carvedilol CR 10 mg daily, titrate to 80 mg daily if tolerated • Metoprolol succinate extended release (Toprol XL) 12.5–25 mg daily, doubling q2wk to 200 mg daily if tolerated
	Loop diuretic* • Patients with NYHA class II–IV HF • Only as needed to correct or maintain fluid balance
	Aldosterone antagonist: monitor serum K^+ and creatinine monthly for 9 mo, q3 mo for 9 mo, and then periodically • All patients with NYHA class III–IV symptoms and who have EF <35%, as long as eGFR >30 mL/min and K^+ <5 mEq/L • Spironolactone 12.5–25 mg daily • Eplerenone 25 mg daily
	Hydralazine/nitrates • Persistently symptomatic African-Americans; NYHC class III–IV despite taking ACE, beta blocker, and aldosterone antagonist • Any patient with current or prior symptoms of HF with reduced ejection fraction (HFrEF) who cannot take or is intolerant to ACE or ARB • Hydralazine/isosorbide dinitrate 37.5 mg/20 mg tid
	Digoxin: may be beneficial in HFrEF to decrease hospitalizations • 0.125–0.25 mg daily (0.125 mg if age >70 yr or impaired renal function)
● D	***Referral to a HF center or cardiologist for management***

* See Tables 8.16 and 8.17 for dosing and precautions.

───────────────

● = *non-urgent referral*

HFrEF especially. With worsening HF symptoms, question the patient about missed medication doses in the preceding week.

G. There is less evidence for how to effectively treat HFpEF.
   1. Focus on BP control because that may slow progression of HFpEF; choose medication based on comorbidities (e.g., ACE with CKD).
   2. ACE/ARB and beta blockers do not seem to decrease mortality as with HFrEF.
   3. Use loop diuretics cautiously because they can worsen symptoms with HFpEF.

PRACTICE PEARLS FOR HEART FAILURE

- Weight gain and the presence of an S3 heart sound are more likely due to worsening HF rather than an acute exacerbation of COPD.
- With edema in HF: ensure patient is on target doses of medications that improve HF outcomes (see Table 8.11); loop diuretics only treat symptoms. If giving both loop and thiazide diuretics, they can be taken at the same time.
- If ordering a loop diuretic, start with furosemide 20–40 mg every morning. Titrate every few days to the lowest dose that achieves fluid balance, up to 80 mg daily before adding a second dose later in the day if needed.
- The three listed beta blockers (in Table 8.11) have been shown to be effective in decreasing the risk of death in HF; this is *not* a class effect.
- For patients taking aldosterone antagonists:
  - Counsel them to avoid foods high in potassium (see Appendix A).
  - Check serum K^+ and renal function 2–3 days after starting the medication, again at 7 days after and then at least monthly for 3 mo, then every 3 mo. Addition of or increase in the dosage of ACE or ARB starts a new monitoring cycle.
- Calcium channel blockers are not recommended as routine treatment for HFrEF; they have shown no functional or survival benefit in patients with HF. Amlodipine may be used for comorbid HTN or ischemic heart disease because it is generally well tolerated and safe.
- Jardiance *is now* approved to reduce the risk of CV death plus hospitalization for adults with HFrEF (as of August, 2021).
- HF with preserved EF (HFpEF)
  - Treated primarily with diuretic(s), especially a thiazide.
  - Avoid using nitrates, spironolactone, and ARBs.
  - Avoid using digoxin in patient > 65 yr of age.
  - Beta blockers do not reduce mortality.
- Statins *should not* be prescribed for HF treatment to improve clinical outcomes but only if otherwise indicated.
- Warn patients to avoid NSAIDs.
- There are *many* other prescription and OTC medications, herbal products and supplements that can adversely affect heart function—review all new medications for possible interactions before prescribing.

HEART MURMURS

I. Definition: turbulent blood flow through the heart as a result of one or more of the following
   A. Stenotic valve
   B. Regurgitant valve (i.e., one that does not stay closed)
   C. Septal defect
   D. Rapid blood flow (e.g., during pregnancy, with fever, and in children)
II. Description of murmurs
   A. Timing (i.e., systolic or diastolic): systolic murmurs are synchronous with the pulse and may or may not be normal; diastolic murmurs are *always* abnormal.

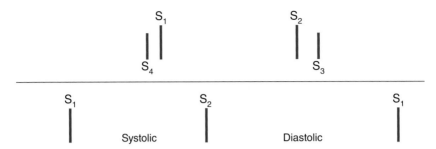

Systolic   Diastolic

B. Quality of sound (e.g., harsh, soft, blowing, or rumbling)
C. Location best heard
D. Radiation of murmur (e.g., to the neck, left axilla, back or across the precordium), which will be in the direction of blood flow
E. Classification of murmurs (see Table 8.12 and Fig. 8.4)
F. Grading
   1/6   Barely audible
   2/6   Audible but soft
   3/6   Easily audible, same loudness as S_1 and S_2
   4/6   Same as 3/6 but with a palpable thrill
   5/6   Audible with only a rim of the stethoscope on the chest; palpable thrill
   6/6   Audible with the stethoscope lifted just barely off the chest; palpable thrill

PRACTICE PEARLS FOR MURMURS

- To differentiate a heart murmur from a carotid bruit, simultaneously palpate the cardiac apex while listening to the bruit; a radiating murmur will be synchronous with the apical impulse, whereas a carotid bruit occurs somewhat later.
- *A new murmur found during a sports physical examination should be evaluated by a cardiologist before allowing the patient to participate in sports.*
- *A new murmur in the setting of an acute MI (AMI) may indicate a ruptured papillary muscle and impending cardiogenic shock; it is a surgical emergency.*
- If the murmur starts with S_1, it is probably associated with mitral or tricuspid valves; if it does not, consider aortic or pulmonic stenosis.

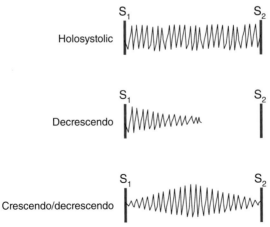

Fig. 8.4 Classification of murmurs.

■ = *not to be missed;* ▲ = *urgent referral*

TABLE 8.12 ■ Classifications of Murmurs

Description	Assessment	Referral Points
Systolic Murmurs		
Physiologic		
Grade 1/6 to 2/6, best heard with the diaphragm Loudest at the middle to lower left sternal border No radiation	May be normal in children or in adults In adults, it is more common with certain conditions (e.g., anemia, hyperthyroidism) No hemodynamic changes	Any previously undiagnosed murmur louder than 2/6 should be initially evaluated by an echocardiogram; **depending on the results, cardiology referral may be indicated** No antibiotic prophylaxis is needed
Aortic Stenosis		
Loud, harsh crescendo-decrescendo murmur Best heard at the second right ICS with the patient leaning forward but may be heard throughout the precordium Frequently radiates to the neck Often associated with a thrill	Ask about fatigue, palpitation, DOE, dizziness, syncope, and angina Radial pulse diminished Pulse pressure may be narrow Sometimes the patient has unexplained gastrointestinal tract bleeding Often associated with aortic insufficiency	Initial evaluation by an echocardiogram; depending on the results, **cardiology referral may be indicated** **Chest pain, dyspnea, or syncope are critical referral points for valve replacement** Antibiotic prophylaxis is no longer recommended*
Mitral Regurgitation		
Holosystolic, blowing, often loud Heard best at the apex in the left lateral position Decreases with inspiration Radiates to the left axilla and occasionally to the back	Symptoms include fatigue, palpitation, dizziness, DOE, syncope, and angina; symptoms range depending on the degree of regurgitation and heart failure Left atrium usually markedly enlarged	Initial evaluation by an echocardiogram; **depending on the results, cardiology referral may be indicated** Antibiotic prophylaxis is no longer recommended*
Mitral Valve Prolapse		
Murmur may or may not be present; sounds like "whoop" A midsystolic click is best heard over the apex with the diaphragm The click and murmur are best heard while the patient is in the sitting or squatting position or with the Valsalva maneuver	Symptoms include dysrhythmias, chest pain, and anxiety Most commonly found in white, Anglo-Saxon women Prognosis for most people is excellent, and treatment may not be indicated Diagnosis is made only with an echocardiogram; not all clicks are significant	Initial evaluation by an echocardiogram; **depending on the results, cardiology referral may be indicated** Antibiotic prophylaxis is no longer recommended* Encourage patients to remain well hydrated, have adequate salt intake, and to avoid caffeine and decongestants
Diastolic Murmurs		
Aortic Regurgitation		
Faint and high-pitched decrescendo, often starts simultaneously with S_2 Heard best with the diaphragm pressed firmly at the left third ICS, with the patient leaning forward and breath held in deep expiration Radiates down	Minor symptoms for years, then rapid deterioration May have associated head bobbing, diaphoresis, carotidynia, and a quick rise, flip, or collapsing arterial pulse Pulse pressure is often widened Apical impulse is displaced down and to left Fingernail bed pressure reveals a pulsating red color	**Obtain an echocardiogram and then refer to a cardiologist** Must be referred early for repair Antibiotic prophylaxis is no longer recommended*

● = non-urgent referral; ■ = not to be missed

TABLE 8.12 ■ Classifications of Murmurs—cont'd

Description	Assessment	Referral Points
Mitral Stenosis		
Diastolic rumble, best heard at the apex with patient in the left lateral position	DOE is common	***Obtain an echocardiogram and then refer to a cardiologist***
Best heard with the bell of the stethoscope		Poorly tolerated in pregnancy
Often associated with an opening snap, and S₁ may be louder than usual		Antibiotic prophylaxis is no longer recommended*

* See BACTERIAL ENDOCARDITIS: ANTIBIOTIC PROPHYLAXIS GUIDELINES, earlier in this chapter.

HYPERTENSION

I. Definition
   A. Diagnosis is made after at least two or more elevated readings at different times (including at the office, at home, or with ambulatory BP monitoring); at each visit, check the BP at least twice with the patient sitting for at least 5 min, with both feet on the floor. Average the readings and classify by the highest reading—systolic or diastolic (see Table 8.13 for classifications).
   B. For pediatric HTN, see Chapter 16, HYPERTENSION.
   C. For HTN in pregnancy, *referral to a high-risk obstetrician.*
   D. Severe HTN: BP $\geq 180/\geq 120$ mmHg or higher
      1. *If presenting with acute, life-threatening complications (hypertensive emergencies), emergent transfer to ED.*
         (a) *Encephalopathy*
         (b) *Retinal hemorrhage or papilledema or severe H/A with vision changes*
         (c) *Acute renal failure*
      2. May be asymptomatic other than possible H/A, with no signs of end-organ damage (hypertensive urgencies); often secondary to nonadherence with therapy or to recent increased salt intake.
      3. Treatment goal: see **IV. B.**

TABLE 8.13 ■ Classification of Hypertension

Stage	BP Range
Normal	<120/<80 mmHg
Elevated	120–129/<80 mmHg
Stage 1	130–139/80–89 mmHg
Stage 2	≥ 140 or ≥ 90 mmHg
Heart failure	Optimal BP not defined; ***consult a cardiologist for recommendations***

Based on American College of Cardiology/American Heart Association recommendations from Guideline for the Prevention, Detection, Evaluation, and Management of High Blood Pressure in Adults, 2017.

● = *non-urgent referral;* ▲ = *urgent referral*

II. Initial workup
  A. Specific history questions
    1. Past medical history
      (a) CV, cerebrovascular, or renal disease; also erectile dysfunction (often a vascular problem)
      (b) DM
      (c) History of HTN (what level, any treatment, and results); especially with BP > 180/120 mmHg, what has been patient's adherence with medical therapy?
      (d) Sleep apnea; is patient using CPAP or BIPAP?
      (e) Current medications (prescription and OTC)
      (f) Additional CV risk factors (e.g., smoking, dyslipidemia, excessive weight, unhealthy diet, low fitness, or eGFR < 60 mL/min) (see Chapter 11, CHRONIC KIDNEY DISEASE)
    2. Social factors: psychosocial stress, work schedules, how to pay for medications, and alcohol intake
    3. FH: HTN, CVA, CHD, HF, renal disease (including polycystic kidneys), DM, pheochromocytoma, cardiomyopathy, and sudden death
  B. Physical examination: main goals are to evaluate for signs of end-organ damage and evidence of an identifiable cause of HTN.
    1. General appearance, including calculation of BMI
    2. Fundoscopic examination
    3. Neck: thyroid and presence/absence of JVD or bruits
    4. CV: heart sounds (including S_4), PMI, breath sounds, edema, and peripheral pulses
    5. Abdomen: liver, presence/absence of bruits in the abdomen and femoral areas, and presence/absence of abnormal aortic pulsation
    6. Neurologic: cranial nerves, DTRs, and sensory changes
  C. Diagnostic tests
    1. Laboratory: CBC, CMP, lipid profile, TSH and free T4, and UA (including albumin/creatinine ratio to estimate proteinuria—see Chapter 15, CHRONIC COMPLICATIONS, I); consider uric acid level
    2. ECG
III. Secondary HTN workup (not needed in every patient with HTN)
  A. Evaluate for secondary HTN with the following
    1. Acute rise in BP with previously stable readings
    2. Onset of HTN in a nonobese patient < 30 yr of age who has no FH of HTN
    3. Excessive end-organ damage (e.g., cerebrovascular disease, retinopathy, LVH, HFpEF and HFrEF, CAD)
    4. Severe HTN > 180/120 mmHg, despite taking three antihypertensive medications (one of which is a diuretic)
    5. Onset of *diastolic* HTN in older adults
    6. Presence of unprovoked or excessive hypokalemia
    7. Increase in serum creatinine of at least 50% within a week of starting an ACE or ARB
  B. Possible causes
    1. Renal artery stenosis/renovascular disease
      (a) Very severe HTN that is resistant to therapy
      (b) Recurrent episodes of flash pulmonary edema
      (c) Unilateral small kidney or renal bruit

(d) Onset before the age of 30 yr or BP ≥ 180 systolic and/or 120 mmHg diastolic after the age of 55 yr

(e) Acute rise (over 50%) in serum creatinine within a week of starting an ACE or ARB

2. Primary hyperaldosteronism (most common cause of drug-resistant HTN)
    (a) Hypokalemia (otherwise unexplained)
    (b) Muscle weakness
    (c) Polyuria

3. OSA
    (a) Daytime somnolence and fatigue
    (b) Loud snoring with apneic periods

4. Medication-induced HTN (e.g., with NSAIDs, steroids/androgens, decongestants, caffeine, MAO inhibitors, some antidepressants [venlafaxine])

5. Alcohol-induced HTN

6. If specific clinical characteristics are present, consider screening for uncommon causes of secondary HTN
    (a) Pheochromocytoma (see Chapter 15, **Adrenal Disorders**, PHEOCHROMOCYTOMA)
    (b) Cushing's syndrome (e.g., moon facies and central obesity, proximal muscle weakness, striae)
    (c) Thyroid disorder (e.g., fatigue and/or anxiety, weight gain or loss, bradycardia/tachycardia)
    (d) Coarctation of the aorta (e.g., arm-to-leg systolic BP difference > 20 mmHg, delayed or absent femoral pulses, murmur)

C. Test for renal artery stenosis (i.e., captopril renal nuclear scan or renal angiography or renal artery duplex Doppler U/S or renal CT angiography) *only if:*

1. There is a moderate or high risk of having renal artery stenosis *and*
2. A corrective procedure would be done if a clinically significant renovascular disease is found.

IV. Treatment of HTN

A. Classification of hypertension (see Table 8.13)

B. For emergency treatment of HTN in office (BP $\geq 180/\geq 120$ mmHg)

▲
1. ***Transfer to ED if the patient is symptomatic with anything other than mild H/A.***
2. Have the patient rest in a quiet room and recheck BP. Consider clonidine 0.2 mg or captopril 6.25–12.5 mg; observe the patient up to a few hours to be sure that BP goes down by at least 20–30 mmHg; use with caution if the patient is tachycardic or has cardiac decompensation.
3. Decrease BP to 160/100 mmHg or less over several hours to days; there is no proven benefit from rapid reduction in an *asymptomatic* patient.
    (a) With previously treated HTN, is the patient taking the medications?
        (i) Increase dose of existing medication or add second one.
        (ii) Restart medications if the patient has been nonadherent.
        (iii) With suspicion of HTN due to high salt intake, add diuretics and reinforce sodium restriction.
    (b) In previously untreated HTN prescribe longer acting medication (i.e., CCB, ACE, or ARB).
    (c) Follow up within a few days.

▲ = *urgent referral*

C. With "white coat" HTN (untreated HTN in the range of 130–159 mmHg/80–99 mmHg), consider home or 24-hr ambulatory BP monitoring before starting medication.
D. Patients with elevated BP are twice as likely to develop HTN as those with normal BP; strongly encourage lifestyle modifications for those patients.
E. Encourage lifestyle changes (the impact of each change is a decrease of 4–5 mmHg in systolic and 2–4 mmHg in diastolic BP).
   1. Weight reduction if overweight; aim for 5%–10% body weight increments
   2. Diet: Mediterranean diet or see Table 8.14 for the DASH diet
   3. Exercise: regular physical activity
      (a) Try a 30-min walk at a rate of 2–3 mph five times weekly (or an equivalent exercise). Consider a structured exercise program.
      (b) Overall increase in physical activity (i.e., 10,000 steps); monitor with pedometer.
   4. Smoking cessation
   5. Alcohol (if used): 3 oz of whiskey, 10 oz of wine, or 24 oz of beer daily; women and thin patients should consume half of these amounts
   6. Sodium restriction < 2.4 g daily and increase dietary potassium (e.g., four to five servings of fruits/vegetables daily)
F. The benefit of pharmacological treatment for HTN is related to ASCVD risk.
   1. To calculate patient's 10-yr risk of a cardiovascular disease (CVD) event, see *http://my.americanheart.org/cvriskcalculator*.
   2. If lifestyle changes are unsuccessful or the patient has an additional risk factor (e.g., DM or CHD), start medication first (or at least simultaneously).

TABLE 8.14 ■ **The DASH Diet***

Food Group & Daily Servings	1 Serving Equals	Examples
Grains and grain products 7–8 servings	1 slice bread ½ cup dry or cooked cereal, pasta, or cooked rice	Whole-grain breads, pita, English muffin, bagel, grits, oatmeal
Vegetables 4–5 servings	1 cup raw leafy vegetables ½ cup cooked vegetables 6 oz vegetable juice	Tomatoes, potatoes, carrots, peas, squash, broccoli, turnip greens, kale, collards, spinach, artichokes, sweet potatoes
Fruits 4–5 servings	8 oz fruit juice 1 medium fruit ¼ cup dried fruit ½ cup fresh, frozen, or canned fruit	Apricots, bananas, dates, grapes, oranges, grapefruit, mangoes, melons, peaches, pineapples, prunes, raisins, strawberries, tangerines
Low-fat and nonfat dairy products 2–3 servings	8 oz milk 1 cup yogurt 1½ oz cheese	Skim or 1% milk, low-fat buttermilk, nonfat or low-fat yogurt, part-skim mozzarella cheese, nonfat cheese
Meat, poultry, fish 2 or fewer servings	3 oz cooked meats, poultry, or fish	Lean cuts with visible fat and skin removed; broiled, roasted, or boiled
Nuts and legumes 1 serving	¾ oz or $^1/_6$ cup nuts 1 tbsp seeds ½ cup cooked legumes	Almonds, filberts, mixed nuts, peanuts, walnuts, pecans, sunflower seeds, kidney beans, lentils

* The Dietary Approach to Stop Hypertension (DASH) diet is low in fat and cholesterol; high in fiber, potassium, calcium, and magnesium; and moderately high in protein. It provides approximately 2000 kcal a day.

3. Start medication(s) for
   (a) Secondary prevention in patients with clinical CVD and an average SBP ≥ 130 mmHg or a DBP ≥ 80 mmHg
   (b) Primary prevention in adults with no history of CVD but with
      (i) An estimated 10-yr ASCVD risk of ≥ 10% and an SBP ≥ 130 mmHg or a DBP ≥ 80 mmHg
      (ii) An estimated 10-yr ASCVD risk of ≤ 10% but with an SBP ≥ 130 mmHg or a DBP ≥ 80 mmHg
4. Initial first-line therapy includes thiazide diuretics, CCBs, ACE inhibitors, or ARBs (see Table 8.15 for additional medication suggestions, depending on comorbidities).
   (a) Stage 1 (see Table 8.13): start with one medication.
   (b) Stage 2 (see Table 8.13): start with two first-line medications of different classes.
   (c) If the patient has known CVD, the recommendation is to follow standard treatment guidelines for previous MI, HFrEF, etc., with the addition of other medications as needed to control BP.
5. Except for additional indications (e.g., rate control with atrial fib), the amount of BP reduction is more important than the choice of medication; see Table 8.16 for Antihypertensive Medications and Dosages and Table 8.17 for Cautions and Contraindications.

G. Follow-up
1. With low-risk adults with elevated BP or stage 1 HTN: recheck after 3–6 mo of lifestyle changes.
2. With stage 1 HTN and 10-yr ASCVD risk ≥ 10%: recheck after 1 mo of lifestyle changes and one antihypertensive medication.
3. With stage 2 HTN: recheck in 1 mo after lifestyle changes and two antihypertensive medications of different classes.

H. If the BP goal is not met at the follow-up visit, stress adherence to medication and lifestyle changes and
1. Increase drug dose by one "step" *or*
2. Substitute another drug ("sequential monotherapy") *or*
3. Add a second agent
   (a) Thiazide, if not already on one, is a good choice.
   (b) If the patient is on a beta blocker (BB), use thiazide or dihydropyridine CCB; ACEs or ARBs may be less effective because beta blocker decreases renin secretion and thus angiotensin II formation.
   (c) Use caution in using a BB in combination with nondihydropyridine CCB (e.g., verapamil or diltiazem) because of an increased risk of bradycardia or AV block.
4. Better response is shown with less side effects if medication is changed or if additional medication is added after a one-step dose increase (instead of the maximum dose before adding another medication).

I. If the BP goal is still not met after 1–2 mo, consider triple therapy with an ACE or ARB, CCB, and thiazide diuretic before using any other class of antihypertensive medication. Most patients will require two or more antihypertensive agents.

J. ***Resistant HTN is diagnosed when the BP goal is not met despite the patient adhering to full doses of a three-drug regimen that includes a diuretic; consultation with a cardiologist should be considered.***

= non-urgent referral

TABLE 8.15 ■ Suggested Antihypertensive Agents (Based on Comorbidities)*

Patient Profile	Suggested Agent*	Agents to Avoid
Angina (stable)	Beta blocker Dihydropyridine CCB	
Asthma, COPD	CCB Central alpha agonist	Beta blocker (except bisoprolol)
Atrial fibrillation	Beta blocker Nondihydropyridine CCB ARB	
BPH	Alpha blocker[†]	
CKD	ACE or ARB Loop diuretics usually needed with advanced disease	
Depression		Beta blockers Central alpha agonist
DM, type 1	ACE or ARB Thiazide diuretic (especially chlorthalidone) Central alpha agonist	Beta blocker with ISA[‡] Alpha blocker
DM, type 2	ACE or ARB CCB	Diuretic at high dose Beta blocker (except carvedilol)

Elderly	Thiazide diuretic
	CCB (dihydropyridine)
		Alpha blocker (use cautiously
		  because of postural hypotension)[†]
		Beta blockers (except with history
		  of MI or HF)

Gout		Loop or thiazide diuretic
HFpEF (diastolic dysfunction)	Diuretic Consider ACE or ARB Beta blocker	Nitrates Spironolactone

HFrEF (systolic
  dysfunction)
	ACE or ARB
	Beta blocker (specifically carvedilol,
	  metoprolol succinate)
	Diuretics (loops)
		Nondihydropyridine CCB

Ischemic heart	ACE (in all patients who have had a STEMI or an anterior NSTEMI) Beta blocker without ISA[‡] CCB	Beta blocker with ISA[‡] Vasodilator
Isolated systolic HTN	Thiazide diuretic CCB (dihydropyridine)	Beta blockers (except with history of MI or HF)
Left ventricular hypertrophy	ARB or ACE CCB	Beta blocker with ISA[‡] Direct vasodilator
Liver disease		Methyldopa
Migraines	Beta blocker CCB	
Osteoporosis	Thiazide diuretic	
Peripheral vascular disease	CCB	Alpha blocker
Tachycardia	CCB (especially verapamil or diltiazem)	

Young or with
  hyperdynamic circulation
	ACE or ARB
	Beta blockers (not commonly used
	  for initial monotherapy)	

* Also see Table 8.16 for dosing guidelines and Table 8.17 for cautions.
† Not as a primary agent but may be useful as an add-on agent, especially in elderly men with symptomatic prostatism.
‡ Intrinsic sympathomimetic activity (i.e., blocks beta$_1$ receptors while mildly stimulating beta$_2$ receptors).

PRACTICE PEARLS FOR HYPERTENSION

- Follow up q1–2 mo, depending on the status, until the BP goal is reached. Once stable, follow-up visits can be at 3–6 mo intervals. In patients > 50 yr of age, SBP is a more important CVD risk factor than DBP.
- Patients ≥ 65 yr of age with HTN
  - Who also have a limited life expectancy or multiple comorbidities: discuss with patient their risks/benefits and preferences regarding antihypertensive therapy, medication choices, and BP goal. Lowering BP is reasonable in many people to prevent cognitive decline and dementia.
  - They may struggle with sodium restriction because they may use more salt to compensate for decrease in taste sensitivity or because they eat more prepackaged foods.
  - Because of physiological changes with aging, BP should be lowered over 3–6 mo, instead of over days, to minimize ischemic symptoms or orthostatic hypotension.
  - If it is difficult to achieve BP ≤ 130/≤80 mmHg (especially if baseline SBP was > 160 mmHg), a reasonable goal may be the best SBP achieved with two or three medications.
- When the patient is on more than one antihypertensive medication, taking one nondiuretic medication at hs may improve BP control (especially with concomitant OSA, DM, CKD).
- With difficulty controlling BP, ask about herbs (e.g., ginseng, bitter orange, guarana, licorice root).
- In black adults with HTN but without HF or CKD (including those with DM): initial antihypertensive therapy should include a thiazide diuretic or CCB; often, two different medications will be needed to obtain BP of < 130/80 mmHg.
- NSAIDs may interfere with the effects of ACE inhibitors, beta blockers, and diuretics.
- Treat with decongestants cautiously; pseudoephedrine has the lowest CV risk profile.
- ACE/ARB
  - Do not give an ACE and ARB simultaneously.
  - Recheck basic chemistry profile 2–3 wk after starting an ACE; if creatinine has increased, recheck again in 2–3 wk. If creatinine level has increased further, stop the ACE.
  - Treatment of HTN with an ARB can help prevent recurrence of atrial fib.
  - Losartan is the weakest ARB and may need to be taken bid; if BP not controlled, try changing to a stronger ARB that can be taken once daily.
- Thiazides
  - Thiazides are more effective than loop diuretics in HTN except when serum creatinine is > 2.5 mg/dL.
  - Chlorthalidone is the preferred thiazide-like diuretic because of a longer duration (i.e., 24 hr) and proven CVD risk reduction; however, the 25 mg tabs are not scored. It also comes in combination only with atenolol, azilsartan, or clonidine.
  - When a stable patient is on a fixed dose of HCTZ or chlorthalidone, the potassium loss occurs only during the first 2 wk of therapy; if the repeat K^+ is normal at 2–3 wk, there is no risk of hypokalemia unless the dose is increased or potassium intake is reduced.
  - Thiazides cross-react with sulfa allergies.
- With normal renal function, approximate equivalent doses are: bumetanide 1 mg = furosemide 40 mg = torsemide 20 mg
- Potential side effects
  - Coughing could be due to ACE (can change to ARB and cough should resolve); if bronchospasms occur, consider the effect of beta blockers; if the patient currently smokes, choose a cardioselective beta blocker.
  - Angioedema secondary to an ACE—there is no pruritus or urticaria.
  - Sexual or erectile dysfunction may occur with alpha blockers, BBs, and central alpha agonists.
  - Edema with amlodipine is not fluid-related, so diuretics *do not* help; try decreasing the dose, adding an ACE/ARB, or changing to a different medication.
  - Diuretics can elevate serum cholesterol and triglyceride levels and decrease HDL levels in patients with diabetes.
  - Olmesartan (Benicar) has been associated with a sprue-like illness (i.e., severe, chronic diarrhea, significant weight loss); the condition resolves when the medication is stopped.
- Potassium supplementation may be needed when taking diuretics (Table 8.18).

TABLE 8.16 ■ Antihypertensive Medication and Dosages

Medication	Initial Dose	Maintenance Maximum
ACE Inhibitors		
Benazepril (Lotensin)*	5–10 mg daily	40 mg daily, in 1–2 doses
Captopril (Capoten)*	12.5–25 mg bid-tid	150 mg tid
Enalapril (Vasotec)*	2.5 mg daily (with diuretics) 5 mg daily (without diuretics)	40 mg daily, in 1–2 doses
Fosinopril (Monopril)*	10 mg daily	80 mg daily
Lisinopril (Zestril, Prinivil)*	5–10 mg daily	40 mg daily
Moexipril (Univasc)*	7.5 mg daily	30 mg daily, in 1–2 doses
Perindopril (Aceon)	4 mg daily	16 mg daily
Quinapril (Accupril)*	10–20 mg daily	80 mg daily, in 1–2 doses
Ramipril (Altace) Capsules may be opened and mixed with applesauce, water, or apple juice	2.5 mg daily	20 mg daily, in 1–2 doses
Trandolapril (Mavik)	1 mg daily	4 mg daily
Angiotensin Receptor Blocker (ARB)		
Azilsartan (Edarbi)*	40 mg daily	80 mg daily
Candesartan (Atacand)*	8 mg daily	32 mg daily
Eprosartan mesylate (Teveten)*	600 mg daily	800 mg daily, in 1–2 doses
Irbesartan (Avapro)*	150 mg daily	300 mg daily
Losartan (Cozaar)*	50 mg daily (25 mg with volume depletion or hepatic impairment)	100 mg daily, in 1–2 doses
Olmesartan (Benicar)*	20 mg daily	40 mg daily
Telmisartan (Micardis)*	20–40 mg daily	80 mg daily
Valsartan (Diovan)*	80–160 mg daily	320 mg daily
Alpha Adrenergic Blocker (Peripheral)†		
Doxazosin mesylate (Cardura)	1 mg qd	16 mg daily
Prazosin (Minipress)	1 mg bid-tid	20 mg daily
Terazosin (Hytrin)	1 mg hs	20 mg daily
Alpha Agonist (Central)		
Clonidine (Catapres)	0.1 mg bid	0.6 mg daily, in 2 doses
Methyldopa (Aldomet)*	250 mg bid-tid	3000 mg daily, in 2 doses
Alpha-Beta Blocker		
Carvedilol (Coreg)	6.25 mg bid	50 mg daily, divided bid
(Coreg CR)	20 mg daily	80 mg daily
Labetalol HCl (Normodyne, Trandate)	100 mg bid	2400 mg, divided bid
Beta Blocker		
Atenolol (recommended *only* with MI, arrhythmia)	25 mg qd-bid	100 mg daily, in 1–2 doses
Bisoprolol fumarate* (recommended *only* with ischemic heart disease, HFrEF, arrhythmia)	2.5–5 mg daily	20 mg daily

TABLE 8.16 ■ Antihypertensive Medication and Dosages—cont'd

Medication	Initial Dose	Maintenance Maximum
Metoprolol tartrate (Lopressor)* Metoprolol succinate (Toprol XL) (both recommended *only* with ischemic heart disease, HFrEF, arrhythmia)	50 mg bid 25–100 mg daily	450 mg daily, in 2 doses 400 mg daily
Nadolol (Corgard)	40 mg daily	320 mg daily
Nebivolol (Bystolic)	5 mg daily	40 mg daily
Propranolol HCl (Inderal)* (Inderal-LA) (both recommended *only* with ischemic heart disease, essential tremor, migraine)	40 mg bid 80 mg daily	160 mg daily, in 2 doses 160 mg daily
Beta Blocker With ISA‡		
Acebutolol (Sectral)	200–400 mg daily	600 mg bid
Pindolol (Visken)	5 mg bid	60 mg daily, in 2 doses
Calcium Channel Blockers (Nondihydropyridines)		
Diltiazem: Cardizem SR Cardizem CD Cardizem LA	60–120 mg bid 120–240 mg daily 180–240 mg daily	360 mg daily, in 2 doses 480 mg daily 540 mg daily
Verapamil (Calan SR, Isoptin SR, Verelan)	120–240 mg daily	480 mg daily, in 1–3 doses (depending on formulation)
Calcium Channel Blockers (Dihydropyridines)		
Amlodipine (Norvasc)	2.5–5 mg daily	10 mg daily
Felodipine (Plendil)	2.5–5 mg daily	10 mg daily
Isradipine (DynaCirc)	2.5 mg bid	10 mg daily, in 2 doses
Nicardipine (Cardene SR)	30 mg bid	40 mg tid
Nifedipine (Procardia XL, Adalat CC)	30–60 mg daily	90 mg daily
Nisoldipine ER (Sular ER)	17 mg daily	34 mg daily
Direct Renin Inhibitor		
Aliskiren (Tekturna)*	150 mg daily	300 mg daily
Direct Vasodilator		
Hydralazine (Apresoline)	10 mg qid	300 mg daily, divided
Loop Diuretics		
Bumetanide (Bumex)	0.5–1 mg daily	Titrated to effective dose; not first-line for HTN
Furosemide (Lasix)	10–20 mg daily	Titrated to effective dose; not first-line for HTN
Torsemide (Demadex)	5 mg daily	10 mg daily
Potassium-Sparing Diuretics		
Amiloride (recommended *only* with HF, to limit K^+ loss)	5 mg daily	10 mg daily, in 1–2 doses
Eplerenone (Inspra)	50 mg daily	50 mg bid
Spironolactone (Aldactone)	25 mg daily	50–100 mg daily, in 1–2 doses

Continued

TABLE 8.16 ■ **Antihypertensive Medication and Dosages—cont'd**

Medication	Initial Dose	Maintenance Maximum
Thiazide Diuretics		
Chlorothiazide (Diuril)	500–1000 mg daily	2000 mg daily, in 1–2 doses
Chlorthalidone (does not come in 12.5 mg tab; 25 mg must be cut)	12.5–25 mg daily	50 mg daily
Hydrochlorothiazide (Microzide)	12.5–25 mg daily	50 mg daily
Indapamide (Lozol)	1.25 mg daily	5 mg daily

See Table 8.17 for cautions and contraindications. Combination agents are not included in this chart.
* Also comes in combination with a diuretic.
† Give the initial dose at bedtime to decrease syncopal episodes; not a first-line blood pressure medication.
‡ Intrinsic sympathomimetic agent (i.e., blocks beta$_1$ receptors while mildly stimulating beta$_2$ receptors).

TABLE 8.17 ■ **Cautions and Contraindications for Antihypertensive Agents**

Medication	Precautions	Contraindications
ACE inhibitors	Monitor serum potassium, BUN, and creatinine at baseline and 2–3 wk after dose increases; stop if creatinine increases by ≥ 1 mg/dL Use cautiously in women of child-bearing age and not on contraception Discontinue therapy if the patient develops angioedema (swelling of hands, face, or tongue), sore throat, or fever (of undetermined origin)	Hypertrophic cardiomyopathy Bilateral renal artery stenosis or stenosis of a solitary kidney Pregnancy (consider urine or serum HCG before use)
ARB	Monitor serum potassium, BUN, and creatinine at baseline Use cautiously if the patient is volume-depleted Use cautiously in women of child-bearing age and not on contraception	Pregnancy (consider urine or serum HCG before use) Renal artery stenosis (as above) CKD (eGFR ≤ 30 mL/min)
Alpha blockers (peripheral)	May have postural BP changes (especially with the first dose or after a missed dose) Elderly patients Cautious use with hepatic impairment (doxazocin)	Hypertrophic cardiomyopathy
Alpha agonists (central)	May have postural BP changes Preexisting bradycardia Concomitant depression Taper slowly because of rebound HTN Severe coronary insufficiency Chronic renal impairment	Active hepatic disease and in elderly patients (methyldopa)
Alpha-beta blockers	Monitor heart rate May have postural BP changes Type 1 or 2 DM COPD Hepatic impairment (mild to moderate) PVD/Raynaud phenomenon Pregnancy Children	Asthma Overt HF (labetalol) Severe bradycardia AV block greater than first degree Severe hepatic impairment

TABLE 8.17 ■ Cautions and Contraindications for Antihypertensive Agents—cont'd

Medication	Precautions	Contraindications
Beta blockers	Monitor the heart rate for bradycardia PVD Type 2 DM or pre-DM (except carvedilol and nebivolol) Dyslipidemia May be less effective in Black patients Taper slowly because of rebound HTN (possible MI or sudden death with sudden stopping)	Type 1 DM Asthma/COPD Sick sinus syndrome or AV blocks Severe PVD Raynaud phenomenon Pregnancy (atenolol)
Beta blockers with ISA*	May accelerate ischemia in CAD Taper slowly because of rebound HTN (possible MI or sudden death with sudden stopping) Asthma/COPD	
CCBs: nondihydropyridines	Monitor heart rate for bradycardia May aggravate CHD and HF Constipation (especially verapamil)	Bradycardia AV blocks Severe left ventricular systolic dysfunction
CCBs: dihydropyridines	May cause lightheadedness, H/A, peripheral edema	
Direct renin inhibitor		eGFR <30 mL/min or creatinine >2 mg/dL (males) or >1.7 mg/dL (females)
Direct vasodilators	May precipitate angina in CAD Pulmonary HTN Severe renal impairment Concomitant treatment with a diuretic or beta blocker may be indicated	Mitral valve rheumatic heart disease
Diuretics: loop	Monitor electrolyte panel plus Mg^{++} Monitor weight May develop tolerance; using staggered dosing may decrease tolerance Ototoxicity may occur with high doses of furosemide Cirrhosis, ascites Hypokalemia (see Table 8.18 for treatment)	Preeclampsia Hepatic coma (bumetanide) Hypertrophic cardiomyopathy (relative contraindication) Sulfa allergy
Diuretics: potassium-sparing	Monitor electrolytes DM Concomitant use of NSAIDs or ACE Use cautiously, if at all, with creatinine >1.5 mg/dL or eGFR <45 mL/min Hepatic impairment (spironolactone)	Preexisting hyperkalemia Acute renal insufficiency: creatinine >2.5 mg/dL (males) or >2 mg/dL (females) Severe hepatic disease (triamterene: no; eplerenone: caution)
Diuretics: thiazide	Monitor electrolyte panel plus Mg^{++} and Ca^{++} before starting and recheck K$^+$ after 3 wk on medication Dyslipidemia (moderate-to-high cholesterol) Type 2 DM or pre-DM Hypokalemia (see Table 8.18 for treatment) Cirrhosis SLE	Sulfa allergy Serum creatinine >2.5 mg/dL (ineffective in severe renal disease) Hypertrophic cardiomyopathy (relative contraindication) Preeclampsia Poorly controlled gout

See Table 8.16 for dosing recommendations.
* Intrinsic sympathomimetic activity (i.e., blocks beta$_1$ receptors while mildly stimulating beta$_2$ receptors).

TABLE 8.18 ■ **Potassium Supplementation**

Dosing	
Prevention	16–24 mEq daily
To correct depletion	40–100 mEq daily
Suggested Products	
8 mEq	Klor-Con 8 or Slow-K
10 mEq	K-Dur 10, K-Tab, Kaon 10, Klor-Con 10
20 mEq	K-Dur 20, 15 mL or Kaochlor 10% liquid
25 mEq	K-Lyte/Cl effervescent
50 mEq	K-Lyte/Cl 50 effervescent

METABOLIC SYNDROME

I. Description: this condition is characterized by insulin resistance and prothrombotic and proinflammatory states; it markedly increases the risk for CHD.
II. Diagnosis: metabolic syndrome is diagnosed when any three or more of the following symptoms are present
  A. Abdominal obesity (waist circumference)
    1. Men: > 40 inches (102 cm)
    2. Women: > 35 inches (88 cm)
  B. Triglycerides: ≥ 150 mg/dL
  C. HDL-C level
    1. Men: < 40 mg/dL
    2. Women: < 50 mg/dL
  D. BP: ≥ 130/85 mmHg *or* on medication for hypertension
  E. FBG level: ≥ 100 mg/dL
III. Management
  A. Reduce and/or treat the underlying causes and conditions.
  B. Encourage dietary changes (e.g., Mediterranean diet) and, if indicated, weight reduction (in 5% increments).
  C. Encourage increased physical activity.
    1. Work up to 30-min walks five times a week (or an equivalent exercise).
    2. Increase overall daily movement (i.e., aim for 10,000 steps daily, monitor with a pedometer).

Peripheral Vascular Conditions

PERIPHERAL ARTERIAL DISEASE

I. Acute arterial occlusion (acute limb ischemia)
  A. Description: usually caused by a thrombus secondary to atherosclerosis; usually found after arterial injury/surgery or with disseminated intravascular coagulation (DIC), sepsis, or hypercoagulability disorders
  B. Signs and symptoms; always examine both extremities
    1. Can occur rapidly or slowly over a few days; may need Doppler to assess pulses
    2. May have decreased or absent posterior tibial (PT) or dorsalis pedis (DP) pulse distal to occlusion (normal pulses on opposite side)

3. Bruit is common if arterial plaque is the source of occlusion
4. Six Ps indicative of occlusion
Pain (starts distally and progresses proximally until sensation lost)
Pulselessness (in affected extremity; if normal on opposite extremity, probable cause is embolism)
Pallor (with mottling and ↓ capillary refill)
Paralysis (indicates advanced ischemia)
Paresthesia (earliest sign is on dorsum of foot)
Poikilothermia (perceived temperature change is early sign)
▲   C. **Treatment is urgent/emergency transfer to ED or a vascular surgeon.**

II. Chronic arterial occlusive disease
A. Description: arterial stenosis causing altered blood flow, normally with exercise (intermittent claudication)
1. With activity, claudication occurs because the metabolic demands of the muscle exceed the available oxygen due to narrowing of arterial lumen.
2. It begins as stenosing lesions that progressively narrow to complete obstruction.
   (a) Pain in foot: tibial or peroneal artery
   (b) Pain in upper calf: usually from superficial femoral artery; pain in lower calf from popliteal artery
   (c) Pain in thigh: common femoral artery, with weak pulses distally
   (d) Pain in buttock or hip: usually from the aorta or aortoiliac arteries; usually also causes erectile dysfunction
3. Is related to smoking, atherosclerosis, HTN (poorly controlled), lack of exercise, obesity, dyslipidemia, and DM
4. People with diabetes are at the highest risk of loss of an extremity because of occlusion of both larger and smaller arteries.
B. Signs and symptoms (may be silent for years)
1. Gradual onset of pain in leg/foot which may proceed to an acute thrombotic event; pain may be constant or intermittent.
2. Intermittent claudication: reproducible cramping pain and fatigue in legs that occurs with exercise and is relieved with rest (within 10 min of rest); severity is graded according to exercise.
   (a) Pain usually progresses to night pain.
   (b) Pain and pallor in feet worsened by elevation and relieved with dangling; patient usually sleeps with feet dangling to decrease pain.
3. Shiny skin with lack of hair on the affected extremity; thickened toenails unrelated to fungus
4. May have small noninflamed and poorly healing ulcer(s) usually found over bony prominences.
5. Vascular bruits; changes in DP and PT pulses at rest and with exercise
C. Diagnostics
1. Buerger's test is an in-office test to assess the adequacy of arterial supply to the legs; both legs are done at the same time, for comparison. If positive, obtain an ABI (see 2, below)
   (a) Have the patient lie supine; elevate the legs to 45 degrees and hold for 1–2 min. Observe the color of the feet (pallor indicates ischemia).
   (b) Then have the patient sit up, with the legs hanging over the side of the table at 90 degrees. As the blood flow returns to the affected leg, the skin (of the foot and lower leg) will become blue and then red.

▲ = *urgent referral*

      2. Portable hand office Doppler ankle-brachial index (ABI) or ABI/segmental Doppler U/S (see calculation of ABI, **IV**, later in this section, and Table 8.19)

      3. CBC, CMP

  D. Treatment

      1. Smoking cessation (most important factor)

      2. Aggressive control of dyslipidemia, HTN, and DM

      3. Exercise program, either at home or outpatient; encourage walking to increase how far the patient can walk before symptoms occur

      4. Close monitoring of skin for nonhealing wounds

      5. Antiplatelet agents

         (a) ASA 81–325 mg daily *and/or*

         (b) Clopidogrel 75 mg daily to decrease the risk of MI or CVA

         (c) Cilostazol 100 mg 1–2 times daily may help alleviate pain and increase walking distance

         (d) Vorapaxar (Zontivity) 2.08 mg daily; give with ASA 81–325 mg or clopidogrel 75 mg

  E. ***Referral to a vascular surgeon for evaluation (especially with an ulcer) and further treatment options***

III. Raynaud phenomenon

  A. Description: recurrent vasospasm of fingers and toes in response to stress or cold exposure

      1. Primary

         (a) No association with any other disease processes

         (b) Symmetrical bilateral involvement of fingers/toes (but usually avoids thumb); absence of necrosis

         (c) Usually found in young females between 15 and 40 yr of age

      2. Secondary: usually associated with an autoimmune disease and is progressive

  B. Pertinent history questions

      1. Are your fingers sensitive to or change color with the cold?

      2. Do your fingers turn white, blue, or both?

  C. Signs and symptoms

      1. Sudden appearance of color change in fingers/toes with cold temperatures

         (a) Changes have a sharp demarcated border between affected and unaffected areas.

         (b) Changes should be reversible when fingers rewarm.

      2. Numbness and pain in the affected fingers/toes

      3. BP normal; peripheral pulses equally palpable

  D. Diagnostics to differentiate between primary and secondary disease

      1. Consider upper extremity Doppler U/S

      2. CBC (may show polycythemia)

      3. CMP (check for possible renal or hepatic involvement, early/late DM); TSH

      4. Antinuclear body/rheumatoid arthritis (ANA/RA) and antiphospholipid antibodies

  E. Nonpharmacological treatment

      1. Avoidance of causative factors

         (a) Cold or rapidly changing temperatures

         (b) Tobacco use or secondhand smoke

         (c) Caffeine, alcohol

         (d) Diet pills, ephedra (herbal), ADHD medications, nasal decongestants, ergotamine

---

● = *non-urgent referral*

2. Wear gloves and warm clothing
3. Avoid repeated trauma to fingers/toes
4. Teach methods to help warm extremity
   (a) Rubbing hands together
   (b) Immerse hands in warm water
   (c) Rotating, whirling, or shaking hands
F. Pharmacological treatment
   1. Medications (to help control symptoms)
      (a) CCB, such as nifedipine SR 30–120 mg daily or amlodipine 5–20 mg daily; monitor BP at home.
      (b) Consider PDEs: sildenafil 20 mg 1–2 times daily or tadalafil 20 mg every other day if CCB ineffective. Contraindicated if using topical nitroglycerin.
      (c) ARB, such as losartan 50 mg daily can be tried, if unable to take CCB; it could also help with BP lowering.
      (d) Fluoxetine 10 mg daily, especially if anxiety is a trigger.
      (e) Topical nitroglycerin (1%–2%) applied to severely affected digits (short-term use—days to weeks); contraindicated if using PDEs.
   2. Medications that may *worsen* the condition
      (a) Beta blockers, clonidine
      (b) Imipramine
      (c) Pseudoephedrine/phenylephrine, weight loss supplements, amphetamines
      (d) Nasal decongestants
      (e) OC and ergots
      (f) Migraine medications
G. ***Referral to vascular specialist for evaluation and treatment***
IV. Calculation of ankle-brachial index
   A. Definition: a diagnostic measure of lower extremity arterial insufficiency (can be done in the office setting or as outpatient); evaluate if
      1. Claudication symptoms are present
      2. There are nonhealing ulcers over bony prominences
      3. Patient is > 65 yr of age or > 50 yr of age with tobacco use and/or DM
      4. Patient also has long-standing or poorly controlled HTN, hyperlipidemia or CHD
   B. Procedure: use a handheld Doppler transducer and place over either the DP or PT artery. The BP cuff is inflated at the ankle; systolic pressure is recorded when the signal reap pears as the cuff deflates. Brachial systolic pressure is recorded in a similar manner.
   C. Calculation: ABI is the highest ankle pressure divided by the highest brachial pressure bilaterally.
   D. Interpretation: normally, ankle systolic pressure exceeds arm systolic pressure.
      1. Ankle pressure does not begin to change until the artery diameter is reduced by at least 50%.
      2. ABI is normal at rest and becomes abnormal with exercise because of stenosis.
      3. Noncompressible arteries can be found in DM and CKD and lead to falsely elevated readings (see Table 8.19 for ABI values).

= *non-urgent referral*

TABLE 8.19 ■ Ankle-Brachial Index (ABI) Interpretation

ABI	Disease Severity
> 1.30*	Noncompressible, calcified vessels; needs further testing
1–1.3	Normal (no disease)
0.91–0.99**	Borderline abnormal
< 0.9***	Diagnostic of occlusive arterial disease: 0.4–0.9: Borderline disease; claudication symptoms are usually present < 0.40: Severe occlusive disease; ischemia, poor healing ulcers, and rest pain common

* Calcified vessels due to diabetes mellitus or end-stage renal disease; suggest toe-brachial index.
** With history of claudication symptoms but the ABI is normal at rest, repeat ABI after exercise.
*** *Referral to a vascular surgeon*.

PERIPHERAL VENOUS DISEASE

I. Acute venous disease
   A. Deep vein thrombosis (DVT) is an acute thromboembolism that occurs unilaterally in the proximal or distal leg but can occur in the upper arm (usually catheter related), with the potential to migrate to the lungs if untreated.
      1. Proximal DVT
         (a) Located in the entire leg and/or calf due to popliteal, femoral, or iliac vein thrombus
         (b) Highest risk for emboli to lungs
         (c) Must be treated with anticoagulation for minimum of 3 mo, with or without acute symptoms (see 6 below)
      2. Distal DVT
         (a) Located below the knee in posterior tibial and peroneal veins (no involvement to popliteal vein)
         (b) Less risk of embolization to lungs
         (c) If acute and symptomatic, needs anticoagulation
      3. Risk factors for DVT
         (a) Medications (e.g., any type of OCs, estrogen replacement or tamoxifen)
         (b) Recent or long-term immobility (e.g., prolonged travel, major surgery, CVA)
         (c) Morbid obesity, varicose veins, smoking and alcohol abuse
         (d) Long-bone trauma or crush injury (especially femur)
         (e) During pregnancy and first postpartum month due to hyperfibrinogenemia
         (f) Increased blood viscosity due to high altitude changes
         (g) Cancer, inheritable thrombophilias, inflammatory bowel disease (IBD), HF
         (h) ≥ 65 yr of age
         (i) PMH or family history (FH) of DVT/PE
      4. Signs and symptoms
         (a) Acute unilateral calf or thigh pain with swelling, redness, and heat to touch; may have aching or cramping in the affected leg that is aggravated by muscle activity, but can occur with rest
         (b) Localized tenderness at site of occlusion with tender cord-like vein

● = *non-urgent referral*

       (c) Circumference of affected leg is larger when compared to other leg (most useful finding); foot and ankle may have pitting edema

       (d) Positive Homan's sign (accurate 30% of time)

       (e) If it occurs in an upper extremity, will see similar swelling in arm and hand with associated pain in neck/shoulder and paresthesia.

5. Diagnostic testing

   (a) Compression U/S with Doppler of entire leg

   (b) Consider labs: D-dimer, CBC, CMP, PT/INR

6. Treatment

▲   (a) ***Transfer to ED if PE or extensive DVT is suspected.***

   (b) May be treated as an outpatient if

      (i) Ambulatory and stable with normal V/S

      (ii) Low risk of bleeding

      (iii) No renal insufficiency

      (iv) Patient (or caregivers) can administer injections (if needed) and maintain oral medication regimen

      (v) Patient (or caregivers) can comply with follow-up testing

   (c) Prescription anticoagulation is the preferred therapy to prevent further thrombosis and complications.

   (d) Initial outpatient anticoagulant therapy recommended for 3–6 mo (first episode) or lifetime if second DVT (see Table 8.22).

      (i) *Monotherapy* with either rivaroxaban (Xarelto) or apixaban (Eliquis) is preferred.

      (ii) If not using rivaroxaban or apixaban, initiate therapy with injectable anticoagulant (Arixtra or Lovenox) *for 5–7 days before starting* dabigatran (Pradaxa), edoxaban (Savaysa) or warfarin.

      (iii) Warfarin therapy requires monitoring with INR for maintenance of therapeutic level; INR goal is between 2 and 3 (see Tables 8.20 and 8.21).

   (e) Recurrent DVT while on anticoagulant therapy—verify adherence, interactions and appropriate dosing

      (i) If on warfarin and INRs erratic, consider changing to DOAC.

      (ii) With DOAC adherence, consider changing to warfarin, since it can be monitored.

      (iii) If the patient is on an adequate dose of DOAC or well controlled on warfarin, consider other causes (e.g., undiagnosed cancer or clotting disorder).

   (f) Stop OC, HRT, or tamoxifen.

   (g) Avoid crossing legs, prolonged sitting/standing, or massaging of extremity.

   (h) Cessation of smoking and alcohol, avoid dehydration.

   (i) Wear graduated compression stockings with minimum compression of 30–40 mmHg for at least 2 yr; this will decrease recurrent thrombosis and post-thrombotic syndrome.

   (j) Repeat compression U/S with Doppler in 3 mo and if DVT has resolved, can stop treatment and use ASA daily; if thrombus still present, repeat U/S again in 6 mo and continue anticoagulant therapy until thrombus resolved.

7. ***Referral to vascular surgeon or hematologist for further evaluation, if not resolving***

▲ = *urgent referral;* ● = *non-urgent referral*

B. Superficial thrombophlebitis
   1. Description: a thrombus in a surface vein causing inflammation and phlebitis
      (a) Usually occurs in the lower leg, but can occur in arm (e.g., IV catheter sites).
      (b) Generally self-limited and benign but if it involves larger veins, can ↑ risk for DVT.
   2. Signs and symptoms
      (a) Presents with more gradual onset of redness along the course of a vein, with swelling, pain, and warmth.
      (b) May be able to see inflamed portions of the vein and may occur with DVT.
   3. Diagnostic testing: compression U/S with Doppler
   4. Treatment if uncomplicated
      (a) Hot or cool moist packs
      (b) Relaxation of the extremity, with elevation above the heart level
      (c) Graduated compression stockings, usually with a pressure of 15–20 or 30–40 mmHg (see COMPRESSION STOCKING THERAPY, later in this chapter)
      (d) NSAIDs if not anticoagulated
      (e) Consider antibiotic therapy for 10 days with cephalexin 500 mg tid or TMP-SMX DS bid (if suspect methicillin-resistant *Staphylococcus aureus* [MRSA])
      (f) Consider anticoagulant therapy for a short period of time, if located near deeper saphenous veins or patient is high risk for DVT
      (g) Smoking and alcohol cessation, weight loss, and increased mobility
      (h) Follow-up in office in 24–48 hr, 2 wk, and again in 1 mo to evaluate resolution
   5. ***Referral to vascular specialist or hematologist if not resolving or if recurring***
II. Chronic venous disease
   A. Varicose veins develop because of valve incompetency that leads to dilated subcutaneous veins
      1. Signs and symptoms
         (a) Usually occurs primarily in one leg, but can involve both legs; can be found from thigh to calf
         (b) Heaviness, fatigue, and aching noted with daily activity; worse toward the end of the day and relief with rest and leg elevation
         (c) Often affected limb is edematous, especially after standing or walking for long periods
         (d) Often has night cramps
      2. Diagnostic testing with compression U/S with Doppler
      3. Treatment
         (a) Periodically rest and elevate legs
         (b) Support or compression stockings (put on before getting out of bed)
         (c) Avoid prolonged standing or sitting; avoid constrictive clothing at the waist and groin
         (d) Avoid OCs or estrogen therapy
         (e) Smoking and alcohol cessation
      4. ***Referral to vascular surgeon for more definitive care***
   B. Venous stasis (also called chronic venous insufficiency): a slow progressive disorder related to chronic vein dilation with venous reflux and skin changes
      1. Associated with edema, thickened skin, and chronic ulceration (see WOUND CARE (CHRONIC), **V**, later in this chapter)

● = *non-urgent referral*

2. Risk factors
   (a) Elderly, smoking, obesity, and varicose veins
   (b) Previous DVT or lower extremity trauma
   (c) History of prolonged standing, sitting, or decreased mobility
3. Signs and symptoms of milder disease
   (a) Leg discomfort and pain, begins unilaterally
       (i) Initially in ankles but later generalized to entire leg
       (ii) Often described as aching, tired, and heavy feeling
       (iii) Worsens with prolonged standing or sitting and improves with elevation of affected extremities
   (b) Swelling
       (i) Unilateral at first beginning at ankles and then will affect both legs with progression of disease
       (ii) Increases with standing/sitting and decreases with elevation and lying down
       (iii) Associated with spider veins, varicosities, and skin color changes
       (iv) Poor response to diuretic
4. Signs and symptoms of stasis dermatitis (more severe disease)
   (a) Red, dry, scaly patches or plaques with chronic swelling in lower legs/ankles
   (b) Pruritus with lichenification due to chronic scratching/rubbing
   (c) Bumpy or cobblestone appearance with thickening of skin ("woody" feeling to leg, known as lipodermatosclerosis) found around entire lower leg(s); it begins slowly on one or both lower legs and ankles
   (d) Hyperpigmentation with brownish color (hemosiderin)
   (e) Weeping and crusting on inflamed skin
   (f) May also have lymphedema and varicosities
   (g) Slow healing tender superficial ulcer(s) with irregular borders, often at medial ankle over an inflamed vein (never on forefoot or above knee)
   (h) Increased risk of cellulitis
5. Diagnostic testing
   (a) Compression U/S with Doppler
   (b) ABI (see PERIPHERAL ARTERIAL DISEASE, **IV**; also, Table 8.19)
   (c) Consider CBC, CMP
6. Treatment
   (a) To control edema
       (i) Weight loss and elevation of legs 3–4 times a day for at least 30 min
       (ii) Short-term use of diuretics (e.g., HCTZ) but they often do not help
   (b) Gradually increase activity with walking, bicycling, or swimming; encourage ankle flexion exercises while sitting.
   (c) Encourage ankle flexion exercises if unable to walk.
       (i) Exercise in chair, doing 10 dorsiflexion each hour (can be sitting or standing)
       (ii) Calf stretches 20 times twice daily
       (iii) "Draw alphabet" with toes twice daily
   (d) Dry, itchy, crusting skin
       (i) Use emollients (e.g., Vaseline) 3–4 times daily to lubricate skin and decrease itching.
       (ii) Can use high- to mid-potency steroid ointments 1–2 times daily for 1–2 wk, for acute redness, pruritus, or oozing lesions.
       (iii) Gentle skin cleansing daily with mild nonfragrant soap (e.g., Aveeno, Dove, Cetaphil), to remove scale (can use soft toothbrush)

(iv) Wet to dry dressings with aluminum acetate (Burow's solution) wrapped around leg(s) for 3–4 hr and changed 2–3 times a day, may help to remove crusts, decrease itch, and decrease bacteria associated with secondary infection.

(e) Compression stocking therapy (see COMPRESSION STOCKING THERAPY, later in this chapter)

(f) Pharmacological treatment (can be used with compression therapy)
  (i) ASA 325 mg daily
  (ii) Pentoxifylline (Trental) 400 mg tid; off-label use for venous leg ulcer
  (iii) Horse chestnut seed extract 300 mg bid to reduce edema and leg pain (use with or without compression)

(g) Aggressive wound treatment if ulcers occur (see WOUND CARE (CHRONIC), **V**, in this chapter)
  (i) Signs of infection: local redness, heat, red streaks up leg, fever
  (ii) If infection suspected: topical (e.g., mupirocin) *or* oral antibiotics (e.g., clindamycin or TMP-SMX) for 7–10 days
  (iii) Wound debridement to decrease bacterial load and enhance healing

● 7. *Referral to wound specialist if worsening or no resolution in 3 mo or to vascular surgeon for further evaluation if potential arterial disease*

ANTICOAGULATION THERAPY

I. Warfarin therapy
  A. Indications
    1. After DVT as a cost-effective means to reduce risk of further embolic events
    2. May be used with atrial fibrillation, cardiomyopathy, and other heart-related injuries or surgeries (e.g., mechanical mitral and/or aortic valves)
    3. Used short term prophylactically after major joint replacement or long term with recurrent disease
  B. Contraindications for starting warfarin are all based on the relative risk of recurrent DVT vs the risk of bleeding.
    1. Severe or active bleeding or within 2 wk of major bleeding event or bleeding that involved brain, eye, or abdominal cavity
    2. Nonadherence to medication monitoring, dementia, high risk of falls
    3. Pregnancy
    4. End-stage renal disease (ESRD)
    5. Uncontrolled HTN (> 180/110 mmHg) or hypotension
    6. Recent surgery (unless joint replacement)
  C. Cautions
    1. There are numerous dosing difficulties and restrictions with foods (e.g., dietary restriction, see Appendix A) and other medications (e.g., OTC and Rx drugs).
    2. Will need to calculate individualized dose and schedule for close monitoring to maintain therapeutic levels and decrease bleeding risks.
  D. Initiating warfarin therapy
    1. Prior to initiating warfarin
      (a) Teach the patient about signs and symptoms of bleeding and precautions to take with ADLs while on warfarin (e.g., using soft toothbrushes and electric razors).

● = *non-urgent referral*

   (b) Review the patient's lifestyle with regard to diet and activity and provide written and oral instructions regarding changes needed while on warfarin; most common reasons for failure to reach therapeutic levels or loss of therapeutic control are poor dietary choices and lack of knowledge about foods high in vitamin K (see **Appendix A**).
   (c) Review the patient's medications, including any herbal or OTC medicines, and teach about drug interactions.
   (d) Diagnostic testing includes PT/INR, CBC, CMP, and urine hCG.
2. Start therapy with enoxaparin 1 mg/kg bid for the first 5–7 days; start warfarin on day 3 while still on enoxaparin
   (a) Check INR on day 3 after starting warfarin; if INR > 2, stop enoxaparin and continue warfarin.
   (b) Recheck INR 3 days later and serially until INR at therapeutic level.
   (c) INR goal depends on the diagnosis for the therapy. Common ranges are
      (i) DVT, A-fib, or PE: 2–3
      (ii) Sole mechanical aortic valve: 2–3
      (iii) Sole mechanical mitral valve or both mechanical mitral and aortic valves: 2.5–3.5
3. Usual starting dose is 5 mg daily (see Table 8.20; also *www.warfarindosing.org* for assistance with dosing); may need a lower dose with
   (a) Elderly
   (b) Malnourished or debilitated
   (c) Hepatic or renal insufficiency
   (d) Increased bleeding risks
   (e) Concomitant use of p450 inhibitor medications
4. Initially, INR will fluctuate and will need to be checked 1–2 times a week until INR normalizes; anticoagulation effect may be seen within 2–3 days.
5. Dose should be taken at the same time every day, preferably evening to allow for INR results to be evaluated and dosing changes made prior to next dose.
6. The majority of warfarin users are elderly.
   (a) Use single-strength tablets for dosing; this is safer than multiples of a dose and easier to remember to take.
   (b) Check with pharmacy or family members if there is a need to cut a dose in half.
E. Dosing changes and INR results (see Table 8.21)
   1. Changes in the dosing schedules are based on the total weekly dose (TWD) rather than the daily dose. Calculate the total dose for the week and make changes by 5%–15% as needed.
   2. Do not make frequent dosing changes for slightly out-of-range results; continue dose and recheck INR in 5 days.
   3. After making a dose change, wait at least 3 days before rechecking INR (unless INR > 6 and treated as outpatient, then recheck in 24–48 hr).
   4. If INR is stable, monitor q4wk.
   5. A good rule of thumb is: *any time a medication is changed or a new medication added, recheck INR within 3 days.*
F. Reasons for INR fluctuations
   1. Change in the diet or lost/gained weight
   2. Any new or discontinued medications, either Rx or OTC; also includes vitamins or supplements

TABLE 8.20 ■ Initiating Warfarin After 5–7 Days of LMWH* Therapy

Day	INR	Warfarin Daily Dose (mg)	Days to Recheck INR
1		5	0
2		5	0
3	<1.5	7.5	3
	1.5–1.9	5	7
	2–3	5	7
	3–3.4	5	3
	>3.5–4	Hold 1 dose, restart at 5	3
6	<1.5	10	7
	1.5–1.9	7.5	7
	2–3	5	7
	3–3.4	5	5
	>3.5–4	Hold 1 dose, restart at 2.5	3
	>5	Hold 2 doses, restart at 2.5	3
9–10	<1.9	10	7
	2–3	5	7
	3–3.4	3.75	5
	>3.5–5	Hold 1 dose, restart at 2.5	3
	>5	Hold 2 doses, restart at 2.5	3
11–13	1.5–1.9	12.5	7
	2–3	5	14
	3–3.4	3.75	7
	>3.5	Hold 1 dose, restart at 2.5	3
	>5	Hold 2 doses, restart at 2.5	3
After 15	Maintain dose if INR in range or increase or decrease by total weekly dose between 5% and 15% of total		

* Low molecular weight heparin.

3. Inadvertent change in the dose
   (a) Confirm the current dose at every visit and when reporting INR.
   (b) Have patient bring current medications in pill bottles and discuss whether the pills have changed in shape, color, or size.
4. Any recent illness (e.g., flu) or new long-term diagnosis (e.g., cancer)
5. Postbariatric surgery
   (a) Dosing changes required due to limited amount of vitamin K in the liquid diet.
   (b) INR should return to baseline in about 3–6 mo.
G. Reversal guidelines for elevated INR level or minor bleeding (e.g., epistaxis, soft tissue hematoma)
   1. The risk of bleeding increases with an INR of >4
   2. If INR is between 3 and 5
      (a) Hold next dose.

TABLE 8.21 ■ **Titrating Warfarin***

INR	Dose Change	Days to Next INR
1.0–1.1	↑ the dose by 15%	3–5 days
1.2–1.5	↑ the dose by 10%–15%	5–7 days
1.5–1.9	Continue the same dose	5–7 days
2.0–2.5	Continue the same dose	5–7 days
2.6–3.0	Continue the same dose	3–5 days
3.0–5.0	Hold the dose for 1–2 days and decrease next dose by 10%	2–3 days
>5	Hold 1–2 doses and consider vitamin K if bleeding risk is elevated (see **ANTICOAGULATION THERAPY, I, Warfarin therapy, G** in this chapter)	1–2 days

Rule of thumb for dosing changes for any INR needing adjustment: calculate the weekly dose and then change by 5%–15%. Example: if total weekly dose is 35 mg (based on 7 days), a 10% decrease would be 31.5 mg for the week and the daily dose would change to 4.5 mg; a 10% increase would give 38.5 mg and the daily dose would be 5.5 mg. Recheck INR in about 3–5 days after making a change. You can also round up or down depending on the stability of INR.

* Start with 5 mg and recheck in 3 days, then follow the table.

    (b) Decrease overall dose by 10% of TWD.
    (c) Recheck INR 3 days.
  3. If INR between 5 and 9 *without bleeding*
    (a) Hold next 1–2 doses.
    (b) Give vitamin K 1–2.5 mg orally once (see 6, below).
    (c) Decrease overall dose by 15% TWD.
    (d) Recheck INR in 3 days.
  4. If INR > 9 *without bleeding*
    (a) Hold warfarin.
    (b) Give vitamin K 2.5–5 mg orally once (see 6, below).
    (c) Recheck INR in 24 hr and repeat vitamin K at same or higher dose if INR not decreasing; repeat INR again in 24 hr.
    (d) Decrease overall dose by 15% TWD and restart warfarin when INR normalizes.

▲ 5. *If bleeding noted and INR > 9; emergent referral to ED*
  6. When using vitamin K
    (a) First dose of vitamin K can be expected to lower INR within 8–24 hr; a second dose may be required at that time to continue lowering INR until the therapeutic range is reached.
    (b) If using high doses of vitamin K (e.g., > 5 mg), beware that this can lead to warfarin resistance for > 1 wk and will increase the risk for thromboembolism. Consider using heparin or enoxaparin to maintain anticoagulation for 5–7 days.
    (c) If tablets are unavailable, the patient is not at risk, and the INR is 4–9 with *no* bleeding, consider eating a diet with foods high in vitamin K (see **Appendix A**).
  II. Other anticoagulant therapies
    A. Indications (see Table 8.22); postbariatric surgery, avoid all DOACs except for apixaban.

▲ = *urgent referral*

TABLE 8.22 ■ Drugs and Indications for Ambulatory Anticoagulation/Antiplatelet Therapy (Excluding Warfarin)

Drug	Dose	Indication
Anticoagulants (DOAC*)		
Apixaban (Eliquis) Oral	10 mg bid × 7 days then 5 mg bid	DVT/PE treatment
	2.5 mg bid	Prophylaxis s/p hip replacement for 32–38 days Prophylaxis s/p knee replacement for 10–14 days
	2.5–5 mg bid	Stroke prophylaxis with nonvalvular AF, start at a lower dose especially for elderly
Dabigatran (Pradaxa) Oral	150 mg bid (if CrCl < 30: 75 mg bid)	Nonvalvular AF; CVA
	220 mg daily	Prophylaxis s/p hip replacement for 10–14 days
Edoxaban (Savaysa) Oral	< 60 kg: 30 mg daily > 60 kg: 60 mg daily	DVT/PE treatment after 3–5 days of IM/SQ anticoagulation
	60 mg	Nonvalvular AF stroke prophylaxis
Rivaroxaban (Xarelto) Oral	10 mg daily	Prophylaxis s/p hip/knee replacement for 10–14 days (hip can be given up to 35 days)
	15 mg bid for 21 days then 20 mg daily	Recurrent DVT/PE *prophylaxis* Nonvalvular AF (prevent VTE/CVA)
	20 mg daily**	DVT/PE *treatment* Stroke prophylaxis
Anticoagulants (Injectable—Short-Term Use, Overlap With Warfarin Therapy)		
Enoxaparin (Lovenox) SQ	1 mg/kg q12h	DVT treatment and prophylaxis STEMI Unstable angina Prophylaxis s/p hip/knee replacement
Fondaparinux (Arixtra) SQ	2.5 mg daily	Prophylaxis s/p hip replacement for 5–9 days, s/p hip fracture surgery for up to 24 days Prophylaxis s/p knee replacement for 5–9 days Prophylaxis s/p abdominal surgery for 5–9 days
	5–10 mg daily (based on weight)	DVT/PE treatment
Heparin	5000 units SQ q8–12h 18 mg/kg/h IV	Thromboembolism prophylaxis Thromboembolism treatment
Antiplatelets		
Clopidogrel (Plavix) Oral	75 mg daily	ACS or recent MI CVA PAD
Prasugrel (Effient) Oral	10 mg daily based on cardiac event	Unstable angina Non-ST-elevation MI STEMI undergoing PCI
Ticagrelor (Brilinta) Oral	90 mg bid[†]	Unstable angina ACS Non-ST-elevation MI STEMI

* Direct acting oral anticoagulants.
** Check renal and hepatic function.
[†] Must limit ASA to < 100 mg daily.

B. Transitioning anticoagulants
1. Transitioning *to warfarin* from
   (a) Enoxaparin (Lovenox) or fondaparinux (Arixtra): overlap warfarin by 5 days or when INR is in therapeutic range for 2 days.
   (b) Dabigatran (Pradaxa): overlap 1–3 days (depending on CrCl).
   (c) Edoxaban (Savaysa): decrease dose by half and overlap 5–7 days (depending on CrCl); check INR weekly and discontinue when INR therapeutic.
   (d) Rivaroxaban (Xarelto) or apixaban (Eliquis): stop dose and start warfarin with no overlap.
2. Transitioning *from warfarin* to
   (a) Dabigatran or apixaban: start when INR is < 2
   (b) Rivaroxaban: start when INR is < 3

III. Duration of anticoagulant therapy
A. Low-risk TIA or minor stroke with CHA2DS2-VASC score < 1 (see Table 8.1): no therapy because of bleeding risk from CVA but may benefit from short-term antiplatelet therapy.
   1. ASA 81–325 mg + clopidogrel 75 mg daily for 3 wk *then*
   2. Stop clopidogrel and continue ASA indefinitely (unless contraindicated)
B. Other chronic cardiovascular diseases based on CHA2DS2-VASC score > 1 (e.g., CVA with bleeding and AF): suggest ASA 81–325 mg + clopidogrel 75 mg daily *or* clopidogrel 75 mg daily alone *or* daily warfarin with an INR range of 2–3.
C. Hypercoagulable state/malignancy or > 2 clots: consider at least 3–6 mo of chronic therapy, or as long as patient is receiving cancer therapy or has active cancer.
D. Status-postarthroscopy (hip or knee): start therapy about 24 hr after surgery and continue for 4–6 wk.
E. Valvular disease: chronic therapy
F. Valvular replacement:
   1. Bioprosthetic: 3–12 mo, followed by ASA 81–325 mg daily indefinitely
   2. Mechanical: chronic therapy

IV. Preprocedural discontinuation (these guidelines are based on general recommendations; physicians may have different protocols)
A. In-office procedures with low bleeding risk (e.g., joint aspiration/injection, superficial aspiration/biopsy, dialysis access): stop DOACs 1 day before but then can restart 4–6 hr after procedure.
B. Hip/knee replacement: stop warfarin 5–7 days before surgery; usually restarted within 24 hr postop.
C. Minor dental procedures: may continue warfarin and ASA but take 4–6 hr after procedure, rather than before it; if needed, can stop 3 days prior and restart 24 hr after procedure if there is no significant risk of thrombosis.
D. Cataract surgery: no need to stop any anticoagulant therapy, but take it 4–6 hr after procedure rather than before it.
E. Elective surgery with no high risk of cardiac event: stop ASA and other anticoagulants about 7–10 days before surgery and restart 24 hr postop when hemostasis is adequate.
F. Colonoscopy: stop all anticoagulants/antiplatelets 3 days before the procedure.
G. Regional anesthesia (may restart ≥ 6 hr after procedure)
   1. Anticoagulants
      (a) Warfarin: stop 5 days before with goal INR ≤ 1.2
      (b) Rivaroxaban/apixaban: stop 3 days before
      (c) Betrixaban/dabigatran: stop 5 days before

2. Antiplatelets
   (a) Cilostazol: stop 2 days before
   (b) Clopidogrel: stop 5–7 days before
   (c) Prasugrel: stop 7–10 days before
V. Complications of anticoagulant/antiplatelet medications
   A. Bleeding
      1. Reversible agents are only available for warfarin and dabigatran (Pradaxa).
      2. Compression to obvious hematomas or active bleeding sites (e.g., epistaxis)
      3. With a serious bleeding episode, stop the medication until bleeding subsides; monitor CBC (and INR, if appropriate).
      4. Nuisance bleeding (i.e., nosebleeds, prolonged bleeding from a small cut)
         (a) Usually not serious or a reason to stop the therapy
         (b) Encourage steps to prevent bleeding (e.g., use saline spray prn to keep nasal mucosa moist; use an electric razor; use a soft toothbrush)
   B. Heparin-induced thrombocytopenia (HIT)
   C. Warfarin-induced skin necrosis

COMPRESSION STOCKING THERAPY

I. Compression stockings are available in OTC and by prescription (see Table 8.23). Any compression higher than 20 mmHg should be custom fitted and applied by a trained individual; document ABI findings (see Table 8.19).
II. Compression stocking application
   A. Length essentially depends on the wearer's preference; measure length before ordering.
      1. Knee-length stockings are preferred; do not pull up to popliteal fossa, which can cause constriction, skin irritation, or discomfort.
      2. Thigh-high stockings are sometimes used after venous surgery and for added support with prolonged travel.
   B. Stockings work best if put on before getting out of bed; if unable to do this, elevate legs for ~20 min prior to donning.
   C. To help with donning stockings (can be difficult for elderly or debilitated patients)
      1. Use baby powder or cornstarch on the legs to help the stockings slide up the leg more easily.

TABLE 8.23 ■ Compression Stockings

Compression	Uses
15–20 mmHg (OTC) No fitting needed; includes TED hose	Minor varicosities Heavy, tired legs Minor leg, ankle, or foot edema
20–30 mmHg (prescription)	Moderate to severe varicose veins Moderate swelling Following vein ablation surgery Phlebitis
30–40 mmHg (prescription)	Severe varicose veins Severe swelling Management of wounds After DVT or after surgical procedures
40–60 mmHg (prescription) Verify no arterial occlusion before ordering	Lymphedema or burn scars

    2. Use rubber gloves to help grip the stockings and with pulling up and smoothing out wrinkles.

    3. Can use a "stocking aide" if patient is unable to pull up stocking.

  D. Stockings can be worn over wound dressings.

  E. Wash stockings daily and hang up to dry; do not use a dryer.

  F. Will probably need new stockings q3–6mo because of stretch.

III. Compressive bandages (applied by trained provider)

  A. Inelastic bandage (e.g., Unna boot) requires more frequent changing because of dressings or edema.

    1. Works better with ambulatory patient

    2. No compression with rest

    3. Can be applied with wounds

  B. Elastic bandages (e.g., Ace wrap) provide less pressure.

    1. May have several layers and will conform to changes in leg size

    2. Works with ambulatory patient

    3. Provides compression with rest

    4. Can be applied with wounds

  C. Intermittent pneumatic compression (IPC)

    1. Most expensive

    2. Requires battery or electrical outlet

    3. Used when at recumbent rest

    4. No bandages necessary

IV. Contraindications to all compression therapy

  A. Peripheral arterial disease or ABI ≤ 0.5 (see Table 8.19)

  B. HF

  C. Acute cellulitis or wounds with necrotic tissue

  D. Contact dermatitis

  E. Use cautiously with poorly controlled DM with neuropathy or poorly healing diabetic wounds

WOUND CARE (CHRONIC)

I. Chronic wounds occur secondary to tissue damage from pressure on the skin over bony surfaces, decreased oxygenated blood for healing or chronic infections, and stasis dermatitis.

  A. *Arterial wounds* commonly occur in patient with occlusive disease that prevents adequate blood flow.

    1. Pressure is not as important as the amount of blood flow to area.

    2. Wounds usually occur more rapidly.

  B. *Diabetic wounds* are usually caused from pressure and the wound is not found early due to neuropathy.

  C. *Venous wounds* commonly occur in bedridden, malnourished, and elderly people.

    1. Amount of pressure is not as important as the length of time the pressure is present over a compromised area, which can be $<2\,hr$ (e.g., surgical procedures).

    2. Wound starts out as redness and then progresses slowly.

II. Documentation

  A. History

    1. What circumstances caused the wound and when did it occur (or was found)?

    2. Ambulatory or nonambulatory patient

    3. Can patient care for wound independently?

    4. Does patient live independently or in facility? Is transportation available if needed for follow-up care?

    5. Incontinent of urine or stools (or both)?

    6. Therapy for the wound up to now

    7. DM control; any other complications related to DM

    8. All known diagnoses (e.g., HTN, malnutrition, dyslipidemia) and comorbidities

  B. Appearance of wound (general documentation)

    1. Description of size, depth, any undermining of wound present

    2. Appearance of the wound surface (wound edges, color) and wound bed; any granulation tissue

    3. Amount of exudate, color, and odor

    4. Tissues surrounding the wound bed

  C. Vascular assessment: poor vascularization is indicated by diminished pulses and capillary refill, thin atrophic skin on extremity with lack of hair, and deformed nails; may also have

    1. Mild to severe pain: rest pain, pain with activity

    2. Edema, cooler temperature of surrounding skin

    3. Color

      (a) Pallor with sitting/standing

      (b) Rubor in dependent position

      (c) Mottling in any position

    4. Intermittent claudication

III. Wound staging

  A. *Deep-tissue pressure injury (DTPI)*

    1. Intact or nonintact skin (there may be a blood-filled blister); persistent nonblanchable discoloration (deep red, maroon or purple); the color changes may be difficult to detect with dark skin

    2. May be due to increased pressure and shear at the muscle-bone interface

    3. The changes may resolve without any damage or rapidly deteriorate to Stages 3, 4, or unstageable wound

  B. *Stage 1 (early localized erythema)*

    1. Nonblanching erythema of intact skin; this is the heralding lesion of skin ulceration usually present over bony prominences

    2. Can be painful, firm localized area with diminished sensation

    3. May be difficult to see on dark skin color

  C. *Stage 2 (red-to-yellow ulcer)*

    1. Partial-thickness skin loss involving the epidermis with exposed dermis

    2. Superficial ulcer that presents clinically as an abrasion, blister, shallow crater, with red or pink wound base without sloughing

    3. Related to skin shear over bony prominences

  D. *Stage 3 (yellow ulcer)*

    1. Full-thickness skin loss involving damage to or necrosis of the subcutaneous tissue that may extend down to but not through the underlying fascia

    2. Ulcer at presentation is a deep crater with distinct ulcer margin with or without undermining or tunneling of the adjacent tissue.

    3. Exudate can be whitish yellow, greenish yellow, or beige.

    4. Slough or eschar may be present, indicating the presence of microorganisms and need for cleaning.

    5. No tendon, ligament, or bone/cartilage is visible.

E. *Stage 4* (black ulcer)
1. Eschar or necrotic tissue present over the wound with full-thickness skin loss and exposed or directly palpable fascia, muscle, tendon, ligament, cartilage or bone
2. Necrotic tissue should be removed as soon as possible because it is an excellent medium for bacterial growth and decreases the wound-healing process (the *exception is heel eschar,* see **V**, B, 5 below).
3. Tunneling and sinus tracts are usually present.
F. *Kennedy terminal ulcer (KTU)*
1. Sudden onset with rapidly developing pressure ulcer(s) that do not respond to treatment; associated with the dying process and can occur weeks to months prior to death.
2. Usually seen on the coccyx/sacrum, buttocks, or other bony areas; can be unilateral or bilateral.
3. Description
(a) Irregularly shaped area that starts out superficially as a red or purple colored area on intact skin and worsens to stage 2 quickly.
(b) Can be horseshoe or butterfly shape.
4. It is usually not associated with neglectful care.

IV. Diagnostic studies (some or all of these may be indicated)
A. CBC, CMP, A1c
B. Wound cultures
C. ABI to determine arterial circulation (see CALCULATION OF ANKLE-BRACHIAL INDEX, earlier in this chapter)
D. Consider X-ray of the area involved; CT or MRI to determine underlying etiology and bone involvement may be needed
E. Compression U/S with Doppler for DVT (especially with unilateral swelling)
F. Bone scan to assess for osteomyelitis
V. Differentiation and treatment of wounds
A. Arterial ulcers
1. Usually chronic and caused by ischemia in the extremity due to
(a) Atherosclerotic changes due to dyslipidemia
(b) Poor control of DM
(c) Injury to already compromised skin from surgery or past wounds
(d) Smoking
2. Signs and symptoms
(a) Claudication with exercise
(b) Acute pain at night and also rest pain; wounds are painful
(c) Skin reddens with dangling and turns pale white with elevation (differentiates arterial from venous wounds)
(d) Wounds are usually found at the end of extremities (e.g., over toe joints on bony prominence, tip of toe), on the dorsal foot, base of heel, and over any pressure areas
(e) Ulcers appear deep (punched out) with uneven edges and a dry, pale-grayish base with nonerythematous borders; there is no granulation tissue; eschar and necrosis may be present.
(f) Shiny, atrophic changes of the skin, with hair loss over the affected extremity
(g) Decreased or absent pulses; prolonged capillary refill > 3–4 sec
3. Treatment
(a) Meticulous wound and foot care

(b) Short course of systemic antibiotics, if infection is suspected (routine antibiotic use is discouraged)

(c) Dressing should maintain a moist wound bed and be changed q1–2d

4. *Referral to a wound care specialist or a vascular surgeon for further evaluation*

B. Diabetic (neuropathic) ulcers (see Chapter 15, CHRONIC COMPLICATIONS OF DM, I)

C. Pressure ulcers

1. Occur with prolonged pressure over bony prominences (e.g., metatarsal heads, calcaneus, sacrum) or as shearing effect (e.g., sliding up or down in bed and turning)

2. Wounds may begin very subtly as reddened areas that progress to avascular white areas and then to skin degradation and ulcer formation

3. Periwound redness with fibrotic changes and eschar

4. Treatment

(a) Remove the cause of pressure, which may resolve any tissue damage; use pillows, supportive limb devices, and off-loading pressure mattresses/beds.

(b) Keep the head of the bed at the lowest effective level to prevent shearing from movement while in bed.

(c) Frequent turning schedules, usually q2h with documented rotation charts.

(d) Manage bowel and bladder incontinence to prevent further skin breakdown and infection.

(e) *If nutritional status in question, consider consultation with dietician for specific suggestions.*

(i) Increase calorie intake (protein, carbohydrates, and fats)

(ii) Supplement with vitamin C, zinc, and multivitamin

(iii) Encourage snacks, double portions of protein, commercial supplements (e.g., Ensure, Boost)

5. Treatment of heel eschar

(a) Dry heel eschar without evidence of infection should be left alone and monitored weekly.

(b) If evidence of infection (e.g., slough, odor, softening), culture wound and start antibiotics.

(c) Use protective wraps to minimize any type of pressure while patient is in/out of bed.

(d) Use air pressure or pressure release beds with cutout heel protectors while in bed.

6. *Referral to a wound care specialist or a surgeon if wounds become resistant to treatment or heel becomes infected.*

D. Venous stasis ulcers: caused by localized edema, varicosities, or stasis dermatitis

1. Wounds are usually found over bony prominences between ankle and knee (e.g., medial/lateral malleolus) and may be circumferential.

(a) Wound has shallow, irregular borders and mild pain.

(b) Edges are pink-red with granulation tissue and moist base with moderate-to-heavy exudate.

(c) Skin around wound has scaling, weeping, and crusting with pruritus.

(d) Surrounding skin has hemosiderin coloring, lipodermatosclerosis with stasis dermatitis.

(e) Feet are warm with normal pulses and sensation.

● = *non-urgent referral*

2. Wound treatment
    (a) Keep the wound bed moist and change dressings appropriately for the amount of exudate; protect the surrounding tissue from maceration.
    (b) Debride
        (i) Necrotic tissue: by surgical, autolytic, or enzymatic methods; short-term use of wet to dry dressings may be effective.
        (ii) Proud flesh: using sharp scissors or scalpel; place parallel to periwound area
    (c) Wound may increase in size and be malodorous and/or have friable granulation tissue with delayed wound healing and tunneling.
    (d) Monitor for infection; obtain tissue C&S and treat aggressively if identified.
    (e) Signs of infection may differ with chronic wounds (especially in elderly) monitor for fever, chills, tachycardia, and leukocytosis.
3. Elevate the extremity after activity.
4. Protect lower extremities by using sheepskin wraps with Velcro to surround the leg from knee to ankle; wraps are warm and nonconstricting.
5. Compression stocking therapy (see COMPRESSION STOCKING THERAPY, earlier in this chapter)
E. Pharmacological treatment of infected wounds
    1. Specific oral antibiotics for 7–10 days (guided by the culture and sensitivity, if possible)
        (a) Clindamycin 300 mg tid
        (b) TMP-SMX DS 1 tab bid
        (c) Cephalexin 500 mg tid
    2. Consider topical antimicrobials for a short period of time (<2 wk) with acute infection
        (a) Iodosorb (cadexomer iodine) decreases bacterial biofilm (i.e., resistant coating of bacteria) and this will stimulate healing.
        (b) Silver-containing dressings may decrease heavy bacterial loads, but may not increase healing; can combine with hydrogels.
        (c) Medical grade honey may be used with sloughing wounds and wounds with infection.
        (d) Topical antibiotics (e.g., mupirocin) used sparingly.
    3. Dressings should be changed q1–2d depending on exudate; wound may need debridement.
    4. As wound improves, treatment will change to promote healing and remove any crusting.
        (a) Can use wet to dry dressing until wound healing and then keep transparent film dressing (e.g., Tegaderm) over wound until healed
        (b) Low adherent dressings to promote healing

CHAPTER 9

Abdominal Conditions

For details regarding complete history and physical examination, see Chapter 1.

ABDOMINAL PAIN (TABLE 9.1; FIG. 9.1)

I. History should include
  A. Location and any radiation
    1. Where did the pain originate and is it still present in same area?
    2. Is the pain referred pain from a different site?
  B. Timing of pain; is it acute or chronic?
    1. Onset
    2. Consistency
    3. Duration
  C. Quality
    1. Sharp, burning
    2. Dull, aching
    3. Spastic (colicky) or cramping
  D. Severity (use pain rating scale)
    1. The elderly may have less intense sensation of pain.
    2. Chronic steroid use will mask pain.
  E. Precipitating or alleviating factors
    1. What makes the pain worse?
    2. What makes the pain better (e.g., change in positions, eating, movement)?
  F. Associated factors (symptoms that have occurred with the pain)
    1. Nausea/vomiting/diarrhea (N/V/D) or constipation, change in stool shape
    2. Fever, fatigue, weight loss, increased thirst, anorexia
    3. Jaundice, urine or stool color changes
    4. Urinary frequency, dysuria, hematuria, polyuria
    5. Cough, SOB, orthopnea
  G. Other history
    1. For women, ask about LMP, whether sexually active and number of partners, menstrual history, contraception usage (current OCP and any missed doses), vaginal discharge, and history of STIs and how treated.
    2. Alcohol use
    3. Travel history
    4. Current medications (e.g., OTC, prescribed or herbals)
II. Types of pain
  A. Parietal pain
    1. Description
      (a) Pain is steady, constant, and described as "sharp," "knife-like," and "constant."
      (b) There will be abdominal tenderness, guarding, rebound tenderness, and rigidity.

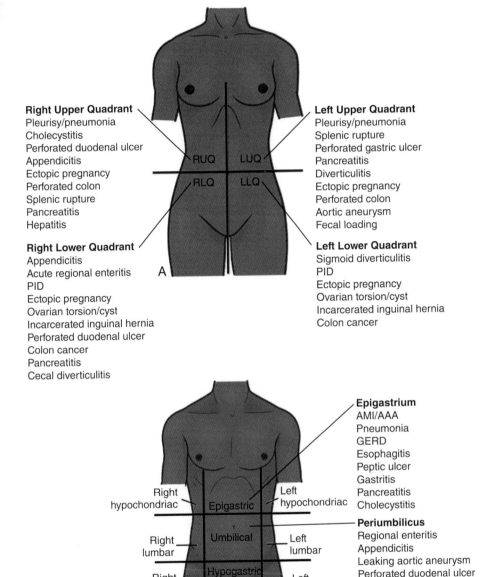

Right Upper Quadrant
Pleurisy/pneumonia
Cholecystitis
Perforated duodenal ulcer
Appendicitis
Ectopic pregnancy
Perforated colon
Splenic rupture
Pancreatitis
Hepatitis

Left Upper Quadrant
Pleurisy/pneumonia
Splenic rupture
Perforated gastric ulcer
Pancreatitis
Diverticulitis
Ectopic pregnancy
Perforated colon
Aortic aneurysm
Fecal loading

Right Lower Quadrant
Appendicitis
Acute regional enteritis
PID
Ectopic pregnancy
Ovarian torsion/cyst
Incarcerated inguinal hernia
Perforated duodenal ulcer
Colon cancer
Pancreatitis
Cecal diverticulitis

Left Lower Quadrant
Sigmoid diverticulitis
PID
Ectopic pregnancy
Ovarian torsion/cyst
Incarcerated inguinal hernia
Colon cancer

Epigastrium
AMI/AAA
Pneumonia
GERD
Esophagitis
Peptic ulcer
Gastritis
Pancreatitis
Cholecystitis

Periumbilicus
Regional enteritis
Appendicitis
Leaking aortic aneurysm
Perforated duodenal ulcer
Aortic aneurysm
Diverticulitis

Hypogastrium
Regional enteritis
PID, UTI
Ulcerative colitis
Colon cancer

Fig. 9.1 Differential diagnosis of abdominal problems depending on pain location. *AMI*, Acute myocardial infarction; *PID*, pelvic inflammatory disease; *UTI*, urinary tract infection. (From Lewis, S. L., Dirksen, S. R., Heitkemper, M. M., Burcher, L. (2014). *Medical-Surgical Nursing* (9th ed.). St. Louis: Elsevier.)

TABLE 9.1 ■ Differential Diagnoses of Abdominal Pain in Young Patients

Infant–12 mo	2–5 yr	6–11 yr	12 yr–Adult
Infantile colic	Gastroenteritis	Gastroenteritis	Appendicitis
Gastroenteritis	Appendicitis	Appendicitis	Gastroenteritis
Constipation	Volvulus	Constipation	Cholecystitis
Intussusception	Constipation	Mesenteric	Pancreatitis
Hirschsprung disease	UTI	lymphadenitis	Constipation
Trauma	Trauma, drugs, toxins	Functional pain	Dysmenorrhea
Testicular torsion	Pharyngitis	UTI	Mittelschmerz
UTI	Mesenteric	Trauma, drugs, toxins	PID
Incarcerated hernia	lymphadenitis	Pharyngitis	Pregnancy
Necrotizing	Diabetic ketoacidosis	Pneumonia	Ovarian torsion
enterocolitis	Henoch-Schönlein	Sickle cell crisis	Testicular torsion
Milk protein allergy	purpura		Diabetic ketoacidosis
			IBD, celiac disease

    (c) Pain is relieved with legs up in the fetal position.

    (d) Pain is aggravated by cough or movement.

  2. Examples of this type of pain

    (a) Abdominal aortic aneurysm (AAA)

    (b) Appendicitis, cholecystitis, pancreatitis

    (c) Diverticulitis, perforation of the gut, peritonitis

  B. Visceral pain

    1. Description: pain is described as dull and poorly localized, cramping, colicky, or gnawing with burning sensation and is usually felt in the midline of the abdomen.

    2. Examples of this type of pain

      (a) Mesenteric ischemia, splenic rupture

      (b) Pancreatitis

      (c) Gastroenteritis (GE)

      (d) Pregnancy, ectopic pregnancy

      (e) Kidney stones, bladder, UTI

      (f) Obstruction in the colon or ileus

  C. Referred pain (see Fig. 9.1)

    1. Description: pain subjectively localized in one region but is due to irritation in another region

    2. Examples of this type of pain

      (a) AAA: pain felt in the back, flank, abdomen, and groin

      (b) Appendicitis: pain felt in the epigastrium, periumbilical region, and RLQ

      (c) Cholecystitis: pain felt in the epigastrium, RUQ, and right scapula

      (d) Ectopic pregnancy: generalized pain felt in the abdomen and either shoulder

      (e) Pancreatitis: pain felt in the epigastrium, abdomen, back, and flank area

      (f) Splenic rupture: pain felt in the RUQ, abdomen, and left shoulder

III. Physical examination techniques used in finding the cause of pain

  A. Observation/inspection

    1. Complete vitals, including temperature and pulse oximetry.

    2. If the patient is lying very still (because of pain): consider peritonitis.

3. If the patient is writhing about on the bed (in pain): consider intestinal, colicky pain from a hollow organ such as kidney stone, gallbladder disease, AAA.
4. If the abdomen is distended and firm: consider bowel obstruction or perforation.

B. Auscultation
1. If bowel sounds are absent: consider peritonitis.
2. If bowel sounds are high pitched or absent: consider bowel obstruction.

C. Percussion
1. Resonant, shifting dullness usually indicates ascites.
2. If percussion causes pain: consider peritonitis.

D. Palpation (examine tender areas last)
1. During palpation, try to visualize which organs are being palpated and the surrounding organs; this will help you identify what abnormalities or masses may be present (see Fig. 9.1).
2. To determine whether a mass involves the abdominal wall or is intra-abdominal, have the patient raise his or her head unsupported.
   (a) A mass in the abdominal wall will become more obvious with tensing of the abdominal muscles and will be more obvious on inspection.
   (b) An intra-abdominal mass will become less obvious because the muscles will push the mass down below the muscle wall.
3. Guarding is voluntary contraction of abdominal muscles and tends to be generalized.
4. Rigidity is involuntary tightening of abdominal muscles and tends to be localized over the inflamed area (rigidity is a positive sign of peritoneal inflammation).

E. Techniques to identify peritoneal signs indicating the need for further evaluation and possible surgical intervention
1. Carnett's sign: have the patient lie flat with the head lifted up and with the chin close to the chest (or shoulders off the bed); this will tighten the abdominal muscles. Pain elicited with this test is usually from the abdominal muscle wall; if pain decreases, this indicates that pain is from intra-abdominal structures.
2. Cullen's sign: yellow-blue discoloration around the umbilicus is suggestive of acute pancreatitis, ectopic pregnancy, or internal hemorrhage.
3. Grey-Turner sign: bruising on the flanks is associated with hemorrhagic pancreatitis, retroperitoneal hemorrhage, or blunt trauma.
4. Kehr's sign: severe left shoulder pain due to blood or pus in the peritoneal cavity, usually due to a ruptured spleen.
5. Markle sign (heel jar test): have the patient stand on toes and then *forcefully* drop down onto heels or have the patient in a supine position on the bed while firmly tapping the heel with the ball of your hand. If pain is elicited, this is suggestive of appendicitis or peritoneal irritation.
6. Murphy's sign: firmly place a hand at the costal margin in the RUQ and ask the patient to breathe deeply. If the gallbladder is inflamed, this will cause pain and the patient will "catch his or her breath" as the gallbladder descends under the hand, indicating inflammation.
7. Obturator test: with the patient supine and his or her knee flexed 90 degrees with the foot on the bed, immobilize the ankle on the bed and internally and externally rotate the hip. If pain is elicited, this would be suggestive of pelvic abscess or appendicitis.

8. Psoas sign: have the patient flex his or her thigh against resistance; or, with the patient lying on his or her left side, extend the right thigh backwards against resistance. If pain is elicited, this would be indicative of peritoneal irritation.

9. Rovsing's sign: palpation in the LLQ causes pain in the RLQ; this is suggestive of peritonitis or appendicitis.

F. Further examination techniques/tests

1. Examination of the anal area and digital rectal examination (DRE) should be included for all patients with abdominal pain (if possible). *Failure to perform rectal examination may be associated with an increased risk of misdiagnosis.*

(a) Observe the anal opening for any obvious hemorrhoids, masses, fissures, or external sources of bleeding.

(b) Check anal ring sensation by stroking each side of the buttocks near the anal area to elicit superficial anal reflex (anal wink). This demonstrates function of L1 and L2.

(c) Using water-soluble lubricant, insert finger into anal opening about 1–2 cm and feel around the ring, then insert finger up to 5–6 cm to check for any masses or abnormalities further up the rectum.

(d) Fecal occult blood testing (FOBT) should be performed with rectal examination.

2. Consider pelvic examination (see Chapter 1, GENITOURINARY (FEMALE), IV) for all women of childbearing age (at the discretion of the examiner) with appropriate testing for sexually transmitted infection (STI); *failure to perform pelvic examination and testing may be associated with an increased risk of misdiagnosis.*

G. Laboratory testing recommended with symptoms of abdominal pain (see Chapter 4 for general lab values)

1. CBC: to rule out infection, anemia/blood loss, platelet disorder

2. Urine

(a) U/A: to identify hematuria, glucosuria, infection

(b) Urine hCG: to rule out pregnancy

3. CMP: to rule out liver or renal disease, electrolyte imbalance, glucose abnormality, calcium disorder

4. ESR and/or CRP: markers for generalized inflammation

5. Amylase/lipase: to rule out pancreatitis

6. FOBT; if diarrhea present, obtain stool cultures for *Clostridium difficile*, leukocytes, O&P, and culture

H. Radiography tests

1. CXR: to rule out pneumonia, masses

2. KUB for constipation, bowel obstruction, and occasionally gallstones or kidney stones

3. Ultrasound (U/S)

(a) Pelvis: to rule out pregnancy, ovarian cyst/tumor/torsion, fibroid tumor

(b) Gallbladder or abdominal/pelvic U/S: to rule out gallstones, masses, and GU system problems

4. CT scan (see Table 4.2)

(a) Abdomen/pelvis: to rule out masses, constipation, aneurysm, pneumonia

(b) Appendix: to rule out appendicitis

(c) Kidney: to rule out kidney stones

5. MRI of the abdomen/pelvis: to check for inflammatory bowel disease (IBD)

> **PRACTICE PEARLS FOR ABDOMINAL PAIN**
>
> - Acute abdominal pain associated with N/V.
>   - With pain persisting for > 6 hr, *followed* by N/V: consider surgical consult.
>   - If N/V occur *before* pain, this is most likely a medical problem.
> - With pediatric patients.
>   - The further the pain is from the umbilicus, the more likely that it is due to acute abdomen; pain at the umbilicus is often associated with constipation or functional abdominal pain.
>   - During the examination, have the child place his or her hand over yours and gently push down while you move your hand to palpate for organs. This allows the child to have some control and reduces fear and ticklishness in the child.
> - With elderly patients.
>   - They will possibly require surgery unless an obvious cause for the pain is found (e.g., UTI or constipation).
>   - Consider intestinal ischemia when pain is out of proportion to physical examination findings, especially with history of CVD.
> - If you think someone is feigning abdominal pain, press into the abdomen with your hands while listening with a stethoscope; if pain is not present with this maneuver, the likelihood of a real surgical problem decreases. Observe for wincing and guarding during examination.

Upper Abdominal Conditions

BARIATRIC SURGERY

   I. Candidates for weight loss *interventions*

      A. BMI 24.9–30 kg/m² *without* comorbidity

         1. Interventions may include:

           (a) Defining weight targets

           (b) Type of diet and/or daily calorie amount

           (c) Physical activity goals

         2. Pharmacological interventions with noncontrolled weight loss medications (e.g., semaglutide or liraglutide, bupropion-naltrexone or orlistat [Xenical Rx or Alli OTC])

      B. BMI > 30 kg/m² *with* comorbidity of CVD, DM, HTN, OSA

         1. Psychological counseling (e.g., behavioral modification techniques)

         2. Diet with weight goals and outside weight management group(s) (e.g., Weight Watchers)

         3. Exercise (with goals of 150 + min/wk)

         4. Pharmacological therapy with non-controlled medications (see A. 2, above)

  II. Candidates for *weight loss surgery* are those who have failed above therapies and have

      A. BMI > 40 kg/m² without comorbidity

      B. BMI 35–39.9 kg/m² with at least one serious comorbidity

         1. DM, CVD, HTN, dyslipidemia

         2. OSA, OHS (obesity hypoventilation syndrome, also called Pickwickian syndrome)

         3. Severe debilitating arthritis, impaired QOL

         4. Venous stasis, asthma, GERD

 III. Most common types of surgery (***referral to bariatric surgery center for evaluation***)

       A. Restrictive: vertical banded gastroplasty, laparoscopic adjustable gastric band, sleeve gastrectomy

---

● = *non-urgent referral*

B. Malabsorptive: jejunoileal bypass, biliopancreatic diversion, biliopancreatic diversion with duodenal switch

C. Combination restrictive and malabsorptive: Roux-en-Y gastric bypass

IV. Follow-up after surgery and in collaboration with bariatric surgery center; they usually follow the patients closely and educate on acceptable forms of OTC and prescription medications. Outside practitioners may need to help monitor comorbidities and treat/follow acute/chronic illness.

A. Medications and supplements need to be liquid or chewable; low in fructose and sorbitol; avoid enteric coated or sustained release medication.

B. Blood levels of fat-soluble vitamins and minerals (including copper and zinc) should be rechecked about 3–6 mo after surgery. If replacements are needed consider

1. Daily chewable (not gummy) multivitamin with 100%–200% daily requirements

2. Calcium citrate or carbonate (with meals)

3. Vitamin D 2000–3000 international units daily

4. Folic acid 800–1000 mcg daily; Fe for *nonmenstruating*: 18 mg elemental daily and if *menstruating* will need 45–60 mg daily

5. Vitamin B_{12} 350–500 mcg daily and thiamine (B_1) 50–100 mg daily

C. Combined oral contraceptives

1. Restrictive surgery (band or sleeve) can take all types of COC

2. Malabsorptive surgery should avoid all types of oral pills and use vaginal ring, patch, IUD, or implants

CHOLECYSTITIS

I. Definition: inflammation of the gallbladder usually caused by gallstones (e.g., acute inflammation) or poor gallbladder function (e.g., chronic inflammation)

A. Most commonly occurs in women of childbearing age, taking OCs and women in the sixth decade of life.

B. More common in obese people.

C. People experiencing rapid weight loss are at higher risk for developing gallstones.

D. Native Americans have a 75% increased risk of gallstones.

II. Signs and symptoms

A. Acute symptoms

1. Pain and tenderness in the RUQ or epigastrium with/without radiation to the infrascapular region, mainly on the right side.

(a) It usually starts within an hour after a fried, fatty, or spicy meal.

(b) It is steady and severe and worsens over 1–2 hr and can last up to 6 hr.

(c) It is lessened if person lies still on table because inflammation has caused parietal peritoneal inflammation.

2. Patient may have fever and malaise with N/V.

3. Jaundice may occur if bile ducts are occluded.

4. Palpation in the RUQ elicits marked tenderness with deep inspiration (+ Murphy sign) with guarding. Elderly patients may have less sensitivity to palpation but should still have + Murphy sign.

B. Chronic disease presents with less severe disabling symptoms and may recur over years, with a history of increased heartburn, belching, or dyspepsia.

III. Diagnostics

A. CBC may show leukocytosis with left shift. U/A to rule out pregnancy (if indicated)

B. CMP, hepatic panel (if not included in CMP), lipase and amylase

       1. Increased amylase, liver enzymes, and bilirubin may be present with or after stone passage.

       2. Alkaline phosphatase and total bilirubin are not usually elevated with acute cholecystitis.

  C. Consider ECG to rule out cardiac origin.

  D. Consider CXR to rule out pneumonia.

  E. U/S gallbladder: if negative and symptoms continue, consider HIDA scan to test for adequate gall bladder function (U/S is the first test because the presence of gallstones must be excluded before performing HIDA, owing to the potential rupture of the gallbladder if the stone is occluding the cystic duct).

   IV. *Referral to a surgeon if gallbladder tests are positive for stones or dysfunction or if symptoms continue after adequate change in diet and weight loss.*

GASTROENTERITIS (ACUTE VIRAL)

   I. Signs and symptoms

  A. Sudden onset of explosive diarrhea accompanied by N/V and abdominal pain/cramping that lasts ≤10 days and is usually self-limiting.

  B. *Dehydration is the most important sign to be aware of and must be treated aggressively; the level of severity will determine treatment* (see Table 16.1, Signs of Dehydration in children); signs of dehydration in adults:

       1. Dry mouth, increased thirst (may lose the sensation of thirst with elderly), decreased skin turgor

       2. Altered mental status (similar to brain fog in COVID patients)

       3. H/A, lightheadedness, dizziness

       4. Decrease in urination and urine becomes concentrated and amber in color

       5. Tachycardia (especially with exertion), hypotension (especially with position change)

       6. Syncope, weakness, and fatigue

  C. Abdomen is usually soft with mild, diffuse tenderness, hyperactive bowel sounds, and increased flatulence.

  II. Diagnostic testing

  A. CBC, basic metabolic profile (BMP), U/A

  B. If diarrhea continues beyond 7 days, may consider stool cultures and stools for O&P (see Lower Abdominal Conditions, DIARRHEA, later in chapter).

  III. Treatment

  A. *Referral immediately to ED with obvious dehydration requiring multiple IV fluids or resuscitative therapies and/or if positive neurologic signs are present along with abdominal pain with N/V and rigidity.*

  B. Note if patient has been hospitalized or taken antibiotics in past 1–3 months (as cause of diarrhea).

  C. If treating as outpatient: monitor closely and follow-up in office in first 24 hr for worsening signs of dehydration.

       1. Home oral rehydration therapy (Table 9.2) should be initiated as soon as possible.

       2. Give minimum of 8 oz of fluids (not coffee or tea) every hr. Use an 8 oz measuring cup for fluids, as this size is less intimidating to patient and will be easier to calculate.

● = *non-urgent referral;* ▲ = *urgent referral*

3. Instruct caregivers on symptoms of worsening condition, especially in the elderly.
4. Encourage bed rest.
5. Diet modification
   (a) Clear liquids for 24 hr; start with 8 oz every hr for first 24 hr.
   (b) After 24 hr, start BRATY diet or soft bland diet (see Appendix A); slowly increase amount and types of foods over next 24–48 hr. If symptoms improving, return to regular diet slowly.
   (c) Refrain from fatty, fried, or spicy foods until symptoms have resolved for at least 48 hr; no caffeine or alcohol for 48 hr.
   (d) No milk or milk products for 1–2 wk.
6. Consider zinc supplements for 2–4 wk to decrease persistent diarrhea and recurrence—can be used for severe acute malnutrition (SAM) associated with diarrhea in underserved populations.
7. Start probiotics daily for 1 mo.

TABLE 9.2 ■ Oral Rehydration Solution Mixtures

Mixture Name	Administration	Special Considerations
Pedialyte Pedialyte advanced care (contains prebiotics)	Give frequent sips, not gulps, q30–60 min	Do not use red drinks Start at first symptoms of diarrhea to maintain hydration Continue breastfeeding
Oral rehydration salts (ORS)	1 packet in 1 L water Give in small amounts q30–60min	There are several similar commercial products on the market Start at first symptoms of diarrhea Continue breastfeeding
Drip drop	Dissolve 1 packet in 500 mL water Do not mix with other solutions	Use with caution in anyone on a salt-restricted diet Give in small amounts at a time Caution under 1 yr of age
Oral rehydration solution (made at home)	Mix 6 tsp sugar with ½ tsp salt in 1 L of water (measure carefully*) OR Mix ½ tsp salt with ½ tsp baking soda with 4 tbsp sugar in 1 L water	Water should be boiled for 15 min or use distilled water Mixture should be cooled before administering Same administration instructtions as above Do not use artificial flavoring Continue breastfeeding
Cereal-based oral rehydration therapy	½–1 cup precooked baby rice cereal or 1½ tsp of granulated sugar with 2 cups water and ½ tsp salt	Should be thin enough to drink Give often by spoonfuls Give even if vomiting Can put in mashed banana or other nonsweetened fruit Mix with a cold product or serve cold; may be more palatable Discard any remaining solution after 24 hr and make new
Homemade mixture	½ tsp salt + ½ tsp baking soda + 4 Tbsp sugar into 1 L of water	Give 6–8 oz every hr Discard every 24 hr

* Watered-down formula does not provide enough calories. Foods high in simple sugars might worsen diarrhea.

8. For N/V
  (a) Ondansetron (Zofran) 4–8 mg q8–12hr (based on age/weight)
  (b) Promethazine: adult: 12.5–25 mg PO/IM q4–6hr
9. Antidiarrheals can be used for up to 2 days (monitor for constipation); bulking agents (fiber products) can be used daily to help bulk stools and slow diarrhea.
10. IV therapy in office with normal saline (if available) may be given to reduce further risk for dehydration.

D. Diarrhea should be resolved within 7 days; if not, may need to look for another cause.

IV. Referral urgently to ED if
  A. *Intractable vomiting with significant dehydration*
  B. *Excessive bloody stools*
  C. *Severe abdominal pain*
  D. *Uncontrolled symptoms > 7 days*
  E. *Patient is ≥ 65 yr of age with dehydration and comorbidities (DM, heart disease, COPD)*
  F. *Altered mental status*
  G. *Unable to maintain fluids at home*
  H. *Pregnancy*

GASTROESOPHAGEAL REFLUX DISEASE (GERD)

I. Definition: reflux of stomach contents into the esophagus due to relaxation of the lower esophageal sphincter (LES)
  A. Common conditions in all ages; can be a chronic with relapses unless treatment started.
  B. *Most concerning if there is new-onset dyspepsia (indigestion)*
    1. Occurring in those ≥ 60 yr of age: recommend EGD (consider cancer or PUD)
    2. Occurring those ≤ 60 yr of age: test for *Helicobacter pylori* disease
    3. *Not to be missed signs,* see VI (later in this section)
  C. Chronic erosive esophagitis is a complication of GERD, which can lead to bleeding, anemia, scarring, and an increased risk of Barrett's esophagus.
  D. *Functional heartburn causes similar pain as GERD but without symptom relief using PPIs.* Affected individuals are considered to be hypersensitive to gastric acid and may need higher doses of PPIs bid or a trial of tricyclic antidepressants (TCAs) or selective serotonin reuptake inhibitor (SSRI).

II. Major risk factors
  A. GERD
    1. Obesity
    2. Cigarette smoking, alcohol use/abuse
    3. Eating full meal late at night; eating large fatty meals
    4. People working night shifts
    5. Chronic illness (e.g., DM slows GI emptying)
  B. GI cancers
    1. Fe deficiency anemia
    2. Hiatal hernia
    3. PMH or FH GI cancer
    4. Cigarette smoking, alcohol use/abuse
    5. Age > 60 yr of age

▲ = *urgent referral;* ▨ = *not to be missed*

    C. Barrett's esophagus more common if
      1. Symptomatic GERD has been present > 5 yr
      2. Age > 50 yr of age, Caucasian, male
      3. Cigarette smoking, chewing tobacco, alcohol use/abuse
      4. Overall obesity and localized central obesity
      5. FH Barrett's esophagus

III. Signs and symptoms
    A. Typical
      1. Heartburn and regurgitation with metallic taste in the mouth (acid brash), belching of fluids or foods; usually occurs about 1 hr after eating and worsens when lying down or bending forward
      2. Anterior chest pain with burning sensation that radiates to the neck
      3. Dysphagia, dyspepsia
    B. Atypical
      1. Chronic nonproductive cough and/or wheezing
      2. Sore throat, hoarseness that is unrelieved with OTC antihistamines or acetaminophen
      3. Frequent throat clearing and globus feeling (sensation of something in the throat)
      4. Noncardiac chest pain
      5. Poor dentition with loss or erosion of enamel
      6. Frequent OM in children

IV. Factors that worsen symptoms (Box 9.1)

V. Factors that aggravate reflux (Box 9.2)

VI. *Not to be missed signs related to precancerous or cancerous conditions.*
    A. *Anorexia; unintentional weight loss; persistent emesis*

BOX 9.1 ■ Factors That Worsen Symptoms by Relaxing the Lower Esophageal Sphincter

Foods	*Medicines*
Chocolate	Theophylline
Peppermint	Anticholinergic medications
High-fat foods	Progesterone
	Calcium channel blockers
	Alpha adrenergic agents
	Diazepam

BOX 9.2 ■ Factors That Aggravate Reflux Symptoms

Foods	*Medicines*
Citrus fruits	Tetracycline
Spicy foods	Quinidine
Tomatoes	Potassium
Coffee	Iron salts
Caffeinated beverages	Nonsteroidal antiinflammatory drugs (NSAIDs) and ASA
	Bisphosphonates

■ = *not to be missed*

■　　　B. **Blood in stools or emesis; iron-deficiency anemia**

■　　　C. **Painful swallowing (odynophagia)**

■　　　D. **Chronic cough or change in sputum production**: consider pulmonary disease/disorders

■　　　E. **Chronic unremitting reflux, hoarseness, and swallowing problems**: consider Barrett's esophagus (highest risk in obese white males > 50 yr of age who smoke)

■　　　F. **New-onset dyspepsia, especially in patients ≥ 60 yr of age**

　　VII. Diagnostic tests

　　　　A. "Clinical history" is a good indicator of disease.

　　　　B. CBC (should be normal); stool for occult blood (should be negative)

　　　　C. *H. pylori* testing if unresponsive to therapy or if the symptoms are suggestive of infection

▲　　　D. **Referral for EGD, urgently if any not to be missed symptoms are present.**

　　VIII. Treatment

■　　　A. If there are no concerning signs (see VI, **not to be missed** signs above) and the clinical history indicates that GERD is the probable cause: initiate lifestyle and dietary modifications first.

　　　　　1. Do not eat meals or drink carbonated beverages within 3 hr of bedtime.

　　　　　2. Decrease the amount of fried, fatty, and spicy foods to decrease gastric acid production.

　　　　　3. Raise the head of bed using 4 to 6-in. blocks, especially if nocturnal symptoms are present.

　　　　　4. Lose weight if indicated; avoid tight-fitting clothing, especially around the waist.

　　　　　5. Decrease factors that aggravate reflux symptoms (see Box 9.2).

　　　　　6. Avoid foods that relax the LES (see Box 9.1).

　　　　　7. Decrease or eliminate NSAID, nicotine, and alcohol use.

　　　　　8. Try chewing gum to help increase salivation to neutralize gastric acid.

　　　　B. Pharmacological therapy (also see Table 9.3, H_2 blockers/PPIs).

　　　　　1. Initial therapy for mild to moderate GERD (e.g., symptoms <2 times/wk, no interference with lifestyle).

　　　　　　(a) Use antacids with symptoms that occur < once a week

　　　　　　(b) If symptoms are predictable, use antacids 1 hr before meals, after meals, and at bedtime; antacids have a rapid onset but short duration

　　　　　　(c) Use OTC H2 blockers bid for 2 wk; if symptoms continue, may need H_2 blockers for another 2–4 wk; if continued failure, then stop H_2 blockers and initiate PPIs daily

　　　　　　(d) Bedtime dosing is useful with nocturnal reflux

　　　　　　(e) When symptoms are controlled, taper down medication to lowest effective dose or discontinue medication

　　　　　2. *If symptoms are intense and predictable* even with treatment

　　　　　　(a) Reevaluate lifestyle and dietary habits.

　　　　　　(b) Use PPIs daily for 8 wk and then *gradually* decrease the dose.

　　　　　　　(i) If symptoms resolve, *gradually* taper dose off (sudden withdrawal may cause rebound acid reflux).

　　　　　　　(ii) If symptoms resolve but then recur, restart PPI at a lower dose for another 8 wk, then change to H_2 blocker daily for 4 wk and then stop treatment.

●　　　　　　(iii) **Referral to gastroenterologist, if symptoms recur again (even without not to be missed signs).**

■ = *not to be missed;* ● = *non-urgent referral;* ▲ = *urgent referral*

TABLE 9.3 ■ H₂ Blockers and Proton Pump Inhibitors

Medication	Dosage
H₂ Blockers	
Cimetidine*	Low dose: 200 mg bid Regular dose: 400 mg bid
Nizatidine	Low dose: 75 mg bid Regular dose: 150 mg bid
Famotidine (OTC,Rx)	Low dose: 10 mg bid Regular dose: 20 mg bid
Famotidine 10 mg/calcium carbonate 800 mg/magnesium hydroxide 165 mg chewable (Pepcid Complete)	1 chewable qd-bid prn heartburn
Proton Pump Inhibitors (PPIs)**	
Omeprazole (OTC, Rx)	Regular dose: 20–40 mg qd High dose***: 40–80 mg qd Ulcer dose: 20–40 mg qd
Lansoprazole (OTC, Rx)	Low dose: 15 mg qd Regular dose: 30 mg qd High dose***: 60 mg qd Ulcer dose: 30 mg qd
Dexlansoprazole	Regular dose: 30 mg qd High dose***: 60 mg qd Ulcer dose: 30–60 mg qd
Rabeprazole	Regular dose: 20 mg qd High dose***: 40 mg qd Ulcer dose: 20 mg qd
Esomeprazole (OTC, Rx)	Regular dose: 20–40 mg qd High dose***: 40–80 mg qd
Pantoprazole	Low dose: 20 mg qd Regular dose: 40 mg qd High dose***: 80 mg qd
Omeprazole + sodium bicarbonate (Zegerid)†	20 mg qd for 4 wk and give 1 hr before a meal

  * Cimetidine can cause confusion in elderly people; always check medications being used.
 ** PPIs should be taken on an empty stomach, half an hour before a meal for peak effect.
*** High doses should be reserved for *H. pylori* resistant symptoms or healing ulcers, used prior to consultation with gastroenterologist.
 † Special considerations for Zegerid.
 • Zegerid dosing is based on omeprazole dose not on bicarbonate dose.
 • Two 20-mg caps or powder packet is *not* bioequivalent to one 40-mg dose.
 • Immediate-release powder can be used for patients who cannot swallow pills (i.e., children and patients with feeding tubes).
 • Children (1–16 yr of age), >20 kg: 20 mg daily.
 • Zegerid is both OTC and Rx (Rx dosing 20–60 mg strength, OTC 20 mg).
 • Zegerid should be taken >1 hr before a meal.

IX. *Referral to a gastroenterologist for endoscopy*
  A. *If any not to be missed signs (see VI.) are present, recommend urgent referral for EGD.*
  B. *If concern for Barrett's esophagus (see II, C)*
  C. *If persistent reflux symptoms are unrelieved with medications after 4–8 wk of full-dose therapy with PPIs and H2 blockers.*

● = *non-urgent referral;* ▲ = *urgent referral*

PRACTICE PEARLS FOR GERD MEDICATIONS

- Recommended short-term (<8 wk) use of PPIs
  - Acute GERD and *H. pylori*
  - Acute new-onset gastric ulcers
  - Stress ulcer prophylaxis (hospitalizations, especially intensive care units)
- Recommended long-term use of PPIs
  - Barrett's esophagus
  - Refractory GERD
  - Erosive esophagitis
  - Zollinger-Ellison syndrome
  - Chronic anticoagulant therapy
  - NSAID-induced ulcers
- Long-term dosing with PPIs can lead to
  - Potential for increased hip fracture risk in postmenopausal women
  - Increased risk of *C. difficile* infection, aspiration pneumonia, and B12 deficiency (consider intranasal or IM replacement with vitamin B12, if deficiency present)
  - Increased risk for kidney damage/disease; use H2 blockers
- Bismuth causes stools to turn black and the patient's tongue may become black on the dorsal side; both should resolve after treatment is stopped.
- Consider sucralfate with GERD related to pregnancy and lactation due to its short half-life.
- Avoid drinking alcohol while taking metronidazole because of vasomotor reactions (e.g., vomiting, flushing, and sweating); this should resolve after treatment is stopped.
- Metronidazole and clarithromycin may cause a metallic taste in the mouth; this should resolve after treatment is stopped. Note the rate of resistance in your area, may not be first-line therapy.
- Clarithromycin has warning against using in patients with heart disease.

HELICOBACTER PYLORI–INDUCED GASTRITIS

I. Definition: most common chronic inflammatory bacterial infection of the stomach
   A. Associated with PUD, chronic gastritis, gastric cancer, gastric mucosa lymphoma.
   B. Infection may be present for years before patient seeks treatment.
   C. Symptoms may be minimal or significant and effect ADLs.

II. Signs and symptoms
   A. Dyspepsia, hunger in the morning, and halitosis
   B. N/V, upper abdominal pain, and anorexia
   C. Increased belching, burping, fullness after a meal and increased bloating
   D. Occasional bowel changes with either constipation or diarrhea

III. Diagnostic tests
   A. CBC (may have microcytic anemia), FOBT (may be positive)
   B. *H. pylori* testing with either blood, fecal antigen, or urea breath test
   C. Endoscopy is indicated if poor response to medical therapy (stop H_2 blockers/PPIs 1–2 wk prior to test if possible).

IV. Lifestyle changes
   A. Increase foods containing flavonoids, such as apples, cranberries, garlic and tea; these may inhibit the growth of *H. pylori*.
   B. Avoid alcohol and smoking.

V. Pharmacological treatment
   A. Triple therapy for 14 days
      1. Clarithromycin 500 mg bid *plus*

        2. Amoxicillin 1 g bid *OR* metronidazole 500 mg tid *plus*

        3. PPI bid (see Table 9.3)

    B. Quadruple therapy for 10–14 days

        1. Clarithromycin 500 mg bid *plus*

        2. Amoxicillin 1 g bid *plus*

        3. Metronidazole (or tinidazole) 500 mg bid *plus*

        4. PPI of choice bid (see Table 9.3)

    C. Bismuth quadruple therapy for 10–14 days

        1. Bismuth subsalicylate 300–524 mg qid *plus*

        2. Tetracycline 500 mg qid *plus*

        3. Metronidazole 250 mg qid *plus*

        4. PPI of choice bid (see Table 9.3)

    D. Levofloxacin triple therapy (if failed above or allergy to above medications) for 10–14 days (off label use); high rates of resistance seen with levofloxacin

        1. Levofloxacin 500 mg daily *plus*

        2. Amoxicillin 1 g bid OR metronidazole 500 mg tid *plus*

        3. PPI of choice bid (see Table 9.3)

VI. Alternate pharmacological treatment (prepackaged, more convenient, more costly, and eradication rates same as others already mentioned)

    A. Pylera (bismuth subcitrate + metronidazole + tetracycline) for 10 days

        1. Three caps 4 times daily *plus* PPI of choice bid (see Table 9.3)

        2. Give after meals and at bedtime.

    B. Prevpac (lansoprazole + amoxicillin + clarithromycin)

        1. 1 dose bid for 10–14 days

        2. Give before meals and swallow doses whole

    C. Helidac (bismuth subsalicylate + tetracycline + metronidazole)

        1. 1 dose qid for 10–14 days

        2. Give with meals and at bedtime.

    D. Voquezna Triple Pak (vonoprazan+amoxicillin+clarithromycin): 1 dose tid × 14 days

VII. Post testing

    A. *H. pylori* post-testing repeated about 4–6 wk after completion of antibiotic with urea breathe test, fecal antigen test or upper endoscopy; 1–2 wk prior to test, *stop* PPI (if possible)

    B. Retreatment with a different antibiotic regimen should be considered if previously positive for *H. pylori* and symptoms return.

▲ **VIII.** *Referral to gastroenterologist if symptoms are not relieved with treatment or they worsen.*

PANCREATITIS

I. Definition: inflammation of the pancreas, with leakage of pancreatic enzymes into the surrounding tissues.

    A. Structural causes

        1. Chronic ingestion of alcohol or obstructing gallstones

        2. Strictures or tumors that block the duct of the pancreas

    B. Hypertriglyceridemia (> 1000 mg/dL)

    C. Common medications that could be implicated

        (a) Diuretics (hydrochlorothiazide)

        (b) Sulfonamides (TMP-SMZ)

        (c) Valproic acid (Depakene)

        (d) Tetracycline

        (e) GLP-1 agonists

▲ = *urgent referral*

II. Signs and symptoms (not all may be present)
  A. *Slow* onset of poorly localized pain: usually caused by metabolic disorder or alcohol abuse; *sudden* onset of severe, localized pain: usually from gallstone pancreatitis
     1. Pain is located in the upper abdomen and may radiate to the back or chest
     2. Persistent pain for hours to days; partially relieved by sitting up or bending forward
  B. N/V, fever, and possible scleral icterus; abdominal distention and/or hypoactive bowel sounds
  C. Signs of intra-abdominal bleeding with ecchymosis in the flanks (e.g., Grey-Turner sign) or periumbilical region (e.g., Cullen sign)
  D. Weight loss (unexplained)
  E. Hypotensive signs: tachycardia, sweating, tachypnea, hypoxemia
III. Diagnostic testing
  A. Amylase >3 times normal has sensitivity of 67%–83%.
     1. Rises in 6–12 hr and
     2. Returns to normal within 3–5 days
  B. Lipase >3 times normal has sensitivity of 82%–100%.
     1. Rises within 4–8 hr and
     2. Returns to normal within 8–14 days
     3. Elevations occur sooner than amylase and are more useful with diagnosis.
  C. CBC (elevated WBC and HCT), elevated BUN, glucose changes, low calcium and magnesium.
  D. Imaging findings (abdominal U/S, CT, or MRI) consistent with pancreatitis.
IV. Treatment
  ▲ A. ***Referral to ED for possible admission.***
  B. Recommendation after discharge
     1. Low-fat diet with smaller portions and eat more often, limit foods high in trans-fats or trans-fat substitutes (e.g., cookies, crackers, cakes, and donuts); this can limit recurrence and also help normalize triglycerides.
     2. Encourage foods high in antioxidants, such as green leafy vegetables, cold-water fish, beans, berries, tomatoes, foods high in vitamins B and C, and iron.
     3. Decrease or eliminate alcohol, caffeine, and tobacco.
     4. Amylase, lipase, and glucose should be monitored every 3 mo until stable and then annually; if hyperglycemia does not normalize, may need to treat for DM.
     5. Supplements for deficiencies related to pancreatitis:
        (a) Multivitamin, omega-3 fatty acids
        (b) Co-Q10: 100–200 mg at bedtime
        (c) Probiotic supplement daily
  C. Suggest counseling for abusive habits leading to episodes of pancreatitis.

PEPTIC ULCER DISEASE

I. Definition: disruption of the mucosal lining of the stomach, duodenum, or both that results in an ulcer
  A. Commonly associated with *H. pylori* disease (either current or past) and chronic ASA/NSAID or steroid use
  B. Risk factors include smoking, alcohol use, and advanced age.
  C. Common in patients between 40 and 60 yr of age but can occur in children under stressful conditions.

▲ = *urgent referral*

II. Signs and symptoms
- A. Pain
  1. Chronic recurrent upper abdominal pain (epigastric or retrosternal) that is burning, gnawing, aching, and described as "hunger pains."
  2. With gastric ulcers: pain occurs with eating and is present until the stomach has emptied; pain is usually absent with fasting; there is early satiety and increased belching, intolerance of fatty foods.
  3. With duodenal ulcers: pain may occur on empty stomach (2–4 hr after a meal or in the middle of the night) and is usually relieved with food, antacids, or liquids such as milk or ice cream.
- B. Guarding is common with palpation.
- C. N/V, constipation and bloating may occur.
- D. Anorexia, weight loss, and feeding difficulties in young children.

III. Complications can occur without prodromal symptoms in the elderly and NSAID users.
- A. Acute perforation with severe abdominal pain and peritoneal signs
- B. Hemorrhage, shock, hypotension

IV. *Not to be missed signs*
- A. *Weight loss; recurrent or intractable vomiting*
- B. *GI bleeding; Fe-deficiency anemia*
- C. *Dysphagia, odynophagia*
- D. *New-onset dyspepsia, especially in patients > 60 yr of age*
- E. *Palpable mass or lymphadenopathy*

V. Diagnostic testing
- A. CBC (may show mild microcytic anemia), stool FOBT (may be positive for blood)
- B. *H. pylori* testing
- C. *Consider referral for endoscopy, especially if symptoms not resolving*

VI. Nonpharmacological treatment
- A. Review all current medications including OTC and herbal products; SSRIs increase the risk of UGI bleed. Stop all ASA/NSAIDs and decrease steroid therapy to the lowest possible dose.
- B. There is a high risk of recurrence, if lifestyle changes are not started; if the ulcer recurs, can use standard dose PPI medications indefinitely.
- C. Stop smoking and decrease or avoid alcohol and decrease caffeine intake.
- D. Diet should be nutritious with frequent small meals; no spicy, fried, or fatty foods or foods that irritate the stomach lining.
- E. Probiotic supplements may speed healing.
- F. Vitamin C 500 mg 2–3 times daily may help healing (no data confirmation, but is not harmful).

VII. Pharmacological therapy (duodenal ulcers for 4 wk; gastric ulcers for 8 wk)
- A. PPIs are the most effective ulcer treatments but antacids can be used more often for minor symptoms (see Table 9.3)
- B. With *H. pylori* testing
  1. If *positive*, treat *H. pylori* (see ***HELICOBACTER PYLORI*–INDUCED GASTRITIS**).
  2. If *negative and the ulcer is not associated with NSAID or steroid use*, begin symptomatic ulcer treatment with PPIs.
  3. If *negative and the ulcer is associated with chronic NSAID use that cannot be stopped,* maintenance treatment will be needed indefinitely
     (a) PPI is first choice (see Table 9.3) at maintenance dose   *or*

_____

■ = *not to be missed;* ● = *non-urgent referral*

       (b) Misoprostol 100–200 mcg (not with pregnancy) qid with food and bedtime *or*
       (c) Sucralfate 1 g bid before meals and bedtime
       (d) Consider switching to celecoxib (Celebrex) for pain
  C. Duodenal ulcers may respond to
     1. Antacids 2–4 tbsp 1 hr before and 2 hr after meals/medications (if not contraindicated) and at bedtime (magnesium antacids tend to cause diarrhea; aluminum antacids tend to cause constipation; use combination products to counteract side effects)
     2. Sucralfate 1 g qid 30–60 min before meals and at hs can be useful
  D. Gastric ulcers
     1. Should be followed by endoscopy because of increased risk of stomach cancer
     2. Usually due to inflammatory process (e.g., alcohol, NSAID use) and tend to heal when triggers are removed
     3. Antacids (e.g., calcium carbonate or magnesium hydroxide)
     4. PPIs (see Table 9.3)
VIII. *Referral to a gastroenterologist for endoscopy and further treatment, with treatment failure, or not to be missed signs or bleeding.*

Lower Abdominal Conditions

APPENDICITIS

  I. Definition: inflammation and/or rupture of the appendix
  II. Signs and symptoms
    A. Begins with vague, constant abdominal discomfort with some cramping and nausea; as time progresses (24–48 hr) pain migrates to RLQ with worsening intensity, anorexia, N/V
    B. Low-grade fever (possibly)
    C. Stooped appearance when walking
    D. Presence of one or more of these signs in adults increases likelihood
      1. Pain worsens with movement (e.g., walking or just moving around in bed), coughing, and deep breathing.
      2. Pain migrates from the periumbilical region to the RLQ usually within 24 hr.
      3. Pain is noted before vomiting.
      4. There is positive rebound and guarding.
      5. Positive psoas sign, Markle sign, and Rovsing's sign (see ABDOMINAL PAIN, III, E)
    E. In children < 5 yr of age, likelihood increases with
      1. Fever ≥ 100.5 °F
      2. Diffuse abdominal pain with eventual migration to RLQ; rebound tenderness and pain to percussion
      3. Irritability, grunting respirations
      4. Refusing to walk and may complain of right hip pain
      5. Pain with cough or jumping
      6. Anorexia, N/V
      7. WBCs > 10,000/µL, Neutrophils + bands ≥ 7500/µL

■ = *not to be missed;* ● = *non-urgent referral*

   III. Diagnostic testing
- A. CBC (may show leukocytosis), ESR/CRP, U/A (usually normal); urine hCG, if childbearing age
- B. Flat and erect abdominal X-ray (may show fecalith)
- C. Abdominal U/S for children (less invasive than CT, but the appendix may not be visualized)
- D. CT abdomen for appendicitis (see Table 4.2) is the gold standard for diagnosis.

   ● **IV.** *Referral to a surgeon or ED for further follow-up if any tests are positive or if the symptoms continue.*

COLON CANCER

  I. Increased risk
- A. Age ≥ 40 yr, Black, male
- B. FH of colon cancer or advanced polyps
- C. Adenomatous polyps on past colonoscopy
- D. IBD, IBS
- E. Sedentary lifestyle, obesity
- F. Fiber-deficient diet, alcohol use, and/or cigarette smoking
- G. Any type of abdominal radiation as a child

  II. Signs and symptoms
- A. Generalized
  1. Overall change in bowel habits unrelated to change in diet/medications
  2. Rectal bleeding, mass
  3. Fe deficiency anemia without obvious rectal bleeding (see Chapter 4, ANEMIA)
  4. Abdominal mass in either LLQ, RLQ, or suprapubic area
- B. Right-sided colon involvement
  1. May be asymptomatic until the tumor causes obstruction
  2. Unintentional weight loss
  3. Anemia; positive FOBT
  4. Crampy, colicky, intermittent abdominal pain
- C. Left-sided colon involvement
  1. Change in bowel habits: diarrhea or constipation alternating
  2. Feeling of fullness after defecation.
  3. Shape of stool changes; bright red rectal bleeding mixed with normal stool
  4. Generalized lower abdominal pain
  5. Unintentional weight loss; anemia
- D. Sigmoid/rectal colon involvement
  1. Obvious rectal bleeding or bleeding mass at anal opening
  2. Mucoid drainage from the anus
  3. Pain with defecation

  III. Diagnostic testing
- A. CBC (may show anemia; see Chapter 4, ANEMIA)
- B. FOBT (stool positive for occult or frank blood); DRE
- C. Abdominal CT may show mass (see Table 4.2).

  IV. Colon cancer screening guidelines according to the CDC, USPSTF, American College of Physicians (ACP)
- A. The preferred colorectal cancer (CRC) *prevention screening for average risk of any race:*

● *= non-urgent referral*

1. Colonoscopy q10yr beginning at 45 yr of age with no interval testing.
2. If unable or patient refuses to have colonoscopy, alternative testing:
   (a) Annual fecal immunochemical test (FIT)
   (b) Stool DNA test (FIT-DNA [Cologard]) testing q3yr
   (c) Computed tomography colonography (CTC) q5yr
   (d) Sigmoidoscopy
       (i) Every 10yr with annual FIT *or*
       (ii) Every 5yr with FIT-DNA q3yr *or*
       (iii) Single test q5–10yr.
   (e) Sensitive FOBT on 3 different samples annually (least effective test)
3. Adults with average risk should continue CRC screening until 75 yr of age; after 75 yr of age, screening is based on patient preference and prior screening history. CRC screening is discouraged after 85 yr of age or if there is < 10 yr life expectancy.

B. *Prevention screening for high-risk* patient (e.g., FH of polyps, first degree relative (FDR) or multiple family members with CRC or advanced polyps): colonoscopy q5yr; if refuses colonoscopy, consider annual FIT or FIT-DNA.
   1. Beginning at 40 yr of age
   2. With a single first-degree relative (FDR) with a documented diagnosis of CRC, screening should start 10yr before FDR diagnosis was made.
   3. Age when patient reaches the age the FDR was diagnosed with an advanced polyp
C. If polyps are noted on colonoscopy, then follow-up is usually q3–5yr or as guided by the gastroenterologist, depending on polyp biopsy.

▲ V. *Referral to a gastroenterologist or surgeon urgently for colonoscopy and biopsy of the lesion.*

CONSTIPATION

I. Rome IV criteria for functional constipation: symptoms present ≥ 3 mo, for at least 25% of bowel movements, with at least two of the following:
   A. Straining during stooling
   B. Lumpy or hard stools
   C. Sensation of incomplete evacuation
   D. Sensation of anorectal obstruction/blockage
   E. Having to do manual evacuation
   F. Three or less spontaneous stools per week
II. Types of constipation
   A. Idiopathic (functional)
      1. Due to slow colonic transit
      2. Dyssynergic movement (inability of anal sphincter muscles to coordinate stool passage)
   B. Secondary constipation due to
      1. Drugs such as anticholinergics, antihistamines, antidepressants, iron supplements, aluminum containing antacids, CCB, opioids
      2. Neurogenic diseases such as DM, Hirschsprung disease and megacolon disorders, Parkinson disease and multiple sclerosis (MS)
      3. Nonneurogenic cause such as aging, hypothyroidism, pregnancy, hypercalcemia, anorexia nervosa
      4. IBS

▲ = *urgent referral*

III. History and physical
- A. How long has this been a problem?
- B. How many stooling events in a week?
- C. Is there a feeling/sensation of uncompleted stooling?
- D. Review all medications (OTC, prescription, and herbals) and reasons for taking.
- E. Other symptoms related to constipation
  1. Changes in stool color, size, shape, consistency, any blood noted
  2. Does patient have to strain, sit on stool for extended lengths of time before stooling?
- F. Focus exam on abdomen and rectal area (see Chapter 1 Focused Examinations, ABDOMINAL PAIN, III. F, in this chapter)
  1. Observe anal area for fissures, hemorrhoids, and laxity of opening.
  2. DRE
     - (a) Test the anal sphincter tone; look for strictures or masses.
     - (b) Internal hemorrhoids
     - (c) Stool consistency and amount of stool in ampulla

IV. Diagnostic tests
- A. CBC (for anemia), CMP
- B. TSH (for hypothyroidism)
- C. Stool for FOBT and DRE
- D. Colonoscopy criteria (see COLON CANCER. IV above):
  1. Patient ≥ 45 yr of age may screen earlier with FH colon cancer.
  2. *Rectal bleeding or iron deficiency*
  3. *Unexpected weight loss*
  4. *Recent or sudden onset of constipation*
  5. *IBD (Crohn or Ulcerative Colitis)*

V. General treatment for idiopathic (functional) constipation in adults (see Chapter 16, Abdominal Conditions, ENCOPRESIS for fecal incontinence in children)
- A. Stop all medications (OTC or prescription) that may contribute to constipation (see II, B, 1, above).
- B. Patient education related to
  1. Importance of reducing daily laxative use while increasing dietary fiber or bulk forming laxatives (see D. 1, below)
  2. Increase dietary fiber to 20–25 g/day (also see Appendix A).
     - (a) Bulk forming cereals (bran, oats)
     - (b) Increase to 4–5 servings raw fruits (e.g., apples)
     - (c) Beans 1–2 servings
     - (d) Vegetables 4–5 servings
     - (e) Prunes 2–4 daily
  3. Increase exercise daily
  4. Increase fluids (noncaffeinated) daily to 2–3 L
  5. Training for routine stooling times (e.g., after a meal)
  6. Constipation can be an ongoing problem for many people or it can be intermittent; medications need to be used based on occurrence.
- C. Home-prepared bulking/motility therapy for chronic constipation
  1. Mix and warm together 60 mL prune juice and 30 mL of milk of magnesia (MOM) and drink while warm.

▓ = *not to be missed*

       2. Mix together 1 cup **P**rune juice, 1 tbsp unprocessed **B**ran and ½ cup **A**pplesauce (PBA) to desired consistency; start with 30 mL daily with breakfast and if necessary, increase weekly to a total of 90 mL tid.

  D. OTC treatment for idiopathic constipation

    1. Bulk-forming laxatives daily

      (a) Psyllium (Metamucil) up to 1 tbsp tid

      (b) Methylcellulose (Citrucel, powdered) up to 1 tbsp or 4 caps tid

      (c) Polycarbophil (FiberCon) > 12 yr of age: 2 tabs 1–4 times a day

      (d) Benefiber 1–3 caps tid

    2. Osmotic laxatives daily or as needed

      (a) Polyethylene glycol 3350 (MiraLAX) > 17 yr of age: 1 capful in 8 oz liquid daily

        (i) May take 1–4 days before onset of action

        (ii) Use shortest effective duration but can be used long-term if needed.

      (b) Lactulose 15–30 mL every other day up to twice daily

        (i) May take 1–2 days before onset of action

        (ii) Can be used daily if needed but usually used for acute constipation.

      (c) Glycerin suppository (Fleet): 1 supp PR daily as needed

        (iv) Rapid onset of action < 12 hr

        (v) Used for acute constipation

      (d) Sodium phosphate rectal (Fleet enema) daily or as needed for some types of secondary constipation with rapid onset of action < 12 hr

        (i) Spinal cord injury: daily bowel program

        (ii) Disimpaction prior to initiation of daily bowel program

        (iii) Can cause atonic bowel secondary to chronic overuse of laxatives

      (e) Magnesium hydroxide (MOM) 1–2 ounces divided 1–2 times daily

        (i) Onset of action ≤ 3 hr

        (ii) Used for incidental constipation

      (f) Magnesium citrate (MagCitrate) 200 mL once daily

        (i) Used for acute constipation with rapid onset of action ≤ 3 hr

        (ii) Watery stools and urgency

        (iii) Monitor for magnesium toxicity with renal insufficiency.

    3. Stimulant laxatives used daily or as needed

      (a) Bisacodyl (Dulcolax) > 12 yr of age: PO 5–15 mg daily; PR 1 supp daily

        (i) Onset of action 6–10 hr for oral and ≤ 1 hr for supp

        (ii) Used for acute constipation

      (b) Sennosides (X-Lax) > 12 yr of age: 8.6 mg 2–4 tabs divided 1–2 times daily

        (i) Onset of action 6–12 hr

        (ii) Comes in combination with docusate

    4. Stool softeners.

      (a) Docusate sodium 50–300 mg 1–2 times a day

      (b) Docusate calcium 240 mg daily

  E. Pharmacological treatment

    1. Lubiprostone (Amitiza) > 18 yr of age: 24 mcg bid; onset of action 1–2 days

    2. Linaclotide (Linzess) > 18 yr of age: 145 mcg daily; onset of action 12–24 hr

    3. Plecanatide (Trulance) > 18 yr of age: 3 mg daily; onset of action 12–24 hr.

    4. Prucalopride (Motegrity) > 18 yr of age: 2 mg daily; onset of action 6–12 hr.

▲ **VI.** ***Referral to gastroenterologist if problems continue; urgent referral with not to be missed signs (see IV, D, above).***

▲ = *urgent referral*

DIARRHEA (SEE TABLE 9.4)

I. Definition:
   A. Acute diarrhea usually presents with three or more loose or watery stools in a 24 hr period lasting < 14 days; usually self-limited but can become chronic lasting > 30 days. It can be infectious or related to food or a medication reaction.
   B. Noninflammatory diarrhea usually presents with watery diarrhea and abdominal cramping but "no blood or fever."
      1. Norovirus/rotavirus
      2. *Clostridioides difficile (formerly Clostridium difficile)* and *Clostridium perfringens*
      3. Protozoan (e.g., Giardia and Cryptosporidium most common)
   C. Inflammatory diarrhea usually has blood or mucus; may be accompanied by fever and abdominal pain and tenesmus.
      1. *Salmonella* (nontyphoidal)
      2. *Campylobacter* spp.
      3. *Shigella* spp.
      4. *Enterotoxigenic E. coli*
   D. Noninfectious acute diarrhea usually seen from
      1. Adverse effects of common medications (e.g., antibiotics, metformin, colchicine)
      2. Cancer
      3. IBD and hyperthyroidism
      4. Food allergies
II. Focus on HPI
   A. Onset of symptoms, has diarrhea slowed down or worsened since onset?
   B. Number of watery or bloody/mucus stools (try to get number and amount of stools per day since diarrhea started); has there been any vomiting?
   C. Any associated symptoms
      1. Fever
      2. H/A, abdominal pain, cramping before or during stooling
      3. Neurologic signs (e.g., paresthesias, loss of use of extremity[s], swallowing difficulty)
   D. Ingestion of suspicious or new foods in last 7 days (see Table 9.4)
      1. Raw or undercooked foods (e.g., sushi for possible salmonella, *E. coli*, *C. perfringens*)
      2. Use of well water or drinking from streams
      3. Picnics
   E. Recent travel (i.e., when and where)
      1. Camping/hiking (possible *Giardia* or *Cryptosporidium*)
      2. International travel (possible Traveler's diarrhea)
   F. Exposure to others with similar symptoms or work in an environment with close quarters (possible virus) or people with poor hygiene (possible infectious diarrhea)
   G. Recent antibiotic use or recent hospitalization (possible *Clostridioides difficile infection, [CDI]*)
   H. Exposure to reptiles or farm animals (possible *Salmonella* or *Campylobacter*)
   I. What treatments have you tried and what treatments are you doing now?
III. Physical examination (see Chapter 1, ABDOMINAL and ABDOMINAL PAIN, III in this chapter for abdominal examination)
   A. Review vital signs including temperature and pulse oximetry and any orthostatic changes.
   B. Mucus membranes for dryness and any ulcerations, skin turgor for any tenting

    C. Abdomen for localized tenderness, distention, bowel sounds, rebound or guarding

    D. Extremities for any swelling

    E. Neurologic examination for any confusion, paresthesia, weakness, dysphagia

IV. Diagnostic testing

    A. Routine stool testing is recommended if diarrhea lasts > 10 days and patient is not improving; stool cultures for specific bacteria or parasite if suspected based on history; routine stool culture if unsure.

    B. CBC, CMP

    C. Urinalysis for hydration status, color

    D. Colonoscopy, abdominal X-rays *are not* usually helpful unless there are other suspected causes such as obstruction, IBD, or cancers.

V. General nonpharmacological treatment (see Table 9.4 for specific treatments).

    A. Prevent dehydration with increase in fluids or ORT (see Table 9.2).

    B. Dietary changes should be very slow.

        1. BRATY diet (see Appendix A)

        2. Boiled potatoes, oats, noodles

        3. Crackers and soup with addition of salt

        4. No dairy products (except yogurt) and no high fat foods

VI. Pharmacological treatment (see Table 9.4 and VII for Travelers diarrhea and VIII for *Clostridioides difficile* [CDI]).

    A. If unsure of cause but is inflammatory diarrhea, consider.

        1. Azithromycin 500 mg daily for 3 days or 1 gm once

        2. Ciprofloxacin 500 mg daily for 3 days or 750 mg once

        3. Levofloxacin 500 mg daily for 3 days

    B. Antimotility agents, antiemetics as needed for < 5 days; taper dose as symptoms improve.

VII. Traveler's diarrhea.

    A. Definition: usually self-limiting bacterial illness

        1. Most common illness affecting international travelers; usually occurs during first week of travel or up to 10 days after returning.

        2. Most cases resolve in 1–7 days without treatment, but some may be severe enough to disrupt ADLs.

        3. Transmission: contaminated food/water (most common with enterotoxigenic *E. coli*)

        4. Consider treatment for high-risk people

            (a) Infants and elderly

            (b) Immunocompromised people

            (c) Presence of IBS/colon disease

            (d) Diabetics

            (e) People on H_2 blockers or antacids

    B. Signs and symptoms

        1. Starts with malaise, anorexia

        2. Followed by abrupt onset profuse watery diarrhea *without* blood, mucus, or foul odor

        3. Positive abdominal pain, cramping, and bloating

        4. Possible low-grade fever; infrequent emesis

    C. Diagnostic testing with stool cultures and stool-specific cultures may be useful if diarrhea lasts > 10–14 days.

        1. Bloody, mucoid diarrhea with abdominal cramping (consider *Campylobacter, Shigella,* or *E. coli*)

2. Upper GI symptoms with bloating, gas, and nausea (consider *Giardia, Cryptosporidium*)

3. Antibiotics within the last 2–3 mo (consider *CDI*)

D. General treatment

1. Traveler's diarrhea does not require antibiotics unless diarrhea is severe. Prompt symptom control is the treatment of choice.

2. Oral rehydration (see Table 9.2) at onset of illness is key; bland BRATY diet may be more palatable and help to bulk stools (see Appendix A). Soups, broth, and fruit juices can be used with mild diarrhea.

3. Antimotility: loperamide (Imodium) 2 mg after loose stools (max dose 16 mg/day); can give with antibiotic therapy; limit use to 48 hr. *do not use with severe bloody diarrhea with fever.*

4. Probiotics for 1 mo or longer if needed

5. Start bismuth subsalicylate 4 tabs q30min up to 8 doses in 24 hr at the start of diarrhea; is slower to act and may cause black discoloration of tongue and stools; *do not use if taking ASA.*

   (a) Bismuth subsalicylate can be used as prophylaxis: 2 tab qid or 2 oz qid for up to 3 wk

   (b) May decrease incidence of traveler's diarrhea (avoid if allergy to ASA)

6. Antibiotic therapy for 1–3 days for moderate to severe diarrhea

   (a) Azithromycin 500 mg daily for 3 days (dosing equivalent for children, pregnancy) and can stop sooner if diarrhea subsides.

   (b) Azithromycin 1 g once

   (c) Levofloxacin 500 mg daily for 3 days or once

   (d) Ciprofloxacin 500 mg bid or 750 mg once

7. If diarrhea persists for > 7 days or dehydration occurs, seek medical care.

8. Follow up in office in 24 hr.

E. *Referral to ED or gastroenterologist (depending on severity of symptoms) if*

1. *Diarrhea worsens*

2. *Dehydration occurs*

3. *Stools are bloody with increased abdominal pain and fever*

F. Prevention

1. Consume only bottled water or canned vegetables; avoid ice, salads, and fruit (unless you peel it); use bottled water to brush teeth.

2. Beware of crowded pools, which could be a source.

3. Consider immunizations appropriate to country visiting (*www.CDC.gov*).

VIII. *Clostridioides (formerly Clostridium) difficile* infection (CDI)

A. Definition: diarrhea caused by broad-spectrum antibiotic use and nosocomial infection from hospitalization; commonly seen in elderly and immunocompromised people.

B. Most common *antibiotics as causative agents*

1. Clindamycin

2. Second- and third-generation cephalosporins

3. Fluoroquinolones

4. Amoxicillin

C. Signs and symptoms

1. Diarrhea within 1–2 wk after antibiotic use or recent hospitalization

2. Stool is watery to semi-formed and has a *foul odor* with no visible blood.

● = *non-urgent referral*

      3. Malaise, anorexia, and weight loss

      4. The person may not consider diarrhea a problem initially.

D. Diagnostic testing

      1. Stool for *C-diff toxins* (cytotoxin assay for *Clostridioides difficile*) and stool culture

          (a) If *C. difficile* positive without symptoms, may be a carrier; no treatment is necessary

          (b) Only liquid stool should be sent!

      2. NAAT for C-difficile toxin

      3. CBC, U/A, CMP (if elderly or diarrhea > 1 wk)

      4. Severity of illness dependent on

          (a) Mild to moderate disease: $WBC \leq 15{,}000/mL$, serum $CR < 1.5\,mg/dL$, serum albumin $> 3\,g/dL$

          (b) Severe disease: $WBC \geq 15{,}000/mL$, serum $CR \geq 1.5\,mg/dL$, serum albumin $\leq 3\,g/dL$

E. Generalized treatment with symptoms

      1. Stop offending antibiotic, which may cause diarrhea to cease in 2–3 days and may require no further treatment.

      2. Evaluate for dehydration and use oral rehydration solutions (see Table 9.2).

          (a) May need hospitalization if significant dehydration is present and the patient is unable to tolerate food or liquids

          (b) May need IV fluids initially

          (c) Follow-up with home health to monitor for dehydration.

      3. Avoid milk and milk products, alcohol, caffeine; start low-residue regular diet.

      4. Antimotility agents may prolong symptoms but if patient is becoming dehydrated from diarrhea, use cautiously for short periods of time.

      5. Strict cleaning of the house and personal items with hot water (120°F); good hand hygiene with soap and water (spores have resistance to alcohol-based hand sanitizers).

      6. Probiotics daily for duration of illness; studies are inconclusive of benefits but no harm has been associated with use.

      7. Discontinue PPIs.

      8. Prevention of initial or subsequent episodes for patient or family

          (a) Minimize use of antibiotics and stop if diarrhea occurs; early detection and testing if indicated.

          (b) Hand hygiene with soap and water and thorough cleaning of all surfaces used by patient; soap and water may be better than alcohol-based products (e.g., spores are resistant to alcohol); consider bleach mixture for cleaning surfaces.

          (c) When considering antibiotic use, choose ones that *infrequently* cause CDI and use for least amount of time.

             (i) Macrolides

             (ii) First-generation cephalosporins

             (iii) Tetracyclines

             (iv) Vancomycin or metronidazole

F. Pharmacological treatment (adults) for 10 days with mild-to-moderate symptoms (e.g., ≥ 3 loose stools/24 hr, positive C. diff toxins and no systemic symptoms)

      1. First episode with WBCs < 15,000 cells/mL, serum CR < 1.5 mg/dL

          (a) Vancomycin 125 mg qid *or*

          (b) Fidaxomicin (Dificid) 200 mg bid

          (c) Alternative: metronidazole 500 mg tid; avoid in very elderly/disabled if diarrhea caused from inflammatory bowel disease (see INFLAMMATORY BOWEL DISEASE in this chapter) and not antibiotics.

2. Recurrence within first 30 days after treatment in a stable patient
   (a) Start *pulsed/tapered* course of vancomycin (if used initially):
       125 mg qid for 7–14 days,   *then*
       125 mg bid for 7 days   *then*
       125 mg daily for 7 days   *then*
       125 mg every other day for 7 days   *then*
       125 mg q3days for 14 days
   (b) If fidaxomicin or metronidazole used initially, give vancomycin 125 mg qid for 10 days; if diarrhea recurs, start vancomycin pulsed/tapered dosing (see above).
3. Subsequent episodes after resolution of diarrhea in a stable patient:
   (a) Vancomycin pulsed therapy (see above)   *or*
   (b) Fidaxomicin for 10 days (see above)   *or*
   (c) Vancomycin 125 mg qid for *10 days* followed by Rifaximin 400 mg tid for *20 days*

IX. *Referral to gastroenterologist or infectious disease specialist if diarrhea persists.*

TABLE 9.4 ■ **Causes of Diarrhea**

Causes of Diarrhea	Transmission	Signs/Symptoms	Treatment*
*Campylobacter*** spp.	Undercooked and cross-contamination of poultry, meat; Unpasteurized milk (cows or goat) Animal contact with puppies, kittens, goats Onset 2–7 days Resolves in ~2–10 days	Frequent regular small volume watery diarrhea with blood and mucus but no foul odor Fever, vomiting Abdominal cramps with or without diarrhea Malaise, H/A Weight loss	Supportive care with oral rehydration solution (ORS)* No antimotility agents Antibiotics (adults) may shorten illness: Azithromycin 500 mg qd × 3 days Erythromycin 250–500 mg tid × 5 days Ciprofloxacin 750 mg bid × 3 days
Clostridium perfringens (food poisoning)	Contaminated, under-cooked or re-heated poultry or meats, home-canned foods, honey Onset symptoms: 6–24 hr Resolves within 1–2 days	Watery diarrhea with abdominal cramping with or without vomiting **Serious symptoms include blurred vision, diplopia, dysphagia, and descending muscle weakness** Can cause necrotic enteritis with bloody diarrhea, vomiting and severe abdominal pain	ORS* or IV fluids with mild symptoms No routine antibiotics Report to health department **Transfer to the ED if serious symptoms present**
Clostridioides difficile (formerly known as *C. difficile*) See Lower Abdominal Conditions, DIARRHEA, VIII			

Continued

■ *= not to be missed;* ● *= non-urgent referral;* ▲ *= urgent referral*

TABLE 9.4 ■ Causes of Diarrhea—cont'd

Causes of Diarrhea	Transmission	Signs/Symptoms	Treatment*
Cryptosporidium (protozoan)	Contact with infected animals or contaminated surface water; person-to-person transmission Onset 2–14 days after exposure Resolves ~5–10 days	Profuse watery diarrhea without blood Abdominal cramping, N/V, Anorexia, weakness, headache, myalgia Dehydration and weight loss	Supportive care with ORS* and rest Nitazoxanide 500 mg (adults) bid × 3 days Antimotility agents for 1–2 days: loperamide (Imodium) or diphenoxylate/atropine (Lomotil) Hand washing with soap and water
Enterotoxigenic *Escherichia coli* (E. coli)	Undercooked beef burgers and similar undercooked foods from restaurants Onset symptoms: 3–4 days	***Acute watery diarrhea followed by bloody diarrhea*** ***Abdominal tenderness*** ***Leukocytosis*** ***No fever*** Severe complication is hemolytic uremic syndrome and pseudomembranous colitis	Supportive care with ORS* and **transfer to the ED** *No antimotility agents* *No antibiotics*
Giardia lamblia (protozoan)	Drinking contaminated water or drinking out of streams or swimming pools, men who have sex with men Onset 7–14 days Resolves in ~5–7 days	Acute onset watery diarrhea that may progress to greasy, foul-smelling stools Abdominal cramps with bloating and flatulence	Supportive rehydration with ORS* Antibiotics: Tinidazole 2 g PO once *or* Nitazoxanide 500 mg bid 3 days (adults) *or* Metronidazole 500 mg bid 5–7 days
Listeria monocytogenes	Deli meats, unpasteurized milk, unwashed raw fruit/vegetables, store-made salads (i.e., chicken, seafood salads), raw or lightly cooked sprouts Seen in infants, elderly and pregnant women Onset in ~24 hr Resolves in ~2 days	Starts with watery diarrhea, fever, N/V, H/A, muscle and joint pain	Supportive care with rest, ORS* If *immunocompetent* and/or <65 yr of age: no antibiotics If *immunocompromised* and/or >65 yr of age: Amoxicillin 500 mg tid or 875 mg bid *or* TMP-SMX DS 1 tab bid Treat for 7 days

■ = *not to be missed;* ▲ = *urgent referral*

TABLE 9.4 ■ Causes of Diarrhea—cont'd

Causes of Diarrhea	Transmission	Signs/Symptoms	Treatment*
Norovirus (usually seen in adults and children) Rotavirus (usually seen in unvaccinated children)	Shellfish, vegetables, fruits, foods touched by infected workers Seen as outbreaks in restaurants, cruise ships, day care, NH and hospitals Onset 24–48 hr Resolves in ~3–5 days	*Abrupt vomiting* and watery diarrhea Low-grade fever Dehydration Myalgias, malaise H/A May have temporary lactose intolerance	Supportive care with ORS*, rest Probiotics Antiemetics if needed No antibiotics Consider zinc 20 mg daily for 14 days Handwashing with soap and water (virus is resistant to alcohol preparations) Antimotility agents (adults only) for 1–2 days: loperamide (Imodium) *or* diphenoxylate/atropine (Lomotil)
*Salmonella*** (non-typhoidal)	Animal/reptile contact, live poultry, and eggs; unpasteurized milk or juice, nut butters Onset 1–3 days Usually lasts 4–10 days	Diarrhea with occasional blood and mucus with foul odor nausea/vomiting at onset Fever, headache Abdominal cramps Weight loss	Supportive rehydration with ORS* No antibiotics unless severe disease/symptoms, then consider for 14 days for adults: Levofloxacin 500–750 mg qd *or* Ciprofloxacin 500 mg bid No antimotility agents Report to health department
*Shigella*** spp.	Ingestion of fecally contaminated water and food or raw vegetables Men who have sex with men Daycare centers Onset 1–3 days May resolve ~1 mo with or without treatment	Painful watery, visibly bloody and/or mucoid stools N/V, abdominal cramping, distention and increased bowel sounds Anorexia, fever	Supportive rehydration with ORS* Prevent malnutrition No antimotility agents Zinc 20 mg qd x 14 days Antibiotics for adults: Levofloxacin 500 mg qd x 3 days *or* Ciprofloxacin 500 mg bid x 3 days *or* Azithromycin 500 mg qd x 3 days *or* Cefixime 200 mg bid x 5 days Report to health department Follow up 1–2 days
Staphylococcus aureus enterotoxin	Improperly handled food and unclean food handlers Onset symptoms: 1–6 hr Resolves ~1–2 days	Starts with vomiting, abdominal pain and nausea, then intermittent water diarrhea without blood/mucus or foul odor, no fever	Supportive care with ORS*, rest No antibiotics No antimotility agents for 1–2 days; if needed loperamide (Imodium) *or* diphenoxylate/atropine (Lomotil)
Travelers diarrhea (see VII, this chapter)			

* See Table 9.2 for oral rehydration solutions.
** Leading cause of inflammatory diarrhea.

DIVERTICULITIS

I. Definition: inflammation and/or infection of a sac-like outpouching of the bowel wall (diverticulosis); microperforation is a possible complication of diverticulosis from trapped food. A small perforation is usually walled-off but may become an abscess and result in free perforation and peritonitis.
   A. Usually involves only one diverticulum
   B. This can progress to a life-threatening illness secondary to an abscess with perforation into the peritoneum, and fistula formation.
II. Signs and symptoms
   A. Recurrent, intermittent LLQ pain and tenderness with increased flatulence; changes in bowel habits (e.g., constipation or diarrhea) can occur.
   B. Acute LLQ pain
   C. Fever, chills, N/V/D (or constipation)
   D. Leukocytosis
   E. Mass in the LLQ can occasionally be palpated.
   F. Decreased bowel sounds
   G. DRE may reproduce pain in the LLQ; stool may be positive for occult blood
III. Diagnostic testing
   A. CBC (usually shows leukocytosis), urinalysis (should be normal)
   B. CMP for any electrolyte or liver enzyme abnormalities
   C. Amylase and lipase if uncertain of diagnosis
   D. If patient is female and of childbearing age, check for pregnancy.
   E. Abdominal U/S (may demonstrate colon wall thickness and fluid collection, which could be abscess formation).
   F. Abdominal CT (with oral and IV contrast) is the diagnostic test of choice (see Table 4.2).
IV. Treatment of nonsurgical/uncomplicated diverticulitis
   A. Bowel rest with clear liquid diet for 48 hr followed with a low-fiber diet and slowly progressing to regular diet over a period of about 10 days; increase fluid intake to maintain hydration.
   B. Avoid laxatives, enemas, and bulk additives such as psyllium in the *acute* phase.
   C. Antibiotic treatment for 7–10 days with Metronidazole 500 mg q8hr *plus*
      1. Ciprofloxacin 500 mg bid *or*
      2. Levofloxacin 750 mg daily *or*
      3. Bactrim DS 1 tab bid *or*
      4. Amoxicillin/clavulanate 875 mg q12hr
      5. If allergic to metronidazole, consider Moxifloxacin (as single agent) 400 mg daily.
   D. Follow up after resolution of diverticulitis with
      1. High-fiber diet (25–30 g/day) (see Appendix A)
      2. Stool softeners
      3. Consider decreased intake of nondigestible foods such as corn, popcorn, and nuts (debatable benefit at this time).
      4. Follow up in office
         (a) In 2–3 days after treatment started
         (b) Weekly until resolved
         (c) 6–8 wk after resolution of symptoms; consider colonoscopy if it has been > 1 yr
▲ V. *Transfer to ED if signs are consistent with perforation of the colon or increased risk factors, such as:*

▲ = *urgent referral*

    A. *High fever > 101 °F, elevated WBC, significant/difficult to control abdominal pain.*

    B. *Patient is > 65 yr of age and cannot care for self at home.*

    C. *Unable to keep fluids down.*

    D. *Immunocompromised or significant comorbidities (DM, HTN, CKD).*

    E. *Failure of office treatment.*

  VI. *Referral to gastroenterologist if symptoms recur; colonoscopy is usually performed 6–8 wk after complete resolution of symptoms.*

INFLAMMATORY BOWEL DISEASES

  I. Crohn disease (regional enteritis)

    A. Definition: chronic recurring immune response and inflammation that may involve *various unrelated segments* of the GI tract from the mouth to the anus

      1. Occurs at any age

      2. Associated with increased risk of GI cancer

    B. Signs and symptoms

      1. Intermittent diarrhea followed by constipation with recurrent episodes of mucoid diarrhea

      2. Colicky or steady abdominal pain located in the RLQ or periumbilical region

      3. Anorexia, flatulence, malaise, and weight loss

      4. Perianal disease with fistula, superficial ulcers, and skin tags

      5. Extraintestinal manifestations may occur in musculoskeletal and dermatologic sites about 10 yr after diagnosis.

    C. Diagnostic testing

      1. CBC (may show macrocytic anemia), ESR/CRP, and CMP (to monitor albumin), iron, ferritin, and vitamin B12.

      2. Stool for occult blood (may be positive), stool cultures, *C. difficile toxins and* O&P

      3. Abdominal CT (see Table 4.2)

      4. Endoscopy (i.e., EGD) and colonoscopy

    D. Treatment

      1. ***Referral to a gastroenterologist or surgeon for management of Crohn disease***

      2. Primary care management

        (a) Stop smoking, limit alcohol intake.

        (b) Stay up to date with immunizations (especially flu and pneumonia).

        (c) Encourage nonresidue diet with high protein, vitamins, and calories; avoid raw fruits and vegetables.

        (d) Patient should continue with annual colonoscopy and endoscopy.

  II. Ulcerative colitis

    A. Definition: inflammation that *involves the colon and rectum*

      1. Primarily in young adults

      2. Associated with increased risk for colon cancer

    B. Signs and symptoms (may wax and wane, and may occur after infectious gastroenteritis)

      1. Frequent episodes of bloody mucus and pus from the rectum

      2. Diarrhea can occur without warning

      3. Cramping abdominal pain is usually mild

      4. Anorexia, malaise, weight loss, and fatigue

      5. Rectal tenesmus

      6. Intolerance of dairy products periodically; consider avoiding during acute flares

---

■ = not to be missed; ● = non-urgent referral

C. Diagnostic testing
   1. CBC (may show microcytic anemia), CMP (may have low K+ and high BUN), ESR/CRP (usually elevated)
   2. Stool for occult blood (may be positive), stool cultures, culture for *C. difficile toxins*, O&P, fecal calprotectin (marker for inflammation)
   3. Abdominal/pelvic CT (see Table 4.2)
   4. Sigmoidoscopy, colonoscopy (if symptoms are not severe)
D. Treatment
   1. ***Referral to a gastroenterologist for management of Ulcerative colitis***
   2. Primary care management
      (a) Stop smoking
      (b) Avoid milk products during acute flare-ups; increase intake of calcium to 1200 mg daily and vitamin D to 800 units daily.

IRRITABLE BOWEL SYNDROME (IBS)

I. Definition: chronic functional GI disorder with altered bowel habits, with no physiologic reason
   A. Cause is unknown but IBS is commonly seen in women between age 20 and 39, with or without a PMH of abuse, depression, post-traumatic stress disorder (PTSD), anxiety, or past episode of infectious gastroenteritis.
   B. Rome IV Criteria for IBS (established at office visit)
      1. Recurrent abdominal pain at least 1 day per week for the previous 3 mo (with onset of symptoms at least 6 mo prior to diagnosis) associated with ≥ 2 signs and symptoms (see also II. below)
      2. Subgroups of IBS
         (a) Constipation (IBS-C): hard, lumpy, pellet-sized stool with mucus discharge; seen more often in women
         (b) Diarrhea (IBS-D): with loose or mushy stools preceded by cramping and urgency, symptoms do not occur at night; more common in men
         (c) Mixed symptoms (IBS-M) with alternating diarrhea and constipation; irregular stool consistency and form
II. Signs and symptoms
   A. Abdominal distention, increased flatulence, bloating with crampy lower abdominal pain
   B. Change in frequency and form of stools
   C. Pain
      1. Poorly localized and often comes and goes
      2. Associated with stool size and frequency
      3. Aggravated by eating and relieved with defecation
      4. Worsened with stressful events
      5. Rectal tenesmus and mucoid discharge
      6. Pain is *not* associated with menstruation, urination, or physical activity
III. Physical exam is usually negative, other than some mild discomfort generalized to abdomen; DRE is usually normal
IV. ***Not to be missed signs***
   A. ***Rectal bleeding and anemia***
   B. ***Men ≥ 50 yr of age***

■ = *not to be missed;* ● = *non-urgent referral*

       C. *FH of colon cancer*
       D. *Weight loss*
       E. *Nocturnal diarrhea; any change in recent bowel pattern*
       F. *Past antibiotic use*
  V. Diagnostic tests (used to rule out more severe illnesses)
       A. CBC, TSH, CMP, ESR, CRP
       B. Stool samples (if diarrhea started after traveling or recent hospitalization)
       C. Colonoscopy
 VI. Nonpharmacological treatment
       A. Exclusion diets that may decrease symptoms; encourage patient to keep a journal of what seems to cause symptoms (e.g., particular foods or situations).
          1. Decrease or stop consuming gas-producing foods
             (a) Beans, onions, celery, carrots
             (b) Prunes, bananas, raisins
             (c) Bagels
          2. Lactose-free diets (especially cow's milk) especially with IBS-D
          3. Diet low in fermentable oligosaccharides, disaccharides, monosaccharides, and polyols (FODMAP)
          4. Diet high in fiber, 25–30 g/day (see Appendix A), especially if IBS-C; supplemental psyllium products may also help
          5. *Referral to dietician*
       B. Lifestyle changes
          1. Increase physical activity to 30 min 5 times a week.
          2. Improve sleep and hours of sleep.
       C. Psychologic counseling to help manage stress and anxiety and to learn relaxation techniques
VII. Pharmacological treatment
       A. Constipation-predominant symptoms
          1. Ground linseeds 6–24 mg/day
          2. Probiotics daily (e.g., *B. infantis* [Align])
          3. Polyethylene glycol 3350 (Miralax) 1 capful dissolved in liquid daily
          4. Bisacodyl (Dulcolax) 1–2 tabs as needed (prn)
          5. For adults > 18 yr of age:
             (a) Plecanatide (Trulance) 3 mg daily   *or*
             (b) Lubiprostone (Amitiza) 8 mcg bid   *or*
             (c) Linaclotide (Linzess) 290 mcg daily
       B. Diarrhea-predominant symptoms
          1. Loperamide (Imodium) 2 mg 45 min prior to meals on regular schedule; maximum 16 mg/day. It can help diarrhea, but not the other symptoms *or*
          2. Eluxadoline (Viberzi) 75–100 mg bid; discontinue if constipation occurs; may be habit forming; caution with hepatitis or renal dysfunction *or*
          3. Bile acid sequestrant (Cholestyramine) 4–36 g daily prn (off label)
          4. Probiotics (*Bifidobacterium infantis*) daily
       C. Abdominal pain and cramping
          1. Dicyclomine (Bentyl) 10–40 mg qid prn before meals *or*

■ = *not to be missed*; ● = *non-urgent referral*

    2. Hyoscyamine (Levsin) 0.25 mg qid prn before meals (max dose 1.5 mg/day) *or*

    3. Peppermint oil caps after meals or prn

VIII. *Referral to gastroenterologist if symptoms continue or any not-to-be missed signs are present*

Liver Disease

JAUNDICE

  I. Definition: Yellow discoloration to skin and sclerae caused by increased bilirubin due to overproduction or inability to conjugate and remove bilirubin (see Chapter 4, LIVER TESTS, I, C).

 II. Conjugated (direct) serum bilirubin > 2 mg/dL often indicates liver disease. Reasons for abnormally elevated bilirubin include:

    A. Hepatocellular pathway (inflamed, infected, or damage to liver; excess conjugated bilirubin); usual finding: AST/ALT ratio > alkaline phosphatase (ALP)

        1. Hepatitis (acute or chronic)

        2. Cirrhosis, liver failure

        3. Drug/toxins (especially acetaminophen and some OTC herbs)

        4. Autoimmune disease

        5. Cancer

        6. Wilson disease and Rotor disease

    B. Post-hepatic pathway (obstructed or inflamed bile duct); usual findings: elevated ALP, ALP > AST/ALT ratio

        1. Gallstones, cholangitis, stricture bile duct

        2. Cancer (pancreas, gallbladder, bile duct)

        3. Pancreatitis

        4. Parasites

    C. Extrahepatic pathway (excess unconjugated bilirubin in blood which the liver cannot bind or excrete); usual finding: ALP > 5 times upper limit of normal (ULN).

        1. Hemolytic anemia, SCA, Thalassemia, G6PD deficiency

        2. Malaria, AIDS

        3. Obstruction of bile ducts, cancer or gall bladder disease

        4. Chronic pancreatitis

        5. Complication after invasive procedures

        6. Gilbert syndrome

        7. Crigler-Najjar syndrome

III. Psuedo-jaundice (carotenemia)

    A. Usually seen in infants and toddlers

    B. Caused by eating foods high in beta-carotene (e.g., eating yellow, orange, or green foods)

    C. Serum bilirubin is normal and no scleral icterus is noted

    D. Resolves spontaneously with decrease intake of green, orange, and yellow foods

IV. History of present illness

    A. Alcohol consumption over last 2 yr

        1. Men > 15 drinks a day

        2. Women > 10 drinks a day

● = *non-urgent referral*

   B. Any type of drug use
      1. Legal medications and amounts taken
         (a) Antibiotics, antiepileptics
         (b) NSAIDs or acetaminophen
         (c) Statins, chemotherapeutics
      2. Herbal supplements
         (a) Chaparral pill/tea, green tea extract
         (b) Ephedra, germander
         (c) Shark cartilage, ji bu huan
      3. Illegal drugs either orally or IV and how often used
   C. Blood transfusion and reason and last transfusion
   D. Type of employment
      1. Food handler
      2. Exposure to environmental toxic chemicals (e.g., mushrooms, vinyl chloride)
   E. History of right-side heart failure; DM, FH liver disease
   F. Any recent travel outside US or lower socioeconomic areas
   G. Military service, tattoos, unprotected sexual encounters
V. Signs and symptoms
   A. Related to hyperbiliruminemia
      1. Icterus to skin and sclerae; starts at head and goes down torso
      2. Pruritus (generalized itching without rash)
   B. Related to liver failure
      1. Abdominal pain and fluid wave/shift
      2. N/V, anorexia
      3. Weight gain in abdomen and wasting of extremities
      4. Swelling of legs, hypotension, confusion (late symptoms)
   C. Related to biliary obstruction
      1. Acute RUQ pain associated with food intake (see CHOLECYSTITIS, earlier in this chapter)
      2. Sweating and anxiety
      3. Change in stool color and character
   D. Related to liver infection (see HEPATITIS, later in this chapter)
      1. Malaise, myalgia, low-grade fever
      2. Anorexia, nausea
      3. Change in urine color
VI. Physical Examination
   A. Monitor vital signs for sepsis (decreased BP and increased HR).
   B. Observe for cachexia, muscle wasting, and overall color and appearance of person.
   C. EENT
      1. Check sclerae and tongue for color.
      2. Kayser-Fleischer rings in iris (usually seen with bilirubin 2–2.5 mg/dL)
      3. Breath odor for fetor hepaticus
      4. Increased jugular vein pressure
   D. Abdomen
      1. Ascites; test for fluid shift/wave
      2. Increased vascularity on abdomen
      3. Palpate for hepatomegaly, pain, tenderness, and masses
      4. Percuss spleen for size
      5. Check for hernias at umbilical and inguinal areas
      6. Check for GI bleeding, either gross or occult

    E. GU: evaluate men for testicular atrophy (e.g., alcoholic cirrhosis) and gynecomastia (e.g., liver disease)

    F. Neuro: check mental status and cognitive status, asterixis, and tremors

    G. Skin: look for palmar erythema, needle tracks, xanthomas (signs of primary biliary cirrhosis), decreased pubic and axillary hair, hyperpigmentation, ecchymosis, petechiae, and purpura

VII. Laboratory/radiologic testing

    A. CBC (looking at number of RBC, platelets and WBC) and peripheral smear (looking at size and shape of RBCs)

    B. CMP (see Chapter 4)

    C. Liver function tests (also see Chapter 4, LIVER TESTS)

        1. ALP (suggests biliary obstruction or alcohol intake)

        2. AST and ALT and AST/ALT ratio

        3. Total and direct bilirubin

    D. Hepatitis panel for hepatitis A, B, C (see Table 9.5)

    E. Gamma-glutamyl transferase (GGT) (liver marker often seen with alcohol abuse or drug reactions)

    F. LDH (high level indicates tissue damage and blood dyscrasias [not specific for liver])

    G. PT/INR (increase bleeding tendencies with liver damage)

    H. Amylase, lipase (elevations with pancreatitis)

    I. Consider acetaminophen level (to determine if an elevated level may be the cause of jaundice)

    J. Urinalysis (see Fig. 4.1); urine is usually brownish colored and frothy when shaken (froth lasts for > 2 min)

    K. U/S RUQ looking for gallstones or fatty liver (90% of all obese people have fatty liver)

    L. HIDA scan (if no stones found in bile ducts) to check gallbladder function

    M. MRI/CT abdomen for masses

VIII. *Referral to hepatologist, gastroenterologist, or hematologist depending on the cause of jaundice.*

    A. Consider repeating any lab values that are suspiciously high.

    B. Stop all known medications that effect the liver.

    C. Stop all alcohol, including oral preparations containing alcohol.

PRACTICE PEARLS FOR LIVER DISEASE

- If you have any concerns of validity, always recheck abnormal lab values before doing further testing.
- Possible diagnosis based on symptoms and liver function tests
  - Acute viral hepatitis in a young person with acute jaundice with viral syndrome and dark frothy urine.
  - Biliary obstruction due to cancer in an elderly patient with painless jaundice, weight loss, abdominal mass, and minimal pruritus.
- ALT is more specific for liver injury than AST.
  - Cholestasis if AST/ALT < 200 U/L and alkaline phosphatase (ALP) is > 3× normal.
  - Hepatocellular dysfunction if AST/ALT ratio > 500 U/L and ALP < 3× normal.
  - Ratio between AST/ALT ratio of < 1 indicates NAFLD; AST/ALT ratio > 2× normal, consider alcoholic liver disease.
  - ALT > AST indicates acute liver damage, chronic liver disease.

= *non-urgent referral*

- AST > 15× normal and ALT > 10,000 could indicate drug-induced acute hepatitis or ischemic hepatopathy.
- GGT > 2–3× normal consider NAFLD, chronic hepatitis C, or alcohol use.
- Cirrhosis indicated with AST > ALT
- Prothrombin is more sensitive than albumin for extrahepatic liver injury.
- Decreased albumin usually more suggestive of liver disease.
- Hepatic failure is significant if mental status is altered and coagulopathy present.
▲ - *If patient has acute hepatitis with elevated prothrombin or mental changes, emergent transfer to hospital.*
- Creatine kinase (CK) increased with muscle damage (e.g., heart or skeletal).
- ALP is found in bile ducts and bone.
  - If ALP and GGT are high, liver damage is more likely.
  - If ALP is high and GGT is normal, bone disease is more likely.

ALCOHOLIC LIVER DISEASE (ALD)

I. Description: Progressive liver damage due to long-term chronic alcohol intake; it occurs in 15%–20% of people who consume alcohol chronically.

II. ALD is the major cause of liver disease in Western countries and is associated with alcohol consumption of ~15 drinks/wk for men and ~10 drinks/wk for women over 2 yr period of time; alcohol consumed with meals *and* outside of mealtimes increases risk up to three times

III. COVID-19 related restrictions have increased/worsened alcohol consumption due to isolation, lack of rehabilitation facilities and have increased hospitalizations for ALD.

IV. Signs and symptoms depend on progress of disease; may be asymptomatic, but in later stages symptoms will worsen.
   A. Initially, symptoms are mild.
      1. Jaundice (see JAUNDICE, A–D)
      2. Weakness
      3. Peripheral edema
   B. Then progresses to alcoholic hepatitis or cirrhosis with
      1. Malnutrition and vitamins A, B, and E and thiamine deficiency
      2. Ascites
      3. Melena or hematochezia
   C. In final stages of cirrhosis/liver failure.
      1. Cognition changes, neurologic deterioration with loss of fine motor control, and gait changes.
      2. Marked hepatomegaly with firmness and nodularity; hepatic bruits.
      3. Weight loss (or gain with ascites), decreased albumin levels.

V. Diagnostic testing.
   A. Elevated AST < 500 international units/mL, ALT < 500 international units/mL; AST > ALT ratio > 2.0, elevated GGT, ALP, and bilirubin.
   B. CBC can indicate macrocytic anemia (MCV > 100 but < 109 unless associated with B12 deficiency); leukocytosis, thrombocytopenia
   C. Albumin (may be decreased), INR, and prothrombin time (may be elevated)
   D. B12 and folate levels (usually decreased)
   E. US RUQ and consider CT abdomen/pelvis if ascites suspected.

▲ = *urgent referral*

    F. EGD (esophageal varices); colonoscopy (colon cancer)

    G. CAGE screening questionnaire

VI. Treatment (see NAFLD in this chapter).

    A. ***Referral to hepatologist and co-management of non-liver issues.***

    B. Fibrosis is not reversible but prognosis can be improved with early intervention of alcohol abstinence, treatment for underlying viral illness, or reversal of metabolic syndrome.

    C. Improve nutrition; vitamin B supplementation (B6 and B12).

    D. Consider milk thistle 100 mg tid and vitamin E 400 international units/mL daily as hepatoprotective agent.

    E. Liver transplant if indicated

    F. Consider hospice for end-stage liver disease.

CIRRHOSIS

    I. Irreversible end-stage liver disease with fibrosis, usually caused by long-term alcoholism but can be caused by NASH, cancer, or viral infections.

   II. Hepatocellular fibrosis leads to diminished function and progresses to portal HTN, esophageal varices, and hepatic failure.

  III. Signs and symptoms

    A. Early symptoms

       1. Fatigue and weakness

       2. Anorexia, nausea, may have weight loss

       3. Dull right upper abdominal pain

       4. Liver enlargement

       5. Telangiectasia on face

       6. In men: impotence, gynecomastia, decreased testicle size

       7. In women: amenorrhea or menorrhagia

    B. Late symptoms

       1. Jaundice and itching

       2. Edema in legs and ascites in abdomen

       3. Venous hum over umbilicus (indicates portal HTN)

       4. Palmar erythema, easy bruising, and abnormal bleeding

       5. Pale or gray-colored stools

       6. Hepatic encephalopathy

       7. Asterixis (flapping tremor)

  IV. Diagnostic testing

    A. CBC with thrombocytopenia, macrocytic anemia, leukopenia

    B. AST/ALT > 1, low albumin, increased bilirubin

    C. Increased INR > 1.5, prolonged PTT

    D. ALP 2–3 times ULN, decreased sodium level, increased serum CR

   V. Treatment

    A. ***Referral to hepatologist***

    B. Liver transplant is only option

    C. Consider hospice care.

⬤ = *non-urgent referral*

HEPATITIS

I. Hepatitis A virus (HAV)
  A. Description
    1. Self-limiting viral illness with incubation period of about 28 days; contagiousness during incubation period and approximately 7 days after jaundice appears; complete resolution of symptoms ≤6 mo.
    2. Transmission route is fecal–oral from contaminated foods/water or person to person (e.g., food handlers or direct contact with stools).
  B. People at risk
    1. Children in day care and preschoolers
    2. Household contacts
    3. Travelers to underdeveloped countries or countries with high risk
    4. IV drug users; men who have sex with men (MSM); homeless populations
    5. People who work with primates
  C. Signs and symptoms
    1. Sudden-onset N/V, fever, malaise, loss of appetite, abdominal pain
    2. Within 1 wk, may see clay-colored stools; dark, tea-colored urine that is frothy if shaken.
    3. Later symptoms include jaundice, icteric color to sclerae, pale stools.
    4. Itching can last up to 2 wk; but earlier symptoms may resolve.
    5. Abdominal pain, liver tenderness, and enlargement with palpation
    6. Aversion to cigarette smoke (occasionally)
    7. Children <6 yr of age may not experience any symptoms.
  D. Diagnostic tests (see Table 9.5)
    1. Hepatitis panel (to screen for hepatitis A, B, C)
    2. AST, ALT (ALT > AST in acute period); serum bilirubin ≤ 10 mg/dL; ALP ≤ 400 U/L
    3. anti-HAV IgM and IgG
      (a) anti-HAV IgM: acute marker of infection, peaks in the first week (before symptoms) and declines within 6 mo of infection.
      (b) anti-HAV IgG (without anti-HAV IgM): marker of remote infection or vaccination; peaks after 1 mo; may persist for years and indicates immunity after infection.
  E. Treatment
    1. Clean surfaces with chlorine, iodine, or bleach 1:100 dilution.
    2. Supportive care with treatment for any of the symptoms
    3. Bed rest with no school or work during acute phase with fever or jaundice; complete recovery noted in ≤6 mo.
    4. Avoid drugs metabolized in the liver (e.g., acetaminophen, alcohol).
    5. Hydroxyzine 10–25 mg tid prn or prochlorperazine 5–10 mg tid prn for nausea or pruritis
    6. Encourage hepatitis A vaccination in all family members and close contacts; encourage patient to get hepatitis B vaccine when the their symptoms are resolved.
  F. Postexposure prophylaxis (PEP)
    1. Healthy persons
      (a) <12 mo of age vaccine not indicated but would receive IG 0.1 mL/kg
      (b) 12 mo to 40 yr of age should receive one dose of Hepatitis A vaccine as soon as possible (within 2 wk of exposure); vaccine is preferred over IG.
      (c) >41 yr of age should receive Hepatitis A vaccine *and* IG 0.1 mL/kg; if noted allergy to vaccine, use *only* IG 0.1 mL/kg.

2. Immunocompromised persons (including children) or with chronic liver disease should receive Hepatitis vaccine *and* IG (0.1 mL/kg).
3. PEP should be offered to all persons who have been exposed to hepatitis A unless they have had previous hepatitis A vaccine or have had hepatitis A in the past.
4. One dose of hepatitis A vaccine is sufficient for prophylaxis but does not provide long-term immunity. Completion of series is recommended.
5. Hepatitis A vaccine and IG can be given on same day but should not be given in same extremity.

G. Prophylaxis for international travel (see CDC's travel page at *https://cdc.gov/travel/yellowbookCh4-HepA.aspx*).

1. Dose of IG is based on possible length of exposure.
   (a) If less than or equal to 1 mo: give one dose of IG 0.1 mL/kg
   (b) If greater than 2 mo: give IG 0.2 mL/kg and repeat q2mo with continued exposure.
2. Older adults, immunocompromised people, people with chronic liver disease or other chronic illnesses and departing within 2 wk should receive both the hepatitis A vaccine and IG 0.1 mL/kg.

II. Hepatitis B virus (HBV)

A. Description

1. Viral illness that has both an acute state with resolution and a chronic state with exacerbations; greater risk for recurrence if patient is < 5 yr of age at time of infection or is immunocompromised; adults may recover without chronic infection.
2. May lead to cirrhosis, hepatic cancers, and progressive liver failure.
3. Transmission route is through blood, blood products, sexual contact, IV needles, perinatal contact, semen, and wound exudate.
4. Incubation period is 60–150 days and symptoms may last for 6 mo.
5. People at risk
   (a) All infants (usually at birth if mother is positive) and children < 19 yr of age (secondary to high-risk behaviors)
   (b) Sexually active adults with exposure to high risk sexual partners
   (c) Men who have sex with men (MSM); illegal IV drug users
   (d) Health care providers, anyone working with blood or blood products and staff working with handicapped or disabled people
   (e) Persons with chronic, immunocompromised illnesses who require daily or chronic medical care
   (f) Persons with chronic liver disease, hepatitis C, or HIV
   (g) Travelers to regions with high endemic rates of infection

B. Signs and symptoms

1. Acute hepatitis B and with exacerbations
   (a) Low-grade fever, profound fatigue, flu-like symptoms
   (b) N/V, anorexia
   (c) Clay colored stools; abdominal pain, RUQ pain
   (d) Dark, tea-colored urine that is frothy if shaken
   (e) Jaundiced and icteric color to sclerae; itching; macular rash
   (f) Liver tenderness, and hepatomegaly
2. Chronic hepatitis B (without exacerbation)
   (a) Spider angioma, palmar erythema
   (b) Gynecomastia, testicular atrophy
   (c) Fatigue
3. Chronic hepatitis B as liver disease progresses
   (a) Hepatic decompensation and encephalopathy

    (b) Somnolence, disturbances in sleep

    (c) Mental confusion, coma

    (d) Ascites, GI bleeding, and coagulopathy

    (e) Glomerulonephritis and kidney failure

  4. Children <5 yr of age may not experience any symptoms.

C. Diagnostic testing (see Table 9.5)

  1. Screening asymptomatic patient for HCV (if born between 1945 and 1965 or was in Vietnam War)

  2. Screening for symptomatic patient

    (a) Hepatitis panel (to detect any coinfection with hepatitis A or C)

    (b) HBsAg (positive with acute infection and indicates patient is infectious; resolves in ~6 mo; if present after 6 mo, considered chronic hepatitis B)

    (c) anti-HBs (appears with resolution of acute illness; indicates immunity and occurs after hepatitis immunizations)

    (d) IgM anti-HBc (positive with acute infection and can remain up to 2 yr and recur with exacerbations)

    (e) IgG anti-HBc (occurs with anti-HBs with resolution of illness; but it can persist into chronic period)

  3. Liver function testing (see Chapter 4, LIVER TESTS)

    (a) ALT > AST

    (b) GGT and ALP elevated but <3 times normal

    (c) Albumin (decreased)

    (d) Bilirubin (increased with acute infection)

    (e) PT/INR (decreased in early stages; may elevate as liver disease progresses).

  4. CBC (leukopenia, lymphocytosis, and thrombocytopenia)

  5. Urinalysis (bilirubin and protein may be present); urine is usually dark and frothy

  6. Screen for TB and HIV

D. Treatment

  1. ***Referral to a hepatologist or gastroenterologist to management and co-manage non-liver issues***

  2. Goals of treatment: reduce inflammation, prevent complications, and reduce further transmission.

  3. Immunize against HAV and give all other pertinent immunizations.

  4. Symptomatic treatment for N/V and malaise (avoid drugs metabolized in the liver)

    (a) Try B6, ginger, or peppermint for nausea.

    (b) Soft, bland diet and oral hydration solutions (see Table 9.2) to prevent dehydration.

  5. No acetaminophen or NSAIDs unless approved by specialist.

  6. Bed rest for as long as symptoms are present

  7. Encourage HBV vaccine for all close contacts.

E. Documentation for immunity.

  1. anti-HBs >10 milli-international units (mIU/mL) indicates protection after hepatitis immunization series of ≥3 doses.

  2. If anti-HBs is <10 mIU/mL after ≥6 doses, person is not protected: then write a letter stating what was done and that the person is not protected against hepatitis B and has a window of 10 days after exposure to get HBIG in order to stay protected.

F. Postexposure prophylaxis (PEP)

● = *non-urgent referral*

1. Determine status of source patient (HBsAg + HCV RNA unless already documented) and exposed person (HBsAg and anti-HBs status) and how many hepatitis B vaccine doses received; determine last tetanus immunization.
2. If exposed person has *completed* hepatitis B series and *anti-HBs* > *10* mIU/mL, no further treatment is indicated.
3. If source patient is negative and *exposed person has anti-HBs* < *10* mIU/mL, no further treatment; *recommend revaccination* if only three-dose series initially.
4. If source patient is positive or unknown and *exposed person has anti-HBs* < *10* mIU/mL *after six doses*, give HBIG 0.06 mL/kg now and in 1 mo with no postvaccination testing.
5. If source patient is positive or unknown and *exposed person has anti-HBs* < *10* mIU/mL *after three doses*, give HBIG 0.06 mL/kg once and repeat three-dose series again and postvaccination testing 2 mo after immunizations has been completed.

III. Hepatitis C virus (HCV)
  A. Description
  1. Viral infection with transmission through blood (primary) or mother to infant and men who have sex with men (MSM). Most acute infections are mild or asymptomatic and become chronic leading to cirrhosis, liver cancer, and liver failure. A small percentage of people will clear the virus.
  2. Incubation is 4–10 wk. Person may be asymptomatic initially and not develop symptoms for > 20 yr; anti-HCV can be detected in blood 2–3 wk after infection.
  3. There is no immunization for hepatitis C.
  4. Screening should be offered to all people 18–79 yr of age *once* with no high-risk behaviors; for people who engage in high-risk behaviors, consider *annual* testing if behaviors continue, such as
    (a) MSM; those coinfected with HIV/HBV
    (b) Those previously (or currently) incarcerated
    (c) Alcohol users or IV drug abusers; needle-stick injury from HCV positive person
    (d) Chronic hemodialysis patients
    (e) Children born to HCV-positive mothers
    (f) Individuals who have received blood or blood products prior to 1987 or solid organ transplants prior to 1992
  B. Signs and symptoms (symptoms similar to chronic hepatitis B)
  1. Fever, fatigue, weight loss, and weakness
  2. N/V, anorexia
  3. Myalgias and arthralgias
  4. Dark urine and clay-colored stool
  5. Jaundice
  C. Diagnostic testing (see Table 9.5)
  1. Hepatitis panel (to detect any coinfection with hepatitis A or B)
    (a) If HCV-positive on screen: order anti-HCV and HCV RNA qualitative and quantitative with reflex genotyping. This will determine the genotype for HCV (genotypes 1 and 4 require longer treatment periods and are associated with a higher incidence of liver damage) and the viral load.
    (b) Positive HCV RNA indicates positive acute infection.
    (c) anti-HCV + HCV RNA indicates chronic infection.
    (d) Negative HCV RNA indicates no infection.
    (e) If anti-HCV reactive and HCV RNA is not detected, there is no current HCV infection or has been cleared with treatment; *a screening anti-HCV will always be positive (reactive) if patient was infected.*

    2. Liver function tests with ALT > AST (see Chapter 4, LIVER TESTS) and CMP and CBC with platelets

    3. Urinalysis; urine hCG, if childbearing age

D. Treatment

    1. ***Referral to hepatologist or gastroenterologist specializing in treatment of hepatitis C and co-manage non-liver issues***

    2. If indicated, administer hepatitis A and B immunizations and do TB skin testing, (see Chapter 7, TUBERCULOSIS), if > 1 yr since last TST.

    3. Stay current with *all* other immunizations.

    4. Encourage stopping all alcohol intake and NSAID use.

    5. Can use acetaminophen up to 2 g/day (if not using any alcohol).

    6. Discourage sharing of any razors, dental care products, toothbrushes; cover any injuries that cause bleeding; *no* blood donations.

TABLE 9.5 ■ Interpretation of Hepatitis Serologic Test Results

Hepatitis A		
anti-HAV IgM	Positive	Acutely infected
anti-HAV IgG	Positive	Remote infection or immunization
Hepatitis B		
HBsAg anti-HBc anti-HBs	Negative Positive Positive	Immune due to natural infection
HBsAg anti-HBc anti-HBs	Negative Negative Positive	Immune due to hepatitis B vaccination
HBsAg anti-HBc IgM anti-HBc anti-HBs	Positive Positive Positive Negative	Acute-phase infection
HBsAg anti-HBc IgM anti-HBc anti-HBs	Positive Positive Negative Negative	Recovery/chronic-phase infection
IgG anti-HBc HBsAg	Positive Negative	IgG anti-HBc will be positive for life after infection Does not indicate current disease, may have history of infection with treatment
Hepatitis C		
anti-HCV	Negative	No infection
anti-HCV HCV RNA	Negative Positive	Acute hepatitis C
anti-HCV HCV RNA	Positive Negative	Anti-HCV will be positive for life if any past infection Negative HCV RNA indicates infection resolved
anti-HCV HCV RNA	Positive Positive	Acute or chronic infection

anti-HBc, antibody to hepatitis B core antigen; *anti-HBs*, antibody to hepatitis B surface antigen; *HAV*, hepatitis A virus; *HBsAg,* hepatitis B surface antigen; *HBV*, hepatitis B virus; *HCV*, hepatitis C virus.

● = *non-urgent referral*

NONALCOHOLIC FATTY LIVER DISEASE (NAFLD)

I. Asymptomatic liver disease with hepatic steatosis can occur without alcohol use or other liver diseases (chronic or acute); may progress to cirrhosis.
   A. Umbrella term for
      1. NAFL (nonalcoholic fatty liver) without inflammation
      2. NASH (nonalcoholic steatohepatitis) with inflammation and apoptosis
   B. NASH can lead to cirrhosis and liver failure more often than NAFL.
II. Commonly associated with metabolic syndrome (see Chapter 8, METABOLIC SYNDROME), and with DM, HTN, and obesity
III. Early signs and symptoms
   A. Malaise, weakness
   B. N/V, anorexia
   C. Dull right upper abdominal pain
   D. Jaundice (late sign)
IV. Diagnostic testing
   A. Hepatitis panel
   B. Elevated AST and ALT > 2–5 times ULN; AST/ALT ratio < 1; albumin and bilirubin normal; ALP 2–3 times ULN; elevated GGT
   C. CMP, CBC with platelets
   D. Elevated ESR, PT/INR (normal initially with elevation/prolongation in later stages)
   E. U/S RUQ
   F. NAFLD fibrosis score calculator for staging fibrosis associated with NASH (*www.nafldscore.com; QxMD; MDCalc*)
V. Treatment
   A. If alcohol is involved, stop drinking.
   B. Hepatitis A and B immunizations; maintain current immunizations.
   C. Treat underlying medical problems.
      1. Increase daily exercise (up to 150 min/wk).
      2. Diet recommendations
         (a) Reduce fatty foods, trans fats in foods, and high fructose corn syrup
         (b) The Mediterranean diet may be beneficial.
         (c) Use olive oil for cooking, salad, etc.
      3. Consider fenofibrates for elevated triglycerides (see Table 8.9).
      4. Control of DM (see Chapter 15, **Diabetes Mellitus**).
   D. Consider adding omega-3 FAs up to 3–4 g daily (associated with some improvement in fatty liver).
   E. Consider silymarin (milk thistle) 100 mg tid and vitamin E 400 international unit/mL daily as hepatoprotective agents; *may* decrease fibrosis.
   F. Consider bariatric surgery for weight loss if indicated.
⬤ VI. *Referral to*
   A. *Hepatologist or gastroenterologist who specializes in liver diseases*
   B. *Dietitian for weight control*
   C. *Consider cardiology to manage any HTN or CAD*
   D. *Consider endocrinology to manage DM*

⬤ = *non-urgent referral*

CHAPTER 10

Gynecologic Conditions

For detailed history and physical examination, see Chapter 1, GENITOURINARY (FEMALE).

Screenings and Pap Smears

SCREENING GUIDELINES FOR WOMEN'S SERVICES (SEE TABLE 10.1)

Interpretation and Management of Pap Smears

  I. If first Pap smear and human papillomavirus (HPV) are *negative*, follow guidelines (see Table 10.1).
 II. If Pap results are *unsatisfactory for any reason*: repeat test in 3 mo and include HPV testing.
   A. Insufficient cells
   B. Obstruction with lubricant or solution particles
   C. Blood in specimen
III. If first Pap smear *positive for low-grade squamous intraepithelial lesion (LSIL), atypical glandular cell (AGC), high-grade squamous intraepithelial lesion (HSIL), or other abnormality regardless of HPV status*, recommend colposcopy.
   A. If repeat Pap smear and HPV continue to be *negative*, repeat in 3–5 yr (based on lifestyle).
   B. If repeat Pap smear *continues to be positive for atypical squamous cells of undetermined significance (ASC-US) and HPV*, recommend colposcopy and annual follow-up with either Pap smear or colposcopy.
   C. If repeat Pap smear continues to be *ASC-US with negative HPV*, recommend annual Pap until ASC-US resolved and then return to q3–5yr Pap screening (repeat ASC-US findings are probably due to inflammation or infection and can be repeated in 3 mo, if needed).

Contraception

CONTRACEPTIVE METHODS

  I. Before prescribing any contraception
   A. Perform initial H&P, which *may* include Pap smear, pregnancy, and sexually transmitted infection (STI) testing; follow-up visit H&P may be based on lifestyle and history.
   B. Discuss with the patient and/or partner/family the following points to ensure the appropriate types of contraception and family planning.
     1. Different types of contraception and/or delivery systems (e.g., pills, patch, insertable or implant)
     2. Length of time they will need protection. Are they wanting reversible or nonreversible contraception?
     3. Intent on starting a family and the time-frame for conception
     4. Any PMH or FH of medical or genetic conditions that might affect choice of contraception

TABLE 10.1 ■ **Screening Guidelines for Healthy Women: Pap Smear, Mammography, and Bone Mineral Density (BMD)**

USPSTF	ACOG
No Pap screen • Age < 21 yr • Age > 65 yr with no increased risk (last two Paps negative within 5–10 yr) • Hysterectomy for noncancerous reasons	No Pap screen • < 21 yr of age • Age > 65 yr of age and if past three screens were negative within 10 yr • Hysterectomy for noncancerous reasons
Pap screen at 21–29 yr of age: q3yr or Pap screen with HPV at ≥ 30 yr of age: q5yr	Pap screen at 21–29 yr of age: q3yr or Pap screen and HPV test starting at 25 yr of age: q5yr *and consider* GC/chlamydia screen at any age with high risk behaviors
Mammography q2yr between 40 and 49 yr of age on *individual basis* at appropriate interval	Mammography q2yr between 40 and 49 yr of age on individual basis
Mammography q2yr between ages 50 and 75; after 75 yr of age, individualize screening	Mammography q2yr between ages 50 and 69; after 70 yr of age, individualize screening
BMD screen if age ≥ 65 yr of age: q2yr	BMD screen at age ≥ 65 yr: q2yr
BMD screen in younger women if fracture risk is equal to or greater than that of a 65 yr of age woman or if high risk (history of fracture and/or one or more risk factors*)	BMD screen women < 65 yr of age: q2yr if high risk for fractures*

*See Chapter 13, OSTEOPOROSIS, **III**.

    C. Consider reviewing or downloading CDC's app for contraceptive selection in all populations and choosing contraception for women with medical conditions: US Medical Eligibility Criteria for Contraceptive Use, 2016 (US MEC) and US Selected Practice Recommendation for Contraceptive Use, 2016 (US SPR).

    D. See Table 10.2 for contraception options for selected medical conditions.

    E. *Document* discussion of pros and cons of contraception and any side effects for contraception. It is important that everyone is in agreement initially with the plan.

▲   **II.** *Urgent referral to ED for any woman, who after starting COCs presents with*

    A. *Severe chest pain*

    B. *Severe H/A or paresthesia*

    C. *Change in vision*

    D. *Pain or swelling in legs, SOB and/or tachycardia*

    E. *Severe abdominal pain*

  III. Barrier methods: diaphragms, cervical caps, sponges.

    A. Advantages

      1. Easy to use and accessible; some benefit in reducing the risk of STIs

      2. 85%–95% effective in preventing pregnancy, especially if spermicide is used

    B. Disadvantages

      1. Pelvic "heaviness" if left in too long; decreases spontaneity of intercourse

      2. May cause vaginal discharge from irritation, spermicide, or latex allergy; may increase vaginal infections

Text continued on page 4

▲ = *urgent referral;* ■ = *not to be missed*

TABLE 10.2 ■ Common Contraception for Selected Conditions*

Conditions or Side Effects	Alternatives
Acne, hair growth, PCOS	OCs with EE 20–30 mcg and lower androgenic activity (desogestrel, drospirenone, norgestimate): Ortho Tri-Cyclen, Yas, Beyaz, Apri-28, Cyclessa
Amenorrhea	Determine cause and correct; may need to change the type of estrogen or progestin
Bariatric surgery	IUDs, patch (if patient's weight < 90 kg), implants or vaginal ring; avoid oral contraceptives unless banding or sleeve procedure was performed, then any type contraceptive can be used
Breakthrough bleeding: • During the first 14 days of the cycle • During the last 14 days of the cycle (before taking inert pills)	OCs with higher endometrial activity: Mircette, Loestrin, Ovcon-35, Ortho-Cyclen, Ortho Tri-Cyclen OCs with higher progestin and/or androgenic activity: Lo-ovral, Levlen, Ortho-Novum-35, Estrostep, Ortho-Cyclen
Breast tenderness	OCs with lower estrogen dose or higher androgenic activity: Loestrin 1.5/30 or 1/20, Levlen, Levora 0.15/30
Controlled DM *without* vascular complication	OCs with lower estrogenic and androgenic activity: Demulen-35, Alesse, Micronor; or use copper IUD
Controlled DM *with* vascular complications	Copper IUD, oral progestins, Depo-Provera, implants, avoid estrogen containing products
Depression	OCs with lower progestin activity: Ortho-Tri-Cyclen, Yasmin, Ovcon-35 Avoid long-acting progestins—may exacerbate depression
Dyslipidemia	OCs with levonorgestrel or, ↓ dose norethindrone: Ortho-Cyclen, Ovcon-35, Desogen Avoid long-acting progestins
Dysmenorrhea	OCs with higher progestational activity: Loestrin 1/10, 1.5/30 or 1/20; Demulen 1/35
Fluid retention	OCs with lower estrogenic activity or estrogen doses: Loestrin 1/20 or 1.5/30
H/A, nausea	OCs with lower estrogenic effects or estrogen doses: Alesse, Mircette, Loestrin Take pill at night to decrease nausea
HTN (controlled)	IUDs or Micronor; No COC[†]
Libido (decreased)	OCs with increased androgenic activity: Alesse, Levlen, Loestrin 1.5/30
Menstrual migraine	If H/A during the last 7 days of pack, consider adding low-dose estrogen on 5/7 of those days. Avoid triphasic OCs
Migraine *with* aura	Copper IUD; Progestin implants/IUD or Micronor; No COC[†]
Migraine *without* aura	<35 yr of age: copper IUD or POPs; if no worsening of H/A can try OCs with lower estrogenic activity or lower estrogen doses: Loestrin 1/10 or Loestrin 1/20, Micronor, Mircette, Sea sonale/Seasonique ≥35 yr of age: copper IUD or POPs, avoid estrogen-containing products Patches may work better for menopausal women; no contraceptive benefits
Postpartum	Non-breastfeeding: avoid estrogen containing products for 42 days, then no restrictions. Breastfeeding: IUDs, POPs

Continued

TABLE 10.2 COMMON **Contraception for Selected Conditions—cont'd**

Conditions or Side Effects	Alternatives
Seizure disorder	Depo-provera and IUDs Avoid oral estrogen and progestins, consider barrier method
Skin rash or pruritus	Usually occurs from inactive ingredients; switch to pills with different inactive ingredients
Smokers <35 yr of age	Consider using pills with ↑ progestin activity such as norethindrone acetate Encourage smoking cessation
Smokers ≥35 yr of age	POPs, IUD, or implants; No COC[†]
Weight gain	OCs with lower estrogenic and androgenic activity: Ortho Novum 1/35, Ovcon-35, Yasmin, YAZ

*OCs are listed by brand names and *it is not an all-inclusive* list.
[†]Combined oral contraceptive (i.e., containing both estrogen and progestin).

3. OTC products such as cervical cap (FemCap) and sponge (Today Sponge) should be used with spermicide to decrease risk of pregnancy but must be used correctly.
4. Diaphragm must be fitted before use, and again if there is any change in body habitus.

IV. Condoms (male and female)
   A. Advantages
      1. Inexpensive and reduce the risk of STIs
      2. 85% effective in preventing pregnancy if used correctly; using spermicide will increase effectiveness.
   B. Disadvantages
      1. May cause skin irritation from latex allergy.
      2. May interrupt foreplay and may rupture during intercourse.
      3. Must be used correctly to prevent semen from escaping into the vagina.

V. Implant (Etonogestrel [Nexplanon]) is long-term contraception method appropriate for women who want reversible contraception and have difficulty remembering to take pills daily.
   A. Advantages
      1. Inserted for 3 yr into the upper inner arm; can be removed and replaced without waiting.
      2. May cause decreased menstrual cycles and decreased blood flow.
      3. If BTB and AUB occur, try NSAIDs (e.g., mefenamic acid 250 mg tid) routinely for 5–7 days or start monophasic low-dose COC, unless estrogen is contraindicated, for 10–20 days for 1–3 mo.
   B. Disadvantages
      1. Does not provide protection from STIs; must be inserted in office setting.
      2. May have decreased efficacy in women with BMI > 30 kg/m$^{2.}$
      3. May cause increased acne or hair growth.
      4. If inserted > 5 days after menses, use back-up contraception or abstain from sexual intercourse for 7 days.
   C. Contraindications
      1. Breast cancer, liver disease, DVT/VTE
      2. Irregular heavy vaginal bleeding

VI. Injectable medroxyprogesterone (Depo-Provera Cl or Depo-subq Provera 104)
   A. Advantages
   1. Requires 1 injection q12wk
   2. Decreases anemia and menstrual pain and bleeding
   3. Can be used with a history of DVT, PE, smoking, CV disease, DM, migraine, seizures
   4. Initial injection should be given
      (a) Within the first 5 days of menstrual cycle   *or*
      (b) Within 5 days postpartum if not breastfeeding   *or*
      (c) Sixth postpartum week if breastfeeding
   5. If > 13 wk since last injection, perform pregnancy test before giving the next injection; use back-up contraception for 7 days.
   6. If BTB or AUB occurs, try NSAIDs (e.g., mefenamic acid 250 mg tid) routinely for 5–7 days.
   B. Disadvantages
   1. Must go to the clinic for injection
   2. *Weight gain* (most common), H/A, depression, irregular bleeding
   3. Bone loss greatest in first 2 yr of use and minimal after that; recovery of BMD occurs rapidly after stopping medication; encourage daily calcium supplementation.
   4. No protection against STIs
   C. Contraindications
   1. Obesity
   2. Suspected pregnancy or abnormal bleeding
   3. Depression
VII. Intrauterine devices (IUDs)
   A. Long-term, reversible method of contraception
   1. Indicated for women who want reversible contraception and/or have difficulty remembering to take pills. Must be inserted in office setting, but no waiting between changes.
   2. Can be used in teens, nulliparous and parous women and at > 6 wk postpartum.
   3. Decreases pelvic pain with endometriosis
   4. Decreases the rate of ectopic pregnancy and can be used as *emergency contraception if contains LNG 52 mg* (see C. below)
   5. Decreases the risk of cervical cancer
   6. Does not protect against STIs, could increase risk of pelvic inflammatory disease (PID)
   7. Breakthrough bleeding (BTB) or abnormal uterine bleeding (AUB) may occur up to 3 mo after insertion; to help control bleeding during this time
      (a) NSAIDs (e.g., ibuprofen, naproxen) 2–3 times daily for 5–7 days
      (b) Tranexamic acid 650 mg tid until bleeding stops (usually 4 days)
   8. If concern regarding switching from one form of contraception to IUD, insert during first 7 days of menses and no back-up birth control needed; *if not* inserted during first 7 days of menses, consider 7 days of back-up contraception or abstaining from intercourse.
   B. Copper-T (nonhormonal) IUD
   1. Inserted for up to 10 yr and no additional back-up required
   2. *Can be used for emergency contraception.*
   3. May increase menstrual bleeding, especially if hx of irregularity; to treat BTB
      (a) Ibuprofen 400 mg tid for 5–7 days
      (b) Tranexamic acid 650 mg tid until bleeding stops
      (c) Mefenamic acid 500 mg tid for 3 days
   4. Reduces risk of cervical cancer

    C. Levonorgestrel-releasing (LNG) IUD
        1. Levonorgestrel 13.5 mg (Skyla); inserted for 3 yr
        2. Levonorgestrel 52 mg (Mirena, Liletta); inserted for 6 yr
        3. Levonorgestrel 52 mg (Kyleena); inserted for 5 yr

VIII. Oral contraceptives (see Table 10.2)

    A. Combined OCs (COCs)
        1. Ethinyl estradiol (EE) is the most common estrogen component and may range from 10 to 35 mcg
            (a) Taking ASA 81 mg daily with COCs may decrease risk of blood clots for all users, but this has not been proven.
            (b) Encourage all women to stop smoking when taking COCs.
        2. Progestin may consist of various types: norethindrone, desogestrel, levonorgestrel, Drospirenone.
            (a) Levonorgestrel + low-dose EE (e.g., 10–20 mcg) has the lowest risk of PE and other arterial thrombosis.
            (b) Drospirenone (and any EE) has the highest risk of PE/DVT/CVA.
        3. Advantages
            (a) Relieves PMS symptoms, decreases menstrual cramping and bleeding, can improve acne, decreases androgen effects (e.g., hirsutism), can increase high-density lipoproteins (HDLs); some pills contain iron supplement to prevent anemia.
            (b) Decreases the risk of breast, uterine, cervical, ovarian and colon cancers and PID.
            (c) May decrease new ovarian cyst formation (high dose estrogen pills) but no effect on current ovarian cysts.
            (d) Can be used to decrease the number of cycles per year depending on the pill pack (e.g., monthly, quarterly, or longer).
            (e) Encourage taking a pill daily to establish routine, even though there may be "dummy" pills at the end of the pill pack.
        4. Disadvantages
            (a) *Should be taken at the same time every day*; long intervals between pills and missing pills increases the chance for pregnancy and BTB, and a back-up method must be used for the remainder of the cycle.
            (b) If started more than 5 days after menses, use back-up contraception for the rest of cycle.
            (c) Missing > 1 pill may cause BTB.
            (d) No protection against STIs; if high risk, consider condoms along with COCs.
            (e) Effectiveness can be decreased with some medications (e.g., antibiotics).
            (f) Estrogen increases the risk of VTE, CVA, and MI.
            (g) The new lower-dose estrogen pills may decrease systemic symptoms of bloating, breast tenderness and nausea, but may increase BTB.
        5. If BTB occurs
            (a) Woman is < 35 yr of age and smokes: try pills with increased progestin or switch to pill with norethindrone.
            (b) Woman is > 35 yr of age and smokes: try POPs, IUD, or implants.
        6. Contraindications
            (a) PE/DVT, HTN
            (b) Migraine with aura
            (c) Breast or cervical cancer

        (d) Smoking after 35 yr of age

        (e) Liver or heart disease, DM

   B. Progestin only pills (POPs)

     1. Advantages

        (a) Norethindrone and norgestrel are common formulations; taken daily with no "dummy pills."

        (b) Can be used during lactation and by women with contraindication to estrogen (e.g., ≥ 35 yr of age who smoke, or have migraines with aura).

        (c) May decrease menstrual cycles and premenstrual syndrome (PMS).

        (d) Decreases the risk of endometrial cancer.

        (e) Fertility is reestablished quickly after stopping pill.

        (f) Initiate on the first day of the menstrual cycle or within the first 5 days of the cycle; using back-up protection is not indicated unless POPs are started at other times during the menstrual cycle, then use back-up contraception or abstain from sexual intercourse or 2 days.

     2. Disadvantages

        (a) No protection against STIs.

        (b) *Must take at the same time every day*; increasing time intervals or missing daily pills decreases effectiveness and increases the risk of pregnancy.

        (c) Unscheduled bleeding episodes may occur and may resolve after 3 mo.

     3. Contraindications

        (a) Breast, uterine, or cervical cancer

        (b) Liver disease, stroke, VTE/DVT

        (c) Irregular or heavy menstrual cycles

IX. NuvaRing (etonogestrel/EE)

   A. Advantages

     1. Patient inserts vaginal ring for 3 wk then removed for 7 days for withdrawal bleeding *or* new ring can be inserted q3wk continuously for 12 mo (this can cause ↑ BTB).

     2. If used correctly, it is 99% effective against pregnancy.

     3. Can be used when BTB occurs on OCs due to more constant hormone levels and no need to remember to take a pill every day; can be used for 3 mo then switch back to oral COC or other forms of contraception.

     4. Can restart > 3 wk postpartum, or > 6 wk postpartum if breastfeeding.

     5. If LMP has been > 7 days or is unknown, use back-up contraception for the first 7 days of ring use.

   B. Disadvantages

     1. May accidently be expelled, and some patients can feel "object in vagina" during intercourse.

     2. May have episodes of vaginitis and leukorrhea.

     3. No protection against STIs

   C. Contraindications: *same as COCs* (see **VIII**, A, above)

X. Annovera (segesterone/EE) ring

   A. Advantages

     1. Reusable ring for up to 12 mo

     2. Inserted for 3 wk then removed for 7 days for withdrawal bleeding. No data for continual use. When removed, wash ring with soap and water and dry.

   B. Disadvantages

     1. Cost

     2. Must keep record of when ring was initially started

     3. Same disadvantages as other combined contraceptives

XI. Patch apply 1 wkly for 3 wk, then off for 7 days
   A. Norgestromin/EE (Xulane or Zafemy)
   B. Levonorgestrel/EE (Twirla)
   C. Advantages
     1. Started within first 24 hr of menstrual cycle; easy to apply and has good adherence.
     2. If used correctly, 99% effectiveness.
     3. When prescribing, add extra patch in case one patch comes off.
     4. Can restart > 4 wk postpartum or > 6 wk postpartum if breastfeeding.
   D. Disadvantages
     1. Caution effectiveness if BMI > 30 kg/m^2 or > 198 pounds.
     2. Patch may irritate the skin and/or may come off unexpectedly.
     3. No protection against STIs
   E. Contraindications: same as COCs (see **VIII**, A, above)
XII. Emergency Contraception (EC) (see Table 10.3)
   A. Back-up protection recommendations
     1. Missed pills (COCs)
       (a) If ≥2 pills are missed *in a row*, take one as soon as remembered, throw out the other pills that were missed, and continue the pill pack. Use back-up birth control for the next 7 days.

TABLE 10.3 ■ Emergency Contraception

Yuzpe Formulation	Brand Name	Dosing (Should Begin Within 72 hr of Unprotected Intercourse)
Levonorgestrel 0.15 mg + ethinyl estradiol 30 mcg	Nordette	4 light-orange pills; repeat in 12 hr
Levonorgestrel 0.1 mg + ethinyl estradiol 20 mcg	Alesse, Aviane	5 orange pills; repeat in 12 hr
Levonorgestrel 0.15 mg + ethinyl estradiol 30 mcg	Seasonique Seasonale	4 light blue-green pills; repeat in 12 hr 4 pink pills; repeat in 12 hr
Levonorgestrel 0.1 mg + ethinyl estradiol 20 mcg	LoSeasonique	5 orange pills; repeat in 12 hr
Levonorgestrel 0.09 mg + ethinyl estradiol 20 mcg	Lybrel	6 yellow pills; repeat in 12 hr
Levonorgestrel 0.15 mg/estradiol 30 mcg	Levora	4 white pills; repeat in 12 hr
Oral Levonorgestrel		
Levonorgestrel 1.5 mg	Plan B (OTC)	1 pill within 72 hr of unprotected intercourse
Progestin receptor modulator		
Ulipristal 30 mg	Ella	1 pill within 120 hr of unprotected intercourse
IUDs		
Copper IUD	Copper IUD	Inserted within 120 hr of unprotected intercourse
Levonorgestrel IUD	Mirena, Liletta, Kyleena	Inserted within 120 hr within 120 hr of unprotected intercourse

      (b) If > 2 pills are missed *in the past 2 wk of the pill pack*, take 1 pill daily until the active pills are finished and then immediately start a new pill pack. No back-up is needed after new pill pack is started.

      (c) If ≥ 3 pills are missed, menses will probably start; continue taking 1 pill daily until the active pills are finished and then start a new pack; use a back-up method for 7 days of the new pack.

  2. If ≥ 1 POP is missed, take it immediately even if it means taking 2 on the same day. Use back-up method of contraception until pills have been taken consistently for at least 2 days. Consider emergency contraception (EC) with unprotected sex.

  3. If > 15 wk from last depo-provera injection, check for pregnancy; if negative, give injection and use back-up method of contraception for the next 7 days.

  4. Use a back-up method of birth control when taking antibiotics (this may not cause decreased efficacy of pill, but if any pills are accidentally missed during illness, then the antibiotic will be blamed for the pregnancy).

  5. COCs need to be taken for at least 7 consecutive days to prevent ovulation; always consider EC with missed pills.

  6. Missing one menstrual cycle while taking OCs is no reason for concern; if two cycles are missed, perform a pregnancy test.

  7. Consider EC if ≥ 2 pills are missed in the first 2 wk of the cycle and the woman had unprotected sex in the 5 days before missing the pills.

B. Formulations for Emergency Contraception (Table 10.3)

  1. Contraceptive method that can be used for prevention of unwanted pregnancy after unprotected sexual intercourse.

  2. Intended for occasional use and back-up use, *not primary contraception.*

  3. ALWAYS perform urine hCG before starting EC; consider pretreatment with anti-emetic 1 hr before dose(s); some types of EC may not be as effective with BMI > 30 kg/m².

  4. Plan B and Yuzpe regimen prevent pregnancy by inhibiting ovulation, not by disrupting the pregnancy; Ulipristal (Ella) and IUDs could affect an established pregnancy (*this is controversial*).

  5. Commercially available emergency contraceptive pills (ECPs) (see Table 10.3)

  6. Yuzpe regimen (see Table 10.3) uses commonly packaged COCs; it is more accessible and provides more privacy to women.

      (a) For effectiveness, *one dose* should equal ethinyl estradiol 100 mcg and levonorgestrel 0.5 mg.

      (b) Take 2 doses, 12 h apart.

      (c) Side effects are nausea and vomiting.

  7. Copper IUD and levonorgestrel IUD (LNG 52) can be used for EC but must be inserted within 5 days; effective with obese women (BMI > 30 kg/m²); can be left in for 5–10 yr based on type inserted.

C. Use barrier method for 14 days or until next period, then resume regular form of contraception.

D. Regular menses may occur earlier after taking EC but if *no* menses in 3 wk, check urine hCG test; *if no menses for 2 mo, refer to gynecologist and order pelvic U/S.*

● = *non-urgent referral*

Menstrual Disorders

PRACTICE PEARLS FOR HORMONE USE

- Elevated FSH and decreased estradiol levels indicate need for estrogen replacement.
- Menopausal hormone replacement therapy.
  - Is *not indicated* for prevention of CV disease; it may worsen lipid profile, and it will not delay dementia.
  - May cause breast cancer (especially if patient is BRCA+); increases risk for DVT/PE, gallbladder disease, and CVA.
  - *Is contraindicated with unexplained vaginal bleeding, liver disease, DVT/PE, cardiac disease or recent MI, concern with varicose veins and past CVA/TIA.*
- Estrogen equivalents: 1 mg 17-β estradiol = 0.625 mg conjugated estrogen = 0.05 mg transdermal patch.
- *Giving estrogen alone (if woman has a uterus) can cause endometrial proliferation and lead to uterine cancer.*
- When using estrogen replacement in menopausal woman (with uterus), add progesterone pills (e.g., MPA, norethindrone or micronized progesterone) to reduce risk of uterine cancer. The progesterone can be taken for 12 days every 1–3 mo, but there is less chance of BTB with daily low-dose progesterone.
- If weaning off estrogen, DO NOT start weaning in the summer months (more likely to have hot flashes anyway). Weaning may take up to 6–12 mo.
- Vaginal estrogen products for dryness have very little systemic effects. Consult with oncologist if considering this option when woman has had breast cancer.
- Decreased libido may be due to vaginal dryness causing pain with intercourse, treat this first with lubricants prior to intercourse *or* routine use of vaginal moisturizers 2–3 times a week. May still need lubricant prior to intercourse.
- Too high a dose of progestins may cause moodiness, irritability, breast pain, and spotting.
- Too high a dose of estrogen may cause breast pain, bloating, missed menstrual cycles, and wheezing.
- Progesterone IUD (LNG 52) can be used for irregular bleeding, dysmenorrhea, contraception, and emergency contraception.
- If giving low-dose COC perimenopausal, stop at approximately 52 yr of age and check FSH and estradiol levels. If menopausal, switch to HRT (estrogen/progesterone combination).
- Transdermal patches.
  - May work better for women with migraines without aura.
  - Applying transdermal patches to the buttocks may increase levels of estrogen.
- *Do not* give thyroid medication at the same time as oral estrogen (e.g., contraception or HRT); separate by 12 hr.
- Caution starting HRT after 60 yr of age and avoid starting HRT after 65 yr of age.

ABNORMAL BLEEDING PATTERNS

I. Definition of bleeding patterns
  A. Normal ovulatory menstrual cycle for adolescents is 21–45 days and for adults is 21–35 days, and has 2 cyclic phases; the menses last approximately 7 days.
    1. Follicular phase is the first half of cycle (prepares for ovulation; rise in estrogen).
    2. Luteal phase is last half (occurs after ovulation; rise in progesterone).
    3. Signs of normal ovulatory cycle
      (a) Regular cycle length
      (b) May have mild PMS/dysmenorrhea
      (c) Changes in cervical mucus from thick to clear and stringy

        (d) May have breast tenderness prior to menses

        (e) May have midcycle pain associated with ovulation

  B. Anovulatory bleeding pattern is heavy, noncyclic bleeding without pathology and may lead to abnormal uterine bleeding (AUB).

    1. Bleeding occurs because of imbalance between estrogen and progestin during monthly cycle. If there is too much estrogen and not enough progestin to cause sloughing of endometrial lining, the bleeding is excessive.

    2. Usually occurs at the extremes of menstrual ages and can occur sporadically during menstrual history.

    3. Causes

        (a) Immature HPO axis is common in first 1–3 yr of menstrual cycles.

        (b) Excessive weight loss; over exercise; eating disorders (results in too little estrogen)

        (c) Polycystic ovarian syndrome (see POLYCYSTIC OVARIAN SYNDROME in this chapter)

        (d) Thyroid disease (see Chapter 15, Thyroid Disorders)

        (e) Hyperprolactinemia (e.g., drug induced or hypothalamic pituitary disease)

        (f) Structural uterine defects (e.g., polyps, fibroids, cancer)

        (g) STIs, endometriosis

        (h) Medication induced (e.g., anticoagulants, contraception use [IUD], illicit drugs, antipsychotics)

        (i) Bleeding disorders (e.g., von Willebrand disease, SLE, ITP)

    4. Signs and symptoms

        (a) Irregular, heavy, prolonged menstrual bleeding occurring intermittently during monthly cycle

        (b) Usually very little cramping or PMS symptoms noted prior to bleeding

II. History should include

  A. Menstrual history

    1. Age at onset of menses and where in the cycle did the irregular bleeding occur

    2. LMP (including first and last day)

    3. Pattern of bleeding

        (a) How many days did you bleed?

        (b) How heavy was your bleeding (i.e., how many pads or tampons used in 24 hr)?

    4. Any symptoms of PMS noted before or after abnormal bleeding (see PREMENSTRUAL SYNDROME, later in chapter).

    5. Any particular events occurring in your life (e.g., weight loss, change in exercise pattern, change in social appearances)?

  B. Do you keep a calendar of menstrual patterns either on paper or on smartphone "apps"?

  C. Estimate amount of blood loss

    1. How many tampons/pads are used in 24 hr?

    2. How often is the product changed and is the product saturated and bleeding through to undergarments?

    3. Are there blood clots and what size, do they occur at beginning of cycle or after cycle has started?

    4. Does it limit ADLs?

  D. Are there any social stressors either at home or school?

  E. Is the patient sexually active and what contraception is used, if any?

  F. Any history of sexual abuse or assault?

  G. Any FH of AUB or bleeding disorders?

III. Diagnostic testing (all ages)
- A. Urine hCG; urinalysis; STI testing (urine or swab)
- B. CBC (anemia is common), coagulation factors (PT, PTT, INR, von Willebrand factor) with heavy bleeding, especially in adolescent female
- C. CMP
- D. TSH, prolactin, FSH/LH (especially if perimenopausal or postmenopausal), estradiol levels (if adnexal mass present)
- E. Pelvic exam and pap, if indicated
- F. Pelvic and transvaginal U/S to evaluate the endometrial lining (thickness of endometrial stripe is dependent on age and menstrual phase)
- G. Endometrial biopsy if AUB is persistent, present in unopposed estrogen setting, with failed medical management or high risk for cancer.
- H. Screen for eating disorder, anxiety, depression (especially female athletes)

IV. Adolescents
- A. Causes of abnormal bleeding
  1. Ovulatory dysfunction is usually due to immaturity of hypothalamic-pituitary-ovarian (HPO) axis.
  2. Stress-induced exercise
  3. Pregnancy; change in contraceptive method
  4. STI or other pelvic infection; endometriosis
  5. Bleeding disorders (e.g., ITP, von Willebrand disease, SLE), which may be undiagnosed until PMH noted.
     - (a) May have had heavy bleeding since onset of menses
     - (b) Increase bleeding with dental procedures
     - (c) Unexplained bruising that does not resolve quickly
     - (d) Unexplained nose bleeds
  6. Medications (e.g., spironolactone, antipsychotics, antidepressants)
- B. Pharmacological treatment
  1. If bleeding is manageable and not effecting ADLs, consider *watchful waiting* until HPO axis has matured.
  2. If *actively bleeding*
     - (a) Monophasic COC with 30 mcg EE/progestin: 1 pill q8hr until bleeding stops, then 1 pill q12hr for 2 days then 1 pill daily for 21 days
       - (i) If bleeding recurs before 21 days, restart q12hr dose for the full 21 days.
       - (ii) If nausea occurs, may need antiemetic.
       - (iii) Can continue COC for 6 mo to 1 yr and then if patient prefers, can stop COC and monitor menstrual cycles.
     - (b) Oral progesterone: Norethindrone 5–10 mg bid for 7 days, if bleeding stops, consider 5 mg hs first 5–10 days each month *(no contraceptive effects)*.
  3. If anemia occurs, start ferrous sulfate 325 mg bid and monitor CBC q6mo as needed until anemia resolves.
- C. Long-term treatment (start after bleeding resolves)
  1. For contraception and control of bleeding with estrogen: low-dose monophasic COC with 30–35 mcg EE for at least 6 mo
  2. For contraception using progestin only
     - (a) POPs
     - (b) Depo-provera
     - (c) Progesterone IUD or implants
  3. *Maintenance progesterone (no contraceptive effects)*
     - (a) Norethindrone acetate 5 mg hs for the first 5–10 days each month *or* micronized progesterone 200 mg first 12 days each mo

       (b) Medroxyprogesterone acetate 10 mg daily for 10 days each month

       (c) Bleeding should occur about 2–3 days after last pill

▲   D. ***Referral to GYN (pediatric, if available) if unable to control cycles or anemia with Hgb <10 g/dL***

V. Women of reproductive age

  A. Causes related to

     1. Regular heavy, prolonged menstrual cycles

       (a) Enlarged uterus secondary to leiomyoma or cancer

       (b) Boggy endometrium secondary to endometriosis

       (c) Bleeding disorders or medications

     2. Regular menstrual cycles with inter-cycle bleeding

       (a) Polyps, cancer

       (b) Recent pregnancy, instrumentation of cervix or uterus or pelvic infection

       (c) Chronic endometritis

     3. Irregular bleeding with longer or shorter intervals

       (a) PCOS, thyroid disorder, hyperprolactinemia

       (b) Cancer

     4. Irregular or heavy bleeding secondary to IUD, HRT, or hormonal contraceptives

     5. Other causes of heavy, prolonged, irregular bleeding

       (a) Trauma (e.g., sexual abuse, straddle injuries, foreign bodies)

       (b) Pregnancy, obesity

       (c) Infection (e.g., PID, endometritis, STI)

       (d) Medications (e.g., anticoagulants, antipsychotics, chemotherapy)

  B. Pharmacological treatment should be focused on physiological cause if known; AUB is commonly caused from ovulatory dysfunction.

▲   1. ***Urgent transfer to ED if bleeding is causing hypovolemia and orthostatic changes or Hgb < 10 g/dL***

●   2. ***If bleeding is related to structural problems (e.g., polyps, fibroids or cancer), consider referral to GYN for possible surgery.***

     3. AUB with *mild* anemia and some disruption in ADLs (e.g., fatigue)

       (a) COCs with EE 30–35 mcg 1 tab qid until bleeding stops or for 5–7 days

       (b) Continuous COC for 1 mo then stop and allow withdrawal bleeding to occur

       (c) Can continue with low-dose COC (has contraceptive effects), cyclic progesterone (no contraceptive effect), or IUD/implant (has contraceptive effects).

       (d) If estrogen is contraindicated, consider

         (i) Norethindrone 5–15 mg daily for 21 days (no contraception)

        (ii) Medroxyprogesterone 10 mg daily for 14 days (no contraception)

        (iii) Levonorgestrel IUD (LNG 52) (contraceptive effects)

     4. If chronic AUB is affecting ADLs but no anemia is noted and patient prefers short-term treatment of < 1 yr, consider

       (a) Low-dose COC in nonsmoking woman, < 35 yr of age, with no HTN and no migraines with aura (has contraceptive effects)

       (b) Cyclic progesterone (e.g., medroxyprogesterone acetate 10 mg daily for 10 days each month) (no contraceptive effects)

     5. AUB without acute symptoms and contraception is needed; consider

       (a) COCs (if not contraindicated) can control bleeding and regulate cycles

       (b) POP

       (c) Depo-Provera or IUD (LNG 52)

● *= non-urgent referral;* ▲ *= urgent referral*

      6. AUB in a woman not wanting to use hormonal therapy or needing contraception, consider

        (a) Tranexamic acid 650 mg tablets, take 2 tabs tid up to 5 days

        (b) NSAIDs started first day of bleeding and continue until bleeding stops

          (i) Mefenamic acid 500 mg tid

          (ii) Naproxen 500 mg initially and then 3–5 hr later followed by 250–500 mg bid

          (iii) Ibuprofen 600 mg daily

      7. *Referral to GYN if symptoms persist and no structural or medical problems found*

VI. Postmenopausal women

  A. *Any bleeding after "menopause"* (no bleeding for > 12 mo after cessation of menses) *is a concern.* Possible causes include

    1. Endometrial hyperplasia and/or cancer (especially if endometrial stripe > 4 mm)

    2. Polyps, fibroids

    3. Hormone replacement therapy (HRT)

  B. Diagnostic testing

    1. CBC, CMP, consider PT/INR

    2. Pelvic and transvaginal U/S

    3. Endometrial biopsy

  C. Treatment after diagnostic testing may include *referral to GYN, oncologist, or surgeon, based on findings.*

AMENORRHEA

I. Primary: absence of menarche by 15 yr of age *with* normal breast development *or* no menarche by age 13 *without* breast or pubic hair development

  A. Causes are usually anatomic or genetic

    1. Genetic (e.g., Turner, gonadal dysgenesis)

    2. Pituitary or brain tumors

    3. Disorders of HPO axis (e.g., hypothalamic or pituitary dysfunction, PCOS).

    4. Anatomic outflow problems (e.g., absence of uterus, cervical blockage or imperforate hymen)

  B. History (includes PMH and FH)

    1. Evidence of stages of puberty present and when development started (see Tanner stages, Box 2.1)

      (a) Breast development or nipple discharge

      (b) Axillary or pubic hair, excess hair growth or early acne

      (c) Acne (at what age) or hirsutism (where is main hair growth).

    2. Any significant problems with birth; increased stress at home or school, bullying

    3. Change in appetite, weight loss/gain; polydipsia, polyuria

    4. Excessive exercise habits (e.g., > 2 hr/day)

    5. Growth problems (e.g., too tall or too short; FH of growth problems or genetic syndromes)

    6. Any drug use (OTC, legal or illegal)

    7. Any problems with H/A, visual changes, fatigue

    8. Did symptoms occur slowly over time or more rapidly?

    9. Sexual history and use of OCP; LMP (if any dates recollected) and how often are menstrual cycles (e.g., monthly, or longer time periods)

● = *non-urgent referral*

C. Physical examination
  1. Height/weight/BMI/growth chart(s); Tanner stages (see Tanner stages, Box 2.1)
  2. Overall appearance in body habitus (e.g., short stature, webbed neck, buffalo hump, striae, goiter)
  3. Skin appearance: early acne and/or increased hair growth (e.g., on face, breast, and lower abdomen)
  4. Inspect breast for general development (see Tanner stages, Box 2.1).
  5. Inspect genitalia for any abnormalities; observe hymen and vaginal opening; speculum exam for presence of cervix and cervical opening (*if appropriate*); bimanual examination to evaluate uterus (*if appropriate*).
D. Diagnostic testing
  1. Urine hCG, urinalysis
  2. FSH/LH
    (a) FSH high: consider genetic abnormality
    (b) FSH low/NL with breast development: consider anatomic abnormality or endocrine disorder (e.g., PCOS or thyroid dysfunction)
    (c) FSH/LH very low/NL without breast development: consider hypothyroidism or congenital abnormality
    (d) FSH low/NL and LH low: consider eating disorder, excessive exercise or stress
  3. TSH, prolactin
  4. Free and total testosterone, estradiol level (E2)
  5. Pelvic U/S for identification of uterus and other structures
E. Treatment
  1. Treat underlying problems (e.g., PCOS, hypothyroidism, malnutrition).
  2. Counsel regarding complications of amenorrhea (e.g., low BMD and increased risk for CV disease).
F. *Referral*
  1. *Geneticist for appropriate tests*
  2. *Gynecologist for appropriate age exam and treatment*
  3. *Nutritionist*
II. Secondary: absence of menses for >3 mo in a woman who previously had normal menstrual cycles or absence of menses >6 mo with history of irregular cycles (<9 cycles/yr)
  A. Causes
    1. Pregnancy
    2. Functional hypothalamic amenorrhea causing anovulation and decreased estrogen levels seen with
      (a) Extreme exercise >2 hr/day
      (b) Severe dietary restrictions in fat
      (c) Eating disorders with extreme decrease in body mass
      (d) Stress
      (e) Pituitary tumors
      (f) PCOS (see **POLYCYSTIC OVARIAN SYNDROME**, later in chapter)
    3. Ovarian failure (e.g., premature or natural menopause)
    4. Structural disorder
      (a) Stenosis of cervix
      (b) Asherman's syndrome (i.e., excessive intrauterine scarring)
    5. Drug induced
      (a) Illegal drug use (e.g., "crack," "meth," cocaine, heroin)

● = *non-urgent referral*

(b) First-generation antipsychotics (e.g., haloperidol)

(c) Herbal products (e.g., black cohosh, ginseng, red clover, DHEA [these products stimulate estrogen receptor sites and may eventually cause excessive bleeding if not opposed with progesterone])

B. History (includes PMH and FH, see I. B, above)

C. Signs and symptoms

1. Weight loss with BMI < 18 kg/m^2 (e.g., eating disorder, extreme exercise)
2. Erosion of tooth enamel; enlarged parotid glands (consider eating disorders)
3. Hirsutism, acne, irregular menses (consider PCOS)
4. H/A, visual field defect, fatigue, galactorrhea, polyuria (consider pituitary tumor)
5. Vaginal dryness, decreased libido, poor sleep habit and obviously pale, dry vaginal tissues (e.g., consider menopause)
6. Abnormal genitalia (consider structural disorder)
7. Breast exam for development, nipple discharge, striae and hair distribution

D. Diagnostic testing

1. Urine hCG (pregnancy most common cause in childbearing age), urinalysis
2. TSH/free T4 (hypothyroidism common cause)
3. FSH, estradiol level (E2)
   (a) FSH increased with low E2: consider menopause
   (b) FSH normal or decreased with low E2: consider functional hypothalamic amenorrhea
   (c) If FSH and E2 are normal: consider evaluation of secondary amenorrhea with progestin challenge (Fig. 10.1)
4. Prolactin (if elevated, consider tumor)
5. Total testosterone, DHEA-S
   (a) Elevated testosterone with normal or ↓ FSH and normal E2 + virilization signs: consider PCOS
   (b) Testosterone > 150 ng/dL or DHEA-S > 700 mcg: consider ovarian or adrenal tumor
6. Pelvic and transvaginal U/S (endometrial lining < 4 mm indicative of hypoestrogenism)
7. Progestin challenge 10 mg for 10 days (see Fig. 10.1) and if no bleeding consider conjugated estrogen (Premarin) 6.25 mg for 35 days and add medroxyprogesterone (Provera) 10 mg days 26 through 35. This will help to determine the cause of amenorrhea.

E. Treat or refer for underlying conditions

1. Prevent/treat osteoporosis (see Chapter 13, OSTEOPOROSIS).
2. Discuss hormone replacement for vasomotor symptoms (see MENOPAUSE in this chapter; see Table 10.4).
3. Lifestyle changes to encourage regular exercise < 1 hr/day, balanced diet, counseling for eating disorders
4. Consider alternative vasomotor control (e.g., SNRIs, antianxiety medications; lifestyle changes with appropriate layered clothing and temperature control).
5. Treat PCOS (see in this chapter); thyroid disorder (see Chapter 15, Thyroid Disorders).

F. *Referral based on findings*

1. *Gynecologist*
2. *Endocrinologist*
3. *Geneticist*
4. *Nutritionist*

⬤ = *non-urgent referral*

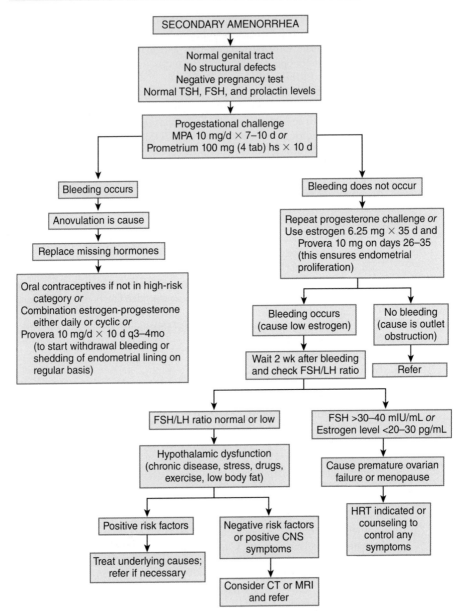

Fig. 10.1 Evaluation of secondary amenorrhea.

DYSMENORRHEA

I. Primary

    A. Painful cramps with menstruation associated with increase in prostaglandins during ovulatory cycles which cause smooth muscle contraction; usually starts within first 1–5 yr of onset of menstrual cycles and *without known pathology.*

    B. Signs and symptoms

        1. Recurrent spasmodic cramping in abdomen/pelvic area with associated lower back pain, and/or leg pain

        2. Occasional diarrhea and low-grade fever

        3. Starts on the first day of the menstrual cycle and decreases as the uterine lining is shed.

        4. May improve with age; may stop or significantly decrease after childbirth.

    C. Treatment

        1. Heating pad to lower abdomen

        2. Vitamin supplements starting 1–2 days before menses and stopping when symptoms resolve or about 3 days within cycle

           (a) Vitamin E 500 units daily or 200 units bid

           (b) Vitamin B6 up to 100 mg daily

           (c) Vitamin B1 (thiamine) 100 mg daily

           (d) Ginger powder 750–2000 mg on first 3 days of menses

        3. NSAIDs should be started at 1–2 days before onset of menses and continued for 3 days into menstrual cycle; if poor response from one NSAID, change to another.

           (a) Ibuprofen 400–600 mg initially then q6hr   *or*

           (b) Naproxen sodium 550 mg initially then 275 mg q6–8hr   *or*

           (c) Mefenamic acid 500 mg initially then 250 mg q6hr   *or*

           (d) Ketoprofen 50 mg initially then 25–50 mg q6–8hr   *or*

           (e) Diclofenac 75–100 mg initially then 50 mg tid   *or*

           (f) Meloxicam 7.5 mg initially then daily   *or*

           (g) Piroxicam 20 mg initially then 10–20 mg daily

        4. Hormonal products

           1. COCs either monthly or continuous (e.g., 3 mo on and 1 wk off)

              (a) Suppresses ovulation

              (b) More predictability with cycles for dosing NSAIDs

           2. Progestin IUD may decrease menstrual cycles and alleviate or eliminate some symptoms.

II. Secondary

    A. Painful menstruation *associated with reproductive disorder*

        1. Endometriosis, fibroids, adenomyosis

        2. Cervical stenosis, scarring from past GYN surgery or PID

        3. Usually begins later in life.

    B. May start several days before onset of the menstrual cycle and may not resolve until the cycle is finished; may worsen over time and occur outside of cycle patterns.

    C. Diagnosis is usually based on physical examination; consider pelvic U/S.

    D. Treatment: **Referral to GYN if symptoms not controlled with previously mentioned treatments.**

● = *non-urgent referral*

MENOPAUSE

    I. *Perimenopause* usually occurs between 40 and 55 yr of age or approximately 4–5 yr before last period.

        A. Menstrual cycle lengthens or shortens and becomes irregular with scant, absent, or heavy bleeding and is associated with

            1. Vasomotor symptoms (e.g., hot flashes and night sweats, change in sleep patterns)

            2. Vaginal dryness, decreased libido

            3. Irritability, mood swings, and fatigue (usually due to lack of sleep)

        B. Diagnostic testing

            1. FSH and LH; TSH, estradiol level

            2. Prolactin level (early morning specimen)

            3. Urine hCG

            4. Consider CMP and lipids.

        C. Lifestyle changes to decrease symptoms

            1. Emphasize weight loss and exercise.

            2. Smoking and alcohol cessation; decrease or eliminate caffeine

            3. Increase milk or milk alternatives (e.g., soy, nut or goat's milk)

            4. Multivitamin; CoQ-10 200 mg daily

            5. Encourage dressing with layers during the day and keeping house slightly cooler and using a fan at night.

        D. Pharmacological therapy *(if woman has a uterus, must give some type of progestin to protect the endometrium)*

            1. If cycles are sporadic and/or heavy with vasomotor symptoms and woman has a low-risk profile and *is not* a smoker

               (a) Low-dose estrogen COC (EE 10–20 mcg pill) *or*

               (b) Estradiol 0.025 mg daily plus micronized progesterone 200 mg first 12 days of each month *or*

               (c) Combination transdermal patch once or twice a week

            2. At 50–52 yr of age, if woman is on low-dose COCs, check FSH on day 5 of pill-free week; if FSH elevated, can switch to low-dose combined HRT (Table 10.4).

            3. If a woman has had partial hysterectomy and is having menopausal symptoms, consider low-dose estrogen replacement therapy (see Table 10.4).

            4. If a woman has increased risk profile or smokes but is symptomatic, can consider: medroxyprogesterone 10 mg daily for 10 days a month; this may help to stabilize cycle and decrease vasomotor symptoms.

            5. Herbal therapies contain products that can stimulate estrogen receptors approximately the same as prescription estrogens; these products may or may not relieve symptoms; any woman with a uterus *must* have both estrogen and progesterone.

    II. Natural menopause (as opposed to surgical) is cessation of menses for ≥ 12 mo after last menstrual bleed; average age at onset approximately 51 yr of age; menopause symptoms that are *more consistent* usually resolve within 2–3 yr of onset.

        A. Signs and symptoms (can be variable in intensity)

            1. Genitourinary

               (a) Vaginal atrophy: decreased tissue elasticity at introitus with thinning and dryness, leading to smaller vaginal opening and pain with intercourse

               (b) Frequent UTIs, urinary frequency and urgency, pelvic heaviness

            2. Hot flashes and night sweats leading to poor sleep hygiene

            3. Neuropsychological

               (a) Mood swings, depression, anxiety, irritability, suicidal thoughts

---

■ = *not to be missed;*

TABLE 10.4 ■ **Hormone Replacement Therapy***

Estrogen Only[†]	Progesterone Only	Combined Estrogen/Progestin
Conjugated equine estrogen: (Premarin) 0.3, 0.45, 0.625, 0.9, 1.25 mg	Medroxyprogesterone (Provera) 2.5, 5.0, 10 mg	Conjugated estrogen/ medroxyprogesterone: (Prempro) 0.625 mg/2.5 mg, 0.625 mg/5 mg, 0.45 mg/1.5 mg, 0.3 mg/1.5 mg
Estradiol: (Estrace) 0.5, 1, 2 mg	Micronized progesterone: (Prometrium) 100 or 200 mg hs	Conjugated estrogen/ medroxyprogesterone: (Premphase) 0.625 mg/5 mg (days 1–14 estrogen alone; days 15–28 both hormones)
Esterified estrogen: (Menest) 0.3, 0.625, 1.25 mg	Norethindrone: (Aygestin, Nor-QD) 2.5, 5, 10 mg	Combined estradiol/norethindrone: (Activella) 1 mg/0.5 mg, 0.5 mg/0.1 mg
Estropipate: 0.75, 1.5, 3 mg		Combined ethinyl estradiol/ norethindrone: (Femhrt) 2.5 mcg/0.5 mg, 5 mcg/1 mg (Jinteli) 5 mcg/1 mg
Estradiol transdermal patches: Vivelle-Dot, Menostar Climara, Alora, Estraderm Dose/application varies from biweekly to once weekly		Estradiol/norethindrone: (CombiPatch) 0.05/0.14 mg; 0.05/0.25 mg twice a week Estradiol/levonorgestrel patch: (Climara Pro) 0.045 mg/0.015 mg once a week
Estradiol vaginal ring:[‡] inserted q90d (Estring) 2 mg (Femring) 0.05 or 0.1 mg		Esterified estrogen/ methyltestosterone (generic only): 1.25 mg/2.5 mg tab; 0.625 mg/1.25 mg tab: 1 tab 21 days on and 7 days off (if uterus, must add progestin)
Estrogen vaginal creams[‡] 1–3 times week (Estrace cream) 2–4 g (Premarin cream) 0.5–2 g		
Estradiol vaginal tablet 2 times a week:[‡] (Vagifem) 10 mcg (Yuvafem) 10 mcg (Imvexxy) 4 or 10 mcg		
Estradiol topical gel/mist daily: (Estrogel) 0.75 mg (Elestrin) 0.52 mg (EvaMist) 1.53 mg (Divigel) 0.25 mg		
Depot estradiol (IM) q1mo: DepoEstradiol 5 mg/mL Delestrogen 10–20 mg		

*This list is *not all inclusive*.
[†]*Must add progesterone for women with a uterus.*
[‡]Useful with atrophic vaginitis, not vasomotor symptoms.

     (b) Fatigue and altered sleep patterns, decreased energy

     (c) Forgetfulness, decreased ability to multitask and decreased ability to concentrate

  4. Breast tenderness, overall fullness of breast tissue is decreased and breasts tend to sag

  5. Weight gain in hips and abdomen

  6. Skin

     (a) Decrease in skin elasticity with dryness and "wrinkling"

     (b) Thinning of axillary, leg, and pubic hair

B. Diagnostic testing: consider

  1. FSH and LH; TSH, estradiol level

  2. Prolactin level (early morning specimen)

  3. Urine hCG

  4. CMP and lipids

C. Lifestyle changes for vasomotor symptoms related to menopause

  1. Emphasize weight loss and exercise; yoga, strength training can help to maintain agility, balance, and muscle mass.

  2. Smoking and alcohol cessation; decrease or eliminate caffeine.

  3. Increase milk or milk alternatives for calcium replacement (e.g., soy, nut or goat's milk).

  4. Multivitamin, CoQ-10 200 mg daily.

  5. Encourage dressing with layers during the day and keeping house slightly cooler, at night and consider overhead or stationary fan.

D. Pharmacological treatment for menopause is best achieved with short-term (<5 yr) hormone replacement therapy (HRT) (see Table 10.4 and PRACTICE PEARLS FOR HORMONE USE [see Menstrual Disorders]); if symptoms are still present after stopping HRT and are affecting QOL, consider restarting HRT at lowest effective dose if less than 2 yr after stopping HRT.

  1. If ≥2 yr post-menopausal *with a uterus* and having vasomotor symptoms that are disrupting QOL, consider oral estradiol 1 mg daily or transdermal patch 0.05 mg 1–2 time a week *with* oral MPA 2.5 mg or oral micronized progesterone 100 mg daily. There are transdermal preparations with both estrogen and progesterone available (see Table 10.4).

  2. If post-menopausal *without uterus* and having vasomotor symptoms effecting QOL, consider estradiol 0.05–1 mg daily or transdermal patch 0.025–0.05 mg 1–2 times a week.

  3. HRT may decrease fatigue and provide overall sense of well-being and improve energy levels; it may also improve some symptoms of vaginal atrophy.

  4. ***Never give unopposed estrogen to any woman who still has a uterus; always balance with progesterone even if considering OTC products.***

  5. Abrupt cessation of HRT may cause sudden onset of vasomotor symptoms or worsening vaginal atrophy; gradual withdrawal over 6–12 mo is recommended if patient has been taking HRT ≥5 yr.

     (a) Suggest dropping one pill every week for 4 wk then decreasing dose by 2 pills a week and continue decreasing until only taking 1 pill a week   *or*

     (b) Decrease pill every other day for 2–4 wk then begin lengthening interval until only taking 1 day/wk then stop.

     (c) If symptoms recur, return to last successful dose schedule.

     (d) Go slow and deal with menopause symptoms as they occur (e.g., irritability, poor sleep habits, fatigue, depression).

  6. Combined estrogen/methyltestosterone (see Table 10.4): only use for post-hysterectomy patients and those who have failed other therapies.

     (a) *May* improve sexual desire (*not guaranteed, not FDA approved*).

■ = *not to be missed;*

(b) Monitor for virilizing characteristics (e.g., deepening voice, hirsutism).

(c) May worsen lipid profile.

7. Compounding hormone products (not FDA approved; they are considered a dietary supplement and are not regulated)

(a) Can be individualized based on dose and route; *if uterus is present, use both estrogen and progesterone products.*

(b) Common compounded products: Biest (20% estradiol and 80% estriol), Triest (10% estradiol, 10% estrone, 80% estrone); can also include progesterone, testosterone, and other products.

(c) A pill containing 1 mg 17 β estradiol + 100 mg micronized progesterone would be sufficient to control hot flashes.

8. Concomitant use of GERD medication (see Table 9.2) can decrease absorption of estrogen product.

E. Vulvovaginitis

1. Signs and symptoms

(a) Vulvovaginal irritation, burning, pain, itching

(b) Dyspareunia, vaginal fissuring and tears with intercourse, vaginal discharge

(c) Urinary symptoms of frequency, dysuria, recurrent UTIs

2. Treatment with OTC lubricants

(a) Use during sexual intercourse (oil-based lubricants can cause latex condom failure).

(b) Examples are Astroglide, Pjur, or Elegance Women's lubricant.

3. Treatment with vaginal moisturizers

(a) Should be used routinely 2–3 days a week.

(b) Examples are Replens, Vagisil, or K-Y liquibeads.

4. Consider mixture of equal portions Vaseline and OTC hydrocortisone cream, applied in *small* amounts topically to vulva (not inserted) q hs to relieve itching; may need to consider increasing strength of topical steroids (see Table 5.3) in short bursts for severe itching.

5. Topical vaginal estradiol preparations (e.g., ring, cream, supp); ***do not use the cream as lubricant for intercourse***.

(a) Estring inserted q90 days

(b) Estradiol vaginal (Vagifem) tab 10 mcg inserted daily for 2 wk, then 1–2 times a week.

(c) Imvexxy 4 and 10 mcg supp inserted daily for 2 wk then twice a week

(d) Premarin cream 0.625 mg or Estrace cream 0.5–4 g daily for 2 wk then twice a week; use lowest effective dose.

(e) *Progestin not needed with lowest dose estrogen topical products*

6. Oral estrogen (see Table 10.4); *not first-line therapy*

7. Ospemifene (Osphena) 60 mg daily (selective estrogen receptor modulator [SERM]) for dyspareunia and vaginal dryness; can increase hot flashes and increase risk for DVT; contraindicated with current or past breast cancer history.

8. Prasterone (Intrarosa) vaginal insert q hs (is converted to estrogen); mainly used for dyspareunia

F. Nonhormonal therapies for emotional lability, change in sleep patterns, irritability, anxiety, and vasomotor symptoms (not FDA approved, but have shown some benefit)

1. SSRIs may help with both emotional and vasomotor symptoms (e.g., fluoxetine 10–20 mg daily).

■ = *not to be missed;*

2. Venlafaxine ER 37.5–75 mg daily
3. TCAs or trazodone may help with sleep disruption
4. Clonidine 0.1 mg bid-tid for hot flashes and anxiety
5. Gabapentin 300 mg hs for sleep disruption and vasomotor

G. Herbal therapies for vasomotor symptoms (hot flashes/night sweats) have not been proven to be effective but may be better than placebo; some products may be harmful if there is a history of breast cancer.
   1. Natural products high in phytoestrogens and isoflavones can relieve some vasomotor symptoms.
      (a) Plant and herbal therapies: soy beans, chickpeas, lentils, tofu, basmati rice, flaxseed (oil or seeds), apples, nuts, and whole grains
      (b) These products must be taken daily to get any benefit.
   2. The following preparations are not prescription, not FDA approved, but may be safe; *should not be taken with breast cancer or during breast cancer treatment.*
      (a) Black cohosh or Remifemin 20–60 mg bid for 4–12 wk for hot flashes, mood swings, vaginitis, sleep disruption
      (b) Evening primrose oil capsules 2–4 cap bid for hot flashes and mood swings
      (c) Vitamin E 800–1000 mg daily for breast discomfort and dry skin
      (d) Soy extract caps 50–100 mg 2–3 times daily for hot flashes

H. Osteoporosis prevention (see Chapter 13, OSTEOPOROSIS)
I. Annual physical examination
   1. Routine screening for dyslipidemia (see Chapter 8, DYSLIPIDEMIA)
   2. Routine screening for colorectal cancer (see Chapter 9, COLON CANCER)
   3. Review mammogram q1yr and BMD q2yr *while on HRT,* otherwise mammogram/BMD as indicated.
   4. Annually review HRT and consider decreasing to the lowest effective dose needed to control symptoms for as long as needed (review MenoPro app from North American Menopause Society [NAMS] to discuss decision making for HRT).
● J. **Referral to gynecologist if unable to regulate menopausal symptoms.**

POLYCYSTIC OVARIAN SYNDROME (PCOS)

I. Description
   A. Hormonal disorder related to ovulatory dysfunction and hyperandrogenism that typically occurs in adolescents and persists into adulthood.
   B. Adolescents may present with late-onset, irregular, or absent menses and during childbearing years, women may have difficulty getting pregnant; if irregular menstrual cycles start after 30 yr of age, PCOS is less likely diagnosis.
   C. Associated with insulin resistance, metabolic syndrome (see Chapter 8, METABOLIC SYNDROME), DM (see Chapter 15, Diabetes Mellitus), CV disease, and obesity and increased risk for endometrial cancer.
II. Signs and symptoms
   A. Oligomenorrhea with irregular, either scant or heavy menses, or with primary or secondary amenorrhea (e.g., no menses or by > 90 days between menses)
   B. Signs of androgen excess
      1. Hirsutism, mainly on the chest, abdomen, face, and nipples
      2. Oily skin and increased acne resistant to treatment
   C. Central obesity (few are underweight)

● = *non-urgent referral*

D. Insulin resistance with
1. Elevated levels of insulin followed by increased glucose
2. Acanthosis nigricans
E. HTN; increased triglycerides with low HDL
F. Infertility or decreased fertility
III. Diagnostic testing (COCs, spironolactone or metformin should be stopped for at least 4 wk before testing)
A. TSH
B. Prolactin (elevated levels indicate pituitary tumor); estradiol levels
C. LH/FSH ratio usually 2:1 (normal ratio does not exclude PCOS diagnosis)
1. Elevated FSH level indicates premature ovarian failure.
2. Elevated LH/FSH ratio indicates anovulation and PCOS.
D. Elevated level of 17-hydroxyprogesterone (> 1000 ng/mL) should be evaluated further as it may indicate congenital adrenal hyperplasia.
E. Total testosterone and DHEA-S are normally elevated with PCOS on random testing; if testosterone > 200 ng/dL or DHEA-S > 800 mcg/dL, this is more indicative of virilizing adrenal tumor.
F. Complete chemistry panel, 2-hr GTT 140–199 mg/dL indicates insulin resistance (> 200 mg/dL indicates DM), lipid panel
G. Pap smear and pelvic examination to identify any structural abnormalities
H. Pelvic and transvaginal U/S (prolonged estrogen stimulation can increase the risk of endometrial cancer)
I. Urine hCG
J. Consider endometrial biopsy (especially if > 45 yr of age)
K. Consider screening tests for depression or anxiety
IV. Treatment goals: decrease testosterone production, reestablish normal hormonal balance and reduce insulin levels
A. Weight loss (even 5%–10% loss can aid in restoring menstrual cycles) and exercise should be initiated immediately
B. Pharmacological therapy
1. COCs are mainstay of treatment to reestablish normal hormonal levels (see Table 10.2)
(a) COCs decrease levels of testosterone and should decrease virilization
(b) Use COCs with EE 20–30 mcg and progestins with lower androgenicity (e.g., desogestrel, drospirenone, or norgestimate). Caution using COC with drospirenone due to increased risk of VTE/PE
(c) Caution using COCs in obese women with BMI > 33 and women > 40 yr of age due to increased risk for VTE/PE
2. For endometrial protection in women who do not wish to use COCs
(a) Medroxyprogesterone 10 mg daily for 10 days every 1–2 mo (will cause withdrawal bleeding about 1–2 days after last dose) *or*
(b) Daily POP *or*
(c) Progestin IUD
3. Metformin for insulin resistance; may also correct anovulation; usual dose is 500–1000 mg bid (no contraception benefits).
4. Antiandrogens may decrease hair growth and improve acne; usually started about 6 mo after COC initiation; *adequate contraception must be established.*
(a) Spironolactone 50–100 mg bid (not FDA approved)
(b) Finasteride 2.5–5 mg daily (not FDA approved)

    C. Hair removal techniques
      1. Electrolysis or waxing)
      2. Eflornithine (Vaniqua) for removal of facial hair
    D. BP on each visit; monitor FBG and A1c annually with lipid profile q1–3yr as indicated.
    E. Monitor for depression and OSA.
  V. *Referral to OB/GYN or infertility specialist if pregnancy is desired.*

PREMENSTRUAL SYNDROME (PMS)/PREMENSTRUAL DYSPHORIC DISORDER (PMDD)

  I. PMS
    A. Cluster of symptoms usually starting between 20 and 30 yr of age, that are both physical and emotional; occurs consistently 5 days before menses starts and resolves 1–2 days after menses; may limit daily activity and decrease quality of work.
    B. Signs and symptoms
      1. Increased appetite, bloating and weight gain (> 2–5 lbs), breast tenderness
      2. Acne, greasy or dry hair
      3. H/A, fatigue
      4. Mood swings with irritability, anger, anxiety, and sadness
    C. Diagnostic testing
      1. Limited to TSH to rule out hyper/hypothyroidism
      2. Screening for dysthymia or major depressive disorder
    D. Treatment is usually supportive, with education, lifestyle changes, and nutritional changes (see PREMENSTRUAL DYSPHORIC DISORDER following).
  II. PMDD
    A. Characterized by more emotional (e.g., depression, anger, irritability, and tension) than physical symptoms (but may see same physical symptoms as PMS), and they do limit daily activity.
    B. PMDD criteria: for most menstrual cycles for the past year, ≥ 5 of the following symptoms occurred during 5 days before menses start and resolved a few days into the menstrual cycle.
      1. Markedly depressed mood with feelings of hopelessness
      2. Marked anxiety, tension, feelings of being "excitable" and "on edge"
      3. Labile mood with mood swings, sadness, and increased sensitivity
      4. Marked irritability, anger, and sense of feeling "out of control"
      5. Decreased interest in usual activity (e.g., work, school, home), lethargy, and lack of energy
      6. Difficulty concentrating, insomnia, and anhedonia
      7. Increased appetite and food cravings with weight gain
      8. May have other physical symptoms (e.g., breast tenderness, swelling in hands, bloating, and H/A)
      9. Symptoms starting later in life (e.g., 40–50 yr of age) are probably related to menopause.
    C. Diagnostic testing
      1. TSH
      2. Screening for depression and alcohol intake

● = *non-urgent referral*

III. Treatment for PMS/PMDD
  A. General
    1. Lifestyle changes
      (a) Relaxation therapy
      (b) Exercise starting with symptoms
    2. Decreased caffeine, alcohol, sugar, and sodium intake at least 2 wk before menses
    3. Regular, frequent, small meals with increased complex carbohydrates
    4. Warm moist heat to the abdomen
  B. Consider herbal supplements daily beginning about 5 days before the start of the menstrual cycle; there are no conclusive benefits but may reduce some of the effects of PMS/PMDD.
    1. Calcium 1200 mg and vitamin B6 up to 100 mg daily
    2. Vitamin E 400–800 IU may decrease breast pain; flaxseed oil or evening primrose oil capsules taken daily *may* decrease hot flashes to some degree
    3. Chasteberry (vitex agnus castus) 20–40 mg daily; improved outcomes with PMS
    4. Magnesium supplements 300–600 mg daily
  C. Pharmacological therapy
    1. Spironolactone 50–100 mg daily may relieve some bloating and weight gain; start before weight increases and stop when menses start.
    2. NSAID of choice (see DYSMENORRHEA, I, C, 3): start 2–3 days before pain is expected and stop about 2–3 days after menses start.
    3. SSRIs (see Table 17.1) can be used in moderate-to-severe cases to improve mood swings, irritability, anxiety, and depression; dose initially may be lower and then increase if needed.
      (a) Daily dosing   *or*
      (b) Intermittent cyclic dosing (i.e., start day 14 of menstrual cycle and stopping 1–2 days after into cycle)   *or*
      (c) Symptom-onset dosing (start at onset of symptoms and continue 2–3 days into cycle)
      (d) If symptoms not controlled, switch to a different SSRI for another cycle; if still failed treatment, try SNRI; anxiolytics are last choice (see 5 below).
    4. Monophasic COCs may stabilize hormonal fluctuations and relieve or eliminate some symptoms.
      (a) Use low-dose COCs with short pill-free period.
      (b) Drospirenone/EE (Yaz or Yasmin) may control symptoms better, but may have elevated risk for DVT.
    5. Anxiolytics or tricyclic antidepressants are used when other therapies have failed and QOL is diminished.
      (a) Start before symptoms and taper off 2–3 days into cycle.
      (b) Commonly used: alprazolam 0.25–2.0 mg daily (start 1–2 days before menses) or buspirone 15–60 mg daily (can start 10 days before menses).
      (c) TCA: clomipramine 25 mg or amitriptyline 25 mg at hs
IV. *Referral to GYN if symptoms uncontrolled and affecting lifestyle*

Gynecologic Infections

BACTERIAL VAGINOSIS (BV)

I. Definition: normal balance of bacteria in the vagina is disrupted, causing overgrowth of certain lactobacilli.

= non-urgent referral

    A. Not considered an STI but is associated with tampon use, douching, and multiple sex partners

    B. Increases chances of acquiring STIs

    C. Recurrences are common due to lower estrogen levels and use of antibiotics.

  II. Signs and symptoms

    A. Foul or fishy smelling vaginal discharge that increases before menses and after intercourse

    B. Thin, gray-white (spilled milk) vaginal discharge

    C. Itching and burning are rare unless coinfection with another pathogen.

 III. Diagnostic testing

    A. Amsel criteria: presence of 3 out of 4 of the following findings is diagnostic of BV.

       1. Copious, thin, grayish-white discharge that coats the vagina

       2. Vaginal pH > 4.5

       3. Positive whiff test (fishy odor of vaginal discharge when 10% KOH is added to sample)

       4. Clue cells on wet prep (> 20% more clue cells than epithelial cells)

    B. If microscopy unavailable: speculum examination findings plus positive whiff test and pH > 4.5 are considered positive.

    C. Commercially available DNA probe for diagnosing BV is available.

    D. Consider STI, HIV, trichomoniasis, and *Candida* infection with repeated BV infections.

  IV. Treatment for symptomatic women (*if the patient is pregnant, referral to GYN*); also see **PRACTICE PEARLS FOR BACTERIAL VAGINOSIS**

    A. Recommended therapy

       1. Metronidazole 500 mg PO bid for 7 days   *or*

       2. Metronidazole gel 0.75% intravaginal applicator once daily for 5 days   *or*

       3. Clindamycin 2% vaginal cream 1 applicator (5 g) hs for 7 days

    B. Alternate therapy

       1. Clindamycin 300 mg bid for 7 days   *or*

       2. Clindamycin 100 mg vaginal supp hs for 3 days   *or*

       3. Tinidazole 1000 mg daily for 5 days *or* 2000 mg daily for 2 days   *or*

       4. Secnidazole (Solosec) 2 g PO once; sprinkle in applesauce and finish within 30 min; do not chew granules.

    C. Recurrent therapy

       1. Tinidazole 1000 mg daily for 5 days   *or*

       2. Metronidazole 0.75% gel 1 applicator intravaginally twice weekly for 4–6 mo   *or*

       3. Metronidazole 500 mg bid for 10–14 days *with*

         (a) *Intravaginal* boric acid 600 mg hs for 21 days; must be stored out of reach of children *(boric acid taken orally can cause death).*

         (b) If in remission by testing approximately 2 days after last boric acid treatment, can start metronidazole gel (intravaginal) 0.75% twice weekly for 4–6 mo.

    D. Follow-up

       1. Treat for any concurrent oral or vaginal *Candida* infection with one dose of fluconazole 150 mg.

       2. Follow up in 1 mo to repeat Amsel criteria (see III, A).

    E. *Referral to GYN if persistent symptoms*

■ = *not to be missed;* ● = *non-urgent referral*

PRACTICE PEARLS FOR BACTERIAL VAGINOSIS

- Avoid douching and use sanitary napkins instead of tampons.
- Limit the number of sexual partners, although there is no need to treat sexual partner.
- Encourage all-cotton underwear and clothing that is not constrictive.
- Avoid alcohol while taking metronidazole and for 72 hr after finishing medication.
- If using clindamycin vaginally, do not use latex condoms/diaphragms for 5 days (clindamycin weakens latex).
- Intravaginal *boric acid* 600 mg at hs 1–2 times weekly may control symptoms *(boric acid taken orally can cause death).*
- Condoms and COCs may decrease risk of recurrent BV and IUDs may ↑ risk of infection.
- Advise cleaning all sex toys.
- Use gloves when participating in digital-vaginal sexual intercourse.

CANDIDIASIS (VULVOVAGINAL)

I. Definition: overgrowth of normal yeast that occurs in vagina secondary to hormonal imbalances or changes in vaginal acidity; not considered STI
   A. Causes
      1. Antibiotic therapy; SGLT-2 inhibitors
      2. New diagnosis of DM or poor control of DM
      3. COCs and post-menopausal HRT
      4. Immunocompromised persons
II. Signs and symptoms
   A. Intense vulvar and vaginal itching and burning; occasional pain with fissuring
   B. Thick, creamy (cottage cheese appearing) nonodorous vaginal discharge
   C. Vulvar erythema causing dysuria and dyspareunia
   D. Balanitis, urethritis, cutaneous lesions/rash on the penis
III. Diagnostic testing
   A. Wet prep with KOH slide shows
      1. Budding yeast with hyphae
      2. No change in lactobacillus count
      3. Vaginal pH 4–4.5
      4. Amine test is negative.
   B. *If recurrent,* check glucose levels or A1c and HIV status.
   C. Consider vaginal culture to determine species if initial treatment failed.
IV. Pharmacological treatment
   A. For *uncomplicated* candidiasis
      1. Topical OTC ($\geq$ 12 yr of age)
         (a) Clotrimazole (Gyne-Lotrimin) 2% cream: 1 applicator hs for 7–14 days   *or*
         (b) Miconazole (Monistat 3) vaginal supp hs for 3 days with topical cream *externally* bid for 7 days   *or*
         (c) Tioconazole (Monistat 1-day) 6.5% ointment: 1 applicator hs once
      2. Topical prescription
         (a) Butoconazole (Gynazole-1) 2% cream: 100 mg/applicator *once*   *or*
         (b) Terconazole (Terazol-3) 80 mg vaginal supp or 40 mg/applicator: 1 supp or applicator daily for 3 days
      3. Oral prescription
         (a) Fluconazole 150 mg tab PO *once*   *or*
         (b) Ibrexafungerp (Brexafemme) 300 mg q12hr for 1 day for azole-resistant infections; not for use during pregnancy or lactation.

■ = *not to be missed*

B. For complicated candidiasis (e.g., severe S/S, and recurrent infection with non-albicans species, pregnancy, or immunocompromised person)
    1. Fluconazole 150 mg every 3 days for 3 doses; *hold statins* when starting dose and for 1 wk after finishing dose   *or*
    2. Clotrimazole, terconazole, or miconazole for 7–14 days bid *and* consider using low-potency *topical* steroid (see Table 5.3) for initial 48 hr until azole starts working.
C. Recurrent candidiasis
    1. Fluconazole every 3 days for 3 doses *followed by* 150 mg weekly for 6 mo   *or*
    2. Consider topical clotrimazole, terconazole, or miconazole daily for 10–14 days followed by topical maintenance therapy twice a week for 6 mo.
D. Treat causes to prevent recurrence; partner should be questioned about symptoms but there is no need to treat partner.
E. Clotrimazole or miconazole can be used in pregnancy; check urine hCG prior to treatment.
F. Topical azoles are considered safe in breastfeeding women.
V. *Referral to gynecologist or dermatologist for uncontrolled symptoms.*
VI. Prevention
A. Wear loose-fitting clothes, all-cotton underwear, avoid panty hose.
B. Remove sweaty or wet clothing as soon as possible.
C. Avoid bubble baths and harsh or use of heavily scented soaps in the genital area.
D. If diabetic, maintain tight control of blood glucose.
E. Use probiotics (especially if on antibiotics).

SEXUALLY TRANSMITTED INFECTIONS

I. Chlamydia Trachomatis (CT)
A. Definition: most common bacterial infection and is the leading cause of infertility, ectopic pregnancy, and PID
B. Signs and symptoms for males and females
    1. Initially may be asymptomatic with only mild dyspareunia and dysuria.
    2. As disease progresses may see mucopurulent cervicitis or vaginal discharge with spotting and inter-cycle bleeding.
    3. Generalized abdominal/pelvic pain or "heaviness"; pain and/or bleeding with intercourse
    4. Exam findings for women
        (a) Positive CMT with purulent discharge from cervix
        (b) Cervix is friable with erosions and irritation.
    5. Exam findings for men
        (a) Prostatitis, proctitis
        (b) Epididymitis with unilateral testicular pain and swelling
        (c) Urethritis with mucoid or watery discharge and/or dysuria
    6. Exam findings that can occur in either male or female
        (a) Conjunctivitis
        (b) Pharyngitis
C. Diagnostic testing should be offered to symptomatic and asymptomatic sexually active persons.
    1. Urine nucleic acid amplification tests (NAAT) for *Neisseria gonorrhoeae*/CT

● = *non-urgent referral*

    2. Urine hCG

    3. NAAT swabs from cervix or urethra; if indicated, from conjunctiva, pharyngeal, anal sites; culture swabs should be plastic or wire shafts with rayon or Dacron tips (*cotton tips are toxic to GC* and CT).

    4. Consider testing for HIV and other STIs.

  D. Recommended treatment first line

    1. Urogenital, rectal, conjunctival, and pharyngeal infection

      (a) Preferred treatment: doxycycline 100 mg bid for 7 days

      (b) Alternative option if pregnant or suspected problems with adherence to full doxycycline treatment: azithromycin 1 g once (observe dosing)

      (c) If treating empirically and suspect *N. gonorrhoeae, also* treat with ceftriaxone 500 mg IM once.

    2. Proctitis: doxycycline 100 mg bid for 7 days and ceftriaxone 500 mg IM *once*

    3. If pregnant

      (a) Azithromycin 1 g PO once

      (b) Erythromycin base 250 mg qid for 14 days (if unable to take azithromycin)

      (c) Amoxicillin 500 mg tid for 7 days

  E. Alternative treatment for 7 days (caution with pregnancy or lactation; for ≥ 18 yr of age).

    1. Levofloxacin 500 mg daily

    2. Ofloxacin 300 mg bid

  F. When treating CT, consider *N. gonorrhoeae* and treat if needed (see D, 1, (c) above).

  G. Consider treating all sexual partners exposed within the last 60 days.

  H. Avoid sexual intercourse until 7 day therapy is completed (or for 7 days after single-dose therapy).

  I. Return for repeat "test of cure" in 3 mo.

  J. Report infection to the health department.

  K. ***Referral to infectious disease specialist if symptoms persist and test of cure is positive.***

II. Genital warts (Condylomata Acuminata) (see Figs. 10.2 and 10.3).

  A. Definition: viral lesion caused by HPV (usually serotypes 6 and 11), asymptomatic and commonly found in anogenital area and spread by direct physical contact.

    1. Increases risk of vulvar and cervical cancers

    2. Most common STI; highly contagious

    3. Condoms decrease the risk but will not be protective because the virus infects areas not covered by condom.

    4. Lesions may occur up to 3–6 mo after exposure and may remain up to 2 yr (with or without treatment).

    5. Can be transmitted vertically during birth.

  B. Signs and symptoms

    1. Usually small, singular, or multiple papules or plaques; with a typical "cauliflower" appearance; can be flat, pedunculated, or rough

    2. Warts can be found on the vulva, in the vaginal or anal opening, under the foreskin of the penis, or on the scrotum; warts may be large enough to limit vaginal, urethral, or anal opening.

    3. Depending on the size and location, warts can be painful and pruritic.

    4. May regress spontaneously.

● = *non-urgent referral*

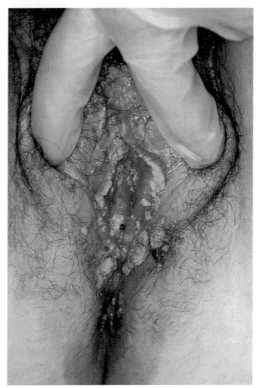

Fig. 10.2 Genital warts. Numerous warts are present on the vulva and vaginal areas. Secondary syphillis may have similar presentation. (From Habif T.P. (2021). *Sexually transmitted viral infections. In Clinical Dermatology: A Color Guide to Diagnosis and Therapy* (7th ed.). Elsevier.)

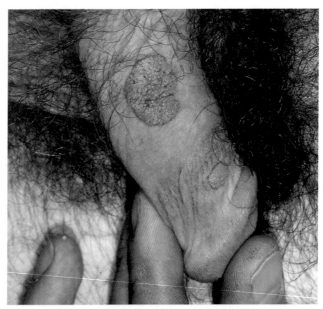

Fig. 10.3 Genital warts. Broad-based wart on shaft of a penis. There are numerous projections on the surface. (From Dinulos, G. H. (2021). *Clinical Dermatology: A color guide in diagnosis and therapy* (7th ed.). Elsevier.)

C. Diagnostic testing
   1. Visual inspection is usually sufficient, but if treating, check urine hCG.
   2. If no resolution after treatment or worsening with treatment, consider biopsy.
   3. If post-menopausal woman has "warty-appearing lesions" in genital area, consider biopsy first (she may have vulvar epithelial neoplasia).
D. Treatment probably does not eradicate HPV infection but can reduce the size and alleviate symptoms, with some wart-free periods.
   1. Warts located on moist surfaces respond best to topical therapies; therapy may take as long as 3 mo to ablate lesions.
      (a) Results improve if < 6 warts.
      (b) If no response to treatment in 3–6 wk, consider switching to another treatment.
   2. Patient-applied therapies (avoid with pregnancy)
      (a) Podofilox 0.5% *solution* (for vulva) or podofilox 0.5% *gel* (Condylox) (for perianal)
         (i) Apply with a cotton swab to visible warts bid for 3 days, followed by no therapy for 4 days.
         (ii) May repeat every week for 1–4 wk.
      (b) Imiquimod 5% (Aldara or Zyclara) cream (for vulva)
         (i) Apply at hs 3 times a week (Aldara) up to 16 wk or Zyclara daily for up to 8 wk; stop if resolution of symptoms occurs.
         (ii) Hand washing with soap and water before application and wash area 6–10 hr later.
      (c) Sinecatechins 15% ointment (Veregen) for vulva area
         (i) Apply to the wart tid until resolution, but not longer than 16 wk.
         (ii) Do not wash off.
         (iii) No sexual contact while the ointment is on the skin.
   3. Provider-applied therapies
      (a) Cryotherapy with liquid nitrogen q1–2wk
      (b) Podophyllin *resin* (Podocon-25) 10%–25% in compounded tincture of benzoin; use ≤ 0.5 mL/treatment.
         (i) The area of application should be small (< 10 cm^2).
         (ii) Apply weekly for 1–4 wk, and only on intact lesions.
         (iii) Apply to each wart and allow to dry before wearing clothes.
         (iv) Wash off after 1–4 hr to reduce irritation.
         (v) Avoid with pregnancy.
      (c) Trichloroacetic acid (TCA) 80%
         (i) Before application, debride area if needed and apply a small amount of Vaseline on the surrounding skin to prevent the acid from touching healthy tissue.
         (ii) For intense pain, neutralize with soap or sodium bicarb (i.e., baking soda).
         (iii) Repeat treatment q1wk up to 4–6 wk.
         (iv) Can be used with *both vulvar and vaginal warts* and in pregnant women.
      (d) Surgical removal with sharp instrument, laser, curettage or electrocautery; will need anesthesia to area.
   4. Patient education
      (a) Sitz baths, loose clothing, acetaminophen for pain
      (b) Avoid sexual intercourse until all lesions are healed; recommend condoms.
      (c) Cervical cancer screening annually especially if anogenital warts.
      (d) Follow up immediately if warts recur.

  5. Recommend HPV immunizations.
    (a) Gardasil 9 (9vHPV) for males and females.
      (i) ≥9 to 14 yr of age: two dose series, 6 mo apart or three dose series at 0, 2, and 6 mo apart
      (ii) 15–45 yr of age and high-risk persons (e.g., immunocompromised, HIV) should receive 3 dose series.
      (iii) If doses are <5 mo between two dose series and <5 mo between first and third dose of 3 dose series, then a booster needs to be given at the appropriate interval.
      (iv) If patient has completed a valid series of any HPV vaccine, no additional doses are required.
    (b) Not recommended during pregnancy but if she becomes pregnant on series, no intervention is required.
  E. *Referral to a dermatologist, plastic surgeon or GYN for possible surgical or laser therapy to excise or ablate multiple lesions*

III. Gonorrhea
  A. Definition
    1. Infection caused by *N. gonorrhoeae,* involving any mucus membrane (e.g., commonly genitalia, but also pharynx, rectum or eyes); may disseminate into joints, endocardium, and meninges.
    2. After exposure, approximately 60%–90% of women become infected.
    3. If untreated, approximately 15% will have PID with increased risk of infertility.
  B. Signs and symptoms
    1. Men and women
      (a) May be asymptomatic
      (b) May see rectal discharge with erythema at anal opening
      (c) Maculopapular rash over body including palms and soles
      (d) Pharyngeal erythema, tonsillar enlargement and discharge with cervical adenopathy
    2. Men commonly have dysuria, urinary frequency, purulent penile discharge, and prostate tenderness.
    3. Women may have purulent vaginal discharge with lower abdominal pain, abnormal menses, and dysuria. *Additional GYN* findings may include
      (a) Positive CMT
      (b) Enlarged Skene's and Bartholin glands
      (c) Red, friable cervix with purulent discharge
  C. Diagnostic testing
    1. Preferred: Urine NAAT (for men); endocervical NAAT swab (for women); alternative is urine for both men and women if unable to do cervical swab.
    2. Urine hCG
    3. Culture of posterior oropharynx, anal orifice, and conjunctiva
    4. C&S (if NAAT unavailable) of any source; use swabs with plastic or wire shafts with rayon or Dacron tips (cotton tips are toxic to *N. gonorrhoeae*).
    5. Consider testing for HIV and other STIs.
  D. Pharmacological Treatment
    1. Recommended therapy
      (i) Ceftriaxone 500 mg IM if <150 kg or 1000 mg IM if ≥150 kg; used for all sites of uncomplicated infection; *one time dose.*

● = *non-urgent referral*

   (ii) If chlamydia not confirmed but possibility, treat with doxycycline 100 mg bid for 7 days.
  2. If pregnant: azithromycin 1 g single dose.
  3. Alternative therapy (if ceftriaxone not available or known allergy)
   (a) Gentamicin 240 mg IM *plus* azithromycin 2 g orally once *or*
   (b) Cefixime 800 mg PO once; if chlamydia possibility, add doxycycline 100 mg bid for 7 days.
  4. Avoid sexual intercourse until therapy is completed (or for 7 days after single-dose therapy).
  5. Encourage sexual partner(s) to get screened, but if unwilling, consider treating sexual partners exposed within the last 60 days if allowed by state law.
   (a) Treat with cefixime 800 mg single dose.
   (b) If unsure of chlamydia infection add either doxycycline 100 mg bid for 7 days (if not pregnant).
  6. Test of cure (retesting after infection)
   (a) If uncomplicated GC and symptoms resolved, retest in 3 mo.
   (b) If *oropharyngeal infection,* retest with NAAT or culture 14 days after treatment.
   (c) If reinfection suspected, obtain culture and repeat with same antibiotic regimen.
   (d) If drug resistance suspected, consider increasing dose of ceftriaxone and adding azithromycin 2 g once.
  7. Report the infection to the health department.
 E. ***Referral to infectious disease specialist if continued positive test of cure or oropharyngeal infection***
IV. Herpes Genitalis (see Figs. 10.4 and 10.5).
 A. Definition: chronic, life-long sexually transmitted viral infection
  1. Many people are asymptomatic and unaware of transmission to others.
  2. Two types: HSV-1 (usually oral-labial, see Fig. 5.16) and HSV-2 (usually genital, see Figs. 10.4 and 10.5); however, either one can infect any mucous membrane; virus remains in the ganglia after infection.
  3. Initial episode may last up to 4 wk if untreated (if treated, may last up to 7–10 days) and recurrent episodes (common) are usually milder and of shorter duration.
  4. Possible triggers after initial infection
   (a) Stress, illness, fever
   (b) Menstrual changes, intercourse, trauma
   (c) Fatigue, poor nutrition
 B. Signs and symptoms
  1. May have "flulike" illness with first outbreak along with inguinal lymphadenopathy, watery vaginal discharge, and dysuria.
  2. Begins with grouped vesicular lesions, followed by an ulcerated area on an erythematous base; vesicles appear "punched-out" on the skin; the surrounding skin may be spared of redness or swelling (see Figs. 10.4 and 10.5).
  3. Prodromal symptoms may include tingling, pain or paresthesias of buttocks, thighs, legs ("boxer shorts" area) or wherever initial infection was seen; *this may be the first sign of recurrent infection.*
 C. Diagnostic testing
  1. Do not screen asymptomatic patients
  2. Urine hCG

● = *non-urgent referral*

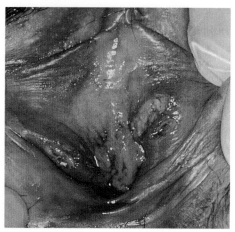

Fig. 10.4 Primary vulvar herpes. (From Johnston, C., Morrow, R. A., Moreland, A., Wald, A. (2010). *Atlas of sexually transmitted diseases and AIDS* (4th ed.). Elsevier Limited.)

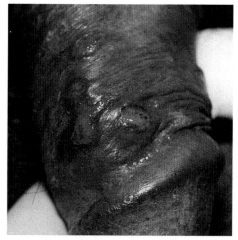

Fig. 10.5 Genital herpes on male. (From Morse, S. A., Holmes, S. A., Ballard, R. C. (2010). *Atlas of sexually transmitted diseases and AIDS* (4th ed.). Elsevier Limited.)

3. Lesion: HSV PCR assay of lesion with typing for HSV-1 and HSV-2 (most sensitive) or viral culture for herpes
4. STI testing for GC/CT, BV and HIV

D. Treatment the same for HSV-1 and HSV-2 in genital area.

1. *Initial outbreak treatment for 7–10 days;* should be started within 72 hr for best results, but do not withhold medications if patient presents after 72 hr; medications can be extended if symptoms present after 10 days.

   (a) Acyclovir 400 mg tid *or* 200 mg 5 times a day
   (b) Famciclovir 250 mg tid
   (c) Valacyclovir 1000 mg bid

2. *Episodic/recurrent therapy* (< 6 episodes/yr with mild symptoms): start within first 24 hr of infection.
   (a) Acyclovir: 800 mg bid for 5 days *or* tid for 2 days *or* 400 mg tid for 5 days
   (b) Famciclovir: 125 mg bid for 5 days *or* 1000 mg bid for 1 day *or* 500 mg once followed by 250 mg bid for 2 days
   (c) Valacyclovir: 500 mg bid for 3 days *or* 1000 mg daily for 5 days
3. *Suppressive therapy* (e.g., for ≥ 6 outbreaks/yr) requires daily therapy.
   (a) Acyclovir 400 mg bid
   (b) Famciclovir 250 mg bid
   (c) Valacyclovir 500 mg or 1 g daily
4. Reevaluate annually and provide the patient with refills for immediate self-treatment.
5. General treatment considerations
   1. Warm, wet soaks to the genital area using vinegar/water; gently pat dry perineal area (do not rub)
   2. Use water spray bottle for cleansing after urination or stooling; gently pat dry perineal area (do not rub).
   3. No feminine hygiene products or douching, no feminine pads; if concerned about discharge, have extra underwear available.
   4. Sleep without underwear or clothing in the genital area.
   5. Wear loose-fitting all-cotton clothing and underwear.
   6. No intercourse while the lesions are active or any symptoms are present.
   7. If symptoms are severe and urination is affected, may need to use topical xylocaine before urination or may consider intermittent or indwelling catheter for short period of time for comfort.
   8. OTC pain medications such as NSAIDs or acetaminophen.
   9. Use condoms for all sexual encounters after symptoms have resolved; this may decrease the risk of transmission.
   10. Advise patients that the virus can spread even without the symptoms being present and that asymptomatic spread is more common in the first year of infection.
   11. Educate about prodromal symptoms (e.g., tingling, paresthesia, and pain) to watch for and when to start treatment. Virus is highly infectious when prodromal symptoms are present.

V. Pelvic Inflammatory Disease
   A. Definition: inflammatory/infective syndrome that affects organs of reproduction and can affect surrounding structures.
      1. Infection usually starts in the vagina and ascends into the fallopian tubes and uterus.
      2. Early diagnosis will minimize long-term complications (e.g., infertility).
      3. Usually caused by *N. gonorrhoeae, Chlamydia trachomatis, Escherichia coli,* group A streptococci, *Mycoplasma genitalium,* or *Gardnerella vaginalis.*
      4. Commonly occurs in younger, sexually active females with multiple partners, prior hx of STI or PID; any instrumentation of the cervix increases risk for PID
   B. Signs and symptoms
      1. Lower abdominal pain of approximately 2 wk with tenderness; worsens with movement and intercourse
      2. Physical exam elicits
         (a) Adnexal tenderness and/or mass
         (b) Cervical motion tenderness (CMT) (highest sensitivity)
         (c) Purulent endocervical exudate (highest specificity)

  3. Additional criteria
       (a) Oral temperature > 101 °F, N/V
       (b) AUB (intermenstrual or after sex)
       (c) Dysuria, urinary frequency
 C. Diagnostic testing
      1. May see elevation in WBC, ESR, C-reactive protein.
      2. NAAT swab for *N. gonorrhoeae (GC)* or *C. trachomatis* (CT); HIV and syphilis
      3. Transvaginal or pelvic U/S may show thickened, fluid-filled tubes or free pelvic fluid.
      4. Urine hCG (*do not miss pregnancy*)
 D. Treatment

▲   1. ***Referral to ED if severe infection (e.g., high fever, N/V) requiring IV antibiotics.***
       2. Outpatient treatment (oral antibiotics are given for 14 days); if suspect PID, treat presumptively to prevent serious reproductive problems.
            (a) Ceftriaxone 500 mg IM once *plus* doxycycline 100 mg bid *plus* metronidazole 500 mg bid   *or*
            (b) Cefoxitin 2 g IM once *plus* probenecid 1 g once *plus* doxycycline 100 mg bid *with* metronidazole 500 mg bid   *or*
            (c) Levofloxacin 500 mg daily *or* moxifloxacin 400 mg daily *or* ofloxacin 400 mg bid *with* metronidazole 500 mg bid; (caution if < 18 yr old); high rates of resistance with fluoroquinolones, use if patient is low risk

▲   3. ***Patient should respond to treatment within 72 hr; if worsening, referral for hospitalization;*** if improving, follow-up in 4–6 wk.
       4. Male partners should be treated for GC/CT if sexual contact has occurred within 2 months of infection.
       5. Consider HIV testing and counseling

▲ E. ***Referral to OB if the patient is pregnant***
 VI. Syphilis.
 A. Definition: systemic disease caused by *Treponema pallidum*
      1. Incubation period is 10–90 days
      2. Recent outbreaks of syphilis have been associated with increases in HIV infection, drug use, and poverty conditions.
 B. Signs and symptoms (may occur at any stage, up to 30 yr after exposure)
      1. Primary syphilis consists of
            (a) Single painless firm, round ulcer (chancre) at site of infection that usually heals in 3–6 wk
            (b) Enlarged lymph nodes
      2. Secondary syphilis consists of
            (a) Nonpruritic rough, reddish brown macular rash on torso, hands, and feet; may have a benign, painless cutaneous lesion in genital area (condyloma lata)
            (b) Raised white lesions in warm, moist areas of mouth or perineum
            (c) "Moth-eaten" alopecia affecting scalp, eyebrows and beard
            (d) Fever, malaise, H/A, myalgias and weight loss
      3. Early latent stage may have no obvious S/S but disease can be transmitted.
            (a) Occurs within first year of infection
            (b) Serology test will be positive

▲ = *urgent referral*

4. Late syphilis (tertiary) and neurosyphilis are usually asymptomatic for years before symptoms occur and include progressive cardiovascular, skin, and neurologic S/S.
   (a) Dementia
   (b) Gradual blindness and deafness
   (c) Loss of coordination, paralysis, numbness
   (d) Aortic dilation and aortic valve regurgitation, ascending aortic arch calcification.
   (e) Skin manifestation with ulcers and elevated round, irregular, serpiginous-shaped lesions (gummas) usually seen in HIV+ person.

C. Diagnostic testing should involve *both* treponemal test (e.g., FTA-ABS or TP-EIA) and nontreponemal tests (e.g., RPR and VDRL) for confirmation.
   1. Treponemal tests remain positive for life. Question patient if they have had syphilis in the past.
   2. Test for HIV, GC/CT, hepatitis B and C at same time.

D. Treatment
   1. Primary stage: benzathine penicillin G 2.4 million units IM once *or* amoxicillin 3 g + probenecid 500 mg PO bid for 14 days
   2. If allergic to penicillin: doxycycline 100 mg bid *or* tetracycline 500 mg qid for 14 days

E. *Referral to infectious disease specialist and health department at earliest opportunity because lifelong follow-up is recommended, even if "cured"*

VII. Trichomoniasis Vaginitis
A. Definition: infection caused by *Trichomonas vaginalis*, flagellated protozoan found in the vagina (see Fig. 1.8); is considered an STI and one of the most common infections causing vaginitis in women and urethritis in men.
B. Signs and symptoms vary from mild to severe
   1. Vulvar redness with yellow-green frothy discharge with foul odor noted at vaginal opening and in vaginal vault; cervix has numerous small hemorrhages (strawberry cervix).
   2. Vulvar itching/burning
   3. Lower abdominal pain, pain with intercourse and bleeding after intercourse
   4. Dysuria, urinary frequency
   5. Symptoms may increase after intercourse or during/after menses.
C. Diagnostic testing
   1. Wet prep of both vaginal secretions and urine may show trichomonads (see Fig. 1.8) (trichomonads can be seen in urine specimen).
      (a) Perform microscopy as soon as specimen obtained.
      (b) *Must keep slide moist and warm for better visualization;* if secretions are dried or cooled on slide, trichomonads are less active and poorly visualized.
   2. WBC > 10/hpf with mixed flora can be seen in urine.
   3. Whiff test may be positive for amine odor.
   4. pH 5.0–6.0
   5. Commercial testing with rapid antigen test vaginal swab (Trichomonas Rapid Test) or NAAT test on vaginal or urine sample (e.g., APTIMA trichomonas test); if testing males, use culture or NAAT swab.
D. Treatment should include partner.
   1. Initial treatment for women
      (a) Metronidazole 2 g orally once *or* metronidazole 500 mg bid for 7 days *or*
      (b) Tinidazole 2 g orally once *or* tinidazole 500 mg bid for 7 days *or*
      (c) Secnidazole 2 g orally once

● = *non-urgent referral*

2. Initial treatment for men
    (a) Metronidazole *or* tinidazole 2 g orally once
    (b) Improved compliance has been noted
3. Recurrent or reinfection usually due to poor compliance with past treatment; consider
    (a) Metronidazole 500 mg bid for 7 days *or* metronidazole 2 g daily for 7 days   *or*
    (b) Tinidazole 2 g daily for 7 days
4. Intravaginal treatment(s) are the least effective.
5. If allergic to "nidazoles," consider desensitization therapy since these are the only drugs effective for trichomonads.
6. Follow up with patient in 2 wk to 3 mo for retest using NAAT.
7. No sexual intercourse for 7 days after treatment; if on metronidazole, no alcohol during and for 5 days after treatment.

E. Prevention
    1. Consistent use of condoms and limiting number of sexual partners
    2. Nonoxynol-9, a spermicidal agent, can decrease the risk of transmission.
F. ***Referral to GYN if symptoms persist or if pregnant***

Breast Disorders

BREAST PAIN (MASTALGIA)

I. Definition
A. Cyclical pain (formerly called fibrocystic breast disease)
    1. Usually caused by hormonal fluctuations; commonly occurs later in the menstrual cycle, usually about 2 wk prior to cycle starting, and resolves when cycle ends.
    2. Pain may be either consistent or cyclic and is usually bilateral and diffuse.
    3. *May* have breast lumps during the same time period.
    4. May be caused from HRT or new or changed OCs.
    5. Pain is an unusual finding in breast cancer; if present, pain is usually unilateral and lumps are usually fixed and nontender.
B. Noncyclical pain (i.e., no association with menstrual cycle)
    1. May be unilateral and diffuse and in different locations.
    2. May be caused by
        (a) Large, pendulous breasts
        (b) High-fat diets, smoking, caffeine
        (c) Breast cysts that do not resolve between menstrual cycles
        (d) Infection in breast (mastitis) or other sites (e.g., axillary infection), pregnancy, or inflammatory cancer
C. Referred pain from
    1. Cervical arthritis
    2. Chest wall from overuse of pectoralis muscle or costochondritis
    3. Trauma
II. HPI
A. Where is the pain located, is it unilateral or bilateral? Describe the pain (sharp, dull, shooting); is it related to your menstrual cycle? Have you started any type of hormonal therapy?
B. Have you been doing any strenuous exercises or repetitive actions?

⬤ = *non-urgent referral*

    C. Do you have arthritis in upper thorax or shoulders?

    D. Are you able to do ADL?

    E. Have you had any trauma recently to chest or upper back?

    F. Any fevers, malaise, breast swelling, redness?

III. Physical examination

    A. With patient in sitting position, describe breasts in relation to symmetry and nipple alignment.

    B. In supine position, palpate breasts to determine where pain is located; document on a valid picture noting quadrants of breast.

       1. Describe location of pain and if diffuse or localized.

       2. Describe texture of breast tissue and any abnormal appearance or feel of skin.

       3. If nodule present: document size, smoothness, and mobility of nodule(s).

       4. Note any nipple discharge and its color, odor, and consistency.

       5. *Note any skin changes (orange peel), bloody nipple discharge, or fixed asymmetrically shaped nodules;* benign nodules are usually of varying sizes and shapes and are well defined and mobile.

IV. Diagnostic testing: Diagnostic mammogram and/or U/S if indicated; consider 3D mammography (if available).

V. Treatment

    A. Decrease or stop caffeine, tea, chocolate, and nicotine.

    B. Wear a good supportive bra.

    C. Apply hot or cold compresses to breast when pain occurs.

    D. NSAID of choice

    E. Vitamin E 1000 IU 1 tab daily and/or vitamin B6 50–100 mg 1 tab daily (may help with pain if started early)

    F. Switch to COCs with lowest estrogenic activity or discontinue use.

    G. Monitor in office q2–3mo for breast pain without obvious reason.

    H. Discuss surgery for breast reduction if pain directly related to large, pendulous breasts.

VI. *Referral to*

    A. *Breast surgeon if nodules are painful or a biopsy is needed*

    B. *Orthopedist for chest wall pain*

    C. *Neurologist for cervical spine issues*

    D. *Plastic surgeon for breast reduction*

MASTITIS

  I. Definition: localized inflammation of breast either from lactation or other disease

 II. Lactational mastitis usually occurs within first 3 mo of breastfeeding and if symptoms continue past 24 hr, stagnant milk has bacteria and infection ensues.

    A. Causes

       1. Blockage of mild duct(s), poor feeding techniques, infrequent feedings

       2. Nipple cracking or swelling; weaning too quickly

       3. Maternal illness, stress, fatigue or malnutrition

    B. Signs and symptoms

       1. Breast is red, hot, and painful with firmness to touch; usually unilateral.

       2. Fever, chills, malaise, purulent discharge from nipple

       3. Pain worsens with nursing and there is a decrease in milk production.

■ = not to be missed; ● = non-urgent referral;

   C. Nonpharmacological treatment for nonsevere mastitis
      1. Continue breastfeeding with complete emptying of breast; if unable, then will need to pump milk routinely until infection clears; consider referral to certified lactation specialist if unresolved.
      2. Cold compresses 3–4 times a day
      3. Increase fluid intake, encourage warm showers and rest.
      4. NSAIDs q6–8hr as needed for pain
   D. Pharmacological treatment for more severe symptoms lasting > 24 hr; antibiotics for 10–14 days to prevent relapse; if rapid response, can decrease to 5–7 days.
      1. Dicloxacillin 500 mg qid   *or*
      2. Cephalexin 500 mg qid   *or*
      3. Erythromycin 500 mg bid   *or*
      4. Clindamycin 300 mg tid; caution due to risk of CDI (see Chapter 9, DIARRHEA, **VIII**, C-difficile)
   E. Follow up in office in 2–3 days; if not responding to antibiotic, switch antibiotics and obtain breast U/S to rule out abscess.
   F. *Candida* infection can cause similar symptoms but with a different presentation.
      1. Pain out of proportion to examination but generally no systemic signs of infection
      2. Shiny, flaky skin on nipple
      3. History of infant with oral thrush or mother with vaginal yeast infection
      4. Pharmacological treatment
         (a) Topical clotrimazole 1% cream or miconazole 2% cream bid; wash off prior to nursing   *or*
         (b) Gentian violet 1% in water: apply to nipples; causes staining   *or*
         (c) Fluconazole (Diflucan) 400 mg day 1, then 200 mg daily × 14 days
         (d) *Treat infant* (if symptoms of thrush present) with nystatin 100,000 units/g, 0.5 mL to each side of mouth qid until resolved
         (e) If candida infection suspected, *all* artificial nipples on bottles or pacifier should be thrown away; purchase new artificial nipples after 48 hr of treatment.
III. Nonlactational mastitis is inflammatory disease of ducts surrounding the areola.
   A. Can occur at any age or in males or females.
   B. Signs and symptoms may be related to an existing mass in breast or areola/nipple ductal blockage.
      1. May have nipple retraction with cheesy discharge
      2. Enlarged, painful axillary lymph node
      3. Red streaks noted from source of infection
      4. Palpable breast mass
   C. Diagnostic testing with
      1. Culture of discharge
      2. Consider U/S and/or diagnostic mammogram
   D. Treatment for 10–14 days; if rapid response to antibiotic, can decrease treatment to 5–7 days.
      1. Amoxicillin/clavulanate 875 mg bid   *or*
      2. Cephalexin 500 mg qid   *or*
      3. Dicloxacillin 500 mg qid
      4. If suspect MRSA infection: TMP-SMX DS or doxycycline 100 mg 1 tab bid
   E. Follow up in 2–3 days; if not improving, obtain breast U/S and diagnostic mammogram.
   F. ***Referral to breast specialist or surgeon specializing in breast disease***

⬤ = *non-urgent referral*

NIPPLE DISCHARGE

I. Physiological causes
   A. Pregnancy and lactation or recent lactation (e.g., bilateral clear to straw colored with early pregnancy)
   B. COC use
   C. Overstimulation of breasts
   D. Cysts (e.g., unilateral discharge, which is usually serous to greenish color)
   E. Nipple piercing
   F. Cloudy/milky appearance may be common in premenopausal women and is usually bilateral and painless.
II. Pharmacological causes include the following
   A. Estrogen products, herbal products with estrogenic effects
   B. Metoclopramide
   C. Psychiatric medications
      1. Clomipramine
      2. Risperidone
      3. Fluphenazine
      4. Haloperidol
III. Pathological causes are usually unilateral, persistent, spontaneous, and localized to a single duct noted on the nipple.
   A. Cancer (e.g., unilateral discharge, usually clear to bloody color)
   B. Pituitary lesion causing hyperprolactinemia
   C. Severe head trauma, extensive thoracic surgery
   D. Mammary duct ectasia (e.g., sticky green-black discharge) or benign papilloma
   E. Infection (usually associated with breast pain)
IV. Pertinent HPI
   A. When was discharge first noticed? Is it from one or both nipples? What is the relationship to menstrual cycles? Is there an increase in discharge with manual manipulation of breast?
   B. What is color, consistency, and any odor related to nipple discharge?
   C. Is there any pain, masses, tenderness, or nipple retraction? Any changes in the texture of the breast tissue?
   D. Are there any new H/As or vision changes?
   E. What prescription and herbal medications are you taking? Have you recently started any new medications?
   F. Are you pregnant, breastfeeding, or recently stopped breastfeeding?
   G. Have you experienced any recent trauma to chest?
V. Signs and symptoms
   A. Noticeable breast pain especially with pressure (when lying on chest)
   B. Lump that is/is not painful with pressure
   C. Discharge noted on bra or with manipulation of breast
   D. Odor
   E. Lymph node involvement in neck, axilla, or chest
VI. Physical examination
   A. Breast examination for nodules and any changes in the appearance of breast (e.g., orange peel, dimpling, or swelling); document any differences in examination noted with position changes.
   B. Observe discharge from nipples for color and if it is unilateral or bilateral ductal discharge.

      C. Other body systems: skin, axillary or supraclavicular lymph nodes, visual field defects, weight gain/loss, liver tenderness

VII. Diagnostic testing

      A. CBC, TSH, prolactin level, urine hCG (if childbearing age)

      B. Diagnostic mammogram, breast U/S, or 3D mammogram if

         1. Bloody or unilateral discharge

         2. Any discharge associated with lump or changes in breast skin appearance

VIII. Treatment

      A. ***Referral to a surgeon for further evaluation if diagnostic testing is abnormal.***

      B. If mammogram is normal or fibrocystic disease is noted

         1. Discourage manual manipulation of breasts.

         2. Follow up in office q3–6mo until resolved.

⬤ = *non-urgent referral*

Urinary Tract Conditions

- Gross hematuria (e.g., pink, red, cola color) and dysuria
  - If at the beginning of urine stream, consider urethral dysfunction.
  - If at the end of urine stream, consider trigone, bladder, or prostate cause.
  - If throughout voiding, consider renal, ureteral, or bladder pathology.
  - If cyclic with menses, consider endometriosis of the urinary tract.
- Microscopic hematuria
  - Defined as positive occult blood in two out of three urine samples, with ≥3 RBCs/hpf.
  - Urine should be collected and tested in the same manner each time.
  - Exclude benign causes of microscopic hematuria such as menstruation, vigorous exercise, sexual activity, viral illness, trauma, or infection.
- If concerned for primary renal disease because of microscopic hematuria, red cell casts, proteinuria, and elevated serum creatinine or if the patient is >40 yr of age: obtain renal U/S and depending on results, **consider referral to a nephrologist or urologist for evaluation.**
- If concerned about bladder disease: assess smoking history, irritative voiding symptoms, or history of recurrent bladder infection; **referral for urology consultation.**
- Chronic WBCs too numerous to count (TNTC) on repeat UAs with negative culture: check CBC (if leukocytes >20,000 mm³, consider **leukocytic leukemia**).
- With complaints of *new-onset* nocturia: consider polyuria associated with DM or HF, bladder irritability from caffeine or other stimulant drugs, or incomplete emptying caused by obstruction from a tumor, stool, or an enlarged prostate. Evaluate the problem and treat as needed.
- Elderly patients
  - Chronic WBCs under the microscope with few to no signs of UTI should be evaluated with a catheter specimen; if elevated WBCs are due to poor midstream UA technique, WBCs will be in the normal range under a microscope.
  - Treatment of *asymptomatic* bacteriuria leads to antibiotic resistance; treat *only* if symptoms are present.
  - Consider UTI or sepsis with acute confusion, lethargy, N/V, or diarrhea; obtain urine specimen as soon as possible.

PSA Guidelines
- Prior to initiating screening, review benefits/concerns regarding findings
- Screening routinely done with PSA; DRE may or may not be indicated for *screening*
- Screening for average risk men
  - ≥50 yr of age
  - >10 yr of life expectancy remaining
- Screening for high-risk men
  - 40–45 yr of age
  - Black men
  - First degree relative with prostate cancer diagnosed <65 yr of age

Continued

■ = *not to be missed;* ● = *non-urgent referral*

PRACTICE PEARLS FOR URINARY TRACT CONDITIONS — CONT'D

- Screening can be done q2–4yr if normal values (e.g., <4ng/mL) and low risk; annually if high risk. *Routine screening* can be stopped after 70yr of age or if life expectancy is <10yr.
- If initial screening PSA is elevated, repeat PSA in 6–8wk and ask the man to refrain from ejaculation or bike riding for at least 2days prior to test; *if still elevated then referral to urologist.*
- If the PSA is elevated on screening and treatment for prostatitis initiated, recheck PSA 6–8wk after symptoms resolve.
- Screen PSA 2wk after any instrumentation and 6wk after biopsy.
- False-positive results for PSA can occur with
  - Acute/chronic prostatitis: usually returns to normal baseline within 8–12wk after symptoms resolve.
  - Prostate biopsy: should start to return to baseline in 2–4wk but do not repeat PSA for at least 6wk.
  - Urinary retention: do not test PSA for at least 2wk after acute episode.
  - Recent ejaculation: can increase PSA results up to 0.8ng/mL within 48hr but should start to return to baseline within 72hr.
  - DRE has minimal effect on PSA but *consider* drawing blood for PSA prior to digital manipulation.
- *Referral to urologist:*
  - *PSA ≥4.0ng/mL after two separate tests 6–8wk apart*
  - *With abnormal prostate exam (e.g., nodules, asymmetry, or induration)*
  - *Elevated PSA with patient taking finasteride or dutasteride*

Disorders in Men and Women

BLADDER CANCER

I. Signs and symptoms
   A. Hematuria (either gross or microscopic) that persists throughout stream and *is not* associated with pain
   B. May have persistent dysuria, urgency, and frequency but no fever or infection noted
   C. May see urinary retention or new onset of urgency/overflow incontinence in a patient who was previously continent; could indicate tumor obstructing urethra
   D. May have palpable mass and/or pain in lower abdomen/suprapubic area
   E. Unintentional weight loss, loss of appetite, and unexplained fatigue
II. Diagnostic testing
   A. Urine dipstick is positive for blood and protein with possible leukocytes
   B. Microscopic examination shows WBCs >2–3/hpf, RBCs >10/hpf, but no RBC casts
   C. Consider renal and bladder U/S
III. *Referral to urologist*

CHRONIC KIDNEY DISEASE

I. Definition: 3mo or longer of documented kidney damage (e.g., albumin excretion >30mg daily or RBC, WBC or fatty casts) or decreased kidney function (e.g., eGFR <60mL/min)

= non-urgent referral

II. CKD staging based on eGFR and albuminuria is used to diagnose and monitor progression of kidney disease
- A. eGFR (estimated with serum creatinine and eGFR equations)
  1. Stage 1: (normal) eGFR >90 mL/min
  2. Stage 2: eGFR 60–89 mL/min
  3. Stage 3a: eGFR 45–59 mL/min and may also see anemia, PAD, and osteoporosis
  4. Stage 3b: eGFR 30–44 mL/min and may also see anemia and osteoporosis
  5. Stage 4: eGFR 15–29 mL/min
  6. Stage 5: eGFR <15 mL/min
- B. Albuminuria is measured with urine albumin/creatinine ratio (UACR) (>30 mg/g is abnormal).
  1. UACR 30–300 mg/g: moderately increased (microalbuminuria)
  2. UACR >300 mg/g: severely increased (macroalbuminuria)

III. Risk factors for CKD
- A. Poorly controlled HTN, DM
- B. Prior injury to kidney, kidney cancer, or transplant
- C. Structural abnormalities such as hydronephrosis, obstruction from renal masses, or renal artery stenosis
- D. Smoking and alcohol abuse

IV. Signs and symptoms
- A. Often asymptomatic stage 1 to stage 3b unless underlying structural damage noted
- B. May present to clinic in early stages with
  1. Hematuria
  2. Edema in face in the mornings and lower extremities in the evening
  3. Increased creatinine and protein in urine
- C. As disease progresses to stage 4 or 5, may see
  1. Fatigue, nausea, anorexia, malnutrition, alteration in taste
  2. Insomnia and cognition changes
  3. Anemia
  4. Pruritus

V. Diagnostic testing with suspected CKD
- A. CBC, iron studies, CMP (to monitor eGFR, creatinine, K^+, BUN, Ca^{2+} and phosphorus, glucose), PTH, lipid profile
- B. Urinalysis, protein/creatinine ratio, urine microalbumin (to monitor progression of ACR)
- C. Bone mineral density (BMD)
- D. Renal U/S and CT with contrast of kidney

VI. Treatment in the primary care setting (often in conjunction with nephrologist, depending on CKD stage)
- A. Aggressive management of HTN (see Chapter 8, HYPERTENSION), DM (see Chapter 15, Diabetes Mellitus, FOLLOW-UP AND TREATMENT)
  1. Initiate therapy with ACE or ARB
  2. Monitor renal function q6mo and *referral to nephrologist if creatinine and eGFR worsening*
  3. Hgb A1c q3mo (with goal of 7.0% or less)
- B. Test for anemia annually starting at stage 3; q6mo at stage 4 and q3mo with stage 5 (if not seeing nephrologist)
  1. If iron deficiency anemia is noted, oral iron supplementation should be started (see Chapter 4, ANEMIA, VII, C).

⬤ = *non-urgent referral*

    2. Recheck CBC and ferritin q3mo
    3. H/H goal is >12/36 and ferritin goal is >100
  C. BMD testing is not usually done unless bone and mineral disorder is present and
     treatment for OP is started; consider BMD at baseline and 2 yr after OP treatment
     initiated (risk of fractures increase in stages 3–5).
  D. Review dietary modifications (based on nephrologist recommendations) to include
    1. Low-sodium diet not to exceed 1500 mg daily; teach patient (and whoever shops/
       cooks, if not the patient) how to read labels for food products and sodium content
    2. Eat primarily fresh or frozen foods, fruits and vegetables and protein in moderation
    3. Eliminate phosphorus/phosphate in diet; no processed foods or dairy
    4. No frozen dinners
  E. Monitor for weight loss at home and in the office
  F. Smoking and alcohol cessation
  G. Avoid all medications that effect kidney function, including NSAIDs and TMP/
     SMZ; may need to adjust dosages of other medication(s) based on eGFR.
  H. Be sure patient has received the appropriate vaccines (influenza annually, covid, and
     pneumonia).
VII. **Criteria for** *referral to nephrologist*
  A. *eGFR <30 mL/min or decline of ~30% in 4 mo without obvious reason*
  B. *ACR >300 mg/g*
  C. *Hematuria that is not related to urological conditions; abnormal urine microscopy with
     presence of fatty casts (which can indicate nephrotic syndrome), WBC, or RBC*
  D. *Complications of CKD that are not responding to treatment or may need more in-depth
     treatment*
  E. *Hereditary kidney disease, SLE, polycystic kidneys*
  F. *Consider referral* with
    1. Serum K^+ >5.5 mEq/L
    2. Difficult to treat HTN
    3. Recurrent kidney stones
    4. Patients <18 yr of age

GLOMERULONEPHRITIS, ACUTE POSTSTREPTOCOCCAL (PSGN)

  I. Definition: acute infection in kidneys *usually* seen in children 5–12 yr of age and adults
     >60 yr of age; caused by *Streptococcus pyogenes*; symptoms usually appear approximately
     1–2 wk after infection, but can manifest up to 6 wk postinfection
 II. Signs and symptoms
   A. Acute-onset oliguria, gross hematuria, smoky/tea colored urine
   B. Edema of hands and face in the morning and feet and ankles in the evening
   C. Malaise, lethargy; back/flank pain
   D. Weight gain; HTN
III. Diagnostic testing
   A. Dipstick urinalysis shows hematuria, proteinuria
   B. Microscopic examination may show the following:
     1. WBCs >10/hpf and RBCs >10/hpf
     2. RBC casts, dysmorphic RBCs (irregularly or oddly shaped RBCs from passage
        through glomerular structures)

● = *non-urgent referral*

3. Proteinuria

C. Serum streptozyme test (can be useful with diagnosis for either past pharyngitis or skin infection)

▲ **IV.** *Transfer to ED if considering this diagnosis*

INCONTINENCE

I. Definition: any involuntary loss of urine not related to spinal cord injury or genitourinary tract trauma/surgery; use history and physical examination to determine the type of incontinence

II. Stress incontinence is loss of urine (without sensation of urgency) with any activity that increases intraabdominal pressure (e.g., physical exercise, sneezing, or coughing) in a person who is usually continent; this is the most common type of incontinence.

A. Symptoms are related to weakness of the pelvic floor musculature and urethral hypermobility

1. Usually seen in women ≥45 yr of age, especially after multiple vaginal births and with obesity

2. Usually seen in men >65 yr of age with BPH or post TURP surgery

B. Physical examination

1. Female: pelvic and rectal examination to evaluate pelvic muscle strength, perineal sensation, and grade of cystocele

(a) First degree: bladder clearly visible

(b) Second degree: bladder seen at introitus

(c) Third degree: bladder protruding from vagina

2. Male: DRE for sphincter tone, any constipated stool and prostate size and shape

C. Diagnostic testing: urinalysis to check for infection or hematuria

D. Nonpharmacological treatment

1. Weight loss, if indicated

2. Change fluid intake pattern to more frequent smaller amounts and no beverages before exercise or within 2 hr of bedtime

3. Timed voiding schedule to avoid full bladder prior to activity, outings, or bedtime

4. Avoid alcohol, caffeine, and smoking

5. Minimize constipation

6. Pelvic muscle (Kegel) exercises up to 100×/day; start slowly and gradually increase

7. Continent devices and supplies

(a) Continence pessaries

(b) Biofeedback with electrical stimulation

(c) Adult-diapers or other incontinence pads

E. Pharmacological treatment *considerations* (there are no specific medications known for treatment)

1. Pseudoephedrine 15–30 mg ~1 hr before exercise

2. Topical estrogen therapy (see Chapter 10, MENOPAUSE, II, E. 7 [Treatment vulvovaginitis])

3. Vitamin E 800–1000 IU daily

F. *Referral to urologist, GYN, or continence specialist if no improvement*

● *= non-urgent referral;* ▲ *= urgent referral*

III. Urge incontinence (UI)/overactive bladder (OAB) is an immediate sensation of urgency without warning; may be unable to reach the bathroom before leakage occurs

A. Caused by overactive, unstable detrusor muscle; leads to uncontrolled muscle contractions and can become a social and health problem

B. Signs and symptoms
   1. Urgency and frequency, as often as q1–2hr
   2. Nocturia with occasional leakage
   3. Perineal skin irritation from urine leakage, wearing pads and from frequent cleansing

C. Physical exam
   1. Female: pelvic and rectal examination to evaluate pelvic muscle strength, perineal sensation, grade of cystocele (if present)
      (a) First degree: bladder clearly visible
      (b) Second degree: bladder seen at introitus
      (c) Third degree: bladder protruding from vagina
   2. Male
      (a) DRE to evaluate anal sphincter tone, constipated stool and prostate size and shape
      (b) If uncircumcised, check for phimosis or balanitis

D. Diagnostic testing
   1. Urinalysis to check for infection or glucosuria; culture if indicated
   2. CBC, BMP

E. Nonpharmacological treatment
   1. Bladder training with planned voiding schedule (e.g., when urge is felt, stop and contract pelvic muscles 2–10 times, relax and repeat until urge subsides, then proceed to bathroom); always void prior to outings
   2. Weight loss, if indicated
   3. Treat constipation if indicated
   4. Spread out daily intake of fluids
   5. Avoid caffeine, alcohol, chocolate, and aspartame (these irritate the bladder wall)
   6. Consider adult diapers or condom catheters, especially at night or for long trips

F. Pharmacological treatment
   1. Avoid if glaucoma, chronic constipation, or urinary retention is present
   2. Avoid with uncontrolled HTN
   3. Monitor for deterioration in mental status or new or worsening signs of dementia
   4. Every 6–8 wk, evaluate treatment and any side effects
      (a) Beta-3 adrenergic agonists
         (i) Mirabegron (Myrbetriq) 25–50 mg daily
         (ii) Vibegron (Gemtesa) 75 mg daily
      (b) Antimuscarinic agents
         (i) Darifenacin (Enablex) 7.5–15 mg daily
         (ii) Trospium IR (Sanctura) 20 mg 1–2 times daily or trospium XR (Sanctura XR) 60 mg daily *on empty stomach*
         (iii) Fesoterodine (Toviaz) 4–8 mg daily
         (iv) Solifenacin (VESIcare) 5–10 mg daily
         (v) Oxybutynin IR 5 mg, 2–3 times a day or oxybutynin XR (Ditropan XL) 5–10 mg daily
         (vi) Oxybutynin transdermal patch (Oxytrol) 1 patch twice weekly to abdomen, hip, or buttock

(vii) Oxybutynin topical gel (Gelnique) once daily to abdomen, thighs, or upper arms

(viii) Tolterodine IR (Detrol) 1 mg bid or tolterodine LA (Detrol LA) 2–4 mg daily

G. *Referral to urologist if no improvement*

IV. Overflow incontinence is

A. Involuntary, intermittent or continual dribbling
   1. Usually due to chronic overdistended bladder from urinary retention or obstruction at meatus from stool or mass
   2. Often occurs more at night and can be a slowly developing process

B. Causes
   1. Bladder outlet obstruction causing occlusion of urethra
      (a) Uterine soft tissue mass (e.g., fibroids)
      (b) Cystocele/rectocele, enlarged prostate
      (c) Pelvic floor surgery causing scarring of urethral tissues
   2. Lack of contraction of detrusor muscle
      (a) Age and lack of estrogen
      (b) Neurologic disease (spinal cord injury, spinal stenosis, multiple sclerosis)
      (c) Chronic overdistention bladder from inability to get to bathroom
      (d) DM, alcoholism, B_{12} deficiency
   3. Reversible causes
      (a) Certain medications (e.g., sedatives, opioids)
      (b) Alcohol, caffeine
      (c) Fecal impaction or constipation

C. Symptoms may be very subtle
   1. Constant dribbling of urine or postvoid dribbling
   2. Incontinence with change in position (volume lost may be small amount)
   3. Sense of incomplete emptying of bladder and of overdistended bladder with pain in suprapubic area; straining to urinate
   4. Ammonia odor and irritation to perineum
   5. Onset of nocturnal enuresis from overflow of urine
   6. Weak urinary stream, frequency

D. Physical examination
   1. Female
      (a) Masses that may be occluding vaginal opening and urethra; cystocele/rectocele
      (b) Check for sensation in perineal area (saddle anesthesia)
   2. Male: DRE for prostate size and symmetry and any large amount of stool
   3. Palpate lower abdomen prior to and after voiding to assess for bladder fullness

E. Diagnostic testing
   1. Urinalysis and possible culture (catheter specimen more accurate)
   2. CBC, CMP, PSA
   3. Postvoid residual with catheter (may see amounts >500 mL)

F. Treatment
   1. If caused from fecal impaction, remove stool and start bowel program
   2. Review current medications and discontinue any that may be causing incontinence
   3. May need to place indwelling catheter initially; then begin bladder retraining
   4. May need intermittent catheterization if neurologic cause

G. *Referral to urologist or urogynecologist if not resolving*

● = *non-urgent referral*

BOX 11.1 ■ Common Causes of Transient Incontinence

Use the mnemonic **DIAPPERS**

Delirium or confusional state (can be caused by any illness or being unaware of need to void)

Infection, acute urinary (asymptomatic bacteriuria does not cause incontinence)

Atropic urethritis or vaginitis (may have vaginal erosions or friability and bladder irritation; may benefit from 3 to 6 mo of topical estrogen)

Pharmaceutical

- Sedatives or hypnotics, especially long-acting agents (may see urinary retention and with eventual overflow)
- Loop diuretics (caused by overwhelming bladder capacity in elderly)
- Anticholinergic agents (e.g., antipsychotics, antidepressants, antihistamines [e.g., diphenhydramine], anti-Parkinson agents, antiarrhythmics, antispasmodics) cause urinary retention with eventual overflow and stool impaction
- α-Adrenergic agonists (causes urinary retention, especially in males) and antagonists (cause relaxation of urinary sphincter)
- Vincristine (can cause urinary retention due to neuropathy)
- Calcium channel blockers and ACE inhibitors (can cause nocturnal diuresis from fluid retention)
- Opioids (can cause urinary retention, stool impaction)
- NSAIDs (cause nocturnal diuresis)

Psychological (depression or behavioral disorders)

Excess urine output (may be due to HF, hyperglycemia, SIADH, caffeine or alcohol)

Restricted mobility with inability to self-toilet (may be due to limited ROM in joints, hypotension, spinal stenosis, poor eyesight, fear of falling, or being restrained in chair or bed)

Stool impaction (causes excess urinary retention by blocking outlet and worsening overflow incontinence)

(Adapted from Resnick, N. M. (1990). Initial evaluation of the incontinent patient. *Journal of the American Geriatrics Society, 38*(3), 311–316.)

V. Transient incontinence is acute onset of involuntary loss of urine in a previously continent patient, usually caused by a reversible problem
   A. See Box 11.1 for Common Causes of Transient Incontinence
   B. ***Referral to urologist or urogynecologist, if no reversible cause is found***

RENAL CALCULI (KIDNEY STONES)

I. Signs and symptoms
   A. Pain
      1. Sudden onset; described as colicky and severe, intermittent, and paroxysmal
      2. *Caused by obstruction and not by movement of the stone;* if pain resolves, obstruction has been relieved, but the stone still may be present
      3. Located in the flank and usually related to obstruction in the upper ureteral or renal pelvic area
      4. Severe enough that most people cannot find a comfortable position and will "pace" to help relieve pain; the patient will frequently comment: "this is the worst pain I have ever had!"
      5. Males: may radiate to the testicle (on the same side) and usually related to lower ureteral obstruction
   B. Gross or microscopic hematuria (RBCs >3/hpf)
   C. N/V
   D. Dysuria and urgency (frequently caused by obstruction in the distal ureter)

● = *non-urgent referral*

II. Diagnostic testing

A. Dipstick urinalysis is usually normal except for blood and protein

　1. Microscopic examination shows RBCs >3/hpf

　2. With pyuria and positive nitrites, consider concurrent UTI

B. Noncontrast helical CT scan ("gold standard") for detection of stones and urinary tract obstruction

C. Consider CBC, CMP with recurrent stones

III. Treatment

▲　A. ***Urgent referral to ED if the pain is uncontrollable, urosepsis or oliguria/anuria are present, or patient is unable to keep fluids down.***

B. Most patients can be conservatively managed with the following:

　1. Pain medications

　　(a) NSAIDs (if not contraindicated) will decrease ureteral smooth muscle tone and alleviate muscle spasm, allowing stone to pass (e.g., ketorolac 10 mg tid day 1, then daily on days 2–3 [if Cr <1.6 mg/dL; do not give >5 days]; can start other NSAIDs after pain controlled (e.g., ibuprofen, diclofenac)

　　(b) Short-acting opioids (see Chapter 14, Therapies for Pain, PHARMACOLOGICAL THERAPIES, VIII) for severe pain, if unable to take NSAIDs

　2. Pharmacological therapy for stone passage in patients with stones >5 and ≤10 mm, with normal kidney function, adequate pain control, and no infection; can be given for 4–6 wk.

　　(a) Tamsulosin 0.4 mg daily

　　(b) Silodosin 8 mg daily (off label)

　　(c) Alfuzosin 10 mg daily (off label)

　3. Increase fluid intake to help passage of the stone (stones <5 mm located in the distal to middle ureter may pass spontaneously)

　4. Use urine strainer for several days after symptoms resolved; if the stone is obtained, send for analysis to help to guide future treatment

C. Prophylaxis based on dietary modifications and pharmacological therapy is lifelong.

　1. Calcium oxalate stones are the most common

　　(a) Increase fluid intake up to 2 L/day; dehydration is common cause of recurrence.

　　(b) Decrease sodium intake to <2 g/day, and *avoid calcium tablet supplementation* (this may increase the risk for further stone formation); intake of calcium foods is recommended.

　　(c) Coffee, tea, and alcohol may be associated with a lower risk of stone formation.

　　(d) Avoid grapefruit, soft drinks, spinach, rhubarb, peanuts, cashews, and almonds.

　　(e) Limit sucrose and fructose in drinks/foods and limit animal protein.

　　(f) Avoid vitamin C intake; this causes increased oxalate excretion which may increase stone formation.

　　(g) Prophylactic pharmacological therapy with thiazide diuretics (e.g., HCTZ 25 mg or chlorthalidone 12.5–25 mg daily) to lower urine calcium.

　2. Uric acid stone is the only stone that can be dissolved

　　(a) Increase fluid intake to 2 L/day

　　(b) Potassium citrate (Urocit-K) mix 15 mEq bid or 10 mEq tid

　　(c) Allopurinol 150 mg bid for hyperuricosuria and recurrent uric acid stones

---

▲ = *urgent referral*

IV. *Referral to urologist* if
1. *Recurrent renal stones with or without recurrent UTI*
2. *Ureteral stone >5 mm that have not passed in 4 wk or poor pain control*
3. *Cystine and struvite stones*
4. *Stones that are located in middle ureter or lower pole calyx*

URINARY TRACT INFECTION (FOR PEDIATRICS, SEE CHAPTER 16, UTI)

I. Acute complicated UTI (*pyelonephritis*) is infection that extends beyond the bladder
  A. Signs and symptoms (patient may present after having symptoms for several days)
  1. Adults
     (a) Fever >99.9°F, chills
     (b) Flank pain or costovertebral angle tenderness (CVAT) may be severe and is usually over the involved kidney but can be bilateral
     (c) Pyuria, dysuria, hematuria, frequency, and urgency
     (d) N/V, malaise, and anorexia
     (e) Male: pelvic or perineal pain with above symptoms; DRE may show painful prostate if infection present
  2. Elderly
     (a) Fever (less common); chills; pyuria
     (b) Mental status changes (common)
     (c) Generalized mental and physical deterioration with increase in falls
     (d) Decompensation in other organ system(s) (e.g., HF)
  B. Diagnostic testing
  1. Urine dipstick will be positive for leukocyte esterase, nitrites, blood (either occult or gross), and protein
     (a) Positive leukocyte esterase and nitrites are good indicators of infection.
     (b) Results may be inaccurate if patient is using any type of oral product that can change the color of the urine (e.g., phenazopyridine).
  2. Urine microscopy: positive for bacteria, WBCs >10–20/hpf, RBCs >3/hpf, and presence of WBC casts (may indicate kidney inflammation)
  3. Obtain urine for C&S to help guide antibiotic treatment
  4. hCG if childbearing age, consider CBC, BMP
  5. Consider plain abdominal films (may show calculi)
  6. Consider renal U/S (may show early scarring)
  C. *Referral urgently to ED if pregnant, or with severe N/V with dehydration or fever >101°F*
  D. Outpatient treatment for *mild to moderate illness: if patient can maintain hydration and pain control with oral intake, and fever is <101°F*
  1. IV fluids in office, if available, and then encourage increased intake of water or oral hydration solution (see Table 9.3) at home
  2. Antiemetics for N/V (e.g., promethazine or ondansetron)
  3. Acetaminophen or ibuprofen routinely, depending on age
  4. Antibiotics:
     (a) Ciprofloxacin 500 mg bid for 5–7 days *or*
     (b) Ciprofloxacin XR 1000 mg daily for 5–7 days *or*
     (c) Levofloxacin 750 mg daily for 5–7 days

● = *non–urgent referral;* ▲ = *urgent referral*

    (d) If allergic to fluoroquinolone, give ceftriaxone 500–1000 mg IM once, then start one of the following:
- (i) TMP-SMZ DS bid for 7–10 days (if the pathogen is known to be susceptible) *or*
- (ii) Amoxicillin/clavulanate 875 mg bid for 10–14 days *or*
- (iii) Cefdinir 300 mg bid for 10–14 days *or*
- (iv) Cefpodoxime 200 mg bid for 10–14 days

E. Follow-up care
1. Recheck in office in 24–48 hr after treatment is initiated to evaluate progress
2. *Referral to*
    - (a) *Urgently to ED if symptoms worsening with fever/pain*
    - (b) **Urologist**
        - (i) *Male with first episode of acute complicated UTI*
        - (ii) *Female with unresolved or recurrent acute complicated UTI*

II. Acute uncomplicated UTI (*cystitis*) is infection limited to bladder
A. Signs and symptoms
1. Young, nondiabetic people w/o structural defects and persons experiencing their first or second uncomplicated UTI (cystitis), may present with
    - (a) Dysuria, frequency, and urgency
    - (b) Hematuria, nocturia, incontinence in an otherwise continent person
    - (c) Afebrile
    - (d) Suprapubic pain, pain in lower back and general malaise
2. Elderly patients may present with different symptoms
    - (a) Somnolence; increased falls
    - (b) Confusion or change in normal behavior
    - (c) Decreased appetite
    - (d) Decreased urine output

B. Diagnostic testing (see Table 4.1)
1. Urinalysis with microscopic evaluation
    - (a) Dipstick results: considered positive if leukocyte esterase and nitrites are both positive, in the presence of symptoms; microscopic evaluation needed if only one is positive
    - (b) Microscopic evaluation is considered positive if
        - (i) WBCs >5/hpf or "too numerous to count" (TNTC)
        - (ii) Presence of bacteria (graded 1+ to 4+ [4+ greatest amount seen])
        - (iii) May see RBCs >3/hpf
        - (iv) If RBC or WBC casts are present, may indicate kidney involvement
2. Urine for C&S should be obtained if this is not the first UTI or in the elderly; considered positive if
    - (a) Colony count >10^5 CFU/mL in an asymptomatic patient
    - (b) Colony count 10^2–10^5 CFU/mL in a symptomatic patient
        - (i) *Escherichia coli* most common bacteria, secondary to cross-contamination.
        - (ii) *Staphylococcus aureus* could be indicative of infection outside of the kidney; check for blood or valvular infections.
        - (iii) *S. saprophyticus, Proteus, Klebsiella*, or *E. coli:* consider CT scan for kidney stones.
        - (iv) *S. saprophyticus* alone: inquire about sexual partners (this is common in young, sexually active women and can be found with vaginal candidiasis).

● = *non-urgent referral;* ▲ = *urgent referral*

   C. Lifestyle changes to help prevent UTI
     1. If using spermicides with diaphragm, consider changing type of contraceptive.
     2. Cranberry juice (sugar free) or pills at night.
     3. Increase water intake and decrease caffeine or carbonated drinks.
     4. Urinate after intercourse.
     5. If postmenopausal, consider topical estrogen products (e.g., Estring, Vagifem, Estrace cream) (see Table 10.4).
     6. Consider probiotics daily.
   D. Pain relief therapy
     1. For adults: phenazopyridine (Pyridium) 100–200 mg tid for 2–3 days
     2. Xylocaine jelly applied sparingly to urethra before urinating (can be used with adults or children)
   E. Pharmacological treatment
     1. Preferred therapy
       (a) Nitrofurantoin ER 100 mg bid for 5 days (CrCl must be >30 mL/min) *or*
       (b) TMP-SMZ DS 1 tab bid for 3 days for women and 7 days for men *or*
       (c) Fosfomycin 3 g; single dose
     2. Alternative therapy (if allergy to above medications)
       (a) Amoxicillin/clavulanate 500 mg bid for 5–7 days *or*
       (b) Cefdinir 300 mg bid for 5–7 days *or*
       (c) Cefpodoxime 100 mg bid for 5–7 days *or*
       (d) Ciprofloxacin 250 mg bid or levofloxacin 250 mg daily for 3 days
     3. In patient with bacteriuria but no symptoms, consider asymptomatic bacteriuria; usually not treated unless patient is going to have invasive procedure or is at high risk for urosepsis
     4. If uncertainty regarding site of infection and no culture results available; treat as acute complicated UTI (e.g., pyelonephritis, I, A earlier in this chapter).
   F. Follow-up
     1. Follow up in office in 48–72 hr and if not improving, obtain urine for C&S (if not done initially) and switch antibiotics.
     2. If improved, repeat urinalysis in 2 wk.
     3. If UTI symptoms return within 2–3 wk after treatment, repeat urinalysis and obtain C&S and restart antibiotics while waiting for culture results.
   G. *Referral to urologist*
     1. *Recurrent cystitis ≥3 in 1 yr (also see III, later in this chapter)*
     2. *Presence of any of the following*
       (a) *Persistent bacteriuria*
       (b) *Recurrent pyelonephritis*
       (c) *History of abdominal/pelvic cancer, outflow obstruction, past/present urologic surgery, or poorly controlled DM*
       (d) *Gross or microscopic hematuria without stones and after antibiotic treatment (especially if hematuria is painless)*
III. Recurrent cystitis (uncomplicated UTI)
   A. Definition
     1. ≥2 times in 6 mo or ≥3 times in 1 yr
     2. Reinfection by same or different bacteria, that occurs >2 wk after treatment
     3. Relapse of infection that occurs with same bacteria *within* 2 wk of treatment

---

● = *non-urgent referral*

       4. Causes can be secondary to sexual intercourse, anatomic causes in GU tract or postmenopausal atrophic changes
- B. Signs and symptoms are same as for acute uncomplicated cystitis (see **II, A**, earlier in this chapter).
- C. Lifestyle changes (see **II, C**, earlier in this chapter)
- D. Prophylactic pharmacological therapy taken for 6–12 mo
  1. TMP-SMZ SS or DS 3 times a wk *or*
  2. Nitrofurantoin 50 or 100 mg daily *or*
  3. Cephalexin 125 or 250 mg daily *or*
  4. Ciprofloxacin 125 mg daily
- E. Prophylactic pharmacological therapy for postcoital cystitis, given once within 24 hr of intercourse
  1. TMP-SMZ SS or DS *or*
  2. Nitrofurantoin 50 or 100 mg *or*
  3. Cephalexin 250 mg *or*
  4. Ciprofloxacin 125–250 mg *or*
  5. Ofloxacin 100 mg
- F. *Referral to urologist for further evaluation if symptoms continue despite treatment.*

Common Disorders in Men

BENIGN PROSTATIC HYPERTROPHY

I. Signs and symptoms usually occur in men >50 yr of age and may have a slow onset
- A. Difficulty in starting or stopping urine stream or having to strain to initiate stream
- B. Decrease in the force of the stream; postvoid dribbling
- C. Nocturia, increased daytime frequency and urgency
- D. Urge or overflow incontinence with urine retention

II. Physical exam
- A. DRE to evaluate size, symmetry, and texture of the prostate
  1. Prostate is usually symmetrically enlarged with palpation but should not be tender
  2. Tenderness may indicate prostatitis
  3. Nodular lesions or asymmetrical firmness may indicate cancer
- B. Abdominal exam for any pelvic masses
- C. Genital exam for any lesions that may be occluding meatus (e.g., warts); testicular exam for swelling or nodules

III. Diagnostic testing
- A. Urinalysis is usually normal (unless UTI present)
- B. Hematuria may be present
- C. PSA (may be normal or high; if elevated, recheck in 1–2 wk)
- D. Creatinine (should be normal)

IV. Nonpharmacological treatment
- A. Limit fluid intake to frequent smaller amounts and decrease after evening meal.
- B. Urinate frequently during the day.
- C. Avoid medications that can cause urinary retention or frequency.
  1. Alpha- and beta-adrenergics, including decongestants
  2. Anticholinergics (see Box 11.1)
  3. Antidepressants (e.g., TCAs and SSRIs)
  4. Diuretics

= *non-urgent referral*

D. Avoid fluids prior to outings or going to bed.
E. Reduce or avoid caffeine and alcohol; smoking cessation.
F. Encourage sitting to urinate and to empty bladder more completely, double void each time.
V. Pharmacological treatment to relieve symptoms that are affecting ADLs
   A. Alpha-1-receptor antagonists: relax smooth muscle in bladder neck, prostate capsule, and prostate urethra; provides benefits within 1 wk; titrate very slowly to reduce orthostatic changes (listed as follows from most side effects to least side effects).
      1. Tamsulosin (Flomax) 0.4 mg daily 30 min after a meal and can increase up to 0.8 mg daily
      2. Alfuzosin (Uroxatral) 10 mg daily; give same time each day after a meal
      3. Silodosin (Rapaflo) 8 mg daily; give same time each day after a meal
      4. Terazosin (Hytrin) 1 mg hs and can increase up to 10 mg hs
      5. Doxazosin (Cardura) 1 mg hs and can increase up to 8 mg hs
   B. 5-Alpha-reductase inhibitor: reduces size of prostate gland; no titration required; effects take up to 6–12 mo to be seen; do not use with irritative symptoms or with erectile dysfunction (ED).
      1. Finasteride (Proscar) 5 mg daily
      2. Dutasteride (Avadart) 0.5 mg daily
   C. Combination 5-alpha-reductase inhibitor + alpha-1-receptor antagonist: dutasteride/tamsulosin (Jalyn) 1 cap daily.
   D. Phosphodiesterase-5 inhibitor (PDE-5): tadalafil (Cialis) 5 mg daily; used predominantly with BPH and ED.
   E. Anticholinergics used predominantly with frequency, nocturia, and urgency symptoms and can be combined with alpha-1 blocker.
      1. Tolterodine (Detrol) 1–2 mg bid or tolterodine ER (Detrol LA) 2–4 mg daily
      2. Oxybutynin extended release (Ditropan XL) 5–10 mg daily
      3. Darifenacin (Enablex) 7.5–15 mg daily
      4. Solifenacin (Vesicare) 5–10 mg daily
      5. Trospium (Sanctura) 20 mg hs or trospium ER (Sanctura XR) 60 mg daily
      6. Fesoterodine (Toviaz) 4–8 mg daily
   F. Beta-3 adrenergic agonists work well when urgency, urge incontinence and frequency related to OAB and detrusor overactivity are present.
      1. Mirabegron (Myrbetriq) 25–50 mg daily
      2. Vibegron (Gemtesa) 75 mg daily
   G. Many of the drugs used to treat BPH are known to lower BP with position changes especially when starting treatment; *patients should be warned to change positions slowly.*
   H. OTC supplement: *Pygeum africanum* (African plum tree) or saw palmetto.
VI. *Referral to a urologist* if
   A. *Symptoms persist after treatment or worsen while on medications; worsening urinary retention*
   B. *Recurrent UTI; recurrent bladder stones or hematuria*
   C. *Pain or suspected prostatitis, with any systemic symptoms (e.g., fever)*
   D. *Renal insufficiency*

EPIDIDYMITIS

I. Signs and symptoms
   A. Tenderness on the posterior side of the affected testis that may radiate to the groin, with induration and scrotal pain and significant swelling in the scrotum

● = *non-urgent referral*

    B. *Positive* Prehn's sign (elevation of scrotum relieves pain)

    C. *Positive* cremasteric sign on affected side (testes elevates with stroking of thigh)

    D. Urinary frequency, hematuria, and cloudy urine

    E. Urethral discharge

    F. May have fever and chills

II. Diagnostic testing

    A. Urinalysis with microscopic exam shows positive bacteria and WBCs >10/hpf

    B. CBC shows elevated WBCs

    C. Obtain urine NAAT for GC/CT or consider culture of penile secretions

    D. Ultrasound of scrotal contents

III. Treatment

    A. Male <35 yr of age and sexually active, suspect GC/CT and treat with

        1. Ceftriaxone 500 mg IM once *plus*

        2. Doxycycline 100 mg bid for 10 days *or*

        3. Azithromycin 1 g PO once

    B. Male >35 yr of age, low-risk sexual activity, suspect *E. coli* or *Pseudomonas*

        1. Levofloxacin 500 mg daily for 10 days *or*

        2. TMZ DS 1 tab bid for 10 days

    C. Men of any age who engage in anal intercourse, suspect *E. coli*

        1. Ceftriaxone 500 mg IM once *plus*

        2. Levofloxacin 500 mg daily for 10 days

    D. Pain management with NSAIDs and/or acetaminophen

    E. Elevation of scrotum and when pain lessens, use scrotal support

    F. Warm-to-hot baths or compresses to scrotum

    G. Follow-up

        1. In 48–72 hr (should see improvement with less pain, no fever, and swelling may be less); *if not seeing improvement (continued or worsening pain, swelling and fever), consider scrotal U/S and referral to urologist*

        2. If positive for GC/CT, retest again in 2–3 mo and encourage partner treatment

ERECTILE DYSFUNCTION

I. Definition: inability to attain or sustain an erection, even with masturbation, sufficient to complete sexual intercourse; may be accompanied with decreased libido and abnormal ejaculation

II. Causes

    A. Drug induced

        1. Antihypertensives, diuretics

        2. Antidepressants, antipsychotics

        3. Recreational drugs and antiandrogens (e.g., progesterones)

    B. Hormone-related deficiency

        1. Decreased circulating testosterone and hypogonadism

        2. Thyroid dysfunction

        3. Cortisol excess or deficiency

        4. Elevated prolactin level, pituitary tumors

    C. Lifestyle

        1. Smoking and alcohol overuse

        2. Obesity and sedentary lifestyle

        3. Bicycling

        4. Aging

⬤ = *non-urgent referral*

    D. Neurologic
       1. Spinal cord and brain injuries
       2. Parkinson disease, dementia
       3. CVA
       4. Multiple sclerosis
    E. Physical deformity of penis
       1. Peyronie's disease
       2. Penile fracture
       3. Any anatomic deviation
    F. Psychogenic
       1. Depression, PTSD
       2. Anxiety, stress with jobs and relationships
       3. Performance stress
    G. Vascular
       1. HTN, CAD, dyslipidemia
       2. DM (uncontrolled or extended history of DM)
       3. Any type of major abdominal surgery or radiation involving perineum or prostate gland

III. HPI
    A. Sexual history
       1. Do you awaken with an erection? (i.e., no morning erection could mean vascular or neurologic damage)
       2. Has the problem occurred over time or suddenly? (i.e., sudden onset could be caused by acute GU trauma [surgery or physical injury] or depression/anxiety)
       3. With stimulation, can you achieve an erection?
       4. Can you maintain an erection long enough to engage in sexual intercourse? (i.e., inability could be related to performance anxiety)
         (a) Prior to penetration
         (b) During intercourse
         (c) Completion of intercourse
       5. Is sexual intercourse satisfactory for you or your partner? (i.e., poor satisfaction could be related to anxiety and depression)
       6. Do you ejaculate at the appropriate time and is this a new occurrence? (i.e., early ejaculation could be genetic or situational)
    B. Consider administering the International Index of Erectile Dysfunction (IIEF) questionnaire to further assist in determining the cause of ED.

IV. Physical examination, with special attention to
    A. Male genitalia (see Chapter 1, Focused Examination, GENITOURINARY (MALE))
       1. Note if there is any localized fibrosis or penile deformity (e.g., Peyronie's disease).
       2. Note size and symmetry of testicles and scrotum.
    B. Palpate abdomen for peripheral and femoral pulses (see Fig. 1.6) and listen for bruits
    C. Hair pattern in genital area, testicular size (see Box 2.1); examine breast for any enlargement
    D. Test cremasteric reflex (e.g., positive if contraction of scrotum and elevation of testis occur with stroking of inner thigh)
    E. DRE to assess prostate status
    F. Test visual fields to rule out pituitary tumors

V. Diagnostic testing
    A. CBC
    B. CMP, lipids, HgA1c
    C. TSH, PSA, free and total testosterone (if testosterone is ↓, check serum prolactin)

  D. Urinalysis

  E. Test for OSA (especially if obese or snores)

  F. Tests for nighttime erection

    1. Postage stamp test

     (a) Place a roll of stamps around the penis at bedtime; if the stamps are broken apart in the morning, erection occurred.

     (b) High sensitivity for differentiating between organic (inability to have an erection) or psychogenic (erection before awakening).

    2. Nocturnal penile tumescence (NPT) testing is usually performed in sleep laboratory to determine number, tumid and rigidness of erections

VI. Treatment

  A. Aggressive lifestyle modification

    1. Smoking and alcohol cessation

    2. Weight loss (if indicated) and increase activity

    3. Aggressive control of secondary disease (e.g., DM, HTN, dyslipidemia)

  B. General pharmacological treatment

    1. If treating depression, change medication to one with less sexual side effects, such as

     (a) Bupropion 100 mg bid and can increase to tid

     (b) Mirtazapine 15 mg hs (caution use in elderly)

    2. If treating psychogenic ED: trazadone 25–100 mg at hs (will not treat depression, but is used for psychogenic ED)

    3. Herbal therapy: yohimbine (an α-adrenergic antagonist touted as aphrodisiac) 15–0 mg, 2–3 times day

    4. Consider testosterone replacement with decreased testosterone levels and/or hypogonadism

  C. Phosphodiesterase type 5 (PDE5) inhibitors:

    1. If currently taking nitrates, combination with PDE5 inhibitors may cause life-threatening hypotension; dose adjustment is required and may need to be off nitrates for up to 5 days

    2. Caution if using with CYP450 3A4 medications

    3. Caution if taking alpha-1 blockers due to hypotensive effect

    4. Pharmacological therapy with PDE5 inhibitors

     (a) Sildenafil (Viagra): start 25 mg and can increase up to 100 mg

      (i) Take on an empty stomach approximately 1 hr before sex; effective up to approximately 4 hr

      (ii) Reduced dosing (25 mg) with renal or hepatic failure

     (b) Vardenafil (Levitra) 10–20 mg

      (i) Take on an empty stomach approximately 1 hr before sex; effective up to approximately 4 hr

      (ii) If $\geq$65 yr of age, start with 5 mg

      (iii) Dose adjustment with hepatic impairment

     (c) Tadalafil (Cialis) 10–20 mg

      (i) Take approximately 1 hr before sex; effective up to 36 hr

      (ii) Can be taken daily (2.5–5 mg) for organic and/or psychogenic ED

      (iii) Dose adjustment for renal and hepatic impairment

     (d) Avanafil (Stendra) 100–200 mg

      (i) Take approximately 15–30 min before sex; effective up to 6 hr

      (ii) Reduced dose (50 mg) if using alpha-1 blockers or has renal or hepatic impairment

VII. *Referral to urologist or endocrinologist for further evaluation if medication does not work*

PROSTATE CANCER

I. Definition
   A. Usually a slow-growing cancer and symptoms may remain undetected for years
   B. Prostate cancer found in younger men (e.g., <55 yr of age) seems to be more aggressive than in men >65 yr of age
II. Signs and symptoms
   A. Localized nodule and pain in prostate area
   B. New-onset impotence or erectile dysfunction
   C. Change in urine stream; new onset of incontinence or UTIs
   D. Unexplained weight loss
   E. Painless gross or microscopic hematuria
   F. Low back pain and pelvic heaviness
   G. Anemia, SOB, and bone pain (usually in later stages)
III. Physical exam
   A. DRE:
      1. Enlarged *asymmetric* prostate (*symmetric* enlargement usually associated with BPH)
      2. Palpable, firm nodule(s) that may be painless
   B. Often difficult to detect prostate cancer with DRE because nodules are usually on the anterior side of prostate and DRE examines the posterior side
IV. Diagnostic testing
   A. Urinalysis and culture if indicated
   B. PSA is usually increased on two different tests, done 1–2 wk apart (see **PRACTICE PEARLS FOR URINARY TRACT CONDITIONS**)
   C. Increased alkaline phosphatase
   D. CBC may show early onset anemia
V. *Referral to a urologist*

PROSTATITIS, ACUTE BACTERIAL

I. Signs and symptoms
   A. Ill appearing male with fever, chills
   B. Malaise, myalgia
   C. Low back, pelvic, or perineal pain; may have referred pain to the end of penis
   D. Dysuria, frequency, urgency, and nocturia; may have palpable bladder distention
   E. Prostate is tender, warm, boggy, and irregular on palpation (do not massage the prostate, may cause bacteremia)
II. Diagnostic testing
   A. Urinalysis with microscopic examination shows WBCs >10/hpf and positive bacteria
   B. Urine for C&S to help guide antibiotic treatment
   C. Gonorrhea/chlamydia (GC/CT) to rule out STI (especially if <35 yr of age, sexually active or has multiple sexual partners)
   D. Elevated WBC, ESR, and PSA (defer PSA *screening* for at least 1 month after symptom resolution)

● = *non-urgent referral*

III. Treatment
  A. For non-GC/CT infection, treat for 4 wk
    1. TMP-SMZ DS 1 tab bid *or*
    2. Ciprofloxacin 500 mg bid *or*
    3. Levofloxacin 500 mg daily
  B. For suspected or confirmed GC/CT infection: ceftriaxone 500 mg IM once *plus*
    1. Doxycycline 100 mg bid for 7 days *or*
    2. Zithromycin 1 g single dose
  C. NSAIDs may be used for pain
IV. Follow up in office or by phone in 48–72 hr after treatment started and then again 1–2 wk later; if positive GC/CT, retest in 3 mo
▲ **V.** *Referral to ED* with
  A. *Symptoms suggestive of bacteremia*
  B. *Inability to care for self at home*
  C. *Acute urinary retention*
  D. *Symptoms worsening within 3 days of treatment*

TESTICULAR CANCER

I. Signs and symptoms usually occur in younger men
  A. The presenting symptom may be gynecomastia with breast nodules
  B. Usually presents as solid, firm, painless, unilateral nodule/mass or swelling in the testicle, with sensation of fullness or heaviness; the testicular mass does not transilluminate
  C. Unexplained weight loss
II. Diagnostic testing
  A. CBC, CMP: consider AFP, β-hCG, LDH
  B. *Urgent* scrotal ultrasound
  C. Consider mammogram/breast ultrasound if breast nodules are noted
▲ **III.** *Treatment is referral to a urologist and/or surgeon (do not delay referral, this is usually an aggressive cancer)*

TESTICULAR TORSION

I. Signs and symptoms usually seen in younger men (e.g., common age range between 10 and 25 yr of age) and *is considered emergency situation*
  A. Sudden onset of severe scrotal pain usually occurring after activity or genital trauma but can occur much later
  B. The scrotum is enlarged, red, swollen with unilateral testicular pain
  C. One testicle is noted to be "high" in the scrotal sac because of shortening of the spermatic cord as it twists (highly sensitive sign for torsion)
  D. N/V
  E. Cremasteric reflex *absent* on the affected side (99% positive sign for torsion)
  F. Prehn's sign *negative* (elevation of the scrotum does not relieve pain)
II. Diagnostic testing should be deferred
▲ **III.** *Emergent referral to ED*

■ = *not to be missed;* ▲ = *urgent referral*

CHAPTER 12

Neurologic Conditions

For details regarding in-depth physical and cognitive assessment, see Chapter 1.

EQUILIBRIUM DISTURBANCES

I. Classification (common causes; not all inclusive)
   A. Dizziness: feeling "off-balance," lightheaded, or unsteady
      1. Parkinson disease
      2. DM neuropathy
      3. Eustachian tube dysfunction
      4. Depression, anxiety
      5. Hypoglycemia
      6. Medication side effect
   B. Presyncope: sense of impending loss of consciousness
      1. Orthostatic hypotension (see III, C)
      2. Vasovagal syncope (see III, D)
      3. Cardiac arrhythmia (see III, A)
   C. Vertigo: spinning or swaying sensation; perception of movement or whirling; can be of self or surroundings; also, see PRACTICE PEARLS FOR DIZZINESS, later in this chapter.
      1. No hearing loss: benign paroxysmal positional vertigo (BPPV), vestibular neuritis, head injury
      2. Hearing loss: Ménière disease, acute labyrinthitis
II. Dizziness
   A. History is most important
      1. Is it brought about by certain movements (e.g., looking up, turning over in bed)?
      2. Is it accompanied by tinnitus or hearing loss?
      3. Is it constant or intermittent?
      4. Any changes in gait?
      5. Any recent trauma?
      6. Are there other symptoms (e.g., H/A, N/V, vision changes, weakness)?
      7. Any new medications?
   B. Examination
      1. VS, including postural VS (see Chapter 1, PHYSICAL EXAMINATION, I, B)
      2. Ears, eyes, nose, and throat (EENT)
         (a) EOMs (also check for nystagmus)
         (b) ENT: check for nasal/sinus congestion, eustachian tube dysfunction
         (c) Hearing evaluation (e.g., 5-foot whisper test, rubbing fingers close to ear)
         (d) Rinne and Weber tests (see Fig. 1.3)
      3. CV, listen for the following:
         (a) Heart rhythm and regularity, murmurs
         (b) Carotid bruits

    4. Neurological
      (a) Cranial nerve (CN) (see Table 1.5)
      (b) DTRs
      (c) Romberg test: the patient will fall toward the affected side with BPPV
  C. Treatment and *Referral*: see **PRACTICE PEARLS FOR DIZZINESS**.

III. Syncope
  A. Cardiac causes
    1. Characteristics
      (a) Sudden onset and resolution and may occur any time (e.g., when supine or during exertion); feels fine subsequently
      (b) May be associated with arrhythmias (i.e., fast [SVT, VT, A-fib] or slow [third-degree AV block with a rate of <30 bpm]) with or without palpitations
      (c) May have a *diagnosis or history* of aortic or mitral stenosis, HF, hypertrophic cardiomyopathy, angina or MI, aortic aneurysm or dissection, or pulmonary HTN
      (d) Consider with medications such as digitalis, beta blockers, calcium channel blockers
    2. Possible diagnostic tests
      (a) Avoid EEG, head CT, and carotid U/S as initial work-up
      (b) Listen for bruits in the neck and abdomen
      (c) Orthostatic VS (see Chapter 1, PHYSICAL EXAMINATION, I, B)
      (d) ECG, Holter or event monitor, echocardiogram
      (e) CXR
      (f) Troponin, complete metabolic profile, CBC; consider BNP
  B. Metabolic causes
    1. Characteristics
      (a) Onset and resolution usually gradual
      (b) Often associated with lightheadedness and paresthesia
      (c) May be associated with infrequent eating (low blood sugar), hypothyroidism, hyponatremia, dehydration, recreational drugs
    2. Possible diagnostic tests
      (a) Avoid EEG and carotid U/S as initial work-up
      (b) Complete metabolic profile, TSH; consider 2-hr GTT
      (c) Consider CT non-contrast of brain (see Table 4.2), if suspecting a mass or CVA
      (d) May be reproducible with hyperventilation
  C. Postural (orthostatic) causes
    1. Characteristics
      (a) Often occurs when standing or sitting up from supine position and is preceded by lightheadedness or dizziness; lying down relieves the symptoms
      (b) May occur as a side effect of many medications (e.g., alpha or beta blockers, diuretics, nitrates, anticholinergics)
      (c) May be associated with vomiting, often with diarrhea (dehydration)
      (d) Consider with DM (autonomic failure) or with a history of anemia (GI bleeding)
    2. Possible diagnostic tests
      (a) Avoid EEG, head CT and carotid U/S as initial work-up of simple syncope in adults
      (b) Orthostatic VS (see Chapter 1, PHYSCIAL EXAMINATION, I, B)
      (c) ECG
      (d) CBC, complete metabolic profile; stool for OB
      (e) Romberg test (see Chapter 1, NEUROLOGICAL, IV, G, 4)

= non-urgent referral

D. Vasovagal causes
  1. Characteristics
    (a) Gradual onset and resolution; patient may feel horrible for up to 1–2 days
    (b) Precipitated by physical or emotional stimuli
    (c) Usually preceded by "vagal" symptoms (e.g., nausea, weakness, yawning, sweating, blurred vision)
    (d) Usually occurs when standing (i.e., in one place for extended time) but can occur when sitting and straining (as with defecation)
  2. Diagnosed primarily by patient's history; avoid EEG, head CT and carotid U/S as initial work-up of simple syncope in adults

PRACTICE PEARLS FOR DIZZINESS

- BPPV
  - Cause: calcium debris (canaliths) within the inner ear
  - Consider BPPV with vertigo lasting < 1 min or occurring with position changes (e.g., turning over in bed, turning or flexing head); often occurs first thing in the morning; associated with nausea and unsteadiness but NO hearing loss or tinnitus.
  - Treatment
    - The Dix-Hallpike maneuver is used to determine which side (i.e., right or left) is affected: with patient sitting on exam table, turn head 45 degrees to one side and lie back quickly with the head extended over the end of the table; a positive test is whichever side causes vertigo *and* nystagmus (which often is a rotating motion of the eyes).
    - Modified Epley maneuver is used for self-treatment of BPPV. It should be done tid until no vertigo for 24 hr. Warn the patient that vertigo and/or nausea may occur with this procedure, at least initially. The steps are:
      - Sit on the bed (with legs extended on bed and a pillow placed so it will be under the patient's shoulders). Turn the head 45 degrees toward the affected side and lie quickly back, with shoulders on the pillow and head on the bed; wait 30 sec.
      - Without raising the head, turn head 30 degrees toward the unaffected side; wait 30 sec.
      - Turn the body and head 90 degrees toward the unaffected side (patient will be "rolled over," with arm underneath body and top leg flexed at the knee and hip); wait 30 sec.
      - Sit up on the side of the bed, with feet on the floor.
    - Sleep in a recliner for 48 hr (allows canaliths to "settle down"), limit movements that cause vertigo.
    - Motion sickness medications are no help and can actually worsen the symptoms.
- ▲ Acute vertigo AND hearing loss: ***primary concern is possible acute labyrinthitis (a very serious infection) or acoustic neuroma; immediately refer to ED***
- Ménière disease
  - Consider with *recurrent* attacks of intense vertigo lasting 20 min to 12 hr; *associated with tinnitus and low-frequency hearing loss.*
  - Treatment
    - Sodium intake, <2 g daily (very helpful to most patients)
    - Limit caffeine (coffee, tea, cola) to 1 beverage daily and alcohol to 1 drink daily
    - With recurrent vertigo episodes, consider HCTZ 25 mg/triamterene 37.5 mg daily
    - For acute vertigo episode: clonazepam 0.25–0.5 mg 2–3 times daily prn
    - May need antiemetic (e.g., ondansetron 4 mg 2–3 times daily prn)
- Syncope and severe lightheadedness can accompany pregnancy.
- Faintness or lightheadedness may be side effects of many medications (e.g., anticonvulsants, antidepressants, antipsychotics, antihypertensives, nitrates, diuretics).
- Consider cerebellar dysfunction or peripheral neuropathy if the patient complains of dizziness plus imbalance, clumsiness, or incoordination; check B_{12} and folate (deficiencies common with alcoholism) and VDRL or RPR (syphilis).

▲ = *urgent referral*

> **PRACTICE PEARLS FOR DIZZINESS—CONT'D**
>
> - Consider carotid sinus hypersensitivity if dizziness or syncope occurs during shaving or when wearing constrictive collars.
> - *Referral*
>   - *Emergent transfer to ED*
>   - *New-onset vertigo accompanied by neurological signs/symptoms* (e.g., diplopia or disconjugate gaze, limb numbness or weakness, slurred speech) or *acute vertigo with new hearing loss*
>   - *Symptoms suggestive of aortic aneurysm/dissection or MI* (see Table 8.5)
>   - *Syncope with unstable VS*
>   - **Neurologist**
>   - CNS signs and symptoms
>   - Progressive, disabling vertigo or dizziness that is resistant to treatment
>   - Patient with BPPV who has neurological signs or does not respond to therapy
>   - **Cardiologist**
>   - Any CV-related cause of dizziness not responsive to therapy
>   - New-onset murmur (obtain echocardiogram before referral)
>   - **Psychiatrist**
>   - Comorbid psychiatric disorder (e.g., panic disorder or depression) that does not respond to reassurance and drug management

FOCAL NEUROLOGIC DEFICIT

I. Bell's palsy
   A. Acute paralysis of the facial nerve; of unknown cause (possibly herpes simplex or zoster infection) (see Fig. 12.1)
   B. Signs and symptoms
      1. Sudden onset (over hours) of unilateral facial paralysis, including eyebrow sagging, inability to close the eye, and mouth asymmetry
      2. May have decreased tearing and/or loss of taste on the anterior two-thirds of the tongue; no real sensory loss on the face, may have tingling sensation
      3. Progressive course with maximal effects ≤3 wk from the first day of weakness (diagnosis is doubtful if *no function* has returned within 3–4 mo)
   C. Diagnostic tests
      1. Forehead muscles are affected by Bell palsy; patient usually CANNOT wrinkle the forehead.
      2. Consider brain MRI with contrast (see Table 4.2) with atypical signs if there is progression after 3 wk or if there is no improvement at 4 mo.
   D. Treatment (medication started preferably within 3 days of symptom onset)
      1. For all patients: prednisone 60–80 mg daily for 7 days
      2. Consider valacyclovir 1000 mg tid for 1 wk in addition to prednisone with severe facial palsy (disfiguring asymmetry with little or no motion in the affected side, incomplete closure of eye).
      3. Eye care
         (a) Artificial tears q1hr while awake and lubricating ophthalmic ointment at hs
         (b) Use protective glasses or goggles; patches can be used, but do not place tape on the eyelid since the patch could slip and abrade the cornea
      4. Follow up in office in 3 wk to confirm the symptoms are improving. About 70% of patients recover spontaneously by 3–6 mo; prednisone therapy (see above) improves the rate of complete recovery to 80%–85%

■ = *not to be missed;* ● = *non-urgent referral;* ▲ = *urgent referral*

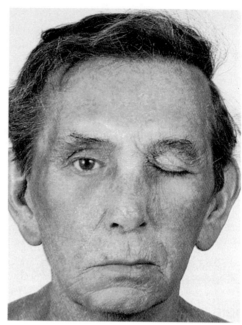

Fig. 12.1 Bell's palsy (Perkins et al., 2011). (From Mosby's Dictionary of Medicine, Nursing and Health Professions (9th ed.). Elsevier.)

    E. *Referral*
       1. *To a neurologist if continues to progress after 3 wk or no improvement by 4 mo*
       2. *Consider Physical Therapy, if needed, for facial muscle weakness or contractures*
 II. Cerebrovascular events (CVA and TIA)
    A. Description
       1. CVA: symptoms last >24 hr
       2. TIA: symptoms last <24 hr
    B. Signs and symptoms (sudden onset)
       1. Carotid circulation
         (a) Hemianesthesia, hemiplegia, neglect
         (b) May have aphasia, visual field defects
         (c) May have H/A, seizures, amnesia, facial paresis
       2. Vertebrobasilar circulation
         (a) Diplopia
         (b) Vertigo, ataxia
         (c) Facial paresis
         (d) Dysphagia, difficulty speaking
    C. Common causes
       1. Circulatory
         (a) Ischemic (e.g., atherosclerosis)
         (b) Hemorrhagic (e.g., aneurysm, artery dissection)
       2. Embolism related to the following:
         (a) Mitral valve disease

= non-urgent referral

(b) Decreased ventricle wall movement (e.g., with MI or HF) with mural thrombus

(c) Dysrhythmia (e.g., atrial fib)

3. Hypercoagulable states, including use of OCs

D. Treatment

▲

1. Depends on the patient's condition (i.e., acute or chronic state): *emergency transfer to ED with acute changes*

2. Counsel for lifestyle changes (at follow-up visits)

(a) Stop smoking

(b) Control risk factors (e.g., HTN, DM, dyslipidemia) and emphasize medication adherence

(c) To improve outcomes after an ischemic stroke:

(i) HTN: long-term goal is <130/80, if possible

(ii) Explain statin benefits, even with no dyslipidemia; prescribe high-intensity statin if patient is <75 yr of age and moderate intensity with older patients

(iii) Antiplatelet therapy should be started within 24 hr of symptom onset (of minor stroke or high-risk TIA). Give clopidogrel 75 mg plus ASA 81 mg daily for 21 days and then change to just one of the agents (usually to ASA).

HEADACHES

I. History (pertinent to H/A) is the most important factor for H/A diagnosis

A. Location: unilateral, frontal and/or bilateral

B. Onset

1. Acute (sudden onset of severe pain)

2. Gradual over hours to days

3. Age at onset

C. Type of pain: aching, throbbing, burning, pressing

D. Radiating: to the eye (e.g., glaucoma), face (e.g., trigeminal neuralgia), neck (e.g., meningitis)

E. Associated symptoms

1. Aura or prodrome

2. Fever, sinus pain

3. N/V, lacrimation (e.g., cluster H/A)

4. Neurologic symptoms

(a) Diplopia, photophobia

(b) Ataxia, paresis

(c) Ptosis

(d) Tinnitus

F. Timing of pain

1. How long does it last (e.g., minutes to hours/days)?

2. Is it continuous or intermittent?

3. Is it chronic?

G. Triggers of pain

1. Food, caffeine, alcohol, chocolate

2. Activity, weather changes (i.e., barometric pressure changes)

3. Postural

▲ = *urgent referral*

    H. Alleviating factors
       1. Lying flat
       2. Dark room
       3. Quiet
       4. Medications
    I. Intensity of pain
       1. Use pain scale
       2. Is H/A the same or is it getting worse?
       3. Is H/A affecting your lifestyle more often?
    J. Past medical history
       1. Is this a similar H/A as in the past with frequency, patterns?
       2. What treatments have been used successfully or unsuccessfully?
       3. Recent or past exposure to environmental toxins; any recent infections?
       4. Any increase in personal stressors; changes in personal life?
    K. Family history of any type of H/A

II. Physical examination (suggested steps to R/O organic causes of H/A)
    A. Head
       1. ENT: look for nasal congestion
       2. Sinus: gently press over the frontal-maxillary area of the face and over mastoid processes and C_2; increased pain suggests sinus congestion
       3. Eyes: gently press on closed eyes; increased pain may indicate glaucoma, but other symptoms would be present
       4. Temporomandibular joint (TMJ): palpate TMJ for pain and crepitus
       5. Scalp: inspect and palpate for point tenderness
    B. Arteries: palpation and also listen for bruits
       1. Tenderness over temporal arteries: if the patient is >50 yr of age, consider temporal arteritis; if younger, consider migraine (if H/A lasting >24 hr)
       2. Carotidynia: tenderness associated with episodic, unilateral H/A
    C. Neck
       1. Meninges: have the patient touch the chin to the chest (flexes low cervical spine) and the chin to Adam's apple (flexes high cervical spine); *if the patient is unable to do these maneuvers, transfer to ED*
       2. Cervical vertebrae: press on spinous processes; head pain is not associated with a lesion below C4; cervical spondylosis is usually C5 or lower
       3. Cervical muscles: palpate for muscle pain and tenderness
    D. Neurologic examination (note if the patient can stand from sitting without any help)
       1. Walking on heels and toes
       2. CN examination (see Table 1.5)
       3. Tandem gait and Romberg test
       4. Symmetry on motor, sensory, reflex, and coordination tests (see Chapter 1, NEUROLOGICAL, IV, E, G-J)
       5. Fundoscopic examination *(transfer to ED with papilledema)*

III. *Not to be missed*
    A. *First or new-type or worst-ever H/A* (possible intracranial bleeding, CNS infection); *immediate transfer to the ED*
    B. *New H/A in patient >50 yr of age* (possible temporal arteritis, tumor, or intracranial bleed)

■ = *not to be missed;* ▲ = *urgent referral*

C. *Worsening or change in pattern compared with usual H/A* (possible mass or subdural hematoma)

D. *Signs/symptoms of systemic illness (e.g., fever, vomiting, nuchal rigidity* [possible CNS infection]); *immediate transfer to the ED*

E. *H/A with exertion (e.g., cough, sneeze, intercourse* [possible increased intracranial pressure])

F. *Focal neurologic signs* (possible CVA, intracranial aneurysm, mass)

G. *Post-traumatic onset or patient taking anticoagulants* (possible intracranial bleeding)

H. *History of neoplasm* (possible metastasis)

I. *H/A during pregnancy or puerperium* (possible preeclampsia or cerebral venous thrombosis)

J. H/A in children
   1. Listen for bruits over the carotid arteries; *if asymmetric or continuous, immediate transfer to the ED*
   2. *If the child has a stiff neck with a severe H/A, immediate transfer to the ED* (possible subarachnoid hemorrhage or meningitis)
   3. Migraine headaches: see Chapter 16, Neurological Disorders, MIGRAINE HEADACHE

IV. Diagnostic studies
   A. Depending on patient history, consider electrolytes, CBC, TSH and free T4, UA, ESR, CRP, toxicology screen
   B. CT or MRI scan (see Table 4.2); CT is sufficient in most patients; it is performed *urgently* for patients with the following:
      1. Recent change in pattern, frequency, or severity
      2. Progressive worsening despite therapy
      3. Focal neurologic signs
      4. *Onset* of H/A at >50 yr of age

V. Classification
   A. Cluster
      1. Characteristics
         (a) More common in men than women, usually after 30 yr of age
         (b) Episodic: intermittent episodes of attacks over weeks to mo, with periods of remission lasting months to years
         (c) Chronic: episodes of attacks continuing >1 yr without a break of at least 1 mo.
         (d) Pain is quick onset, exquisitely severe, non-throbbing, and unilateral in the head and face with pain in, around, or behind eye
         (e) Occurs up to 8 times a day; often cyclical, occurring at the same time of day; lasts 10 min to 3 hr; the episodes can last for 2 mo or longer
         (f) May worsen when lying still and is associated with pacing, rocking, and agitation
         (g) Triggers: ETOH, tobacco, histamines, vasodilators, and seasonal allergies
      2. Associated symptoms: only during attacks and are ipsilateral to pain
         (a) Lacrimation, ptosis, and conjunctival injection
         (b) Nasal congestion and rhinorrhea
         (c) Facial flushes, sweating
      3. Treatment
         (a) CT/MRI with initial attack (see Table 4.2); no labs are helpful

---

▲ = *urgent referral;* ▥ = *not to be missed*

(b) Start acute and preventative meds as soon as possible

(c) *Acute*

　(i) O_2 at 12–15 L/min using nonrebreathing mask, with the patient sitting upright; use for 15 min, even if the pain subsides before then. Do not use if patient has severe COPD.

　(ii) Sumatriptan 6 mg IM or 20 mg intranasal (intranasal form is administered contralateral to the side of the H/A); intranasal does not work as fast as injectable. More than 2 doses per day may be needed until the preventative medication has taken effect.

　(iii) Prednisone 60–100 mg daily for 5–14 days; taper by decreasing the dose 10mg daily. This is best used for patients with episodic clusters lasting <2 mo or as an adjunct for the first 2 wk of verapamil administration (since it takes a relatively long time to titrate med to an effective dose).

(d) *Preventative*: start ASAP at onset of a cluster episode and taper medication after expected duration of episode passes. For patients who respond to the preventative medications, consider a trial of dose reduction q3mo; restart at lowest effective dose if headaches recur

　(i) Verapamil 240 mg daily, increasing daily dose by 80 mg q10–14days, often up to 480–960 mg (regular release form given in 3 divided doses daily and sustained release given in 2 divided doses); benefit of verapamil is usually seen within 2–3 wk (may also use prednisone during the first 2 wk)

　(ii) Galcanezumab (Emgality) SQ qmo; not a first line preventative medication and can be very expensive

　(iii) Consider lithium for chronic cluster H/A if other medications are ineffective or contraindicated

(e) There is no evidence of benefit with botulinum injections or hyperbaric O_2

B. Migraine

1. Most patients have a family history of H/A; rarely starts after 50 yr of age

2. Migraine *without* aura: at least five H/A meeting the following criteria:

　(a) Lasts 4–72 hr

　(b) At least two of the following: unilateral, pulsating, moderate-to-severe intensity, worsened by routine physical activity

　(c) At least one of the following during H/A: nausea, vomiting, photophobia, phonophobia

　(d) H&P and neurologic examinations do not suggest underlying organic disease

3. Migraine *with* aura

　(a) Attacks include transient, reversible symptoms (aura) that gradually develop over 5–20 min and last <60 min with:

　　(i) Visual: flickering lights, spots, lines; loss of vision

　　(ii) Sensory: pins and needles, numbness

　　(iii) Speech disturbance

　　(iv) Brainstem involvement: diplopia, vertigo, tinnitus

　(b) Has features of migraine without aura, and H/A develops during or within 60 min of aura

4. Menstrual migraine

　(a) For ≥3 cycles, cyclical migraine associated with menses, starting 2 days before menses and lasting 2 days into the cycle; associated with drop in estrogen.

　(b) Can occur with or without aura; other symptoms are similar to chronic migraine.

(c) *Abortive* migraine treatment as needed (e.g., NSAIDs or triptan); menstrual migraines tend to be more severe and less responsive to abortive therapy.

(d) *Preventative*

(i) If menses are predictable: start scheduled NSAID (e.g., naproxen 500 mg bid) or triptan (e.g., frovatriptan 2.5 mg daily or bid, naratriptan 1 mg bid, or zolmitriptan 2.5 mg bid) a few days before menses and continue for 5–6 days total.

(ii) If menses are unpredictable or patient desires contraception: consider contraceptive with estrogen. To decrease frequency of menses, give extended-cycle OC or continuous use of low-dose monophasic combo OC (include directions "for continuous use" in the Rx for 28-day products to limit callbacks from the pharmacy).

(iii) May use beta blocker or tricyclic if needed (see under *Preventative*, 5 (c) and Table 12.2).

5. Treatment

(a) Lifestyle measures may help to control migraines

(i) Get adequate sleep and regular physical exercise.

(ii) Eat at regular times, with a protein source at each meal; limit caffeine intake and drink adequate amounts of water.

(iii) Encourage patient to prioritize obligations to create a sense of control; find healthy ways to deal with stress.

(iv) Avoid possible triggers (see Table 12.1).

(v) Have patient keep a headache diary, including medication usage.

(b) *Abortive*

(i) Usually more effective when taken at onset of H/A.

(ii) Try one medication for at least three H/A before deciding it will not help.

(iii) *Mild-to-moderate H/A*, not associated with vomiting or severe nausea (to avoid medication overuse [rebound] H/A, limit use to <10 days/mo)

(a) Combination: naproxen 500 mg q12hr OR ibuprofen 600 mg q6hr AND acetaminophen 650 mg q6hr OR 1000 mg q8hr

(b) Excedrin Migraine 2 tabs

(c) Naproxen or ibuprofen with a triptan (see below for list)

(iv) *Moderate-to-severe H/A*, not associated with vomiting or severe nausea

(a) Combination sumatriptan and naproxen 550 mg (individually or as combined agent, Treximet)

(b) Triptans (may repeat dose once in 2 hr if needed); if one triptan is ineffective, a different one may work. Dosed orally unless noted otherwise
Almotriptan (Axert) 6.25–12.5 mg
Eletriptan hydrobromide (Relpax) 20–40 mg
Naratriptan (Amerge) 2.5 mg
Rizatriptan (Maxalt) 10 mg PO or orally dissolving tablet
Sumatriptan (Imitrex) 6 mg SQ or 50–100 mg PO or 20 mg nasal spray
Zolmitriptan (Zomig) 2.5–5 mg PO or 2.5 mg dissolving wafer

(c) CGRP antagonists may be used if the patient has a contraindication to or inadequate response to 2 or 3 triptans
Rimegepant (Nurtec ODT) 75 mg PO once in 24 hr
Ubrogepant (Ubrelvy) 50–100 mg PO; may repeat in 2 hr if needed

(v) Injected or nasal sumatriptan may be needed with vomiting or severe nausea.

(vi) Ketorolac 30–60 mg IM once, in place of oral NSAID (30 mg dose if patient is >65 yr of age, <50 kg, or has renal impairment).

TABLE 12.1 ■ **Potential Migraine Triggers**

Triggers	Avoid or Limit*	Allowed
Beverages	Red wine, beer Coffee, tea, caffeinated colas Chocolate or cocoa	Whiskey, scotch, vodka, fruit juices, and sauterne and Riesling wines No more than 1 cup coffee, 2 cups tea, 2 cola drinks daily Noncola soft drinks, flavored waters, decaffeinated drinks
Dairy products	Milk, buttermilk, cream Sour cream, yogurt Hard (aged) cheeses: cheddar Brie, processed cheeses	Low-fat or skim milk No more than ½ cup yogurt Cottage cheese, cream cheese Butter, margarine, cooking oils
Meats/poultry	Processed meats: hot dogs, bologna Aged, cured, smoked, marinated meats Organ meats: liver	Fresh or frozen meats Limit eggs to ≤3/wk
Fish	Dried, smoked fish, pickled herring	Fresh or frozen fish, canned tuna or salmon
Vegetables	Most beans and peas Onions Pickles, olives, sauerkraut	String beans Asparagus, beets, carrots, spinach, tomatoes, squash, corn, zucchini, broccoli, lettuce, potatoes
Grains, breads, cereals	Yeast breads (white), sourdough breads	Rice, pasta Whole wheat and rye breads English muffins, Melba toast, bagels Most cereals
Soups	Soups containing MSG or yeast Soups from bouillon cubes	Homemade soups
Fruits	Citrus fruits, bananas, figs, raisins, papaya, kiwi, plums, pineapples, avocados	Limit citrus and bananas to ½ to 1 daily Apples, prunes, cherries, grapes, apricots, peaches, pears
Desserts, snack foods	Chocolate Ice cream Cookies or cakes made with yeast Potato chip products Nuts, seeds Peanut butter	Sugar candies Sherbet, ices, sorbets Cookies or cakes made without yeast Pretzels Jam, jelly, honey
Additives	MSG (may be in Chinese foods) Seasonings and spices Soy sauce	Salad dressings (in small amounts) White vinegar
Miscellaneous nonfood triggers	Oral contraceptives Air travel Stress Weather (low-pressure system)	

*Although there is little evidence that avoiding known "triggers" prevents migraines, including MSG, chocolate, tyramine, and sulfites

(vii) Dexamethasone 10–25 mg IM or IV as a single dose, in addition to standard abortive treatment, reduces risk of early H/A recurrence.

(viii) May need medication for nausea (e.g., promethazine, ondansetron).

(ix) Opioids and butalbital-containing compounds are discouraged and are associated with higher rate of rebound H/A.

TABLE 12.2 ■ **Suggested Preventative Migraine Agents**

Patient Conditions	Suggested Medication(s)
HTN *but* <60 yr of age *and* nonsmoker	Metoprolol, propranolol, or timolol
HTN *but* >60 yr of age *or* smoker	Verapamil
Depression or mood disorder	Amitriptyline or venlafaxine
Insomnia	Amitriptyline
Obesity	Topiramate
Raynaud phenomenon	Verapamil
Seizure disorder	Valproate or topiramate

(c) *Preventative*
  (i) Consider with >4 H/A month or lasting >12 hr; medication used is based on side effects, other conditions, and cost (see Table 12.2). Evaluate effectiveness in 4–6 wk (may continue to increase over 3–6 mo).
  (ii) Beta blockers (first line)
    (a) Metoprolol 25 mg bid and titrate to 100–200 mg daily
    (b) Propranolol 20 mg bid and titrate to 40–160 mg daily
    (c) Timolol 5 mg daily and titrate to 20–30 mg daily in 2 divided doses
  (iii) Anticonvulsants (first line)
    (a) Topiramate 25 mg daily; may increase by 25–50 mg qwk up to 100 mg bid
    (b) Valproate 500–1500 mg daily (not recommended in women of child-bearing age)
  (iv) Antidepressants (second line)
    (a) Amitriptyline 10 mg hs; titrate to 20–50 mg hs
    (b) Venlafaxine 37.5 mg and titrate to 75–150 mg daily
  (v) CGRP antagonists
    (a) Expensive; not much data comparing to efficacy of first line agents, but often used for patients when other therapies have failed
    (b) Avoid use in patients with high cardiovascular risk (e.g., uncontrolled HTN)
    (c) Injectable monthly or quarterly, depending on medication
    (d) Medications include erenumab (Aimovig), fremanezumab (Ajovy), and galcanezumab (Emgality)
  (vi) OTC products
    (a) CoQ10 100 mg tid
    (b) Melatonin 3 mg hs
    (c) Riboflavin 400 mg daily
    (d) Not found to be effective: magnesium (in adults), butterbur, feverfew
  (vii) Opioids and butalbital-containing products should not be used for migraine prevention
C. Tension-type headache
  1. Characteristics
    (a) Bilateral, non-throbbing, dull, "tight band" around head (there is often tenderness of muscles in head, neck, or shoulders)

        (b) Mild-to-moderate intensity (not disabling) and can last 30 min to 7 days

        (c) Often related to stress or mental tension; not aggravated by physical exertion

        (d) There are no associated auras, N/V, photophobia, or phonophobia

    2. Treatment

        (a) Naproxen 500 mg, IBU 200–400 mg, or ASA 650–1000 mg (NSAIDs are less likely to cause medication overuse H/A than other analgesics)

        (b) OTC pain reliever with or without caffeine

        (c) Combinations with opioids or butalbital are not recommended unless the other options are ineffective or contraindicated; do not prescribe >18 tablets a month

        (d) For prevention, consider amitriptyline 10 mg hs and increase the dose by 10–12.5 mg q2–3wk as tolerated, until H/A improves or dose reaches 125 mg nightly

        (e) Lifestyle changes may help: regulation of sleep, exercise, and meals (e.g., decrease red meat, sugar, and chocolate); stress reduction, biofeedback, stretching exercises

VI. Temporal arteritis (also, giant cell arteritis [GCA])

  A. Characteristics

    1. Classical: unilateral temporal area; exquisite tenderness or burning, throbbing

    2. May progressively worsen or wax and wane

    3. Associated with jaw pain on chewing, fatigue, fever, weight loss; may have vision loss

    4. May have tender, engorged vessels across the forehead and temporal area

  B. Treatment

    1. Obtain ESR or CRP (usually elevated, but this does not definitively diagnose GCA)

    2. Steroids: start once diagnosis is strongly suspected, even before confirmed; prednisone 40–60 mg daily in a single dose, at least until the biopsy results are back

    3. May need opioids for pain

  C. *Referral*

▲   1. *Urgent to a surgeon for possible biopsy;* do not withhold steroids before biopsy is performed (it can be done up to 4 wk after starting high-dose steroids)

    2. *Referral to a rheumatologist for further care*

PRACTICE PEARLS FOR HEADACHES

- Inform the patient to treat H/A in early stage so that it will not become disabling.
- A H/A diary can be useful to monitor triggers (also see Table 12.1) and treatment effectiveness.
- If the complaint is H/A, consider migraine first.
- Patient must *stop daily use of analgesics* to prevent rebound H/A; overuse of medications for even a few months can make H/A worse or chronic:
  - To break the cycle, stop the medicine (may need to wean if using opioid or butalbital multiple times daily).
  - Reinforce to use *preventive* therapy and to not use acute therapy >2 times a week.
- *Referral to H/A specialist*
  - *Patient with complex medical or psychiatric conditions* (e.g., CV or renal disease, DM, bipolar disorder).
  - *If treatment options have not helped.*

● = *non-urgent referral;* ▲ = *urgent referral*

MENINGITIS

   I. *Viral* signs and symptoms
     A. Fever, H/A (usually severe), nuchal rigidity
     B. Drowsiness, fatigue, photophobia
     C. May have negative Brudzinski and Kernig signs (see III)
  II. *Bacterial* signs and symptoms
     A. Fever, H/A (usually severe), nuchal rigidity, altered mental status
     B. Drowsiness, fatigue, seizure
     C. With meningococcus: purpura, red papules; may be faint pink macules
     D. Positive Brudzinski and Kernig signs (see III)
 III. Physical examination signs
     A. Brudzinski sign: passive flexion of the chin on the chest causes spontaneous hip flexion
     B. Kernig sign: positive (abnormal) response is inability or reluctance to fully extend the leg at the knee with the thigh flexed at the hip to 90 degrees; may be performed with the patient supine or sitting
▲ **IV.** Treatment: ***immediate transfer to ED***

MOVEMENT DISORDERS

   I. Parkinson disease
     A. Description: chronic, progressive, neurodegenerative disorder usually diagnosed at or after 50 yr of age
     B. Signs and symptoms
       1. Early stages
         (a) Tremor: observed best in relaxed extremity; usually begins unilaterally in the finger and thumb (pill rolling); stops during voluntary movement
         (b) Rigidity: detected earliest in neck muscles; cogwheel rigidity on passive motion; have the patient stand with arms at sides: when the examiner twists the patient's shoulders side to side, the patient's arms will not swing freely
         (c) Bradykinesia: slow, fluid movements; gait disturbances (i.e., shorter, shuffling steps); difficulty initiating voluntary movements (e.g., performing tasks like buttoning clothes, double clicking on a computer mouse, or standing up from a chair)
       2. Later stages
         (a) Postural instability
         (b) Akinesia (difficulty initiating movement), rigidity, ataxia, festinating gait (i.e., quicker, shorter steps like running a race), and stooped posture
         (c) Excessive salivation, dysphagia, and constipation
         (d) Low volume, pitch monotony, and dysarthric speech (difficulty speaking)
         (e) Expressionless face and decreased blinking
         (f) Confusion, hallucinations, and dementia
     C. Diagnosis
       1. Based on clinical findings; can be confirmed only on autopsy
       2. There are no radiology or lab tests for diagnosis
     D. Treatment: ***Referral to a physician (preferably neurologist) for initial diagnosis***; may comanage with the physician

---

● *= non–urgent referral;* ▲ *= urgent referral*

II. Seizures
    A. Definition: paroxysmal, disorderly discharge of neuronal impulses and spread of these impulses throughout brain tissues
        1. May be an isolated event with or without an obvious precipitating cause or may be recurrent.
        2. Epilepsy is diagnosed when seizures recur over a period of time without obvious precipitating events.
    B. Classification

PRACTICE PEARLS FOR SEIZURES

- With a seizure (especially if the first one), check blood glucose level.
- *Consult a physician if seizures are different, new-onset, or refractory (i.e., do not respond to therapy);* may comanage with the physician.
- Treatment is based on the seizure type and tolerability of side effects; monotherapy is the treatment of choice when possible.
- Never stop anticonvulsants abruptly; wean over 2–6 mo; if the patient is taking >1 drug, withdraw sequentially, not simultaneously.
- Educate the patient on the importance of medication adherence; many treatment failures are due to poor compliance.
- Febrile seizures
  - Usually occur in children 6 mo to 6 yr of age and with fever >101°F (rate of fever increase not a factor).
  - Unknown cause; CNS infection/inflammation or systemic problem should be excluded.
  - Simple: occurs once in a 24-hr period, lasts <15 min with no focal features; complex: occurs more than once in a 24-hr period, lasts >15 min, or has focal features or postictal paresis.
  - Occurrence does not mean that the affected child has a seizure disorder/epilepsy.
- Driving restrictions vary from state to state; driving requirements can be found at www.epilepsyfoundation.org/resources/drivingandtravel.cfm.

III. Tremors
    A. *New-onset tremor often warrants referral to a neurologist;* obtain a TSH and free T4 before the neurologist sees the patient. The most important diagnostic distinction is between parkinsonian and essential tremors.
    B. Action tremors: typically increase with muscle activity and are reduced or absent at rest
        1. Physiologic
            (a) Characteristics
                (i) Most evident in hands and fingers; worsen with fine motor tasks
                (ii) Little functional impairment
                (iii) May be enhanced by increased sympathetic activity (e.g., medications such as SSRIs, TCAs, amphetamines; anxiety, excitement or fright; hypoglycemia; thyrotoxicosis; fever)
            (b) Treatment
                (i) Reassure the patient that no disease is present
                (ii) Avoid caffeine and other stimulants
                (iii) Anxiolytics may be *occasionally* used in stressful situations
        2. Essential
            (a) Characteristics
                (i) Most evident during use of affected muscles; may involve extremities (mainly upper) or head/neck and voice.
                (ii) May cause significant functional impairment; affects writing skills.
                (iii) Family history of this disorder in up to 70% of patients.

● = *non-urgent referral*

(b) Treatment
   (i) Avoid nicotine and other stimulants; worsened by stress, hypoglycemia, and fatigue
   (ii) Propranolol 20 mg tid, increase as needed and tolerated and/or primidone 12.5–25 mg hs and increase to 250 mg daily in divided doses; giving both medications may be more effective than either alone
   (iii) Consider P.T. or O.T. consultation for lifestyle changes needed due to tremors
C. Resting tremor: typically most noticeable when the involved extremities are at rest and is relieved or absent during activity
1. Characteristics
   (a) Most commonly seen with Parkinson disease but can occur with other neurologic diseases
   (b) May be asymmetric, involving the extremities but not usually the head/neck (although it can affect the tongue, lips, and chin)
   (c) Typical movement: alternating forearm pronation and supination or "pill rolling"
2. Treatment: stop or reduce any drugs that might exacerbate parkinsonism
3. *Referral to a neurologist if Parkinson disease is suspected*

NEUROMUSCULAR DISORDERS

I. Guillain-Barré syndrome
   A. Signs and symptoms
      1. Progressive (over approximately 2 wk), fairly symmetric muscle weakness, usually with ascending paralysis; may develop paraplegia or quadriplegia
      2. Acute onset of hyperalgesia or myalgia
   B. Treatment: *immediate transfer to ED*
II. Multiple sclerosis
   A. Signs and symptoms
      1. Sensory symptoms present in most patients sometime during the disease: numbness, tingling, "pins and needles," tightness, coldness, or sensation of swelling of limbs or trunk; may have intense itching (especially unilaterally in cervical dermatomes)
      2. Pain is common: trigeminal neuralgia, dysesthesia (unpleasant sensation when touched)
      3. Fatigue unrelated to the amount of activity performed; may be improved by rest
      4. Coordination: vertigo, gait imbalance; may have intention tremor in limbs and head
      5. Bowel and bladder dysfunction (may be intermittent in early stages)
   B. Treatment: *referral to a neurologist*; may comanage care
III. Myasthenia gravis
   A. Signs and symptoms
      1. Cardinal: fluctuating muscle weakness, often with muscle fatigue; commonly worse late in the day or after exercise; as the disease progresses, symptoms are continually present but fluctuate from mild to severe
      2. Dysphagia, jaw fatigue with chewing
      3. Ptosis, diplopia
   B. Treatment
      1. *Referral to a neurologist*; may comanage care
      2. *Emergency transfer to ED for myasthenic crisis (abrupt worsening of symptoms plus possible HTN, respiratory distress, incontinence)*

● = *non-urgent referral;* ▲ = *urgent referral*

CHAPTER 13

Musculoskeletal Conditions

Introduction

I. A chief complaint ascribed by the patient to a joint may originate elsewhere. Bones and joints can be affected by systemic diseases and by local problems.

II. Elicit all factors of the chief complaint and associated symptoms and obtain a careful review of systems.

III. One of the most important points is to determine whether the symptoms are due to structural damage or inflammatory joint disease (Table 13.1).

PRACTICE PEARLS FOR MUSCULOSKELETAL COMPLAINTS

- Pain *without* injury: consider arthritis (see General Musculoskeletal Disorders, OSTEOARTHRITIS, later in this chapter), infection, or metastatic cancer (primarily in the spine and/or ribs).
- Presence of pain in the absence of obvious joint disease: consider neuropathy.
- Limp *with* pain: consider neuromuscular involvement; *without* pain: consider muscle disease.
- Fatigue (i.e., weariness or exhaustion from work, exertion, or stress) and malaise (i.e., a vague, indefinite feeling of infirmity or lack of health) can be associated with other conditions (Table 13.2).
- Paired joints usually provide a comparison, and both should be examined; perform thorough assessment above and below the area of complaint. Consider comparison X-ray of both joints.
- Remember that joint pain may be referred or radicular (resulting from nerve compression or injury).
- Inspection and palpation are the primary assessment techniques; percussion is occasionally used to elicit point tenderness, which may indicate a fracture.
- Ask the patient to touch with one finger the spot that hurts the most (localizes the problem and helps to narrow possible diagnoses).
- Knowledge of surface anatomy is critical to musculoskeletal examination; dermatomes are illustrated in Fig. 13.1.
- Without appropriate findings for arthralgias/myalgias, there is no need to test for Lyme disease unless there is a history of exposure or visit to an endemic area.
- Evaluate muscle strength on a scale of 0–5 (Table 13.3).

TABLE 13.1 ■ Comparison of Structural and Inflammatory Joint Conditions

Structural Lesion	Inflammatory Joint Disease
Pain occurs on use, improves with rest	Morning stiffness, especially for >30 min
Usually involves weight-bearing joints	Also involves nonweight-bearing joints
No acute exacerbations	Often has flare-ups
No systemic symptoms	Systemic symptoms common

TABLE 13.2 ■ Possible Causes of Fatigue and Malaise

Associated Symptoms	Possible Diagnosis	Diagnostic Tests
Fever, lymphadenopathy, weight loss	Malignancy	CBC, ESR Possibly CXR, CT, or MRI (see Table 4.2)
Increasing fatigue over time	Malignancy or anemia	CBC, ESR, chemistry profile Probably CXR Possibly CT or MRI (see Table 4.2)
Daytime somnolence, snoring (especially if increased), obesity	Sleep apnea	Sleep studies
Flat affect, appetite or sleep changes, possibly sexual dysfunction	Depression	None, if no other history findings suggest a physical cause
Change in skin or hair texture, heat or cold intolerance, weight changes	Thyroid disorder	TSH and free T4
Fever, cough; sometimes sore throat and lymphadenopathy	Infection	Treat empirically or obtain lab work and X-rays as indicated (e.g., CBC, strep screen, Monospot, CXR)
Weight loss but no fever or signs/symptoms of infection	Malignancy, poor nutrition, malabsorption syndromes	CBC, chemistry panel Consider X-rays
Pallor	Anemia	See Chapter 4, ANEMIA Stools for occult blood if indicated
Weight loss, polydipsia, polyuria	Diabetes mellitus	FBG (usually with a chemistry panel) Possibly A1c

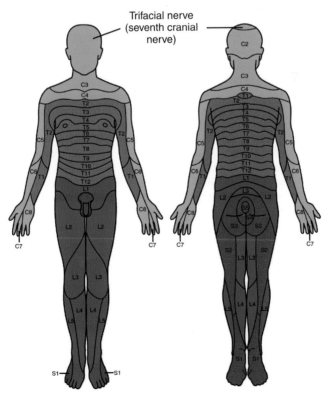

Fig. 13.1   Dermatomes. (From Nagelhout, J. J., & Plaus, K. (2014). *Nurse anesthesia* (5th ed.). St. Louis: Elsevier.)

TABLE 13.3 ■ Evaluating Muscle Strength

Score	Description
5 (Normal)	Has complete joint ROM with full or normal resistance
4 (Good)	Weak but able to resist the examiner
3 (Fair)	Moves against gravity but cannot resist the examiner
2 (Poor)	Moves but unable to resist gravity (passive ROM only)
1 (Trace)	Has muscle contraction but limited or no joint motion
0 (None)	Has no evidence of muscle function

General Musculoskeletal Disorders

FIBROMYALGIA SYNDROME

I. Description

A. Fibromyalgia is a common cause of chronic musculoskeletal pain; it is a chronic centralized pain sensitivity syndrome, characterized by diffuse, multifocal, migratory, waxing and waning pain, primarily described as arthralgia and myalgia (suggestion: share this with the patient and then explain it in more common words; it lets them know it is not all in their head).

B. There are minute changes (of unknown cause) in specific parts of the brain that lead to chemical changes and subsequent symptoms.

1. Dysregulation of the thalamus, hypothalamus, and amygdala
2. Hyperactive sympathetic and endogenous opioid systems (taking opioids makes the pain and other symptoms worse)
3. Neurotransmitter changes
   (a) Increased substance P, glutamate, and others—leads to increased pain
   (b) Decreased epinephrine and norepinephrine, serotonin and dopamine; this negatively affects mood, sleep, and energy (leading to "fibro fog," fatigue, and nonrestful sleep)

C. Because of the previously described changes, pain signals are amplified and inhibitory signals are reduced.

1. Hyperalgesia: things that hurt, hurt more (e.g., one pin stick feels like multiple ones; getting bumped with shopping cart feels like hit by a truck)
2. Allodynia: things that normally do not hurt, now do (e.g., a hug, a heavy blanket)
3. Global sensory hyperresponsiveness: patient is hypersensitive to almost everything (e.g., perfume, light, sounds, medications)

D. Autonomic dysfunction can result in multiple physical symptoms.

1. Dizziness, lightheadedness, presyncope
2. Tachycardia, dyspnea, cold and/or bluish discoloration of hands and feet
3. Temperature dysregulation
4. Bowel and bladder symptoms
5. Hair thinning/loss, fingernail changes

II. Diagnosis
- A. Do not be afraid to make the diagnosis; it gives the patient a sense of relief and allows them to "get off the fence" and move on to living with the condition.
- B. Criteria to help with diagnosis of fibromyalgia
  1. ACR 1990 criteria (specific tender points) is no longer used because the tender points could not be standardized and the criteria did not take into account the other symptoms.
  2. ACR 2010 criteria (revised in 2016) includes a widespread pain index (WPI) and symptom severity scale (SSS); these can be used to follow symptom severity over time.
     - (a) Generalized pain, present in at least 4 of 5 regions (this helps to exclude regional pain disorders)
     - (b) Symptoms have been present at least 3 mo
     - (c) Diagnosis of fibromyalgia is likely with a WPI ≥7 (out of 19) *and* SSS ≥5 (out of 12) OR WPI 4–6 *and* SSS ≥9 (these scales can be found at www.fmnetnews.com)
  3. AAPT 2019 criteria (both of the following must have been present for at least 3 mo)
     - (a) Multiple site pain (MSP) in 6 or more sites (out of 9 possible sites) (see Fig. 13.2)
     - (b) Moderate to severe sleep problems or fatigue
- C. Fibromyalgia often worsens with the following
  1. Anxiety and stress
  2. Temperature changes
  3. Humidity and weather changes (barometric pressure)
  4. Fatigue, poor sleep
- D. Detailed history and examination are most helpful; X-rays, CT and MRI scans, and EMG studies are unnecessary unless some other diagnosis is suspected
- E. Diagnostic studies help to rule out other causes and reassure the patient of diagnosis; there are no confirmatory tests or biomarkers for fibromyalgia at this time
  1. ESR, CRP, creatinine kinase (CK), RF/CCP, ANA, liver enzymes (muscle disease or rheumatologic condition like PMR, RA, SLE)
  2. TSH, CMP, AM cortisol level (drawn before 8 a.m.) (thyroid, renal, hepatic, or endocrine problem)
  3. CBC (chronic infection)
  4. Consider celiac serology (higher incidence with fibromyalgia)
  5. Overnight sleep study (sleep apnea and restless leg syndrome [RLS])

III. Treatment
- A. Multidisciplinary team works best because there is no known cure; an individualized, holistic treatment plan offers the best chance for management and improvement of symptoms
  1. PCP: to overall manage the patient's conditions (fibromyalgia is now more of a PCP condition and not rheumatology); subsequent visits:
     - (a) Be honest and open, "We do not cure fibromyalgia."
     - (b) Review current therapy and address new concerns; DO NOT focus on the pain or fatigue (symptom focused behavior is not helpful).
     - (c) The goal is to improve function; "Don't tell me what you cannot do, tell me what you can and want to do."
     - (d) Review medications every visit for compliance and tolerability.
  2. Physical therapy: increased functional ability and tolerance (target most painful issues over multiple treatments of a long time)

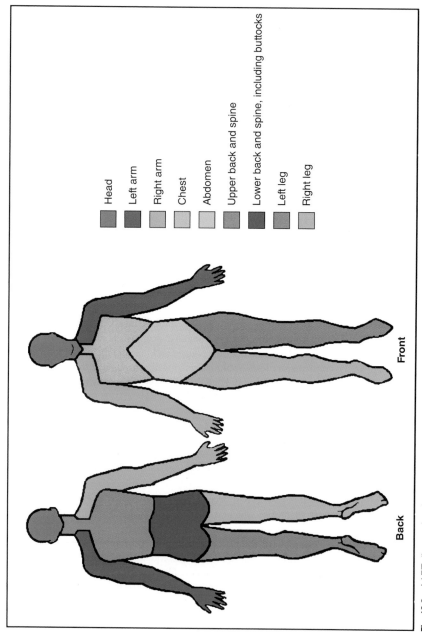

Fig. 13.2 AAPT diagnostic criteria for fibromyalgia (2019). (From Arnold, L. M, Bennett, R. M., et al. (2019). *The Journal of Pain, 20*(6). St. Louis: Elsevier.)

3. Occupational therapy: help with endurance, "brain fog," and ADLs (lifelong therapy)
4. Cognitive behavioral therapy or biofeedback therapy
5. Psychology or psychiatry: for any concomitant diagnosis
6. Massage therapy: NOT deep tissue but superficial Swedish-type (ongoing, often monthly)
7. Acupuncture therapy: licensed therapist to focus on what is worse at the time (ongoing)

B. Nonpharmacological care (some patients respond to these without needing medication)
1. Education: diagnosis and treatment of fibromyalgia, the cause, the importance of treating mood and/or sleep disorders, and patient's role in their own treatment; reassure patients that this is a real illness and not "in their heads."
2. Gentle, low-impact aerobic exercise tailored to meet specific needs; suggestions include walking, biking, swimming, or water aerobics, slowly and consistently (e.g., 5 min) on alternate week days and increasing 5 min q2wk with a goal of 20–30 min, 3–5 times every week by the end of the first year
3. Yoga and/or Tai Chi
4. Weight modification (excess weight can be proinflammatory and is hard on joints)
5. Smoking cessation
6. Adequate nutrition and sleep (including patient education on the importance of good sleep and adverse effects of poor sleep on pain)
7. Encourage the patient to prioritize time and activities (e.g., work, leisure, ADLs)

C. Pharmacological therapy (symptomatic; no treatments are curative)
1. "3 rules" of medications (tell the patient: "My job in the beginning is to not hurt you, because you are more likely to be hypersensitive.")
   (a) Start at very low doses, so low they probably will not help much.
   (b) Increase doses very gradually, over weeks or often months.
   (c) If side effects occur, back down to previous dose and retry later.
2. Opioids and corticosteroids are *ineffective.*
3. FDA approved
   (a) Duloxetine (pain + mood), start at 10–20 mg daily and may increase to 60 mg (weeks to months).
   (b) Milnacipran (pain + mood), start at 12.5 mg daily and may increase to 50 mg bid (weeks to months); may need up to 100 mg bid.
   (c) Pregabalin (pain + sleep + paresthesia), start at 25 mg daily and may increase to 50–75 mg bid (weeks to months); may need up to 300–450 mg in bid split dose.
4. Non-FDA approved but helpful
   (a) Gabapentin (pain + sleep + paresthesia), start with 100 mg hs and then bid after 2 wk
   (b) Amitriptyline 10 mg hs; may increase by 5 mg q2wk till maximum relief of symptoms is achieved without unacceptable side effects (usually 35–50 mg daily)
   (c) Cyclobenzaprine 5–10 mg hs (to help with muscle tightness and cramping, primarily in the evenings); can be titrated to 30–40 mg in split dose
   (d) Acetaminophen or NSAIDS (can help with peripheral pain)
   (e) Memantine (Namenda) 10–20 mg daily (can reduce pain and increase the pain threshold)

GOUT

I. Description: clinical syndrome resulting from urate crystals deposited in the tissue, with inflammation and potential destruction of the tissue or joint. All patients with gout will have hyperuricemia at some point, but most people never experience a gout attack.
   A. Primary hyperuricemia: no coexisting disease or drug that alters uric acid production or excretion
   B. Secondary hyperuricemia: excessive urate production or diminished renal clearance (see risk factors, below)
   C. Can affect several different joints but usually only one at a time; often involves the big toe (MTP joint). Very rarely affects the spine.
   D. Other than gout, hyperuricemia can result in urate nephropathy and nephrolithiasis (uric acid stone, not calcium oxalate stone).

II. Risk factors
   A. Male sex
   B. Certain ethnic groups: Taiwanese, Pacific Islander, and New Zealand Maori
   C. Living in high-income countries (specifically, North America and western Europe)
   D. Dietary: diet rich in red meat and some seafood/fish (sources of purine); for men, drinking ≥2 sugar-sweetened soft drinks a day, foods high in fructose (e.g., apples, grapes, watermelon, asparagus, zucchini) or any fruit juices
   E. Alcohol (men especially): beer is a higher risk of gout compared to distilled spirits
   F. Medication: diuretic (loop or thiazide)
   G. Comorbid conditions: HTN, DM, obesity or weight gain, dyslipidemia (cholesterol and trigs), CKD

III. Signs and symptoms
   A. Acute stage: affected joint is red, warm, and very tender (even the sheets hurt); reaches maximum inflammation within 24 hr. There is no fever or leukocytosis.
   B. Chronic gout: may have large, painless nodules (tophi), especially over the MTP or MCP joint
   C. May have kidney stone(s)

IV. Diagnostic tests
   A. Consider CBC, ESR (if unsure of diagnosis).
   B. Serum uric acid: not recommended during an acute attack because the level may be low; the most accurate time for baseline level or monitoring therapy is at least 2 wk after resolution of acute flare.
   C. "Gold standard" is seeing urate crystals in joint fluid aspirate (recommended only if the diagnosis is uncertain; usually done by a rheumatologist).

V. Treatment
   A. Acute flare: most effective when started within several hours of symptoms; consider comorbidities before choosing treatment.
      1. NSAIDs: indomethacin 50 mg tid or naproxen 500 mg bid; may taper as symptoms improve but continue until pain free, up to 1 wk; consider using PPI while taking NSAIDs.
      2. Prednisone 30–50 mg daily until the symptoms begin to resolve; then taper over 7 days.
      3. Colchicine 1.2 mg PO and then 0.6 mg 1 hr later; no repeat dose.
      4. If patient is on an anticoagulant, may use colchicine or prednisone.
   B. Recurrent or chronic gout
      1. After second or third attack, check uric acid levels and consider prophylactic therapy (which is usually continued indefinitely).

      (a) Start with allopurinol 100 mg daily (with normal renal function) and increase by 100 mg weekly; may take up to 800 mg daily. Doses >300 mg per day are given in divided doses with meals. With renal insufficiency, start with 50 mg daily and titrate more slowly.

      (b) Also give colchicine 0.6 mg 1–2 times daily *or* NSAIDs daily for 6 mo to prevent gout flares.

      (c) If an acute flare occurs, treat as described previously; if using prednisone, may need to extend taper to 10–14 days.

      (d) Continue urate-lowering therapy during the attack.

    2. Instead of allopurinol, may use febuxostat (Uloric) 40–80 mg daily.

    3. Uric acid goal is <6 mg/dL; it is recommended to lower the uric acid no more than 1–2 mg/dL per month, to reduce risk of a flare.

VI. Address prevention between gout attacks (most patients have second attack within 2 yr).

  A. Lifestyle changes to reduce risk factors

    1. The DASH diet has been associated with lower risk of developing gout (see Table 8.14).

    2. Reduce sugar-sweetened drinks and foods; avoid fructose-containing foods and alcohol.

    3. Encourage diet higher in low-fat dairy and plant sources of protein; more complex carbs instead of refined carbs; less saturated fat.

    4. Cherries and cherry juice have been associated with less frequent gout attacks.

    5. Weight loss if overweight; increased exercise.

  B. Managing comorbid diseases

    1. Consider stopping possible aggravating medications.

    2. For patients needing antihypertensive therapy, losartan has a uricosuric effect (start at 50 mg daily).

  C. Instruct the patient to start NSAIDs *when acute symptoms start*, without waiting to consult the provider each time.

VII. *Referral: to a rheumatologist if not responding to therapy.*

LEG CRAMPS

I. Causes

  A. Most leg cramps are idiopathic; most patients do not have a fluid or electrolyte imbalance.

  B. There are many medical conditions that can be associated with nocturnal leg cramps.

  C. Structural/mechanical causes include flat feet, wearing shoes of different styles or different heel heights, prolonged sitting, or working on a concrete floor.

  D. Potential aggravating medications (e.g., LABA inhalers, K+ sparing or thiazide diuretics)

II. There is little evidence that many of the leg cramp remedies are effective.

  A. Nonpharmacological therapies

    1. Daily stretching the calf muscles

    2. Using hot or cold packs; may also use a hot shower or warm tub bath

    3. Encourage patient to drink 8 oz water before hs, in addition to staying hydrated during the day; avoid caffeine and alcohol

    4. Tonic water, apple cider vinegar, or pickle juice may help some people

  B. Pharmacological therapies (try for at least a month)

    1. OTC supplements and medications

      (a) B-complex vitamin, containing 30 mg B6, tid

● = *non-urgent referral*

        (b) Magnesium or calcium might help with pregnant woman or if patient is deficient.

        (c) Iron may help if patient also has iron deficiency anemia.

        (d) If vitamins are ineffective, try diphenhydramine 12.5–50 mg hs.

    2. Prescription medications

        (a) If diphenhydramine is ineffective, try diltiazem 30 mg or verapamil 120–180 mg q evening.

        (b) Gabapentin 600–900 mg, divided between dinner time and hs, may help.

III. Therapies to avoid

    A. Quinine (due to possible severe side effects, including death, and cost)

    B. Homeopathic products are not proven safe or effective.

IV. *Referral to sleep specialist if therapy is ineffective.*

OSTEOARTHRITIS (OA)

    I. Description: degenerative changes in joints related to past trauma, aging, and/or obesity

        A. Common in weight-bearing joints (e.g., hip, knee, spine) and DIP/PIP joints and base of the thumb

        B. Joints usually spared: wrist, elbow, ankle (unless previous fracture)

    II. Signs and symptoms

        A. Joint stiffness on rising, lasting <30 min; occurs more by the end of the day. The joint damage may not correlate with the severity of joint pain and disability.

        B. Affected joints are irregularly shaped but *not* red or warm; pain is dull, achy, worse with activity, and improves or relieved with rest.

        C. May have nontender Heberden (DIP) and Bouchard (PIP) nodes.

        D. There are no extra-articular manifestations but consider sleep and mood disturbances because of the pain and change(s) in ability to do desired activities.

    III. Diagnostic tests: consider especially with knee or hip pain or symmetric pain in hands

        A. Lab: ESR, RA factor

        B. X-ray of the affected joint(s)

    IV. Treatment

        A. The goals of treatment are to minimize pain, optimize function, and modify joint damage

        B. Patient education is essential to get the best results

        (1) Discuss the cause(s) of the arthritis and the expected prognosis.

        (2) Help patient to set realistic goals and positively reinforce achievements (e.g., start with walking 10 min 3 times a week with eventual goal to be 30 min 3 times a week by 3 mo).

        C. Nonpharmacological therapy (tried first or in conjunction with medication)

        (1) Weight loss of at least 10%, if indicated.

        (2) Rest joint 12–24 hr with acute pain, then resume ROM and exercise (especially aquatic exercise).

        (3) Consider P.T. for suggestion of specific aerobic and strengthening exercises and O.T. for help with ADLs. Tai Chi has been shown to help with knee pain, function, and less analgesic use.

        (4) Use of items such as cane, knee brace, thumb splint.

        D. Pharmacological therapy (use only when symptomatic; none are disease-modifying)

        (1) With hand and/or knee OA: topical NSAIDs (e.g., diclofenac gel 2–4 times a day over affected joints) have similar efficacy to oral NSAIDs and have less GI and renal effects.

● = *non-urgent referral*

(2) With pain in multiple joints and/or hip OA: oral NSAIDs at the lowest dose needed to control the pain, used on a prn basis

(3) With OA in multiple joints and contraindications to oral NSAIDs: duloxetine 30 mg daily for a week, then may increase to 60 mg daily

(4) Acetaminophen is no longer recommended as first-line treatment due to safety concerns and negligble effects on pain.

(5) Consider opioids only for short-term use with severe symptoms unresponsive to other treatments (e.g., while awaiting a scheduled surgery).

  E. Alternative treatments that may be effective for pain relief and decrease inflammation

(1) Curcumin (turmeric) 500 mg bid

(2) *Boswellia serrata* extract may help with pain, stiffness, and function.

(3) Glucosamine *sulfate* 1500 mg daily may be of some help, especially with weight-bearing joints; shellfish allergy is not a problem with this. It may take up to 3 months for effects to be seen.

  F. *Referral to an orthopedic surgeon with no response to therapy or functional limitations and pain at rest or at night*

OSTEOPOROSIS

I. Types

  A. Primary: occurs in postmenopausal women (estrogen deficiency) or in men and women >75 yr of age (due to subtle, prolonged imbalance between bone resorption and formation or reduction in vitamin D synthesis)

  B. Secondary: due to extrinsic conditions such as chronic liver or kidney disease, IBD, malabsorption, COPD, hyperparathyroidism, premature menopause

II. Signs and symptoms

  A. Backache or pain, acute and chronic

  B. Kyphosis or scoliosis, atraumatic fractures

  C. Loss of height (>2 cm since last seen or >4 cm loss over lifetime)

  D. No peripheral bone deformities

III. Risk factors for fracture(s)

  A. Dietary

1. Inadequate calcium
2. Excessive phosphate
3. Inadequate vitamin D intake in elderly people

  B. Physical

1. Immobilization or sedentary lifestyle
2. Previous fracture
3. Low body weight
4. Older than 75 yr of age

  C. Social

1. Alcohol abuse, current cigarette smoking
2. Caffeine >16 oz daily (e.g., coffee, tea, caffeinated soda, energy drinks)

  D. Medical

1. Chronic diseases (e.g., liver or renal problems, ulcerative colitis, history of gastric bypass)
2. Medications: glucocorticoids (e.g., patient with COPD, Addison disease); many chemotherapy agents; progesterone and DMPA; SSRIs; chronic PPI use

---

  ● = *non-urgent referral*

3. Excess thyroid hormone replacement or hyperthyroidism
4. Males: androgen deprivation therapy for prostate cancer (e.g., Lupron)
5. RA

IV. Diagnostic tests

A. Bone mineral density (BMD) is the primary test; dual-energy X-ray absorptiometry (DEXA) is the most thorough

1. Initially ordered in women >65 yr of age *or* postmenopausal women <65 yr of age with clinical risk factors for fracture (see III, earlier in this chapter). Consider BMD for men >70 yr of age or sooner with loss of 1.5-in. height or with risk factors for fracture (see III, earlier in this chapter).

2. Results (if not normal)
   (a) Osteopenia: 1–2.5 standard deviations (SD) below the expected bone mass
   (b) OP: >2.5 SD below the expected bone mass

B. X-ray of vertebrae not necessary unless vertebral fractures are suspected.

C. Consider labs with significant decline in BMD *while on therapy*: CBC, ESR, possibly protein electrophoresis (to rule out multiple myeloma and leukemia); TSH and free T4, serum calcium and possibly PTH, and FBG (to rule out endocrine disease).

V. Treatment

A. Nonpharmacological therapy

1. Activity
   (a) Maintain weight-bearing exercise (e.g., walking at least 30 min 3 times a week); consider resistance training 2 times a week.
   (b) There is no evidence that high-intensity exercise (e.g., running) is a greater benefit than low intensity (e.g., walking).
   (c) Consider physical therapy measures for back muscle spasm.
   (d) Prevention of falls.

2. Diet
   (a) Calcium intake of 1200 mg daily total (food and supplement)
      (i) Food sources (see Appendix A)
      (ii) Calcium supplements 500–600 mg bid with meals
   (b) Avoid excess phosphate (e.g., carbonated beverages)
   (c) Encourage daily vitamin D: 600 units (if <70 yr of age), 800 units (>70 yr)
      (i) Supplements (e.g., with calcium or in a multivitamin)
      (ii) Food sources: seafood, eggs, organ meats, fish liver oils, vitamin D-fortified dairy products

3. Smoking cessation (cigarette smoking accelerates bone loss)

B. Pharmacological therapy: prescribed for patients with OP or at high risk for fracture/OP

1. Indications
   (a) Postmenopausal women (and men ≥50 yr) with history of hip or vertebral fracture OR with T-score worse than −2.5
   (b) Consider treatment for postmenopausal women with T-score between −1 and −2.5 AND a 10-yr probability of hip fracture of ≥3% (can be calculated on the FRAX website)

2. Medication options (all patients should have a normal serum calcium and vitamin D levels before starting therapy; they should take calcium and vitamin D if dietary intake is not adequate)
   (a) Bisphosphonate therapy is first-line therapy (decreases hip and vertebral fractures). With poor dentition, have the patient see a dentist before starting bisphosphonates
      (i) Alendronate (Fosamax) 70 mg qwk (can also be given 10 mg daily)

   (ii) Risedronate (Actonel) 35 mg qwk or 150 mg qmo (also 5 mg daily)
   (iii) Ibandronate (Boniva) 150 mg PO qmo or 3 mg IV q3mo
   (iv) Zoledronic acid (Reclast) 5 mg IV yearly
   (b) Anabolic medications: teriparatide (Forteo) or abaloparatide (Tymlos) SQ daily stimulate bone growth and are used mainly for patients with a very high fracture risk or those who had a fracture while on a bisphosphonate. Use for a maximum of 2 yr, then restart bisphosphonate to help maintain bone density.
   (c) Denosumab (Prolia) IV q6mo is used instead of an anabolic medication, for patients with a very high fracture risk or if intolerant to oral bisphosphonates. It is associated with increased infection risk; also, stopping or delaying a dose can lead to rebound vertebral fractures due to rapid bone loss. Change to bisphosphonate or raloxifene after medication is stopped.
   (d) Raloxifene (Evista) 60 mg daily, for menopausal women with OP and no history of fragility fracture, who do not tolerate bisphosphonate or denosumab; if hot flashes occur, stop medication until symptoms stop and then "wean up" (e.g., 1 day in week 1, 2 days in week 2, 3 days in week 3, etc., until taking daily).
C. Therapies not found to be beneficial
   1. Giving more than one medication
   2. Calcitonin
   3. Calcitriol
   4. Vitamin K or B_{12}, folate, or fluoride
   5. Androgen therapy
   6. Isoflavone supplements
   7. Tibolone
VI. Follow-up
   A. Annual chemistry screening, breast examination, and mammography (as indicated)
   B. Repeat BMD in 1–2 yr after initiating therapy
      1. If stable or improving, repeat less frequently.
      2. If worsening, verify medication adherence (including calcium and vitamin D supplements) or the development of a disease or disorder that could affect the bones and repeat in 1–2 yr. If the decline is >5%, consider changing from oral bisphosphonate to zoledronic acid, denosumab, or teriparatide or abaloparatide.
   C. Bisphosphonates may be stopped after 5 yr of use for most patients (those with no previous vertebral fractures and for whom BMD is stable); recheck BMD q2yr after stopping medication.
   D. Patient education
      1. Fall prevention, balance
      2. Body mechanics
      3. Alert the patient taking bisphosphonates to report any vision loss or eye pain.

RESTLESS LEG SYNDROME

   I. Description: RLS (also called Willis-Ekbom disease [WED]) is a syndrome characterized by an overwhelming urge to move the legs; it occurs at rest and is relieved by movement.
   A. Although long remissions are possible, the condition is generally chronic or recurrent.
   B. The cause of RLS/WED is unknown but often occurs in association with iron deficiency, multiple sclerosis, end-stage renal disease, pregnancy, and possibly Parkinson disease and essential tremor.

    C. A positive family history (FH) of RLS/WED is present in 40%–60% of patients.

    D. May be triggered by smoking, fatigue, sleep deprivation, or by stopping or starting certain medications. These medications include the following:

      1. Antidepressants: mirtazapine, TCAs, SSRIs, SNRIs

      2. Antihistamines: fexofenadine, loratadine, diphenhydramine

      3. Major tranquilizers: haloperidol, quetiapine, thorazine

      4. Metoclopramide

II. Diagnostic criteria

    A. The almost irresistible desire to move legs usually associated with paresthesias (e.g., sensations described as creepy, crawling, or drawing; not usually burning or pins-and-needles feeling)

    B. Symptoms are worse or present only at rest and are at least partially or temporarily relieved during activity. They are worse in the evening or at night.

III. Additional findings that may be present

    A. Sleep disturbances (e.g., difficulty falling and remaining asleep, exhaustion)

    B. Involuntary movements (e.g., periodic jerking)

    C. Normal neurological examination

IV. Treatment

    A. Check serum iron and ferritin levels, and, if low, give iron supplement (e.g., ferrous sulfate 325 mg) with vitamin C 100–200 mg daily to get ferritin levels to >50 mcg/L; recheck ferritin level after 3–4 mo of therapy and then q3–6mo until serum ferritin is >75 mcg/L.

    B. Nonpharmacological remedies may help

      1. Hot baths or heat or ice pack to legs

      2. Leg massage

      3. Regular exercise

      4. Avoid aggravating factors (i.e., sleep deprivation, caffeine, nicotine, ETOH)

    C. Pharmacological therapy (if the first medication is ineffective or not tolerated, try a medication from another class)

      1. Dopamine agonists

        (a) First-line therapy; take ~2 hr before RLS/WED symptoms start. The doses for RLS/WED are lower than those used to treat Parkinson disease.

        (b) Medications

          (i) Ropinirole 0.25 mg daily, in the evening; may increase by 0.25 mg q4–7days until symptoms are controlled (up to 4 mg daily).

          (ii) Pramipexole (Mirapex) 0.125 mg daily, in the evening; may increase by 0.125 mg q4–7days until symptoms are controlled (up to 1 mg daily).

          (iii) Rotigotine (Neupro) once-daily patch; start with 1 mg/24 hr and titrate weekly up to 3 mg/24 hr if needed; rotate application sites to lower the risk of skin reactions.

        (c) Evaluate the patient every 6 mo for effectiveness of therapy and also for augmentation (e.g., increased symptoms despite dose increase, earlier onset in the afternoon/evening, shorter action of the medication, or spread of symptoms to the trunk and/or arms).

        (d) If augmentation occurs

          (i) Recheck ferritin level

          (ii) Try splitting the medication dose to bid or modestly increase the dose *or*

          (iii) Start an alpha-2 ligand (e.g., pregabalin), and wean off the dopamine agonist.

2. Alpha-2 ligands
   (a) A first-line therapy for many patients (especially with comorbid painful peripheral neuropathy, insomnia or sleep disturbance, or Parkinson disease)
   (b) Not associated with augmentation.
   (c) May be associated with increased risk of suicidal thoughts and behavior.
   (d) There is potential for misuse and abuse of these medications.
   (e) Medications
      (i) Gabapentin enacarbil 600 mg in the early evening (i.e., ~5 pm)
      (ii) Pregabalin 150–450 mg daily, in the evening; start at 50–75 mg and titrate weekly
      (iii) Gabapentin 100–300 mg daily, ~2 hr before hs; titrate slowly up to effective dose (may be 900–2400 mg daily; if over 600 mg, divide the dose with one-third in the AM and two-thirds 2 hr before hs)
3. If the above therapies are ineffective or cause augmentation or adverse effects, tramadol may be used. Start at 50–100 mg at hs; after 1–2 wk, if helping but not lasting through the night, consider extended-release tramadol 100 mg (may increase to 200 mg at hs after 1–2 wk if needed).

V. *Referral: to a sleep specialist or neurologist if therapy is not as effective as the patient would like*

RHEUMATOID ARTHRITIS (RA)

I. Description: symmetric, inflammatory polyarthritis of unknown etiology; it affects at least three joints, including small joints of hands and feet; does not affect DIP joints or thoracic/lumbar spine

II. Signs and symptoms
  A. Joint stiffness on rising, lasting >1 hr; often improves with activity
  B. Affected joints are red, swollen, and warm
  C. Ulnar drift or deformities of fingers (swan neck, boutonniere) are often present
  D. Malaise and/or fatigue are often present
  E. May have extra-articular manifestations but not early in the disease (e.g., pleural effusion, HF, A-fib, anemia, vasculitis, neuropathy)

III. Diagnostic tests
  A. Lab: RA factor (high sensitivity), ESR or CRP, ANA, CBC, CMP, UA; consider anti-CCP (high specificity), serum uric acid, UA
  B. Consider X-rays of painful joints (e.g., hands)

IV. Treatment
  A. *Referral: to a rheumatologist*
  B. Monitor patients taking immunosuppressive agents for signs of HF and skin cancers
  C. *No live vaccines* (e.g., for shingles) if taking biologic DMARD agents (e.g., Enbrel, Humira)
  D. Consider O.T. referral for splinting and help with ADLs
  E. Paraffin baths can help with hand and foot pain

● = *non-urgent referral*

Location-Specific Musculoskeletal Disorders

NECK

I. Inspection: observe for any deformities and abnormal posture
II. Palpation: assess for tenderness and/or muscle spasm
   A. Cervical spine processes
   B. Trapezius and sternocleidomastoid muscles
   C. Muscles between scapulae
III. Muscle testing
   A. ROM: Ask the patient to perform the following:
     1. Touch the chin to the chest (flexion); abnormal if <60 degrees
     2. Touch the chin to each shoulder (rotation); abnormal if <90 degrees
     3. Touch each ear to the respective shoulder without raising the shoulder (lateral bending); abnormal if <45 degrees
     4. Tip the head back and look toward the ceiling (hyperextension); abnormal if <75 degrees
   B. Spurling maneuver (may be called "axial compression"): patient seated with head rotated slightly to one side and chin flexed toward the chest; the examiner presses gently down on the head; if the patient tolerates this well, repeat with the head rotated slightly to the side and have them look up. Positive test with radicular symptoms beyond the shoulder: ipsilateral side—consider compression; contralateral side—consider muscle tension. Perform this on the unaffected side first and then on the affected side.
   C. Assess for bilateral shoulder shrugs (against resistance) and grip strength.
IV. Sensory testing of C-spine (see also DTRs [Chapter 1, NEUROLOGICAL, IV, J] and Fig. 13.1)
   A. C4–C5: numbness in the deltoid region and diminished biceps reflex
   B. C5–C6: numbness in the dorsolateral areas of the thumb and index finger; diminished biceps and brachioradialis reflexes
   C. C6–C7: numbness in the index and middle fingers and back of the hand; diminished triceps reflex

---

PRACTICE PEARLS FOR NECK PAIN

- Pain not caused by injury and not relieved by rest or is progressive: consider cancer or infection
- No treatment has been shown to change the natural course of mechanical neck pain; management is toward patient comfort until it resolves. Consider P.T.
- Possible causes of referred neck pain (i.e., absence of physical findings, including neck tenderness, loss of motion, or pain with motion) include the following:
  - Shoulder (bursitis, tendinitis, arthritis)
  - Reflex sympathetic dystrophy
  - ***Thoracic outlet syndrome***
  - ***Bronchogenic cancer***
  - ***CAD, aortic dissection***
  - Peptic ulcer disease, pancreatitis, cholecystitis
- Possible neck pain diagnosis (Table 13.4)

■ = *not to be missed*

TABLE 13.4 ■ **Neck Pain**

Finding	Possible Cause(s)	Additional Points
Acute pain with neck movement, localized and episodic; often present when waking and usually lasts 1–4 days. There is muscle tenderness	Neck sprain	Pain relief with relative rest, NSAIDs or acetaminophen, muscle relaxers, and hot and/or cold packs If neck tenderness persists and is associated with other tender areas in the body, consider fibromyalgia
Involuntary rotation or lateral bending of the head; usually associated with tender muscle spasm, pain with neck movement, and limited ROM	Torticollis	May be acute or chronic
Acute or recurrent pain, more severe and lasts longer than a stiff neck; may be associated with whiplash injury or sudden movement; symptoms increase with ipsilateral rotation and contralateral bending of the neck. May have limited ROM	Cervical strain	Neurological examination of the upper extremities is normal; *if related to trauma or an accident, obtain C-spine X-ray with oblique view and referral to or consult with a physician*
Neck pain with radiation: pain similar to cervical strain but with sharp, burning, or tingling pain to the shoulder, back, or arm(s). May have muscle tenderness and/or spasm, limited ROM, and extremity weakness	Herniated cervical disc DJD with a bone spur	*Referral; consider X-ray and MRI of C-spine first*

SHOULDER

I. With shoulder pain, attempt to answer the following questions:
   A. Is ROM normal or abnormal? Is it painful?
   B. Are any structures tender (Fig. 13.3 and 13.4) and does palpation reproduce the pain?
   C. Is neurologic examination of the arm and shoulder normal?

II. Inspection for swelling, deformity, inequality, and muscle atrophy
   A. Anteriorly: shoulders (including shoulder height) and shoulder girdle
   B. Posteriorly: scapula and related structures

III. Palpation for tenderness and crepitus
   A. Site where the patient locates pain
   B. Sternoclavicular joint
   C. Acromioclavicular (AC) joint: consider AC joint strain or osteoarthritis (OA)
   D. Subacromial area (between the humeral greater tubercle and the acromion process)

IV. Muscle testing
   A. ROM (designate by degrees): examine the patient from behind and ask the patient to perform the following:
      1. Raise arms forward and then overhead with palms touching (elevation, flexion).
      2. Keep elbows at the side, swing forearms out: perform with and without resistance.
      3. Place each thumb between scapulae: "back scratcher" (adduction, extension, internal rotation).
   B. Muscle strength: have the patient
      1. Flex the elbow to 90 degrees, then abduct the arm to 90 degrees; have the patient resist as you press down on the distal arm (evaluates deltoid and rotator cuff).

● = *non-urgent referral*

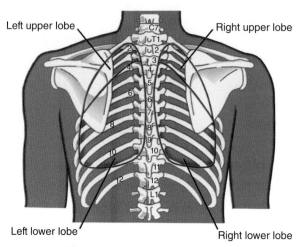

Fig. 13.3   Upper spine and landmarks.

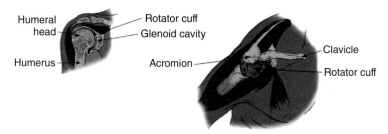

Fig. 13.4   Anatomy of shoulder. (From Pfenninger, J. L., & Fowler, G. C. (2011). *Pfenninger and Fowler's procedures for primary care* (3rd ed.). Philadelphia: Elsevier.)

2. Raise arms straight out to the side (abduction, extension) with thumbs up and then rotate thumbs down (evaluates rotator cuff): perform with and without resistance.
3. Flex the elbow to 90 degrees while you support the elbow; have the patient resist as you press against the distal forearm, attempting to internally rotate the arm (evaluates rotator cuff).

C. ROM testing results
1. ROM full, symmetric, and painless: check for referred pain (Table 13.5)
2. Active ROM is painful or impaired: perform passive ROM. If passive ROM is normal with abnormal active ROM, it is probably muscle/tendon weakness or neurogenic weakness; the most common causes are rotator cuff tear and cervical spine disorders causing deltoid weakness.
3. Active and passive ROM both limited: try to localize the restriction. Restrict scapula movement by placing the heel of your hand over the upper scapula and your fingers over the shoulder; feel the shoulder as active or passive abduction of the arm is attempted.
   (a) Restriction seems inflexible: bony (e.g., degenerative joint disease)
   (b) Restriction "gives away" with pressure and is due more to pain and muscle spasm: periarticular (e.g., tendinitis, bursitis, muscle spasm or strain)

D. Determine what degree of shoulder motion causes pain or limitation (Fig. 13.5)
1. All directions of movement: glenohumeral joint itself (e.g., arthritis of the joint)

TABLE 13.5 ■ Referred Shoulder Pain

Site	Possible Causes	Additional Points
Trapezius ridge	Diaphragmatic Pleuritis Pericarditis Subdiaphragmatic disease Ruptured organ (e.g., ulcer) Ectopic pregnancy Splenic rupture	Perform cardiorespiratory and abdominal examinations Check for postural hypotension
Acromioclavicular area	Diaphragmatic or subdiaphragmatic disease (e.g., cholecystitis)	
Lower scapula	Gallbladder disease	Check Murphy sign (see Chapter 9, **ABDOMINAL PAIN III**, E, 6,)
Back of the neck, interscapular area, and posterior shoulder	Cervical spine disease (most common site for referred pain)	Perform neck examination
Deltoid area	Articular and periarticular disorders of the shoulder (e.g., arthritis, bursitis)	
Mid-humerus (brachial insertion site)	Rotator cuff problem	

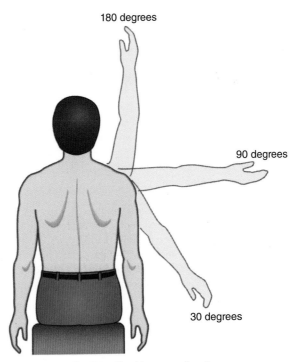

180 degrees

90 degrees

30 degrees

Fig. 13.5 Shoulder range of motion.

2. Initial 30 degrees of abduction impaired: rotator cuff muscles
3. Initial 90 degrees of abduction impaired but 90–180 degrees normal: rotator cuff muscles, tendons, or bursae
4. Initial 90 degrees of abduction normal but 90–180 degrees impaired: AC joint disorders
5. Internal and external rotation impaired: rotator cuff muscles, other muscle spasm, impingement syndrome (most common cause of shoulder pain)

V. Sensory testing
   A. ROM of neck
   B. Muscle testing
     1. Shoulder shrug against resistance (cranial nerve XI or cervical [C] nerves 3–5)
     2. Scapular retraction: "stand at attention" against resistance (C5)
     3. Motor strength of biceps, triceps, and wrist extensors and flexors (see Table 13.3)
     4. Deep tendon reflexes: biceps, brachioradialis, triceps
     5. Sensory examination using light touch along dermatomes and peripheral nerves (see Fig. 13.1 for dermatome distribution)

VI. Elevated arm stress test (EAST) for thoracic outlet syndrome
   A. Patient stands with the back to a wall and abducts both arms at least 90 degrees and then opens and closes fists at a moderate speed for 3 min
   B. Results (***with positive test, referral to vascular surgeon***)
     1. Positive test: reproduction of neurologic and/or vascular symptoms
     2. Negative/inconclusive test: only a sense of fatigue in the arm

VII. Treatment of common shoulder problems
   A. Rotator cuff tendinitis
     1. Treat with rest and ice for acute pain; may take NSAIDs at full strength for 3–4 wk.
     2. Restrict overhead reaching, any movement with the elbow away from the body, and sleeping on the involved side.
     3. Once pain has improved, begin gentle ROM movements of the shoulder; perform to "stretch" and not pain.
     4. Discourage use of a sling, which may hasten development of a frozen shoulder.
     5. ***Referral: if no improvement after 3 wk.***
   B. Rotator cuff tear: ***referral to an orthopedic surgeon***
   C. AC strain
     1. The goal is to allow ligaments to reattach.
     2. Activity is limited for 30 days
       (a) Avoid sleeping on either side.
       (b) Do not reach overhead or across the chest.
       (c) Lift close to the body, but do not lift more than 20 lb.
     3. Apply ice (see RICE mnemonic, Table 13.13).
     4. Shoulder immobilizer, probably for 3–4 wk.
     5. ***If no improvement in 2 wk, consult or referral to a physician.***
     6. Patient education: if treatment recommendations are ignored, the ligament may not reattach, leading to persistent symptoms.

● = ***non-urgent referral;*** ■ = ***not to be missed***

PRACTICE PEARLS FOR SHOULDER CONDITIONS

- Acute symptoms for <2 wk: often an injury such as a fracture, rotator cuff tear, or biceps tendon rupture
- Biceps tendon rupture: ask the patient to make a "Popeye arm" or "show their guns." There will be an abnormal bulge in the mid-humerus area with the tendon rupture. This can be acute or chronic; often can be surgically repaired if found early.
- Night pain is often worse with bursitis and rotator cuff inflammation.
- With burning, constant pain: consider a neurogenic cause.
- Bilateral shoulder pain after 50 yr of age: consider polymyalgia rheumatica.
- Consider MRI or CT prior to referral to an orthopedic surgeon (with acute pain, but not with chronic).
- Common chronic shoulder pain
  - Pain on top of the shoulder and worsened by touching the opposite shoulder with the hand of the affected side: consider AC joint arthritis or separation.
  - Pain in the lateral deltoid area and worsened by overhead activities: consider bursitis, frozen shoulder, or rotator cuff problem.
  - Shoulder pain relieved by placing the forearm on top of the head: consider cervical nerve root problem.
  - Pain along glenohumeral joint lines: consider degenerative arthritis of the joint.
  - Aching pain and paresthesias radiating from the neck to the shoulder and/or down to the hand, associated with intermittent swelling and discoloration of the arm and worsened by overhead activities: consider thoracic outlet syndrome.
  - *Consider referral to physical therapy (PT) before orthopedist because much of the time, PT with or without a steroid injection will be the initial treatment.*
- If the condition does not respond to nonsurgical therapies after 3 wk, *referral to an orthopedic surgeon*
- See Table 13.5 for referred shoulder pain.

ELBOW

   I. Inspect and palpate
      A. For nodules, swelling, or tenderness of extensor surface of the ulna, lateral and medial epicondyles, and olecranon process (including the groove on each side)
      B. For muscle wasting of interossei and hypothenar eminence
  II. Muscle testing
      A. ROM: ask the patient to perform the following:
         1. Bend and straighten elbows; if checking ROM against resistance, the examiner applies resistance at the wrist, not the hand.
         2. Rest arms at the side with the elbows flexed, then pronate and supinate the hands with and without resistance (Fig. 13.6).
         3. Flex the elbows and rest the forearm on a flat surface; have the patient resist wrist flexion and extension.
      B. Determine what type of elbow motion causes pain or limitation
         1. With flexion/extension: consider ulnar-humeral joint problem
         2. With forearm pronation/supination: consider problem with the proximal radial and/or ulnar joints (e.g., "tennis elbow" or "golfer's elbow")
 III. Sensory testing
      A. Tinel test (for cubital tunnel syndrome): firmly percuss over the ulnar nerve in the ulnar groove at the palm and elbow; *positive test* with paresthesias in the ring and little fingers

---

● = *non-urgent referral*

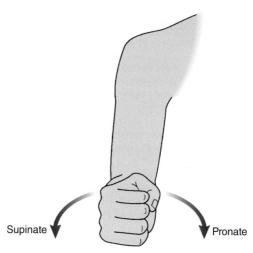

Fig. 13.6   Elbow range of motion test.

TABLE 13.6 ■ Common Elbow Disorders

Finding	Possible Cause(s)	Additional Points
Swelling over the olecranon process (can move without difficulty and is not painful)	Olecranon bursitis	Pull-on elbow brace may help Aspiration of the bursa for specific diagnosis and then apply a fairly tight neoprene sleeve and/ or consider consultation with a physician Often recurs
Pain or tenderness over the lateral epicondyle, aggravated by resisting wrist extension	Epicondylitis (tennis elbow)	Caused and aggravated by hand and wrist movements; splint the wrist to prevent movement and take NSAIDs for 7–10 days A tennis elbow band may prevent recurrence Modify or eliminate causative activities
Pain or tenderness over the medial epicondyle, aggravated by resisting wrist extension	Epicondylitis (golfer's elbow)	Caused and aggravated by hand and wrist movements; splint the wrist to prevent movement and take NSAIDs for 7–10 days Modify or eliminate causative activities
▲ Pain in the elbow and limited ROM	Nursemaid's elbow Dislocation	**_Referral: to ED_**

    B. Sensation in all finger tips and radial and ulnar sides of hands, front and back

    C. If the pain history indicates a radicular source (e.g., tingling, numbness), examine the cervical spine (see NECK examination)

  IV. Common elbow disorders: see Table 13.6

▲ = *urgent referral*

PRACTICE PEARLS FOR ELBOW PAIN

- Acute pain
  - After injury: consider fracture, dislocation, or tendon/ligament rupture
  - Conditions within the joint may cause acute synovitis (e.g., swelling, tenderness, limited motion): consider RA, gout, or **septic arthritis** (especially with IV drug abusers); **refer urgently to ED with suspected septic arthritis**
- Chronic pain
  - Commonly associated with overuse injuries (work or sport)
  - May be OA or inflammatory condition (i.e., RA or gout)
  - **If pain persists despite treatment: consider X-rays, P.T. evaluation, orthopedic referral**
- A patient with an elbow overuse injury frequently also has rotator cuff tendinitis.
- Referred pain can be from the following:
  - **Angina**
  - Cervical radiculopathy
  - Carpal tunnel syndrome

WRIST AND HAND

I. Inspection
   A. Inspect for swelling, redness, nodules, deformity, and muscle/thenar atrophy.
   B. Have the patient make a fist and look at the knuckle (MCP) profile for symmetry.
   C. Inspect nails for pitting and other signs of systemic disease.
II. Palpation of the following for swelling, bogginess, or tenderness
   A. Medial and lateral aspects of each DIP and PIP joint (Fig. 13.7)
   B. MCP joints just distal to and on each side of the knuckle (use your thumbs for examination)

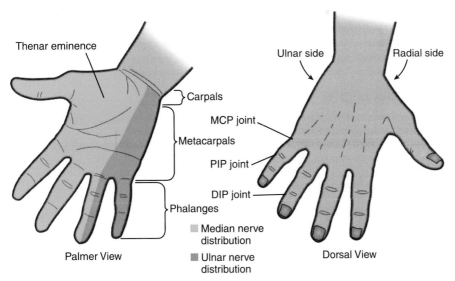

Fig. 13.7 Anatomy of hand and nerve distribution.

▲ = *urgent referral;* ■ = *not to be missed;* ● = *non-urgent referral*

     C. Wrist joint (your thumbs on the dorsal side and your fingers beneath it)

     D. Capillary refill and radial and ulnar artery pulses

III. Muscle testing (take into account the dominant hand)

     A. ROM: ask the patient to perform the following:

       1. Make a fist, with the thumb across the knuckles.

       2. Extend and spread fingers 3 times.

       3. Touch each finger with the thumb of the same hand (thumb-finger opposition).

       4. With palms down, move the fingers laterally (ulnar deviation) and medially (radial deviation).

       5. Flex and extend wrists with and without resistance.

     B. Assess grip strength bilaterally (see Table 13.3)

     C. Finkelstein test for de Quervain tenosynovitis: the thumb is held in the palm with a closed grip; the wrist is ulnarly deviated; a *positive (abnormal)* result is pain from the radial styloid to the "snuff box"

IV. Sensory testing

     A. For carpal tunnel syndrome (CTS)

       1. Phalen maneuver: have the patient press the backs of hands together (flexes wrists at 90 degrees) for 60 sec; positive (abnormal) results are numbness and tingling in the thumb and first two fingers.

       2. Tinel sign: hyperextend the wrist and firmly percuss over the median nerve on the palmar side approximately 1 cm proximal to the wrist; positive (abnormal) results are tingling or shock-like sensations across the palm, thumb, and first two fingers.

     B. Remember that hand or wrist pain may be referred from cervical nerve roots, brachial plexus, or peripheral nerves; "radicular," or nerve pain, is often described as tingling, burning, or numbness and follows dermatomes (see Fig. 13.1) or peripheral nerve distributions; if such pain is present, check DTRs and sensory status; the following sensory areas are to be tested (also see Fig. 13.7):

       1. Tip of the index finger (median nerve)

       2. Tip of the little finger (ulnar nerve)

       3. Dorsal first web of fingers (radial nerve)

       4. Dorsal-ulnar surface of the hand (dorsal branch of the ulnar nerve)

  V. Common wrist and hand conditions: see Table 13.7

PRACTICE PEARLS FOR WRIST AND HAND PAIN

- *Refer all patients with fractures early to an orthopedic surgeon or to ED if same-day orthopedic follow-up is not accessible.*
- If pain persists despite immobilization for 3 wk, repeat X-rays to check for carpal fracture or osteonecrosis, which may not be evident on initial films.
- Localization of pain
  - Radial side: consider trauma, de Quervain tenosynovitis, or arthritis
  - Ulnar side: consider cartilage tear (with trauma) or tendinitis
  - Palmar side: consider CTS, ganglion cyst, or tenosynovitis
- For CTS, nonpharmacologic strategies that can help
  - Have the patient hold the elbow next to the body and using the other hand, forcefully extend the wrist for 10 sec, 10 times tid; this stretches the carpal tunnel.
  - Wear a wrist splint at night.
  - Vitamin B6 100 mg bid may help with paresthesia; use NSAIDs prn for pain.

● = *non-urgent referral*

TABLE 13.7 ■ **Common Hand and Wrist Disorders**

Finding	Possible Cause(s)	Additional Points
Hand or finger swelling, pain, or deformities	OA or RA, gout Trauma	See the specific conditions, earlier in this chapter Consider CBC, CRP, ESR Consider X-rays
Thenar atrophy	Carpal tunnel syndrome	*Referral to an orthopedic or hand surgeon*
Painless swelling (cyst) on the dorsum of the hand or wrist	Ganglion	No treatment necessary unless painful; may attempt aspiration with an 18-g needle, compressing cyst as it gets smaller
Pale fingers and slow capillary refill	Raynaud phenomenon Ulnar or radial artery lesion	See Chapter 8, **PERIPHERAL ARTERIAL DISEASE, I)** *Consult with physician; referral immediately to the ED if the problem is acute*
Loss of resistance against extension or flexion	Cervical nerve root lesion	*Referral to a spine specialist or neurologist*
Passive ROM normal with absent active ROM; may or may not have pain	Peripheral nerve lesion (e.g., radial, median, ulnar) Brachial plexus lesion	*Referral to an orthopedic surgeon or neurologist*
Unable to flex the DIP or PIP joint		*Referral to an orthopedic or hand surgeon*
Asymmetric knuckle profile	Metacarpal fracture Degenerative joint disease	X-ray, *referral if fracture is present*
Finger "locks" or jumps with flexion	Trigger finger OA, trauma	*Referral to an orthopedic or hand surgeon*
Digital mucous cyst		Soft cyst, usually between DIP and nail bed; treatment is aspiration if it is bothersome

HIP AND LOW BACK PAIN

   I. History: in addition to the usual questions, ask every patient about the following signs and symptoms, which are *red flags (not to be missed) warranting immediate referral:*
   A. *Bowel or bladder incontinence*: consider lower disc disease or cauda equina syndrome
   B. *Numbness in the "saddle area"*: consider cauda equina syndrome
   C. Pain suggestive of dissecting aortic aneurysm (*severe "tearing" pain*) or cancer (*back pain, especially if worse while supine, and history of cancer*)
   D. *Fever and/or weight loss* (particularly in a patient with immunosuppression, DM, or history of substance abuse or recent spinal surgery)
   E. *In a patient <20 yr or >55 yr of age with no prior history of back pain*: consider ankylosing spondylosis, osteoporosis (OP), infection, or tumor
   F. *Unrelenting night pain (or no relief with bed rest) and/or difficulty in finding a comfortable position*
   G. *Risk factors for spinal infection*
      1. Known infection elsewhere

■ = *not to be missed;* ● = *non-urgent referral;* ▲ = *urgent referral*

2. IV drug use

3. Systemic signs and symptoms, including fever

4. Lab evidence, including elevated WBC count and ESR

II. Physical examination (inspection/palpation/neuromuscular)

A. Watch the patient walk (abnormal gait often indicates hip disease); have the patient walk on heels (L5) and then on toes (S1); if the patient is able to do this, cauda equina syndrome is ruled out

B. Patient standing

1. Look at thigh muscles for atrophy.

2. Look at the patient's back for deformities (e.g., kyphosis, scoliosis) or lateral curves.

3. Look for height difference in shoulders, iliac crests, and skin crease below buttocks.

4. Palpate for levelness of iliac crests (not level: probably pelvic tilt).

5. Check ROM forward, backward, and to both sides

(a) Forward flexion decreases pain in spinal stenosis and increases pain in sciatica.

(b) Look for flattening of the lumbar curve.

6. Press for tenderness along the sacrum and lateral buttocks.

C. Patient sitting

1. Look again for atrophy of thigh muscles.

2. Palpate for point tenderness; may percuss the vertebrae for pain.

3. Palpate paravertebral muscles for tightness or bulge.

4. Have the patient flex the hip upward (i.e., raise thigh) as you resist by pressing down on the distal thigh.

5. Check DTRs.

6. The examiner extends each knee individually until the leg is straight (passive straight leg raise [SLR]).

D. Patient supine

1. Look for differences in leg length (may indicate a somatic dysfunction for which chiropractic or osteopathic manipulation may help).

2. Auscultate and palpate the abdomen (to check for bruits and aneurysm).

3. Palpate for pain along the anterior-superior iliac crest, over the greater trochanter, and over lateral fibular heads.

4. Flex the patient's knee and hip and check internal and external rotation in relation to pain.

5. Abduct and adduct the straight leg (testing hip ROM).

6. Have the patient bend each knee (individually) up to the chest and pull firmly against the abdomen; the opposite thigh should remain on the table, fully extended.

7. Check motor, sensory, and circulatory status (e.g., flexion of the great toe against resistance, sensation along dermatomes [see Fig. 13.1 for dermatomes], capillary refill).

8. Passive SLR bilaterally with the foot dorsiflexed: note the degree of elevation causing pain (15–30 degrees in severe cases, 30–60 degrees in milder cases) and any radiation of pain down the leg; pain *must* extend below the knee to be a positive test

9. If suspecting piriformis syndrome: have the patient lie supine; internal and external rotation of the foot will reproduce piriformis pain.

III. Hip and low back pain diagnosis (see Tables 13.8–13.10)

PRACTICE PEARLS FOR HIP AND LOWER BACK PAIN

- Plain X-rays showing osteoarthritis do not necessarily rule out other causes of hip pain.
- *A phrase to help remember which type of CA metastasizes to the bone*: "BLT with Mayo and a Kosher Pickle" (breast, lung/lymphoma, thyroid, multiple myeloma, kidney, prostate).
- Disc disease and myofascial pain are most common in adults <50 yr of age.
- A patient with an acute herniated disc prefers to stand.
- Spinal stenosis, cancer, and Paget disease usually occur in adults >50 yr of age.
- Spinal stenosis also involves numbness and/or weakness in legs with standing; improves or resolves with sitting or bending forward.
- Gabapentin is *not* effective in radicular low back pain. Consider a 3 mo trial of amitriptyline 25 mg daily (research has shown a decrease in disability at 3 mo).
- Facet pain is only in the back; have patient lean back and then to the right and left; pain will be in one side or the other, in an area approximately 6-in. diameter. *Consider referral for possible nerve or facet injection(s) or radiofrequency nerve ablation.*
- Treatment for mechanical low back pain
  - Advise the patient to avoid bed rest (including sitting in bed) and to simply limit painful activities; improvement usually occurs within a few weeks.
  - Encourage cold packs; the patient may alternate cold and hot packs.
  - NSAIDs are given for pain; adding muscle relaxers has *not* been shown to help.
  - Exercise is the key to treatment (e.g., walking, swimming, cycling).
    - Start as soon as possible, starting with 5–10 min and working up to 20–30 min daily.
    - Abdominal (core) and back strengthening exercises may help to prevent future problems (although not consistently proven in research).
  - Instruct regarding lifting and carrying techniques.
  - Recheck if not improved in 1 wk.
  - Additional therapeutic modalities for cervical, thoracic, and lumbosacral strains
    - Spinal manipulation (e.g., osteopathic, chiropractic)
    - Myofascial release, deep massage
    - PT for commonly used modalities
    - Trigger point injections with saline, Marcaine, or Xylocaine.
- Bilateral hip pain that starts with walking and is relieved with rest: consider vascular or neurogenic claudication.
- *Young adolescent with hip or knee pain but no physical findings (except maybe a limp):* suspect *slipped capital femoral epiphysis* until ruled out with X-rays (AP and frog-legged view); *if present: emergent orthopedic referral*
- Referred pain to the hip may be from the following:
  - *Testicular torsion (urgent referral to ER)*
  - Lumbar spinal problem
  - Disorder of the pelvic cavity
  - Vascular or neurogenic claudication
- *Referral: all patients with positive neurological findings, for consultation and further diagnostic studies; often, specialists may want MRI of the area done before patient's appointment.*
- Treatment for *chronic* low back pain
  - Nondrug strategies: staying active, P.T., acupuncture, and/or tai chi can help
  - NSAID at lowest effective dose, for shortest time necessary
  - Duloxetine 60 mg daily if patient also has neuropathy, depression, or anxiety
  - Consider tramadol or other opioids as last result for severe pain, at the lowest dose and shortest time possible
- Hip osteoarthritis points
  - Helpful: exercise, weight loss of at least 10% (if needed), Tai Chi, steroid injection
  - May be helpful: patient education, acetaminophen or tramadol, acupuncture
  - Not recommended: glucosamine, vitamin D or fish oil, methotrexate, stem cell injections, intraarticular hyaluronic injections (e.g., Synvisc), TENS

■ = *not to be missed;* ● = *non-urgent referral;* ▲ = *urgent referral*

TABLE 13.8 ■ Common Hip Disorders

Finding	Possible Cause(s)	Additional Points
Unequal leg length	Fracture or dislocation	Painful internal or external rotation is also present ***Transfer to ED after examination***
Limited ROM	Arthritis Fracture Dislocation	With arthritis, internal rotation is lost early
Active hip and knee flexion of one leg results in passive flexion of the other leg	Flexion deformity of the passive hip	***Consult an orthopedic surgeon or physiatrist***
Pain radiates to the lateral knee	Iliotibial band syndrome	Often found in joggers Treat with NSAIDs and hip adduction stretching exercises
Tender to palpation along the lateral knee/greater trochanter	Trochanteric bursitis	Treat with NSAIDs and stretches; possibly steroid injections
Limited ROM and progressive limp	Aseptic necrosis (osteonecrosis) of the hip	Usually associated with a dull ache or throbbing pain in the groin, lateral hip, or buttock area ***Referral to an orthopedic surgeon***

TABLE 13.9 ■ Common Low Back Pain Examination Findings

Finding	Possible Nerve Compression	Muscle Spasm
"Radicular" pain	X	
Pain radiates below knees	X	
Asymmetry on inspection or palpation		X
Limited ROM	X	X
Paravertebral muscle bulge		X
Positive SLR	X (usually at 40–60 degrees)	Possible
Asymmetric DTRs	X	
Asymmetric motor or sensory findings	X	
Unequal sacroiliac joints, sacral spines, or leg lengths		X

TABLE 13.10 ■ Comparison of Lumbar Nerve Roots

Finding	L4	L5	S1
Pain	Lateral hip and anterior leg	Mid buttock to lateral buttock, lateral leg	Mid buttock, posterior leg, lateral foot
Numbness	Distal anterior thigh and knee	Lateral calf	Posterior calf and lateral foot
Motor weakness	Quadriceps extension	Dorsiflexion of the great toe	Plantar flexion of the foot
Reflexes	Diminished patellar reflex	—	Diminished Achilles tendon reflex
Screening examination (unable to perform)	Squat and stand	Walk on heels	Walk on toes

● = non-urgent referral; ▲ = urgent referral

KNEE

I. History
  A. Pain related to mechanical use (e.g., brought on by walking, climbing, bending)
    1. Sharp, stabbing pain: consider mechanical problem
    2. Dull, aching pain: probably degenerative and overuse problems
    3. Localization of pain can significantly narrow possible diagnosis
      (a) Worse with repetitive flexion-extension movement with weight bearing (e.g., going up or down stairs or squatting and then standing): stress on extensor mechanism
      (b) Worse with pivoting: meniscus or patella
      (c) Increases during the day: degenerative arthritis
      (d) Decreases during the day: inflammatory conditions (e.g., arthritis, tendinitis)
  B. "Clicking": common and does not imply disease; may be associated with a torn meniscus, arthritis, or chondromalacia
  C. Buckling (i.e., knee "gives away")
    1. True: the patient cannot bear weight; associated with anterior cruciate tear, torn meniscus, patellar dislocation.
    2. Pseudo: transient; often a disorder of the extensor mechanism (e.g., patellofemoral disorder or weak quadriceps muscles, especially in elderly or sedentary individuals) or injury of the lateral or medial collateral ligament.
  D. "Locking" of knee
    1. Acute: usually related to trauma
    2. Recurrent: usually due to a torn meniscus but may be degenerative arthritis
  E. Swelling
    1. What area of the knee? Is it associated with redness and/or increased warmth?
    2. Constant or recurrent (what seems to cause it)?
II. Inspection
  A. With the patient undressed below the waist, compare both knees during the examination (Fig. 13.8).
  B. Watch the patient walk; evaluate symmetry of gait.
  C. Patient in the supine position with legs extended and relaxed, look for the following:
    1. Atrophy of quadriceps muscles
    2. Effusion (loss of normal knee hollow on the sides of the patella)
    3. Alignment of knees (e.g., normal, varus, valgus)
III. Palpation: examine the uninjured knee first; with the legs extended and relaxed, evaluate:
  A. For thickening or swelling above and on the sides of the patella; to identify a large effusion, perform ballottement
    1. Firmly grasp the thigh just above the patella (forces fluid into the space between the patella and femur); using two fingers of the other hand, push the patella sharply back against the femur.
    2. Positive (abnormal) result is a palpable click.
  B. Patellofemoral compartment
    1. Move the patella side to side.
    2. Push the patella distally and ask the patient to tighten the knee against the table (contracts quadriceps muscles); note pain (patellar grind) or crepitus (crepitus alone has little significance).
IV. ROM
  A. Incomplete extension is the most subtle limitation.
  B. Limited ROM may be due to joint effusion, pain, or a mechanical problem of the joint, menisci, or ligaments.

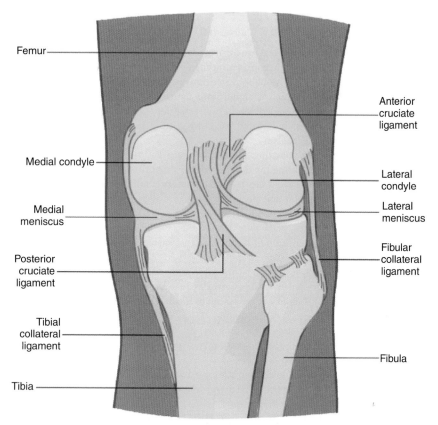

Fig. 13.8 Left knee. (From Rutter, P., & Newby, D. (2008). *Community pharmacy: symptoms, diagnosis, and treatment.* (2nd ed.). Hamilton, Australia: Elsevier.)

    C. Test the integrity of the collateral ligaments
        1. Medial: with the leg extended, exert pressure on the lateral side of the knee and medial side of the ankle
        2. Lateral: with the leg extended, exert pressure on the medial side of the knee and lateral side of the ankle
        3. Positive (abnormal) result is pain and "opening up" of the knee toward the side being tested
    D. Perform McMurray test
        1. Flex the knee while holding the heel of the foot in your hand, with the ball of the foot resting on your wrist.
        2. Place your other hand on the joint line of the knee.
        3. Rotate the foot laterally and extend the leg: checks the medial meniscus; rotate the foot medially and extend the leg: checks the lateral meniscus.
        4. Positive (abnormal) result is a palpable, painful click of the knee.
    E. Tibiofemoral joint: flex the knee to 90 degrees with the foot on the examination table
        1. With your thumbs, press into the joint space on either side of the patellotibial tendon and let your fingers surround the sides of the leg (resting on top of the collateral ligaments and menisci); palpate for tenderness or irregular bony ridges along the joint space.

2. Palpate the extensor mechanism for tenderness: quadriceps tendon on the superior patella and patellotibial tendon on the inferior patella.
3. Palpate the medial and lateral areas of the knee for tenderness.
4. Palpate the posterior surface of the knee for hamstring muscles (knee flexors).
5. In an adolescent with knee pain, press on the tibial tuberosity and note swelling or tenderness.

F. Test the integrity of the cruciate ligaments (drawer tests)
1. Knee flexed with the foot flat on the table; sit on the foot and grasp both sides of the tibia at the knee.
2. Pull the tibia forward: tests the anterior cruciate ligament.
3. Push the tibia back: tests the posterior cruciate ligament.
4. Positive (abnormal) result is movement of the tibia away from the joint.

V. Common knee disorders: see Table 13.11

PRACTICE PEARLS FOR KNEE PAIN

- With knee problems, also examine the hip, spine, and back because referred knee pain may be from the following:
  - Adults: herniated disc, muscle strain, hip injury
  - Children: hip pathology
- MRI is rarely needed as part of the initial evaluation of knee complaints.
- Patella fractures may result from injuries such as falls; fracture of tibia or femur is usually due to major trauma.
- Older patients with degenerative meniscal tears can be treated with quadriceps and hip abductor strengthening exercises, rather than surgery.
- Knee osteoarthritis points
  - Helpful: exercise, weight loss of 10% (if needed), Tai Chi, splints, diclofenac tablets or topical gel, intraarticular steroid injections
  - May be helpful: patient education, taping, acetaminophen or tramadol or duloxetine; Questionable: intraarticular hyaluronic injections (e.g., Synvisc)
  - Not recommended: glucosamine, TENS, stem cell injections (although more research is currently underway)
- *If the condition does not respond to nonsurgical therapies, referral to an orthopedic surgeon*

TABLE 13.11 ■ **Common Knee Disorders**

Finding	Possible Cause(s)	Additional Points
Loss of knee "hollows"	Effusion Synovial thickening	Warm and tender: may be synovitis Nontender: OA Positive bulge sign or fluid wave with effusion
Positive patellar ballottement	Large effusion	See above ***Consult or referral to an orthopedic surgeon***
Crepitus or pain with quadriceps tightening	Osteoarthritis Patellofemoral syndrome (PFS)	PFS is the most common knee problem: treat with NSAIDs and decreased knee stress until improvement is seen with quad strengthening exercises ***Referral: to P.T. if no improvement after 3–4 wk***

● *= non-urgent referral*

TABLE 13.11 ■ Common Knee Disorders—cont'd

Finding	Possible Cause(s)	Additional Points
Pain and abnormal movement when testing collateral ligaments	Tear of the medial or lateral collateral ligament	*Referral to an orthopedic surgeon*
McMurray test: positive results	Torn meniscus	*Referral to an orthopedic surgeon*
Pain with palpation of the tibiofemoral joint	Damaged menisci or collateral ligament(s) Bursitis	Positive results from McMurray test or weakness of the medial or lateral collateral ligament Pain more over the tibial tubercle Locking or "giving out" of knee with weight bearing
Bony ridges along the tibiofemoral joint	Osteoarthritis	
Swelling or pain over the tibial tuberosity	Osgood-Schlatter disease	Normal quadriceps strength and ROM of knee
Positive result from drawer tests	Cruciate ligament tear	*Referral to an orthopedic surgeon*
Posterior knee pain	Hamstring strain or tendinitis	*Referral to P.T.*
	Baker cyst DVT	*Referral to an orthopedic surgeon* Venous Doppler
Pain over the lateral femoral epicondyle	ITB syndrome	*Referral: to P.T.;* NSAIDs routinely for 7–10 days
Severe pain in the extremity out of proportion to what would be expected; sensation of tightness and swelling; worsened by passive stretching	Possible acute compartment syndrome	*Emergent transfer to ED*

FOOT AND ANKLE

I. The foot is not often a site of referred pain; most significant structures are either palpable or easily tested during physical examination; try to localize the problem to the forefoot, midfoot, or hindfoot (Figs. 13.9 and 13.10).

II. Inspection and palpation

A. Beginning away from the area of maximal pain, inspect and palpate all surfaces for swelling (unilateral [i.e., localized] or bilateral [i.e., systemic]), deformities or nodules, calluses or corns, or point tenderness.

1. Ankle joint: over the anterior aspect, lateral and medial malleoli, and ligaments
2. Achilles tendon
3. MTP joints
   (a) By "squeezing" the forefoot with your thumb and fingers just proximal to the distal ends of the first and fifth metatarsals

● = *non-urgent referral;* ▲ = *urgent referral*

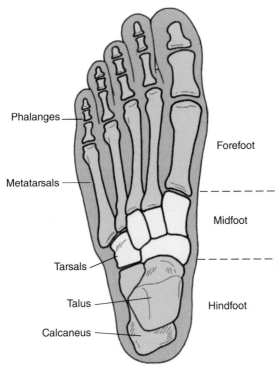

Fig. 13.9 Areas of foot. (From Benzon, H. T., Rathmell, J. P., Wu, C. L., Turk, D. C., & Argoff, C. E. (2008). *Raj's practical management of pain* (4th ed.). Philadelphia: Elsevier.)

        (b) Palpate the distal end of each metatarsal individually using your thumb and index finger.
    4. Plantar surface: for plantar warts, ulceration, tenderness on pressure over the heel or ball of the foot
  B. While you observe the patient from behind, have the patient stand on toes barefooted; ***verify that both heels rotate inward; unequal with posterior tibial tendon problem, referral to an orthopedic surgeon if present***
  C. With ankle injuries, to evaluate for ***Achilles tendon tear***, squeeze the sides of the calf (tibia-fibula "squeeze test"); *if the foot does not move, the test is positive (see Table 13.12).*
III. ROM: perform actively or passively or both
  A. Dorsiflexion (point the foot toward the patient)
  B. Plantar flexion (point the foot away from the patient)
  C. Inversion (twist the sole of the foot inward)
  D. Eversion (twist the sole of the foot outward)
  E. Flexion of toes
IV. Common foot and ankle disorders: see Table 13.12

■ = *not to be missed;* ● = *non-urgent referral*

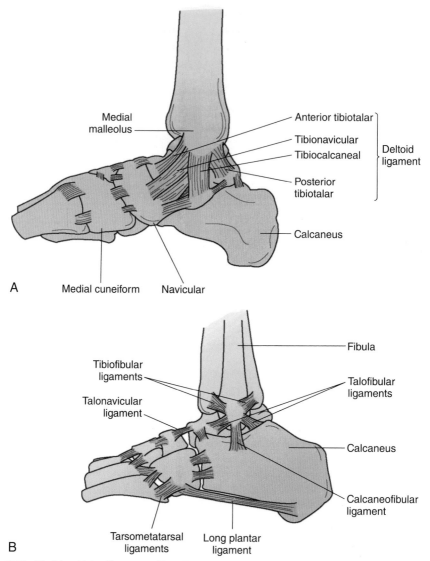

Fig. 13.10 Medial and lateral ligaments. (From Fritz, S., & Grosenbach, J. (2008). *Mosby's essential sciences for therapeutic massage* (3rd ed.). Philadelphia: Elsevier.)

TABLE 13.12 ■ Common Foot and Ankle Disorders

Finding	Possible Cause(s)	Additional Points
Heel pain	Plantar fasciitis Bone spur Tendinitis	Treat with rest, NSAIDs, heel pad, or orthotics Local steroid injection may help Roll arch of the foot over a frozen juice can **Referral: if no improvement** (it often takes 6–12 mo for symptoms to resolve)
Pain with palpation	Sprain or fracture	Consider consultation
Ankle pain with tibia-fibula "squeeze test"	Fracture	**Referral to an orthopedic surgeon**
Unable to bear weight immediately after an accident	Severe sprain or fracture	**Urgent referral to an orthopedic surgeon**
Unable to plantar flex foot or walk on toes; with the patient prone, squeeze the calf muscle and the *foot will point if the tendon is intact*	Rupture of Achilles tendon (if the foot does not move as described)	**Urgent referral to an orthopedic surgeon**
Unable to dorsiflex foot	Injury to the tibiotalar joint	**Referral to an orthopedic surgeon**
Pain at the base of toes increases with squeezing the forefoot while pressing upward on the sole between the third and fourth metatarsal heads	Morton neuroma	Shoes with good support or extra padding NSAIDs **Referral to an orthopedic surgeon or podiatrist if no improvement**

PRACTICE PEARLS FOR FOOT AND ANKLE PAIN

- To distinguish warts from calluses: warts have interruption of skin lines, blood vessels in the core, and tenderness with squeezing the sides of the lesion.
- Medical conditions that may affect the feet include DM, peripheral vascular disease (PVD), neuropathy, inflammatory arthritis, or gout.
- With bilateral foot pain, consider a systemic or spinal cause.
- Forefoot problems in women are often caused by high-heeled and/or ill-fitting shoes. Initial treatment always includes shoe modification (i.e., low heels, wider or longer shoes).
- Plantar fasciitis is the most common cause of heel pain. *If treatment modalities* (see Table 13.12) *do not help, consider X-ray of the foot and referral to a podiatrist or orthopedic surgeon.*
- *The following findings suggest severe ankle injury, and the patient should be referred soon to an orthopedic surgeon*:
    - *Eversion injury* (more serious: medial support is stronger)
    - *Immediate diffuse swelling* (often indicates bleeding)
    - *Unable to bear weight immediately*
    - *Positive tibia-fibula "squeeze test"* (Achilles tendon tear)
    - *Positive drawer test*
    - *X-ray examination shows avulsion fracture or fracture of the foot*
- *Consider acute Charcot neuroarthropathy in any obese patient 40yr of age or older with diagnosis of neuropathy and who presents with acute swelling of foot with no trauma and little or no pain.*
    - If X-ray and CBC are normal, MRI or CT scan of foot should be done.
    - *If is suspected, immobilize the foot/ankle and urgently refer to foot and ankle specialist*

● = *non-urgent referral;* ▲ = *urgent referral;* ■ = *not to be missed*

STRAINS AND SPRAINS

   I. Strain: excessive stretch or tear of the muscle fibers
     A. Common sports injury seen in activities such as jumping, running, and kicking
     B. A complete tear of a muscle is called a rupture
   II. Sprain: excessive stretch of the ligament with disruption of its fibers
     A. Commonly occurs in the knee, ankle, or wrist during physical activity
     B. *Uncommon in children with open growth plates or in a patient with significant OP* (bone injury or fracture more likely to occur in these cases)
     C. See Table 13.13 for clinical findings and treatment of sprains

TABLE 13.13 ■ **Comparison of Sprains**

Grade of Sprain	Clinical Findings	Suggested Treatment
I	Mild stretching of the ligament Pain and tenderness with little or no swelling; no joint instability Able to bear weight with minimal pain	Symptomatic treatment only: RICE* NSAIDs around-the-clock, not prn, for 48 hr When pain is resolved, begin active or passive ROM 3–4 times qid
II	Significant but incomplete tearing of the ligament Moderate pain, swelling, and ecchymosis with slight-to-moderate instability "Pop" felt and often heard with injury; defect palpable Weight bearing and walking are painful	Immobilization: posterior splint, air cast, or soft brace and non–weight bearing with crutches until able to walk with normal gait RICE* NSAIDs around-the-clock, not prn, for 48 hr When pain is resolved, begin ROM 3–4 times qid May need opioids for pain
III	Complete ligament tear Marked pain, swelling, tenderness, and ecchymosis with significant instability Unable to bear weight or walk	***Referral to an orthopedic surgeon*** Symptomatic treatment is controversial Posterior splints and crutches NSAIDs around-the-clock for 48 hr and opioids for prn use

* RICE is an acronym for the treatment of many joint injuries:
R Rest: avoidance of activities that cause pain; the length of time varies with the injury.
I Ice: 20 min qid, usually for 2–3 days; a convenient ice pack is a bag of frozen peas or corn, which can "mold" around an injury and be refrozen as often as necessary (caution the patient to somehow mark the bag so that the vegetables are not accidentally eaten after being thawed and refrozen).
C Compression: use of ACE bandage to provide support and limit swelling.
E Elevation: keep elevated as much as possible for 24–48 hr.

PRACTICE PEARLS FOR STRAINS AND SPRAINS

- With strains, try to gently stretch the injured muscle while palpating for a defect in the muscle.
▲ • *If the patient is unable to contract the muscle to move a joint, consider complete rupture or severe pain as the cause. Immobilize the joint and referral urgently to an orthopedic surgeon or ED.*
- Order X-rays with suspected fracture, pain over malleoli or midfoot areas, or inability to bear weight immediately after injury.

● = *non-urgent referral;* ▲ = *urgent referral*

CHAPTER 14

Pain

INTRODUCTION

I. History related to pain
    A. Have the patient describe the pain, as well as factors that worsen or improve/relieve it.
    B. Does the patient take any prescription pain medications regularly? If so, how often and for what kind of pain? Are they effective?
    C. Does the patient take any medications for psychiatric conditions (e.g., anxiety, depression, bipolar D/O)?
    D. Does the patient use marijuana or illicit/street drugs (currently or in the past)?
    E. With chronic pain, what is the impact on the following:
        1. Overall quality of life and functioning (e.g., socializing, relationships, mood and anxiety, sleep, exercise, and occupation)
        2. Basic ADLs and activities required to live independently (e.g., shopping, preparing meals, doing housework, managing finances and medications)
II. PMH related to pain
    A. Ask about prior evaluations and treatment of pain
    B. Current and past providers (including alternative practitioners) and reasons for visits
    C. Past medications prescribed, OTC meds, or alternative methods, and the effects
    D. Any tests/imaging studies done in the past 10 yr?
    E. Was pain associated with trauma, surgery, or illness?
    F. Is there any litigation pending?
III. For patients who can communicate, a common method for identifying pain is to use a rating scale (e.g., 0–10, with 0 being no pain and 10 being the worst pain imaginable)
IV. Consider the following when a patient cannot communicate in a meaningful way:
    A. Attempt to obtain a self-report (consider https://wongbakerfaces.org/)
    B. Ascertain what behaviors the patient may exhibit with pain (i.e., from family, past clinicians)
        1. Patients with dementia or other disabilities may or may not be able to accurately report pain and may exhibit confusion, irritability, loss of appetite, or frequent falls (see Table 17.1).
        2. Children may have aggressive outbursts, become withdrawn, eat excessively, or have a poor appetite.

ACUTE PAIN

I. Description
    A. Results from trauma, surgery, or acute illness (e.g., kidney stone); the pain is well localized and may be described as sharp, aching or throbbing
    B. Expected to be self-limiting, usually improving as the injury heals; may last up to 3 to 6 mo

C. Set realistic goals for pain relief and function (e.g., return to normal life balance, ADLs); total pain relief may not be realistic (e.g., after major surgery or severe injuries)

D. The goals of the treatment(s) chosen are to help minimize
  1. Physiologic responses, such as immobility, muscle spasms, and shallow breathing
  2. Anxiety, depression, and fear
  3. Progression to chronic pain

II. Treatment
  A. Medications (also see **PHARMACOLOGICAL THERAPIES**, later in this chapter)
    1. NSAIDs
    2. Acetaminophen when NSAID is indicated but not desirable
    3. Oral opioid (e.g., hydrocodone)
    4. Agents NOT preferred
      (a) Codeine (metabolized to morphine; genetic metabolism may result in poor response or toxicity)
      (b) Tramadol (many drug interactions and lowers seizure threshold)
      (c) Fentanyl patch (risk of respiratory depression)
  B. **NONPHARMACOLOGICAL THERAPIES** (see Therapies for Pain, later in this chapter) can be used in conjunction with medications, based on the cause and severity of the pain

CHRONIC PAIN

I. Description
  A. Definition: pain persisting 3 mo or longer beyond the expected normal healing time
  B. May be continuous, intermittent, or a combination of both
  C. Often associated with sleep or appetite disturbances, irritability, social withdrawal, depression
  D. Often, there is a disparity between examination and/or diagnostic tests and the level of patient complaints (e.g., patient rates pain as a 10 and no pain is elicited on examination)
  E. General treatment
    1. Should be multidisciplinary and not focus on medications alone. The pain experience and treatment options can be impacted by the patient's socioeconomic status, culture, access to healthcare, geography, and availability to exercise.
    2. *Offer hope and potential for pain improvement;* often, there is not a cure. Key goals in chronic pain management include improvement in satisfaction and quality of life and to improve overall physical functioning as compared to baseline.
      (a) Help patient set realistic functional goals (e.g., able to cook meals, returning to work, taking a walk with someone). Reassess at each visit (see Box 14.1); modify if needed.
      (b) Focus on being able to complete daily self-help goals rather than focusing on the pain. This helps the patient to see improvement in their condition.
    3. Evaluate for and treat concomitant depression and anxiety.
    4. Evaluate for and treat insomnia or sleep apnea (adequate, restful sleep often improves quality of life and satisfaction with treatment).
    5. Keep in mind that therapies previously tried and "failed" may be related to
      (a) Inadequate dose or duration or timing

BOX 14.1 ■ PEG* Scale†

Q1: What number from 0–10 best describes your *pain* in the past week?
    0 = "no pain" to 10 = "worst pain you can imagine"
Q2: What number from 0–10 describes how, during the past week, pain has interfered with your *enjoyment of life?*
    0 = "not at all" to 10 = "complete interference"
Q3: What number from 0–10 describes how, during the past week, pain has interfered with your *general activity?*
    0 = "not at all" to 10 = "complete interference"

---

* *Pain, Enjoyment of life and General activity.*
† Average three individual question scores; 30% improvement from baseline is clinically meaningful.

    (b) Side effects that could have been avoided with slower titration or use of alternate medication in the same category
    (c) Poor communication between provider and patient regarding the value and rationale of proposed treatment(s) (e.g., referral to psychologist, psychiatrist, pain management specialist, or PT)

II. Classification
  A. *Neuropathic pain* involves damage of peripheral or central nerves (onset may be weeks to months after acute nerve injury). Trigeminal neuralgia has peripheral and central components
    1. Peripheral pain
      (a) Caused by PHN, DM neuropathy, and peripheral nerve damage
      (b) Described often as *"pins and needles," "on fire,"* or *"electric shocks."* May also be aching, crushing, paroxysmal stabbing
    2. Central pain
      (a) Caused by post-CVA, MS, radiculopathy, spinal cord injury pain
      (b) Described as a loss of sensation with brief bursts of sharp pain, steady burning sensation, allodynia (i.e., pain due to a stimulus not normally painful, such as temperature or physical stimuli)
    3. Treatment
      (a) Medications (also see **PHARMACOLOGICAL THERAPIES**, later in this chapter)
        (i) Tricyclic antidepressants (TCAs), SNRIs, pregabalin, gabapentin; lidocaine 5% patch or gel has also been shown to be effective.
        (ii) Consider opioids *only* if preceding measures are insufficient (see **PRESCRIBING OPIOIDS FOR CHRONIC PAIN**, later in this chapter).
      (b) Consider **NONPHARMACOLOGICAL THERAPIES** such as cognitive behavioral therapy, PT, exercise, relaxation, acupuncture.
    4. *Referral for possible other interventions (e.g., nerve blocks, spinal cord stimulation, surgery)*
  B. *Nociceptive (peripheral) pain* due to peripheral tissue damage
    1. Chronic pain (also called somatic pain) that is usually associated with degenerative joint disease and/or chronic overuse

---

◉ = *non-urgent referral*

(a) More continuous, achy, and dull; does not resolve but the patient may manage with medications and lifestyle changes

(b) Examples are back pain, myofascial pain syndrome, OA

(c) Treatment

(i) Should focus on behavioral modification and physical rehabilitation (e.g., TENS unit, PT, acupuncture, massage, or trigger point pressure or injection may help).

(ii) NSAIDs (oral or topical) can help; consider trials off of the NSAID to avoid unnecessary use and adverse effects.

(iii) Acetaminophen is not an NSAID but can provide pain relief to some patients.

(iv) Opioids should be used chronically *only* if the preceding recommendations have failed to provide adequate pain relief *and* improvement in function (also see **PRESCRIBING OPIOIDS FOR CHRONIC PAIN**, later in this chapter).

2. Inflammatory pain is associated with chronic inflammation in joints or infection that destroys the musculoskeletal surface areas.

(a) Pain is caused by innocuous stimuli without trigger; there may be obvious deformity or swelling of the area.

(b) Described as a sharp or dull pain in the deformed-appearing joint.

(c) Examples are rheumatoid arthritis, recurrent gout attacks, or psoriatic arthritis.

(d) Treatment includes NSAIDs, disease-modifying antirheumatic drugs (DMARDs), and nonpharmacologic therapies such as light exercise, heat, and OT/PT.

C. *Visceral pain*

1. Is diffuse, poorly localized, and noxious

2. May be dull, aching, deep, cramping, and squeezing

3. Examples are renal calculi or any type of damage to internal organs

4. Treatment is alleviation of the underlying cause of pain and may require opioids, antispasmodics, benzodiazepines, and NSAIDs (also see **PHARMACOLOGICAL THERAPIES**, later in this chapter)

D. *Centralized sensitization pain*

1. No identifiable tissue or nerve damage but there is neuronal dysregulation

2. CNS is the origin and amplification of the pain

3. Fibromyalgia is the common example, but there can be other pain conditions as well (see Chapter 13, **FIBROMYALGIA SYNDROME**)

Therapies for Pain

NONPHARMACOLOGICAL THERAPIES

I. Often helpful in giving patients some control over their pain (acute and chronic); combination therapies have been shown to be more effective than any single approach for managing chronic pain

II. Environmental

A. Comfortable lighting and temperature

B. Positioning with pillows, blankets, etc.

III. Distraction techniques (e.g., music, puzzles, or games)

IV. Educational programs pertinent to diagnosis

V. Self-hypnosis, psychotherapy, relaxation techniques, or cognitive behavioral therapy
VI. Physical modalities
   A. Chiropractic
   B. Massage, therapeutic touch
   C. Physical therapy (including TENS unit, ultrasound therapy, heat therapy)
   D. Acupuncture
   E. Exercise programs (yoga has been shown to decrease some pain significantly after 12 wk of regular exercise)
VII. Herbal products (not exclusive); caution patients to research all of them on reliable websites, not on social media platforms
   A. Comfrey topical preparation for bruises, pulled muscles, or sprains; do not use on broken skin, for >6 wk, or if pregnant
   B. Aloe topical gel or spray for burns
   C. Witch hazel *topically* to treat skin inflammation; not intended for oral use
   D. Arnica gel may help with OA pain. *Do not* take orally or use if pregnant or nursing

PHARMACOLOGICAL THERAPIES (ALSO SEE TABLE 14.1)

I. Explain to patient that it will take 2–3 wks to adequately evaluate the therapy; some medications take longer than that to see the full effect
II. Acetaminophen
   A. Analgesic, antipyretic (no antiinflammatory properties)
   B. Using with NSAID (e.g., acetaminophen 500 mg with ibuprofen 200–400 mg q6hr prn) may provide better pain relief
   C. Cautions
      1. Chronic use may be associated with hepatotoxicity, CKD, HTN, chronic daily H/A and PUD. Consider periodic CMP and CBC (hepatic and renal function evaluation).
      2. With chronic liver impairment, be aware of other OTC medications that the patient is taking; many may contain acetaminophen (maximum dose is 3000 mg daily).
      3. Possible serious skin reactions (e.g., Stevens-Johnson syndrome, TEN).
III. Anticonvulsants (for peripheral and central neuropathic pain)
   A. Gabapentin
      1. May or may not be more effective than pregabalin but is less expensive and insurance may want it to be tried first.

TABLE 14.1 ■ Suggested Therapies for Pain

Pain Level	Neuropathic Pain	Nonneuropathic Pain
Mild-to-moderate pain (1–4 out of 10)	Adjuvant therapy ± mixed opioid analgesic*	Mixed opioid analgesic ± adjuvant therapy
Moderate pain (4–7 out of 10)	Adjuvant therapy ± weak opioid analgesic[†]	Weak opioid analgesic[†] ± adjuvant therapy
Severe pain (7–10 out of 10)	Adjuvant therapy ± strong opioid analgesic[‡]	Strong opioid analgesic[‡] ± adjuvant therapy

*See **VIII**, Opioids, C., 2.
[†]Weak: acetaminophen with codeine or oxycodone or hydrocodone, butorphanol.
[‡]Strong: morphine, oxycodone, fentanyl, hydromorphone.

2. With immediate release (IR) form: start at 100–300 mg hs and increase by 100–300 mg weekly; target dose is 1200–3600 mg daily, divided tid

3. With extended release (ER) form: start with 300 mg daily and gradually increase to a maximum dose of 1800 mg once daily (usually hs)

4. Requires renal adjustment dosing.

B. Pregabalin

1. Indicated only for DM peripheral neuropathy, fibromyalgia, and PHN.

2. Start at 125–150 mg daily, in 2—3 divided doses; the dose is based on efficacy and tolerability; titrate slowly after 1 wk if needed, up to maximum daily dose which depends on diagnosis—300 mg [DM], 300–450 mg [fibromyalgia], 600 mg [PHN].

3. Requires renal adjustment dosing.

C. Carbamazepine for trigeminal neuralgia: initially 100 mg IR bid or 200 mg XR daily; titrate daily to effect, to maintenance dose of 200–1200 mg daily, in divided doses

IV. Antidepressants

A. SNRIs (duloxetine, venlafaxine)

1. Used with neuropathic pain with DM or MS, chemotherapy-related neuropathy; duloxetine also used with fibromyalgia and chronic low back pain.

2. Consider for patients with comorbid depression.

3. Duloxetine: start at 30 mg daily and increase by 30 mg weekly; target dose is 60 to 120 mg daily

4. Venlafaxine ER: start at 37.5 mg daily and increase by 37.5 mg weekly; target dose is 150–225 mg daily

B. Tricyclics (e.g., amitriptyline, nortriptyline, or desipramine)

1. Used with peripheral and central neuropathic pain; consider also with pain-related insomnia. Amitriptyline is only TCA with proven benefit in migraine prevention.

2. Nortriptyline and desipramine are better tolerated (i.e., less sedation and anticholinergic side effects).

3. Start with 10–25 mg daily and increase by 10 mg weekly; target dose is 10–150 mg once daily or divided bid. Educate patient that it can take 6 to 12 wk for an adequate trial of the medication.

4. Combination of nortriptyline plus gabapentin works better for DM neuropathy than either medication alone.

V. Cannabis and cannabinoids

A. Their use for chronic pain is controversial, with mixed results shown in efficacy; also, the legal status of these products is mixed and varies between locations.

B. Used for spasticity with MS, chemotherapy-induced N/V or neuropathic pain.

C. There is concern with misuse and psychiatric (e.g., anxiety, depression, hallucinations, paranoia) and cognitive effects (e.g., abnormal thinking, cognitive impairment).

D. Use cautiously in patients with cannabis use or prior/current substance use disorder. Consider stopping cannabis used for pain relief when it has not reduced pain or improved function and quality of life.

VI. Muscle relaxers

A. Uses

1. Muscle spasms: associated with current or prior injuries (e.g., bursitis, herniated disc, excessive stretching)

2. Spasticity: muscle fibers do not relax well; often associated with a permanent condition (e.g., head injury, CP, CVA, spinal cord injury)

B. Types

1. Centrally acting

(a) Relieve symptoms of spasm (although it is likely due to the sedation effects)

(b) Includes cyclobenzaprine, orphenadrine, metaxalone, and methocarbamol
    (i) Because of sedation, use cautiously with weakness, ataxia, and lightheadedness.
    (ii) Carisoprodol is no longer recommended because of lack of efficacy and high rates of physical dependence.
2. Peripherally acting
    (a) Used for spasticity
    (b) Includes baclofen, Botox, and tizanidine
    (c) May cause sedation, confusion, increased weakness, nausea, and dry mouth
C. Cautions
1. *Monitor for weakness and gait disturbance in elderly patients taking muscle relaxers (all of them are on the Beers list).*
2. *Consider periodic liver and renal function tests if using long term.*
3. *Some of them may cause a dangerous withdrawal if stopped suddenly.*

VII. NSAIDs

A. Antiinflammatory and analgesic properties and are most effective for mild-to-moderate pain (e.g., acute conditions such as postsurgical pain or dental surgery or musculoskeletal injury); NSAIDs can also be used to treat chronic pain.
B. If one NSAID is not effective or tolerated, consider trying a different one.
C. Improved efficacy when given with acetaminophen (e.g., acetaminophen 500 mg with ibuprofen 200–400 mg q6hr prn).
D. Ibuprofen 800 mg has *not* been shown to be much more effective than 400 mg.
E. Consider topical NSAID (e.g., diclofenac gel) for acute musculoskeletal injury.
F. Cautions
1. GI toxicity (e.g., gastritis, GI bleeding, ulcers)
    (a) Consider daily PPI to decrease GI risk.
    (b) Oral diclofenac, indomethacin, and ketorolac are not more effective than other NSAIDs, but they do *cause more GI problems.*
2. *May significantly affect renal function, especially with comorbid HTN or in elderly patients; if NSAID is used in patients also taking ACE, ARB, or diuretic, consider checking serum creatinine and K+ weekly for several weeks.*
3. All prescription NSAIDs have a Black Box warning regarding cardiovascular (CV) effects; consider naproxen or celecoxib if chronic NSAID use cannot be avoided (they are less likely to elevate BP).

VIII. Opioids

A. Acute moderate-to-severe pain
1. Can be used when NSAIDs are ineffective or contraindicated but they are not proven to be more effective than ibuprofen 400 mg for pain relief.
2. Use a low dose of a short-acting medication, for 3–7 days (e.g., hydrocodone APAP 5/325 mg 1 tab q6hr; this will be giving 20 morphine milligram equivalents [MME] daily).
3. Advise patient not to expect complete pain relief and to wean off the opioid to OTC pain medications as soon as possible.
4. Do NOT use codeine or tramadol in children <18 yr of age or in breastfeeding women (increased risk of respiratory depression and death).
B. Chronic use—see **PRESCRIBING OPIOIDS FOR CHRONIC PAIN**, later in this chapter
C. Types
1. Opioids with or without acetaminophen

■ = *not to be missed*

2. Mixed mechanism opioid (not fully related to opioids but binds to the same receptor)
   (a) Tramadol with or without acetaminophen
   (b) Tapentadol (ER formulation is the only opioid with FDA approval for painful DM neuropathy)
3. Buprenorphine (buccal film, sublingual tablet or film); some products are available for chronic pain (*dosed in mcg*), some for opioid dependence, and some for opioid use disorder (*dosed in mg*).

D. Cautions
1. May cause drowsiness, oversedation, confusion, hallucinations, decreased ability to make accurate judgments.
2. When prescribing opioids for longer than a few days, initiate a prophylactic bowel regimen to prevent constipation.
3. Use cautiously with COPD or other acute/chronic respiratory illnesses because of possible respiratory depression.
4. *Avoid concurrent use of opioids and moderate- or high-dose gabapentin (nearly 60% higher risk for opioid-related death compared with opioids alone).*

IX. Topical preparations
A. Capsaicin (e.g., Zostrix OTC cream)
1. Used for localized peripheral neuropathic pain (e.g., PHN); it has been used for HIV or DM neuropathy and also OA affecting one or a few joints.
2. *While wearing gloves*, apply to the affected areas at least tid–qid (less often decreases efficacy).

B. Lidocaine 5% patch
1. Used for localized peripheral neuropathic pain (e.g., PHN); possibly effective for DM neuropathy.
2. Apply 1–3 patches in a single application and may leave in place for up to 12 hr in any 24-hr period.
3. If the Rx patch is too expensive or not covered, consider OTC lidocaine patches 4% or ointment/cream (have patient follow the OTC box directions).

X. Adjuvant therapies: for enhancing analgesics and managing other symptoms associated with chronic pain
A. Injectable
1. Trigger point injections (alone or with steroid)
2. Steroid joint injections
3. Epidural steroid injections

B. Oral medications
1. Insomnia: trazodone 25–150 mg hs, diphenhydramine 25–50 mg hs, amitriptyline 25–50 mg hs
2. Steroids (e.g., prednisone, dexamethasone) for inflammatory pain (dose individualized)

C. Neurostimulator implants are options for back pain
D. Psychological counseling should be done routinely as part of chronic pain care

PRESCRIBING OPIOIDS FOR CHRONIC PAIN

From U.S. Department Health and Human Services, CDC guidelines 2017:
I. Guidelines for PCP treating adults >18 yr of age with chronic pain ≥3 mo, excluding cancer, palliative, and end-of-life care

■ = *not to be missed*

II. When considering long-term opioid therapy
  A. Set realistic goals for pain and function (e.g., walk around the block vs total pain relief).
  B. Opioid therapy should always be initiated as a trial, with the understanding the medication will be stopped if harms outweigh benefits or the goals of therapy are not being met.
  C. Check that nonopioid therapies have been tried and optimized (see **PHARMACOLOGICAL THERAPIES**, earlier in this chapter).
  D. Discuss benefits and risks (e.g., addiction, OD) with patient.
  E. Evaluate risk of harm or misuse.
    1. Discuss risk factors with patient.
      (a) Illegal drug use; prescription drug use for nonmedical reasons
      (b) Personal and family history for ETOH or drug use disorder and personal history of psychiatric disorders (e.g., depression, anxiety)
      (c) Sleep-disordered breathing
      (d) Concurrent benzodiazepine use
    2. Check prescription drug monitoring program (PDMP).
    3. Check urine drug screen (to confirm presence of prescribed substances and for undisclosed prescription drug or illicit substance use).
  F. Set criteria for stopping or continuing opioids.
  G. Assess baseline pain and function (e.g., PEG scale; see Box 14.1).
  H. Prescribe short-acting opioid using the lowest dose on product labeling; match duration to follow-up appointment.
  I. Schedule initial reassessment within 1–4 wk.
III. If renewing *without* patient visit, check that follow-up visit is scheduled ≤3 mo from last visit
IV. When reassessing at follow-up visit, continue opioids only after confirming clinically meaningful improvements in pain and function without significant risks or harm
  A. Assess pain and function (e.g., PEG, see Box 14.1) and compare results to baseline.
  B. Evaluate risk of harm or misuse (also see **II, E, 1**, earlier in this chapter).
    1. Observe patient for signs of oversedation or OD risk; if yes, taper dose.
    2. Check PDMP.
    3. ***Check for opioid use disorder if indicated (e.g., difficulty controlling use); if yes, referral for treatment.***
    4. Consider checking urine drug screen (see **II**, E, 3 earlier in this chapter).
  C. Check that nonopioid therapies are optimized.
  D. Determine whether to continue, adjust, taper, or stop opioids (see **V**, following); to taper—a decrease of 10% of original weekly dosage is reasonable starting point and further tapering (dose, time frame, and intervals) are based on monitoring the patient and their feedback.
  E. Calculate opioid dosage MME (see Table 14.2).
    1. If ≥50 MME/day total (e.g., ≥50 mg hydrocodone; ≥33 mg oxycodone), increase frequency of follow-up and consider offering naloxone.
    2. ***If ≥90 MME/day total (≥90 mg hydrocodone; ≥60 mg oxycodone), consider specialist referral.***
  F. Schedule follow-up at regular intervals (≤3mo).
V. Discontinuing opioid therapy
  A. Therapy may be stopped because the medication did not help, intolerable side effects occurred, the pain got worse (opioid-induced hyperalgesia), opioid use disorder (OUD) developed, or there was medication diversion.

───────────────

● = *non-urgent referral*

B. Before stopping opioids (unless diversion occurred), develop a "weaning" schedule with the patient and taper the opioid appropriately.
C. Continue to offer nonopioid or nonpharmacological therapies for the chronic pain.
D. Consider discontinuing the opioid if it has not appreciably improved pain and function, if increased doses have not helped, or if the side effects have reduced quality of life or function.
E. *Patients who develop OUD should be referred to a provider trained to treat OUD.*

TABLE 14.2 ■ Morphine Milligram Equivalent

Prescribed Medication	Daily Dose = 50 MMEs*	Daily Dose = 90 MMEs
Morphine	50 mg	90 mg
Hydrocodone (Vicodin)	50 mg	90 mg
Oxycodone	35 mg = 52.5 MMEs	60 mg
Hydromorphone (Dilaudid)	13 mg = 52 MMEs	23 mg = 92 MMEs
Oxymorphone	17 mg = 51 MMEs	30 mg
Fentanyl (transdermal)	25 mcg/h = 60 MMEs	37.5 mcg/h = 90 MMEs
Codeine	340 mg = 51 MMEs	600 mg = 90 MMEs
Methadone**		

MME, Morphine milligram equivalent.
*Unless noted otherwise. Doses ≥50 MME/day doubles the risk of death from opioid OD compared to <20 MME/day.
**Methadone: Because methadone potency increases with repeated dosing, conversion ratio with other opioids can vary widely, depending on the baseline opioid (MME) use, and thus, many commonly used equianalgesic dosing tables do not apply..

PRACTICE PEARLS FOR TREATMENT OF PAIN

- Use a stepwise approach for pain medications (see Table 14.1 for suggested therapies).
- "Opioid Analgesic REMS Education Blueprint for Health Care Providers Involved in the Treatment and Monitoring of Patients with Pain" from the FDA contains core educational information for caring for patients with pain; also includes nonpharmacologic treatments and nonopioid medications for pain.
- With chronic noncancer pain, opioids should be reserved for when it is adversely affecting function and/or quality of life *and* when the benefits outweigh potential harms.
  - Start with immediate- or short-acting (IR/SA) medication at the lowest effective dose. If a higher dose is needed, consider calculating the total daily dose and increase in 25% increments. Establish a maximum daily dose, and adjust the dose at the next monthly visit.
  - If there is not much benefit from a given dose, consider alternative medications.
- Consider prescribing naloxone for all patients who receive opioids (especially if the dose >50 MME or if the patient is also taking benzodiazepines).
- Patients who do not have relief at 1 month are not likely to have relief at 6 mo.
- Chronic opioid therapy
  - Extended release/long-acting (ER/LA) opioids should be used only for management of cancer pain, used in palliative care, or with conditions associated with severe continuous

● = *non-urgent referral*

PRACTICE PEARLS FOR TREATMENT OF PAIN—CONT'D

pain (disabling and associated with significant functional impairment); start only if patient has been taking opioids for at least a wk.
- There is no evidence that ER/LA meds are more effective than IR/SA meds, and the risk of OD and misuse are higher with ER/LA opioids. They are not indicated for prn use.
  - To convert to ER/LA form of the same medication (e.g., morphine IR to ER), give the same total daily dose in 2–3 divided doses.
  - Methadone and fentanyl should only be prescribed by providers familiar with these medications.
- Patients on stable opioid doses should be seen at least every 3 mo; see patient more frequently after dose change or changing to ER/LA form (increased risk of OD in first week after changes).
- See Table 14.2 for MME chart.
- With chronic noncancer patient, consider nonopioid or nonpharmacological options for breakthrough pain, rather than prescribing an IR/SA opioid.
- Long-term use of opioids can cause hypogonadism, immunosuppression, and increased risk of MI.
- Opioid contracts
  - Initiate when prescribing chronic opioid therapy. Signed by the patient and provider.
    - Specify *all* opioids and other potentially addictive medications (i.e., tramadol, butalbital, benzodiazepines).
    - Include that patient will obtain scheduled medications from only one provider and one designated pharmacy.
    - The patient is responsible for the written prescription and medication (i.e., if either is lost, they will not be replaced), and for obtaining refills during regular office hours.
    - Include consequences if the agreement is not followed (i.e., no further controlled substances will be prescribed).
  - The patient agrees to random urine drug screens.
    - Used to verify appropriate use (i.e., the prescribed drug should be present) and to see if any other drugs are being taken.
    - Shows substance(s) used in previous
      - 1–7 days: phencyclidine (PCP), ketamine
      - 3 days: amphetamines, cocaine, opioids
      - 3–10 days: methadone
      - 7 days: marijuana (detectible up to months, with moderate-to-heavy use)
    - False-positive results secondary to drug interactions with specimen solution may occur (Table 14.3); a positive screening test may be confirmed with a more specific test.
    - False-negative results may occur if the wrong screening panel is used; let the lab know what you are looking for so that they screen for the appropriate drug.
      - Medications taken as a patch will not show up in a drug screen.
      - Many commonly abused drugs are not detected by many commonly used screening tests (e.g., GHB [gamma hydroxybutyrate], LSD, designer amphetamines [e.g., ephedrine, mephedrone, MDPV], and tryptamines [e.g., DMT, MEO, DeoMT]).
    - If the patient admits to past substance use/abuse, consider increased frequency of random urine drug screens and before refills.
- *"Opioid use disorder" has replaced the older terms of opioid abuse and dependence.* Discussion of this condition is beyond the scope of this book. See *DSM, 5th edition,* for the diagnostic criteria; *consider referral to a pain management specialist who prescribes medication-assisted therapy (e.g., buprenorphine).*
- *Referral to a pain specialist if the symptoms are debilitating or do not respond to initial therapies or for increasing need for pain medication.*

= non-urgent referral

TABLE 14.3 ■ **Possible False-Positive Test**

Substance/Medication Taken	False-Positive Result
Vicks inhaler	Amphetamine/meth
Pseudoephedrine, ephedrine, phenylephrine Some beta blockers (e.g., propranolol, atenolol) Levodopa and carbidopa	Amphetamine
Sertraline	Benzodiazepine
NSAIDs, Marinol Hemp containing food products	Cannabinoid/marijuana
Fluoroquinolone (levofloxacin, ofloxacin), ranitidine Poppy seeds	Opioid
Venlafaxine, tramadol	Phencyclidine (PCP)
Dextromethorphan	Phencyclidine (PCP), opioid

CHAPTER 15

Endocrine Conditions

Adrenal Conditions

ACUTE ADRENAL INSUFFICIENCY (ADRENAL CRISIS)

I. Description: results from lack of cortisol as caused by the following
   A. Too rapid cessation of steroid therapy
   B. Stress, trauma, infection, surgery, or prolonged fasting in a patient with Addison disease (i.e., insufficient amount of steroid therapy)
   C. May occur as a result of pituitary destruction, bilateral adrenalectomy, or trauma to adrenal glands.
II. Signs and symptoms
   A. *The predominant feature is shock.*
   B. The patient often has nonspecific symptoms such as
      1. H/A and lassitude
      2. N/V, anorexia
      3. Fever
      4. Hypotension and/or dehydration out of proportion to current illness
      5. Skin hyperpigmentation (with long-standing adrenal insufficiency)
      6. Weakness, fatigue, lethargy
      7. May have confusion or coma
III. Treatment
   A. *Transfer immediately for emergency treatment*
   B. After acute crisis, maintenance doses of corticosteroids (may comanage with the physician)

CHRONIC ADRENAL INSUFFICIENCY (ADDISON'S DISEASE)

I. Description: autoimmune destruction of adrenal cortices results in chronic cortisol, aldosterone, and adrenal androgen deficiency
II. Signs and symptoms
   A. Hallmark signs are hypotension and hyperkalemia at the time of diagnosis (resolves with treatment).
   B. Other signs may include
      1. Increased skin pigmentation and diffuse tanning (especially over flexor surfaces, palm creases, and areolae)
      2. Volume and sodium depletion
      3. Generalized weakness and/or fatigue, worse with exertion and better with bed rest; chronic malaise
      4. Anorexia, N/V, diarrhea
      5. Scant pubic and axillary hair in women
      6. May also have memory impairment, depression, or psychosis

▪ = *not to be missed;* ▲ = *urgent referral*

   III. Diagnostic tests

      A. CBC: WBC shows moderate neutropenia, lymphocytosis, elevated eosinophils

      B. CMP: hyperkalemia, hyponatremia, hypoglycemia

      C. A rapid ACTH stimulation test (drawn between 6 and 8 am) will establish or exclude adrenal insufficiency.

   IV. Treatment

▲   A. ***Referral urgently to an endocrinologist***

      B. Replacement glucocorticoids and mineralocorticoids for life (by endocrinologist)

      C. Education (by the endocrinologist) on how to manage minor illnesses and major stresses and when and how to inject glucocorticoids for emergencies

      D. The patient should wear an ID band stating they have Addison disease.

CUSHING'S SYNDROME AND DISEASE

   I. Description

      A. *Cushing syndrome:* caused by adrenal hyperplasia or tumors, extra-adrenal malignancies, or chronic glucocorticoid use

      B. *Cushing disease:* generally caused by ACTH hypersecretion due to pituitary adenoma

   II. Signs and symptoms (none are diagnostic and many are nonspecific)

      A. Central (truncal) obesity

      B. Moon face, buffalo hump, supraclavicular fat pads

      C. Protuberant abdomen with purple striae; wasted-appearing extremities

      D. Oligomenorrhea or amenorrhea, impotence

      E. Weakness, especially in the upper arms, legs, and hips

      F. Acne; thin skin with easy bruising and poor wound healing

      G. Excessive coarse hair on face, chest, and back

      H. Labile mood swings to psychosis

   III. Treatment

      A. ***Referral to an endocrinologist if you suspect the condition***

      B. If appropriate, the patient should wear an ID band stating they have Cushing syndrome or disease.

PHEOCHROMOCYTOMA

   I. Description: caused by tumor in the adrenal glands or sympathetic chain

   II. Signs and symptoms

      A. Triad of attacks of H/A (mild to severe), generalized sweating, and tachycardia (paroxysmal), but *many patients do not have these together*

      B. Paroxysmal HTN

      C. Weakness

      D. Anxiety, tremor

      E. *Patients who have paroxysmal HTN and tachycardia during diagnostic procedures, anesthesia, or surgery or with foods containing tyramine should be evaluated for pheochromocytoma.*

   III. Diagnostic tests: 24-hr urine for fractionated catecholamines, metanephrines, and creatinine; if all elevated, consider abdominal CT with and without oral and IV contrast and pelvic CT without contrast

   IV. Treatment: *referral to a surgeon with positive test results*

● *= non-urgent referral;* ▲ *= urgent referral*

Diabetes Mellitus

SCREENING

I. Adults
   A. Age > 45 yr of age: if normal, repeat testing q3yr
   B. Age < 45 yr of age, if overweight (BMI ≥ 23 kg/m²) AND one or more risk factors
      1. First-degree relative with DM: parent, sibling, child
      2. Member of a high-risk ethnic population: non-Hispanic Black (e.g., someone from Caribbean island or Africa), Hispanic, Native American, Asian American, or Pacific Islander
      3. Has delivered a baby weighing > 9 lbs or has been diagnosed with GDM
      4. Previously documented pre-DM
      5. HTN: BP > 140/90 mmHg
      6. HDL levels < 35 mg/dL or triglyceride levels > 250 mg/dL or both
      7. Habitual physical inactivity
      8. History of vascular disease
      9. Has other clinical conditions associated with insulin resistance (e.g., acanthosis nigricans, PCOS)
   C. Screening is recommended in some asymptomatic patients
      1. Taking antipsychotic agents for schizophrenia or severe bipolar D/O
      2. Chronic glucocorticoid use
      3. Sleep disorder along with glucose intolerance
   D. Elderly patients may have atypical signs and symptoms; consider screening for DM with
      1. Altered mentation, behavior changes, sleep disturbances
      2. Incontinence (new onset or suddenly worsening), anorexia, weight loss, falls
      3. Earlier warning signs may include shin spots and recurrent skin infections (especially yeast infections)

II. Children
   A. Remains controversial because there are no data from controlled studies showing that earlier diagnosis improves long-term outcomes
   B. The American Diabetes Association (ADA) recommends: screening q3yr in children (starting at 10 yr of age) if overweight (BMI > 85th percentile for age and sex) *plus* at least one of the following risk factors
      1. First- or second-degree relative with type 2 DM
      2. Member of a high-risk ethnic population: non-Hispanic Black, Hispanic, Native American, Asian American, or Pacific Islander
      3. Signs of or conditions associated with insulin resistance (e.g., acanthosis nigricans, HTN, dyslipidemia, or birth weight small for gestational age)
      4. Mother had DM or GDM during child's gestation
   C. Diagnostic criteria values are the same as for adults (see Table 15.1)

III. Screening in pregnancy
   A. Screen between 24 and 28 wk gestation; give 50 g oral glucose load and obtain plasma glucose 1 hr later (fasting not necessary); a value of > 140 mg/dL indicates the need for fasting 3-hr GTT.
   B. Screen as early as the first prenatal visit in women with a high risk of GDM (e.g., marked obesity, past history of GDM, glycosuria, or strong FH of DM); if this screening has negative results, repeat at 24 to 28 wk gestation.
   C. If the patient does have gestational DM (according to criteria in Table 15.1), a regular 2-h GTT with 75 g glucose load is done 6 wk postpartum to see if blood sugars have returned to normal or remain elevated.
   D. If a woman has GDM, lifelong testing at least q3yr is recommended, regardless of BMI.

TABLE 15.1 ■ **Criteria for Diabetes, Prediabetes, and Gestational Diabetes**

DM	Pre-DM	Gestational DM
FBG levels ≥ 126 mg/dL on at least two occasions* (preferred test)	FBG levels 100–125 mg/dL on at least two occasions* (preferred test)	After receiving a 100-g glucose load: positive test result if two values meet or exceed the following:
Random blood glucose ≥ 200 mg/dL[†]	2-h value during GTT is 140–199 mg/dL (impaired glucose tolerance)	FBG levels: 95 mg/dL
2-h value during GTT > 200 mg/dL	A1c 5.7%–6.4%	1-h GTT: 180 mg/dL
A1c > 6.5%		2-h GTT: 155 mg/dL
		3-h GTT: 140 mg/dL

* Oral GTT is not necessary if fasting glucose levels are elevated on two occasions.
[†] Order FBG and A1c to verify.

DIAGNOSIS

I. Diagnosis of DM and pre-DM should be based on blood glucose values by laboratory determination or A1c values and not by capillary blood glucose monitors.

II. Diagnosis is based on the criteria set by the ADA; see Table 15.1 for specific criteria.

III. Be aware of common terminology that can cause patients to feel judged, shamed, or labeled; consider replacing them with positive terms that send a message of hope.

Instead of	*Consider*
Diabetic	Person with DM
Test	Check
Control	Manage
Suffering with DM	Living with DM
Good/bad/poor levels	Target levels

IV. Classification (for treatment, see **FOLLOW-UP AND TREATMENT**, later in chapter)

A. Insulin resistance

1. Consider diagnosis with one or more of the following

(a) Presence of PCOS

(b) Presence of acanthosis nigricans (see Figs. 15.1 and 15.2) around the neck or under the arms; it usually improves with treatment

(c) Weight gain

(d) Dyslipidemia

(e) Systolic BP elevated after eating

(f) Presence of diastolic dysfunction

(i) S_4 heart sound

(ii) Possible HF

(iii) Echo shows stiff left ventricle (secondary to free fatty acid [FFA] deposits)

(a) Presence of nonalcoholic fatty liver disease (NAFLD)

(b) Clotting abnormalities

(c) Gout (increased FFA deposits in kidneys interfere with uric acid excretion)

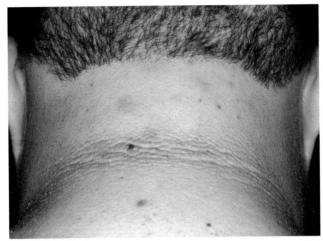

Fig. 15.1 Acanthosis nigricans of the neck. (From Dinulos, James G.H. (2021). *Habif's Clinical dermatology*, 6th ed.)

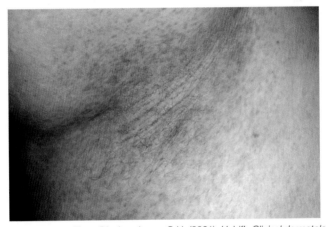

Fig. 15.2 Acanthosis nigricans. (From Dinulos, James G.H. (2021). *Habif's Clinical dermatology*, 6th ed.)

    2. Evaluation
        (a) Elevated 2-hr value during GTT (140 to 199 mg/dL), which indicates either impaired glucose tolerance or prediabetes
        (b) There is no validated clinical test to measure insulin resistance directly.
  B. Prediabetes: fasting and/or 2-hr glucose higher than normal but not high enough to meet the criteria for DM
    1. Impaired fasting glucose: FBG 100 to 125 mg/dL
    2. Impaired glucose tolerance: 2-hr glucose 140 to 199 mg/dL on GTT or A1c 5.7%–6.4%
  C. Type 1 DM: the pancreas produces no insulin (also see Table 15.2)
  D. Type 2 DM: insulin resistance; eventually insulin production decreases (also see Table 15.2)
    1. DM or impaired glucose tolerance may develop as a result of the following
        (a) Pancreatic disease (e.g., cystic fibrosis or chronic pancreatitis)
        (b) Endocrinopathy (e.g., Cushing syndrome, acromegaly, or pheochromocytoma)

TABLE 15.2 ■ **Overview of Type 1 and Type 2 Diabetes**

Characteristic	Type 1	Type 2
Usual age at onset	Usually around puberty but 25% present after 35 yr of age	Older than 30 yr of age*
Associated with obesity	Not usually	Frequently
Classic signs and symptoms	Polyuria, polyphagia, polydipsia Weight loss Fatigue, weakness Feeling edgy, moody Approximately ⅓ patients present with DKA (> 50% in child < 3 yr of age)	Relatively few classic symptoms Repeated or hard-to-heal vaginal yeast or bladder infections May have blurred vision, tingling in extremities, poor wound healing May have acanthosis nigricans (see Figs. 15.1 and 15.2) Consider in children with Usually > 10 yr of age Usually BMI ≥ 95th percentile Insulin resistance **(DIAGNOSIS, IV)** Positive FH of type 2 DM May present symptomatically (e.g., polyuria, polydipsia, nocturia)
Etiology	Beta-cell destruction because of autoimmune disease Genetic and environmental triggers	Genetic and environmental factors appear to be important Usually arises because of insulin resistance combined with relative insulin deficiency
Ketosis prone	Yes	No, except in periods of acute stress
Dependent on insulin to sustain life	Yes	No, but may eventually require insulin therapy to control hyperglycemia

* More children, even as young as 10 yr of age, are being diagnosed with type 2 DM; this is probably related to lifestyle changes (i.e., increased fast food intake and decreased activity).

    (c) Drugs and chemical agents (e.g., thiazide diuretics primarily at doses > 25 mg HCTZ daily or equivalent, glucocorticoids, atypical antipsychotics)
2. Gestational DM (GDM): develops during pregnancy (usually at 24 to 28-wk gestation) owing to increased amounts of glucocorticoids and other hormones released from the placenta; usually disappears when pregnancy ends but does increase risk for type 2 DM later in life.

COMPREHENSIVE MEDICAL EVALUATION (INITIAL VISIT)

    I. History.
        A. Symptoms of DM (see Table 15.2)
        B. PMH
            1. Diabetes related
                (a) Eating patterns, nutritional status, weight history; growth and development in children and adolescents

(b) Current treatment: medications, meal plan, self-monitoring of blood glucose (SMBG), and patient's use of data

(c) Prior A1c results

(d) Previous DM treatment, including nutrition and self-management education

(e) Patient may complain of xerostomia or a burning sensation in the mouth.

(f) Frequency, severity, and causes of acute complications (e.g., DKA, hypoglycemia) and prior or current infections (especially GU, skin, foot, and dental)

(g) Symptoms and treatment of chronic complications of DM (see later in this chapter)

  2. History and treatment of other conditions, including eating and endocrine disorders and risk factors for atherosclerosis (e.g., smoking, HTN, dyslipidemia)

  3. Gestational history and contraception

C. Social history

  1. Exercise history

  2. Tobacco, ETOH, and/or controlled substance use

  3. Lifestyle, cultural, psychosocial, educational, and economic factors that may influence DM management

D. FH of DM and other endocrine disorders

II. Physical examination

A. Height and weight (growth chart for children and adolescents), vital signs

B. Fundoscopic evaluation

C. Oral examination: candida infection, gingivitis, and/or periodontitis

D. Thyroid palpation.

E. Cardiovascular, including auscultation for bruits and palpation of pulses

F. Abdominal examination

G. Skin examination (for acanthosis nigricans, see Figs. 15.1 and 15.2)

H. Foot examination (including sharp and dull sensations and monofilament for neuropathy) (Fig. 15.1 and also **CHRONIC COMPLICATIONS OF DM, IV**, later in this chapter)

III. Diagnostic evaluation

A. Fasting complete chemistry panel, A1c, and lipid profile

B. *If uncertain whether patient has type 1 or 2 DM, obtain a C-peptide level (C-peptide is produced when insulin is available, so low or no C-peptide means insulin is required to treat the DM).*

C. UA for glucose, ketones, protein, and evidence of microalbuminuria or infection

D. ECG (adults) at initial evaluation and then as indicated

IV. Counseling

A. Recommend DM self-management education for all patients at diagnosis.

B. Emphasize that DM is a chronic disease and management of it involves four equal components; review at each DM follow-up visit.

  1. Meal plan

    (a) Diet management is of utmost importance; poor eating habits will lessen or negate efforts to achieve lower blood glucose levels.

    (b) Weight reduction when indicated

      (i) Any degree of weight loss is likely to improve blood glucose levels and/or decrease the need for medications; sustained weight loss $\geq 7\%$ is optimal.

      (ii) Can also improve liver function in NAFLD, which is associated with insulin resistance and type 2 DM

    (c) See also **CURRENT DIETARY RECOMMENDATIONS.**

■ = *not to be missed*

2. Lifestyle changes
   (a) Exercise (see **EXERCISE AND DIABETES**, later in the chapter)
   (b) Quit smoking.
   (c) Noncardiac benefits may include reduction in urinary incontinence, OSA, and depression; may also improve mobility and physical conditioning.
3. Monitoring
   (a) Blood glucose goals
       (i) 70–130 mg/dL fasting or pre-prandial; < 180 mg/dL hs or 1–2 hr post-prandial (PP)
       (ii) A1c: should be tailored by balancing lower risk of complications with the risk of hypoglycemia; reasonable is < 7% (or < 6.5% if done safely) but in older patients or those with limited life expectancy or comorbid conditions, strive for < 8%.
   (b) Maintain BP < 140/90 mmHg.
   (c) Control dyslipidemia if necessary; suggested priority is as follows
       (i) LDL (see Chapter 8, **DYSLIPIDEMIA**; a statin is recommended for all patients with DM and < 75 yr of age; may consider if over 75 yr of age)
       (ii) HDL > 40 mg/dL (males) or > 50 mg/dL (females)
       (iii) Triglycerides < 150 mg/dL
4. Medications (if needed)
C. Recommended immunizations
   1. Pneumonia: see Chapter 3, **PRACTICE PEARLS FOR RESPIRATORY SYSTEM**, for current recommendations.
   2. Hepatitis B, three-dose series: all unvaccinated adults 19 to 59 yr of age, with DM; consider for adults ≥ 60 yr of age
   3. Discuss COVID-19 vaccine.
V. Discuss treatment goals and plan (see **FOLLOW-UP AND TREATMENT**, for specifics).
VI. *Referrals* (if indicated)
   A. *Diabetes Education Program, if available (this is a standard of care for DM, recommended by the ADA and American College of Endocrinologists).*
   B. *Dietitian consultation (especially if the patient is newly diagnosed); if someone else in the home does meal planning and cooking, encourage that person to attend the appointment; this is recommended if it is not part of the Diabetes Education Program or as a follow-up visit for further teaching or clarification.*
   C. *Ophthalmologist or optometrist for an annual dilated eye examination.*
   D. *Podiatrist for orthotics or evaluation/treatment of abnormal foot exam.*
   E. *Consider referral to bariatric surgeon (with BMI ≥ 40 kg/m2 regardless of glycemic control or BMI 35 to 39 kg/m2 with inadequately controlled hyperglycemia).*

CURRENT DIETARY RECOMMENDATIONS

I. Nutritional goals
   A. *Consider referral to an individualized medical nutrition therapy program or dietician.*
   B. Promote and support healthy eating habits, emphasizing a variety of nutrient-dense foods and appropriate portion sizes in order to
      1. Improve overall health
      2. Attain glycemic, BP, and lipid goals
      3. Delay and/or prevent DM complications

= non-urgent referral

    C. Provide adequate calories to achieve and maintain a healthy body weight; to calculate the desired body weight ($\pm$ 10%, depending on frame size)
       1. Women: 5 feet = 100 lbs; add 5 lbs for each additional inch of height and subtract 5 lbs for each inch less than 5 feet
       2. Men: 5 feet = 106 lbs; add 6 lbs for each additional inch
    D. If weight loss is indicated (BMI $\geq$ 25 kg/m^2), encourage the patient to set a goal of losing 5% of the body weight (not so overwhelming as a goal of losing $\geq$ 50 lbs).
       1. Calorie restriction (e.g., 500 fewer calories daily) will result in short-term blood glucose improvement.
       2. Long-term blood glucose control also requires weight loss; sustained weight loss $\geq$ 7% is optimal.
       3. There is no general consensus on the best weight loss plan; some examples include counting calories, the low-carb diet (although benefits tend to not be maintained), Mediterranean diet, and intermittent fasting.

II. Meal planning strategies
    A. Emphasis should be on healthful eating habits, with nutrient-dense foods (e.g., vegetables, fruits, legumes, low-fat dairy, lean meats, nuts, seeds, and whole grains) more of the focus than specific nutrients (e.g., protein, carbs, fats).
       1. Choose whole foods over processed foods; minimize refined grains.
       2. Minimize added sugars (in foods and drinks) and artificial sweeteners.
       3. Examples of possible food plans include the Mediterranean diet, the DASH diet (see Table 8.14), vegetarian or vegan diets.
    B. The plan should be appropriate for the patient's lifestyle and should provide day-to-day consistency in calorie and mealtimes; update as needed for changes in growth or lifestyle; encourage these guidelines
       1. Eat three balanced meals daily, 4 to 5 hr apart.
       2. Eat at the same time daily whenever possible.
       3. Include a bedtime snack, especially if taking insulin.
    C. The point system, carbohydrate counting, plate method (Fig. 15.3), and others may be used.
    D. For patients taking insulin, the most important dietary component is for the patient to learn to estimate the amount of carbs eaten at any meal or snack.
    E. SMBG data should be used to make adjustments in food intake or insulin dosages.

III. ADA additional recommendations
    A. Reduce intake of refined carbs and added sugars.
    B. Noncaloric sweeteners approved by the FDA are acceptable; sugar alcohols (e.g., sorbitol) have a low glycemic effect but may cause diarrhea.
    C. Fats: avoid trans fats; replace saturated fats with unsaturated fats
    D. Protein (individualized)
       1. 20%–30% of total calories daily (if no significant renal insufficiency)
       2. 0.8 g/kg body weight daily (with early stages of CKD)

IV. Alcohol
    A. Avoid in patients with poor metabolic control, those attempting weight loss, or with elevated triglycerides, or with nephropathy, and in pregnant women.
    B. Moderate intake (1 to 2 servings per day for men; 1 per day for women) is acceptable; 1 drink = 12 oz beer = 5 oz wine = 1.5 oz 80-proof liquor.
    C. Can contribute to hypoglycemia in patients taking insulin or sulfonylureas; for this reason, recommend that the patient eat protein when drinking alcohol.

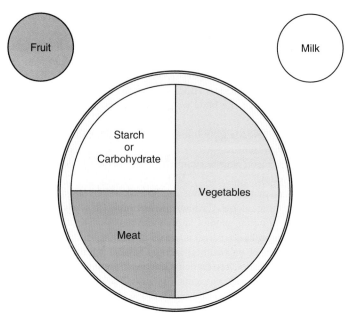

Fig. 15.3 The plate method. (Using a standard size dinner plate.)

V. Micronutrients
   A. Sodium: < 2300 mg daily
   B. Vitamin B12 deficiency may occur with metformin.
VI. Supplements
   A. Vitamins and minerals are generally not needed unless the patient has underlying deficiencies.
   B. There is insufficient evidence to support using micronutrients such as cinnamon and chromium.
VII. Fasting and DM medications
   A. Fasting for morning labs: usually no adjustments
   B. Fasting 12 hrs or more (e.g., for Yom Kippur or Ramadan; some intermittent fasting diets)
      1. Medications that rarely cause hypoglycemia (i.e., metformin, TZD, DPP-4 inhibitors, GLP-1 inhibitors)—OK to continue for intermittent or religious fasts.
      2. SGLT2 inhibitors—consider holding up to 2 days before religious fasts (concern about dehydration).
      3. Insulin or sulfonylureas
         (a) Hold prandial insulin or sulfonylureas once the patient stops eating.
         (b) Consider holding sulfonylureas 24 to 36 hr before a fast lasting 24 hr or more.
         (c) Basal insulin—consider giving 50% of the usual dose if DM is well controlled or patient is higher risk for hypoglycemia (e.g., elderly, CKD); otherwise, consider reducing the dose by 30%.
            (i) NPH or long-acting (e.g., glargine, detemir): reduce at the start of the fast

(ii) Degludec: start the reduced dose the day *before* the fast
4. Instruct patient to break the fast for blood glucose < 70 mg/dL or if they have symptoms with blood glucose < 80 mg/dL.

EXERCISE AND DIABETES

I. Weight loss and exercise work together to decrease insulin resistance, which is a primary problem in type 2 DM.
II. Exercise can also delay progression of impaired glucose tolerance to type 2 DM.
III. Pre-exercise evaluation
  A. Routine testing is not recommended for asymptomatic patients.
  B. Perform a good history; assess for cardiovascular risk factors and atypical presentation of CAD.
  C. Assess for conditions that might be contraindications to certain types of exercise or predispose to injuries (see Exercise Restrictions, **IV**, below).
IV. Exercise restrictions
  A. Avoid exercise in extreme heat or cold and during periods of poor glycemic control.
  B. With *active proliferative retinopathy*
    1. Try walking, water aerobics, cycling.
    2. Avoid vigorous intensity aerobic exercise or any type of resistance training (e.g., free weights or weight machines).
  C. With *peripheral neuropathy*
    1. With a foot injury or open sore, avoid weight-bearing activities (e.g., running, prolonged downhill skiing).
    2. Consider workout machines that engage arms and legs without weight bearing (e.g., recumbent bike or stepper), swimming or water aerobics, tai chi, and yoga.
    3. With all exercise, be sure to wear proper footwear.
  D. With *autonomic neuropathy*: because of increased risk for cardiovascular death and silent ischemia, patient should undergo cardiac evaluation before starting physical activity more intense than usual.
V. Individualize the exercise plan according to the patient's level of fitness, lifestyle, and motivation.
  A. Warm up and cool down for 5 to 10 min (walk at a comfortable pace; gentle stretching).
  B. Keep moving (i.e., aerobic activity) for 20 to 30 min; the patient may have to work up to this. The goal is 30 min 5 days a week.
  C. Adults should participate in resistance exercise 2 to 3 times a week, on nonconsecutive days.
  D. Older adults: flexibility and balance training recommended 2 to 3 times a week (e.g., yoga, tai chi).
  E. Children and adolescents should participate in moderate- or vigorous-intensity exercise for at least 60 min daily.
VI. Exercise points for patients using insulin (Table 15.3)
  A. Do not exercise if the blood glucose level is < 60 mg/dL or > 250 mg/dL.
  B. Always begin exercise at least 1 hr after the last insulin injection and avoid exercise during the time of peak insulin action.
  C. Encourage the patient to have a quick snack readily available (see foot note for Table 15.6).
  D. If hypoglycemic symptoms occur during exercise, *stop immediately* and check blood glucose levels.

TABLE 15.3 ■ Food and Insulin Adjustments for Exercise

Variable	Management and Adjustment
Blood Glucose Levels	
< 100 mg/dL	Add a snack and recheck glucose in 15–30 min
≥ 250 mg/dL	Adjust insulin Delay exercise until glucose decreases
Exercise	
Moderate exercise for < 30 min	No snack unless blood glucose level is < 80 mg/dL
Exercise for > 30 min	A snack every 30–60 min The snack should be ~ 10–15 g of carbohydrates for every 30 min of exercise (see footnote for Table 15.6)*
Strenuous exercise for > 45–60 min	May require < 20% decrease in the corresponding insulin component Do not inject insulin into the exercising extremity.
Prolonged rigorous exercise	May require large decreases in insulin ($^1/_3$ to ½ of the usual dose).

* The snack size may vary from patient to patient and with the duration and intensity of exercise.

MONITORING

I. SMBG (self-monitoring blood glucose)
    A. Monitoring may vary with the following
        1. Level of glycemic control desired
        2. Medication regimen variations
        3. Propensity for hypoglycemia
        4. More frequent testing is necessary when the usual daily schedule is changed (e.g., travel, surgery, hospitalization) or during periods of illness or stress.
        5. Type of DM (e.g., SMBG is not necessary if not on insulin, but the patient may want to check sugars periodically anyway—see B.1., following)
    B. Tips for effective SMBG
        1. 1- or 2-hr postprandial (PP) testing may be helpful 2 to 3 times a week (allows the patient to see the effects of a particular type of food on blood glucose levels).
        2. Patients with nocturnal hypoglycemia should test 1.5 to 2 hr after the evening snack or between 1 and 3 a.m. once or twice a week.
        3. The patient should record all test results. Recording insulin doses (when applicable) along with the blood glucose results is also helpful; be sure that the patient knows that they must separately enter routine doses and compensatory doses (e.g., according to a "sliding scale").
        4. Teach the patient to record results in a method that allows quick comparison of day-to-day results so that the patterns are easily recognizable. Even when the blood glucose meter maintains a record, it can be helpful to also keep a paper record for ease of seeing the "big picture."
        5. Continuous blood glucose monitoring may be considered for patients with type 1 DM or some type 2 DM (e.g., patients on insulin with hypoglycemia unawareness).
            (a) Has been shown to increase the time within the targeted blood glucose range; BG between 70 and 180 mg/dL for 70% of the time results in an A1c of ~ 7.

(b) It is not associated with increased severe hypoglycemia or DKA with type 1 DM.

(c) Can improve quality of life for the patient and caregiver(s)

    (i) Decreased emotional distress and fear of hypoglycemia

    (ii) Increased quality and quantity of sleep

    (iii) Improved treatment satisfaction and feelings of self-efficacy

(d) Results can be used to guide lifestyle or medication changes.

II. Glycosylated hemoglobin (A1c)

  A. Assesses long-term glucose control because it reflects mean blood glucose concentration over the preceding 8 to 12 wk (previous month accounts for ~ 50% of the A1c value).

    1. An A1c of 6 corresponds to an average blood glucose of 125 mg/dL.

    2. Every increase in A1c of 1 point (e.g., change from 6 to 7) corresponds to an increase in average blood glucose of 30 mg/dL.

  B. Not affected by glucose at the time the specimen is drawn, so fasting is not necessary

  C. With discrepancies between SMBG and A1c, consider

    1. Inaccurate testing technique or machine malfunctioning

    2. A1c represents an average blood glucose concentration, so fluctuations in blood glucose levels may result in near-normal A1c levels.

    3. Fabricated SMBG results

      (a) A1c < 7.3%: postprandial (PP) sugars account for 70% of result

      (b) A1c > 7.3%: PP sugars account for 50% of the result

    4. Hemoglobinopathies (e.g., sickle cell anemia lowers results; hemoglobin F may elevate results)

FOLLOW-UP AND TREATMENT

I. Prediabetes and insulin resistance

  A. Monitor for progression to type 2 DM annually with A1c and FBG (at minimum).

    1. Patients < 70 yr of age can decrease risk of developing DM by 60% with consistent lifestyle changes.

    2. Patients > 70 yr of age are likely to regress to normal blood glucose with healthy eating (but not as restrictive with foods) and being as active as possible—no drastic lifestyle changes.

  B. Recommended lifestyle changes

    1. The best results follow changes in eating, similar to DM; it is a good idea to have the patient meet with a dietitian knowledgeable about DM.

    2. The Mediterranean diet has the strongest evidence for preventing type 2 DM.

    3. Encourage the patient to work up to walking 30 min, 5 times a week; it can be split into two 15-min walks if this is more feasible. Walking should be faster than a casual stroll, but the patient is still able to carry on a conversation without difficulty.

    4. Weight reduction is an important goal (see **CURRENT DIETARY RECOMMENDATIONS, I**, earlier in the chapter).

    5. Medicare Diabetes Prevention Program is a 16-session program designed to help people with prediabetes make long-term lifestyle changes to prevent or delay development of type 2 DM; see cdc.gov/diabetes/prevention for further information.

  C. Currently, no medications are recommended, although some research has shown reduction in development of DM, especially if the BMI $\geq$ 35 kg/m^2 and patient < 60 yr of age, with metformin, pioglitazone, or liraglutide.

II. Type 1 DM

    A. Overall management goals

        1. Avoid excessive hypoglycemia and hyperglycemia, especially when accompanied by ketoacidosis.

        2. Balance food intake with insulin and exercise (see Table 15.3 and **EXERCISE AND DIABETES**, earlier in the chapter).

        3. Maintain an appropriate weight and provide optimal nutrition.

    B. Follow-up appointment q3mo

        1. History

          (a) Frequency and cause(s) of hypoglycemic and hyperglycemic episodes

          (b) Any changes by the patient in the treatment plan; problems with adherence

          (c) Symptoms suggesting development of complications of DM

          (d) Current medications

          (e) Psychosocial issues (e.g., quality of life issues, depression, ability to pay for medications or tests)

        2. Physical examination

          (a) Height and weight, vital signs

          (b) Oral examination for periodontal disease

          (c) Cardiovascular examination including bruits and pulses

          (d) Foot examination: inspect the feet at every visit; also see **CHRONIC COMPLICATIONS OF DM**, IV, for neurologic examination.

        3. Laboratory and other testing

          (a) Complete chemistry profile (at least q3–6mo)

          (b) A1c q3mo

          (c) Annual fasting lipid profile, urinalysis for protein and albumin/creatinine ratio (ACR), TSH (as indicated)

          (d) Annual dilated eye examination by an ophthalmologist or optometrist

        4. Counseling

          (a) Discuss treatment goals and plan; individualize the goals, taking into account the patient's ability to understand and carry out the treatment regime and understand the risk of hypoglycemia.

            (i) Consider need for "refresher" self-management education and support annually and when complications arise.

            (ii) Consider recommending the American Diabetes Association (ADA) website for additional information and resources.

          (b) Review food plan (see **CURRENT DIETARY RECOMMENDATIONS**, earlier in the chapter).

          (c) Discuss exercise and weight reduction plan (if indicated) (see also **EXERCISE AND DIABETES**, earlier in the chapter).

          (d) Review medications.

    C. Treatment includes insulin and dietary management.

        1. Indication: to provide a physiologic insulin profile to cover basal insulin secretion and PP glucose excursions

        2. The blood glucose goals are as follows

          (a) Fasting and pre-prandial glucose

            80–130 mg/dL   (ADA)

            70–110 mg/dL   (American Association of Clinical Endocrinologists [AACE])

(b) 2-hr PP glucose

< 180 mg/dL	(ADA)
< 140 mg/dL	(AACE)

(c) A1c: should be tailored by balancing improved complications with the risk of hypoglycemia; reasonable is < 7% (or < 6.5% if done safely) but in older patients or those with limited life expectancy or comorbid conditions, strive for < 8%.

3. Initiating insulin (also see Table 15.4): which one is prescribed is often based on patient preference and the payer (e.g., which insurance, if any, the patient uses).

(a) Most patients should be treated with multiple daily injections (basal 1 to 2 times a day [depending on insulin given], plus short- or rapid-acting insulin pre-prandial) or continuous subcutaneous insulin infusion (CSII). Either of these is considered intensive insulin therapy.

   (i) Most type 1 patients will be on 0.4 to 1 unit/kg/day (may increase during puberty, pregnancy, or illness).

   (ii) Consider starting with 50% total daily dose (TDD) being basal insulin and 50% TDD divided over the pre-prandial bolus insulin injections. This method decreases A1c with less weight gain and hypoglycemia episodes than other methods.

   (iii) With glargine U-100 or insulin detemir, twice daily injections may give better glycemic control (total dose split between injections).

   (iv) Insulin degludec U-100 or U-200 can be administered once daily, any time of day. It also can be mixed with rapid-acting insulins (whereas glargine U-100 and detemir insulins cannot).

(b) Consider educating the patient to adjust prandial insulin dose according to pre-meal blood glucose and expected carb intake.

   (i) Rapid-acting insulins can be injected 10 to 15 min before or up to immediately after meals.

   (ii) Regular insulin should be injected 30 to 45 min or more before meals.

If blood glucose is:	Adjust premeal insulin by:
> 180 mg/dL	+ 3 units
140–179 mg/dL	+ 2 units
80–99 mg/dL	− 1 unit
60–79 mg/dL	− 2 units
< 60 mg/dL	− 3 units

(c) Advantages of intensive insulin therapy
   (i) Increased flexibility in the timing of meals
   (ii) Adjustments for the size of meals are readily made.

(d) Disadvantages of intensive insulin therapy
   (i) Requires frequent SMBG
   (ii) Fear of hypoglycemia
   (iii) Weight gain is more likely.
   (iv) CSII requires an expert DM management team and availability of 24 hr support.

(e) When on multiple doses of insulin or insulin pump, verify the patient knows how to respond appropriately to SMBG results by making adjustments in the diet or insulin regimen; the goal is to achieve and maintain blood glucose levels within the desired range individualized for each patient. Suggested SMBG checks

   (i) Before meals and snacks and at hs; occasionally PP

  (ii) Before exercise

 (iii) When hypoglycemia is suspected or after treatment for low blood glucose (until glucose levels are normal)

 (iv) Before driving or operating machinery

  (f) Continuous blood glucose monitoring (CGM) may be useful for patients with frequent or severe hypoglycemia or who have developed hypoglycemia unawareness. CGM does not totally eliminate SMBG (e.g., if symptoms do not match the blood sugar reading or when the machine needs calibration). For tips on effective SMBG, see **MONITORING** (earlier in chapter).

    4. Currently NOT recommended for type 1 DM treatment: amylin analogs, GLP-1 RA, SGLT2 inhibitors, or metformin

    5. Sick day management (see **ACUTE COMPLICATIONS OF DM, III**)

  D. Switching insulin products (see **III**. Type 2 DM, G)

TABLE 15.4 ■ **Pharmacokinetics of Insulin**

Type of Insulin	Blood Glucose Affected	Approximate Duration (hr)
Rapid- or Short-Acting (Prandial)		
Insulin lispro (Humalog, U-100, U-200) or (Admelog U-100) Insulin lispro-aabc (Lyumjev)[†]	postprandial	4–6
Insulin aspart (Novolog, Fiasp)	postprandial	4–6
Insulin glulisine (Apidra)	postprandial	4–6
Regular (Novolin R, U-100) or (Humulin R, U-100 or U-500)	2–4 hr after taking	8
Basal		
Intermediate-Acting		
NPH (Humulin N, Novolin N)	a.m. dose: before dinner p.m. dose: fasting	12
Longer-Acting		
Detemir (Levemir)	Peaks at 3–9 hr	up to 24*
Glargine U-100 (Lantus, Basaglar) Glargine U-300 (Toujeo)	No pronounced peak	up to 24 up to 32
Insulin glargine-yfgn U-100 (Semglee)[††]	No pronounced peak	~24
Ultra-Long-Acting		
Degludec U-100, U-200 (Tresiba)	No pronounced peak	> 24

* Shorter than glargine but slightly longer than NPH. At doses ≥ 0.8 units/kg, the duration is less variable and closer to 24 hr.
† New insulins, classified as a biologic (also see **PRACTICE PEARLS FOR INSULIN THERAPY**).
†† New insulins, classified as a biosimilar (also see **PRACTICE PEARLS FOR INSULIN THERAPY**).
Combination insulins are also available; their pharmacokinetics depend on the individual components:
- 70/30 (NPH and Humulin regular)
- 75/25 and 50/50 (lispro protamine and insulin lispro)
- 70/30 (aspart protamine and insulin aspart)

E. With poorly controlled DM, consider the following
   1. Overeating (specifically simple carbs)
   2. Inadequate exercise and/or activity
   3. Over-insulinization (usually in patients with marked "glucose bounces")
   4. Incorrect insulin injection (technique and/or sites; see **PRACTICE PEARLS FOR INSULIN THERAPY**)
   5. Overeating carbs at night in response to minor hypoglycemia symptoms
   6. Chronic ETOH use with an underlying hepatic disease
   7. Eating disorders
   8. Depression and/or anxiety disorders
F. *Referral to endocrinologist for management, but especially with*
   1. *Concurrent illness (e.g., infection or dehydration requiring hospitalization), DKA*
   2. *Recurrent hypoglycemia*
   3. *Unable to obtain glycemic control*
III. Type 2 DM
A. Overall management goals
   1. Eliminate symptoms
   2. Improve quality of life
   3. Reduce the risk of microvascular and macrovascular complications through glycemic control
B. Follow-up visit every 3 mo if DM is uncontrolled, every 6 mo if controlled.
   1. History
      (a) Frequency and cause(s) of hypoglycemic and hyperglycemic episodes
      (b) Results of SMBG (if the patient does them)
         (i) Frequency depends on glycemic goals and treatments used
         (ii) May motivate the patient to make lifestyle changes but is expensive
         (iii) May not be needed for patients who are managed with diet and/or oral agents not associated with hypoglycemia
         (iv) For tips on effective SMBG, see **MONITORING** (earlier in chapter).
      (c) Any changes by the patient in the treatment plan; problems with adherence
      (d) Symptoms suggesting development of complications of DM
      (e) Current medications
      (f) Psychosocial issues (e.g., quality of life issues, depression, ability to pay for medications or tests [which is often a big problem if patient is uninsured or on MCR or MCD])
   2. Physical examination
      (a) Height and weight, vital signs
      (b) Oral examination for periodontal disease
      (c) Cardiovascular examination including bruits and pulses
      (d) Foot examination: inspect the feet at every visit; also see **CHRONIC COMPLICATIONS OF DM**, IV, for neurologic examination.
   3. Laboratory and other testing
      (a) Complete chemistry profile (at least q3–6mo)
      (b) A1c every 3 to 6 mo
      (c) Annual fasting lipid profile, urinalysis for protein and albumin/creatinine ratio (ACR), TSH (as indicated)
      (d) Annual dilated eye examination by an ophthalmologist or optometrist

---

● = *non-urgent referral*

4. Counseling
  (a) Discuss treatment goals and plan; individualize the goals, taking into account the patient's ability to understand and carry out the treatment regime and understand the risk of hypoglycemia.
     (i) Consider need for "refresher" self-management education and support annually and when complications arise.
     (ii) Consider recommending the American Diabetes Association (ADA) website for additional information and resources.
  (b) Review food plan (see **CURRENT DIETARY RECOMMENDATIONS**, earlier in the chapter).
  (c) Discuss exercise and weight reduction plan (if indicated) (see also **EXERCISE AND DIABETES**, earlier in the chapter).
  (d) Review medications.
C. Treatment involves lifestyle changes plus medication (*if diagnosis of type 1 or 2 DM is uncertain, obtain a C-peptide level* [*C-peptide is produced when insulin is available, so low or no C-peptide means insulin is required to treat the DM*]).
  1. Instituting treatment early in the course of DM, before A1c is significantly elevated, is associated with improved glucose control and decreased long-term complications.
  2. Stress the importance of lifestyle changes as the base for all treatment for DM (see **CURRENT DIETARY RECOMMENDATIONS** and **EXERCISE AND DIABETES**, both earlier in the chapter).
D. Pharmacological therapy (also see Table 15.5)
  1. Initially, based on A1c
    (a) ≥ 7.5%: consider starting metformin
    (b) ≥ 1.5% above goal: consider metformin *plus* additional agent (see 3., below)
    (c) ≥ 10% and symptomatic: consider starting insulin (with or without additional agents)
  2. Metformin should be continued in combination with other agents, including insulin, if tolerated and not contraindicated.
  3. The choice of additional agent(s) is based primarily on the presence of ASCVD, CKD or HF (particularly HFrEF).
    (a) If *established ASCVD disease (or high risk for it)* predominates
      (i) Add a GLP-1 receptor agonist (RA) or SGLT2 inhibitor with proven CVD benefit.
      (ii) If the A1c remains above goal after 3 mo, a medication from the opposite category should be added. Other options include a DPP-4 inhibitor (if the patient is not taking a GLP-1 RA), basal insulin, a low-dose TZD, or a sulfonylurea.
    (b) If *CKD or HF (especially HFrEF)* predominates
      (i) Give an SGLT2 inhibitor with HF and/or CKD benefits; if contraindicated or not tolerated, give a GLP-1 RA with CV benefit.
      (ii) If the A1c continues above goal, add a GLP-1 RA with CV benefit to the SGLT2 inhibitor. Other options include DPP-4 inhibitors (except saxagliptin, *and* if the patient is not taking a GLP-1 RA), basal insulin, or a sulfonylurea.

■ = *not to be missed*

    (c) *With no significant risk factors for CV disease and no established ASCVD, CKD, or HF*: the choice is based on which of these is most concerning to the patient: cost, weight gain, or risk of hypoglycemia (see E. Noninsulin hypoglycemic agents and Table 15.5).

       (i) Cost: add either a sulfonylurea or TZD; if the A1c remains above goal, add a medication from the other category as the third agent.

      (ii) Weight gain: add either an SGLT2 inhibitor or GLP-1 RA; if the A1c remains above goal, add a medication from the other category as the third agent.

     (iii) Risk of hypoglycemia: add a DPP-4 inhibitor, GLP-1 RA, SGLT2 inhibitor, or TZD; if the A1c remains above goal, a second or third agent from these medications can be given (*do not* prescribe both a DPP-4 inhibitor and a GLP-1 RA).

  4. If a fourth agent ("quadruple therapy") is needed, consider a sulfonylurea or basal insulin (see F. below).

E. Noninsulin hypoglycemic agents (also see Table 15.5)

  1. Oral hypoglycemic agents (OHAs)

    (a) Are ineffective unless a DM food plan, weight loss (as appropriate), and exercise are part of the management plan; in reality, these are more effective than OHAs for decreasing insulin resistance.

    (b) Taking an "extra" dose to cover excess food intake is ineffective and may be harmful; this should be emphasized to patients.

    (c) Reinforce that OHAs are not oral insulin and do not work like insulin.

    (d) When one OHA is being changed for another, a delay between regimens is not necessary.

  2. In patients intolerant to or unable to take metformin or sulfonylureas, repaglinide and pioglitazone are reasonable alternatives.

  3. Dosing with renal insufficiency

    (a) Metformin is safe with eGFR > 30 mL/min.

    (b) Dose modification with DPP-4 inhibitors, meglitinides

    (c) Cautious use with SGLT2 inhibitors

    (d) No restriction with thiazolidinediones (TZD), GLP-1 RA, sulfonylureas

  4. Possible causes for noninsulin agent failures

    (a) Overeating and weight gain

    (b) Poor compliance

    (c) Lack of physical activity

    (d) Stress or concurrent illness (e.g., surgery, trauma, infection)

    (e) Decreasing beta-cell function or increasing insulin resistance

    (f) Inadequate drug dosage

    (g) Concomitant therapy with diabetogenic drugs (e.g., corticosteroids)

  5. Management of noninsulin agent failures

    (a) Address possible causes before altering therapy.

    (b) Combination therapy (e.g., with metformin) may be more successful than monotherapy.

    (c) Insulin may "tune up" insulin receptors initially, after which, use of an OHA may be effective.

Text continued on page 456

TABLE 15.5 ■ Noninsulin Hypoglycemic Agents

Medication	Action	Glucose Target/A1c Reduction*	Weight Effect	Comments and Contraindications
Alpha-Glucosidase Inhibitors				
Acarbose (Precose) Miglitol (Glyset)	Slows intestinal carbohydrate digestion and absorption	Reduces PPG A1c: 0.6%–0.7%	Neutral	High incidence of GI side effects (e.g., diarrhea, flatulence, cramping), especially with high-carbohydrate meal or if drug is started at a comparatively high dose Delays absorption of *sucrose but not glucose*; if patient is also taking insulin or sulfonylureas and experiences hypoglycemic symptoms, give glucose tabs or gel; candy, soda, or sugar-sweetened juices *will not* help Contraindications Ketoacidosis Inflammatory bowel disease Intestinal obstruction Cirrhosis Serum creatinine > 2 mg/dL
Biguanides				
Metformin	Decreases hepatic production of glucose Increases insulin sensitivity in muscle and fat	Reduces FPG and PPG A1c: 1%–1.5% (monotherapy)	Neutral or weight loss Counters insulin-associated weight gain	May cause gastric distress or diarrhea, but these decrease with time Stop drug 48 hr before surgery or any test with an iodine contrast dye Hold drug with N/V or dehydration (increased risk of lactic acidosis) May reduce CV mortality, especially in obese patients Can be started with eGFR ≥45 mL/min; contraindicated if <30 mL/min. If already on metformin and the eGFR is 30–45 mL/min, weigh benefits and risks of continuing prescription Can lower vitamin B12 levels; check with anemia, if symptoms of peripheral neuropathy develop, or if patient is PPI user or a vegetarian Contraindications Type 1 DM eGFR <30 mL/min Pregnancy and lactation Alcohol abuse Acute or chronic metabolic acidosis

DPP-4 Inhibitors

Alogliptin (Nesina)[†]
Linagliptin (Trajenta)[†]
Saxagliptin (Onglyza)[†]
Sitagliptin (Januvia)[†]

Slows degradation of natural GLP-1, thus stimulating insulin secretion when glucose levels increase. Decreases gastric emptying and increases satiety	Reduces PPG A1c: 0.7%	Neutral

Consider pancreatitis with severe abdominal pain with/without vomiting
May cause severe joint pain (stop medication if occurs)
May cause or worsen HF (saxagliptin, alogliptin)
Dosage modification with renal impairment
Do not use with GLP-1 receptor agonists

GLP-1 Receptor Agonists

Dulaglutide (Trulicity)
Exenatide (Byetta, Bydureon, Bydureon BCise)
Liraglutide (Victoza, Saxenda)
Lixisenatide (Adlyxin)
Semaglutide (Ozempic, Rybelsus)
Tirzepatide (Mounjaro)

Stimulates insulin secretion when glucose levels increase. Decreases gastric emptying. Increases satiety	Reduces PPG primarily A1c: ~1%	Weight loss

May cause nausea, diarrhea (less with low dose start and titrate as tolerated)
Consider pancreatitis with severe abdominal pain with/without vomiting
Many in this class, if used in patients with high CV risk or disease, may reduce death from CV causes and any cause; they also help prevent progression of CKD
Most are injected drugs—pay attention to dosing frequency (varies from bid to weekly)
Semaglutide also comes in oral form
Contraindications
FH of thyroid cancer or multiple endocrine neoplasia syndrome
Do not use with DPP-4 inhibitors

Meglitinides

Nateglinide (Starlix)
Repaglinide (Prandin)[†]

Stimulates insulin release (glucose dependent)	Reduces PPG A1c: 0.7%	Weight gain

Do not use nateglinide with impaired renal function
May cause hypoglycemia (less risk with repaglinide)
Flexible dosing—can skip a dose if meal skipped
Contraindications
Ketoacidosis
Type 1 DM
Pregnancy
Gemfibrozil used with repaglinide

Continued

TABLE 15.5 ■ Noninsulin Hypoglycemic Agents—cont'd

Medication	Action	Glucose Target/A1c Reduction*	Weight Effect	Comments and Contraindications
SGLT-2 Inhibitor				
Canagliflozin (Invokana)† Dapagliflozin (Farxiga) Empagliflozin (Jardiance)† Ertugliflozin (Steglatro)†	Increases urine excretion of glucose	Reduces FPG and PPG A1c: 0.7%–1%	Weight loss	Consider avoiding use with following conditions because of increased risk: Frequent UTIs or genital yeast infections Low BMD and high risk for falls or fractures Foot ulceration (e.g., foot deformity, neuropathy, PVD, Hx of previous foot ulcers) Predisposed to DKA (e.g., ketosis-prone DM, drug or alcohol addiction) Possible other adverse effects: hyperkalemia, bladder cancer, dehydration (use with caution if patient also taking NSAID, ACE/ARB, or diuretic; decrease dose of diuretics), acute pancreatitis, and Fournier gangrene Recurrent genital infection involving the penis and/or foreskin and it does not resolve promptly with treatment, have patient evaluated for a cancerous lesion Recurrent genital infections may be *more common in summer months.* May cause ketoacidosis *without significant* hyperglycemia; consider obtaining anion gap with symptoms (e.g., dyspnea, vomiting, fatigue). Do not rely on urine ketones to diagnose DKA To decrease DKA risk, stop med 3 days before surgery and hold it until oral intake is back to normal May cause acute kidney injury requiring dialysis; check creatinine 1–2 wk after starting or dose increase; stop medication with 30% increase All SGLT2 inhibitors decrease hospitalizations due to HF and CKD progression Empagliflozin and canagliflozin are associated with decreased CV mortality Contraindications Prior history DKA eGFR <30mL/min (canagliflozin), <45mL/min (dapagliflozin, empagliflozin) or <60mL/min (ertugliflozin)

Sulfonylureas (Second Generation)

Drug	Action	Effect	Adverse Effects	Notes
Glimepiride (Amaryl)[†] Glipizide (Glucotrol, Glucotrol XL) Glyburide (DiaBeta, Micronase)	Effective only with endogenous insulin secretion Increases insulin production and secretion Effective for 7–10 yr in most patients	Reduces FPG A1c: 0.8%	Weight gain	Stop when starting basal plus prandial insulins May cause severe hypoglycemia (less with glimepiride); remind patient to not skip meals If patient is >65 yr of age, start with 2.5 mg qd Contraindications Type 1 DM Pregnancy or lactation Major surgery Severe infection, illness, trauma History of severe reaction to sulfa Over 65 yr of age: glimepiride and glyburide (because of increased risk of prolonged hypoglycemia)

Thiazolidinedione (TZD)

Drug	Action	Effect	Adverse Effects	Notes
Pioglitazone (Actos)[†] Rosiglitazone (Avandia)	Increases insulin sensitivity in muscle and fat	Reduces FPG and PPG A1c: 0.8%	Weight gain (especially at higher doses)	Increased risk of hypoglycemia if used with insulin or sulfonylureas FDA boxed warnings re: potential to cause or worsen HF; stop the drug at the first signs Increased fracture risk Contraindications Active liver disease History or diagnosis of HF Type 1 DM

* When added to metformin.
[†] Also comes in combination with metformin or another antidiabetic agent.
FPG, Fasting plasma glucose; PPG, postprandial glucose.

F. Many patients eventually require insulin therapy after 10 to 15 yr of OHA therapy because of declining beta-cell function.
   1. Indications
      (a) Newly diagnosed with A1c > 10% (allows the beta cells to "rest" and after about 6 mo, may be able to start noninsulin agent(s) and stop the insulin)
      (b) Hyperglycemia and unable to achieve glycemic goals, despite lifestyle changes and noninsulin agents
      (c) Pregnancy
      (d) During periods of stress, illness, or injury; steroid injections (either joint or back)
      (e) Marked and otherwise unexplained recent weight loss and/or presence of moderate-to-heavy ketonuria
      (f) Onset of chronic complications
   2. Goals of insulin therapy are as follows
      (a) Fasting and pre-prandial glucose
          80–130 mg/dL   (ADA)
          70–110 mg/dL   (American Association of Clinical Endocrinologists [AACE])
      (b) 2 hr PP glucose
          < 180 mg/dL   (ADA)
          < 140 mg/dL   (AACE)
   3. Optimal insulin therapy requires an understanding of insulin pharmacokinetics (Table 15.4).
   4. Initiating insulin (also see Table 15.4 and **PRACTICE PEARLS FOR INSULIN THERAPY**, later in the chapter).
      (a) Assess lifestyle, willingness to start insulin, and ability to monitor glucose levels. Educate patient on insulin titration (if needed) and avoidance and treatment of hypoglycemia.
      (b) A common combination is once-daily insulin added to an existing noninsulin regimen.
          (i) Start basal insulin at 10 units or 0.1 to 0.2 units/kg daily.
          (ii) Suggested titration: adjust the insulin dose by 3 units every 3 days, based on the FBG values, until the FBG goal is reached or daily dose is 0.5 units/kg.
      (c) If the basal insulin is titrated to acceptable FBG *or* if the dose is > 0.5 units/kg/day *and* the A1c is not at goal, consider
          (i) Continue basal insulin at bedtime *and add* GLP-1 agonist or SGLT2 q a.m. (this is associated with less weight gain or even weight loss and less frequent hypoglycemia episodes than adding mealtime insulin.)
          (ii) Continue basal insulin daily *and add* rapid- or short-acting insulin with the largest meal of the day (prandial dose); start with 5 units once daily (see Adjusting insulin, 5. below, for titration).
          (iii) If on long-acting insulin, change to NPH insulin bid (split the dose 50:50 or ⅔ total dose before breakfast and ⅓ before dinner or at bedtime).
          (iv) Stop the basal insulin and start injections of premixed insulin before breakfast and dinner.
          (v) If one regimen is not effective in reaching glycemic goals, consider switching (see G. Switching insulin products, below).
      (d) When starting more than 1 injection daily, stop all oral diabetic agents except metformin (simplifies medical regimen and cost).
   5. Adjusting insulin
      (a) Before changing the insulin dose, determine the cause of hypoglycemia or hyperglycemia if possible.

(b) Usually, adjust the insulin dose based on the average of 3 days' readings; teaching the patient self-titration can get better glucose control.

    (i) Basal insulin: adjust by 3 units every 3 days until 0.5 units/kg/day or FBG is at goal

    (ii) Pre-prandial insulin: adjust by 2 units twice a week

(c) If on more than one insulin injection daily with consistent elevations of blood glucose levels at the same time daily for 3 consecutive days that cannot be explained by changes in the diet, activity, illness, or stress: adjust the insulin component relevant to that time period (see Table 15.4).

(d) Intensive insulin therapy is *contraindicated* when

    (i) The patient cannot comply with the regimen.

    (ii) The patient is insensitive to signs of hypoglycemia.

    (iii) The patient has a compromised mental status or comorbid neurological conditions (e.g., seizures, CVA or cerebrovascular disease).

G. Switching insulin products (which insulin is prescribed is often based on patient preference and the payer [e.g., which insurance, if any, the patient uses]).

1. Converting *NPH to longer-acting insulin*

    (a) To detemir *(Levemir):* convert unit for unit; give detemir once daily or divided bid

    (b) To glargine *(Lantus, Basaglar, Toujeo)*

        (i) From NPH once daily: convert unit for unit and give long-acting insulin once daily

        (ii) From NPH bid: reduce total daily dose by 20% and give long-acting insulin once daily

    (c) To degludec *(Tresiba):* convert unit for unit and give once daily

2. Converting *longer-acting basal insulin to NPH*: convert unit for unit and give NPH bid

3. Converting *one long-acting to different long-acting basal insulin*

    (a) Glargine *(Lantus)* to/from glargine *(Basaglar):* convert unit for unit

    (b) Glargine U-100 *(Lantus, Basaglar)* to glargine U-300 *(Toujeo)*: convert total daily dose unit for unit and give Toujeo once daily

    (c) Glargine U-100 *(Lantus, Basaglar)* to detemir *(Levemir):* convert unit for unit and give once daily or divided bid

    (d) Glargine U-300 *(Toujeo)* to glargine U-100 *(Lantus, Basaglar)* or detemir *(Levemir):* reduce total daily dose by 20% and give once daily

4. Converting between *long-acting basal* and *ultra-long-acting insulin*

    (a) Detemir *(Levemir)* or glargine *(Lantus, Basaglar, Toujeo)* to degludec *(Tresiba):* convert unit for unit and give once daily

    (b) Degludec *(Tresiba)* to NPH, detemir *(Levemir)* or glargine *(Lantus, Basaglar, Toujeo)*

        (i) Limited information; consider converting unit for unit

        (ii) Give glargine *(Lantus, Basaglar, Toujeo)* once daily; give detemir *(Levemir)* once daily or divided bid; give NPH divided bid (split the dose 50:50 or ⅔ total dose before breakfast and ⅓ before dinner or at bedtime)

5. Converting *one rapid-acting (Humalog, Novolog, Apidra) to another rapid-acting insulin*: convert unit for unit

6. Converting *rapid-acting (Humalog, Novolog, Apidra) to regular insulin (Humulin R, Novolin R):* convert unit for unit

7. Converting *regular (Humulin R, Novolin R) to rapid-acting insulin (Humalog, Novolog, Apidra)*: convert unit for unit
8. Converting *between premixed insulins (Humulin 70/30, Novolin 70/30, Humalog Mix 75/25, NovoLog Mix 70/30)*: convert unit for unit

---

PRACTICE PEARLS FOR INSULIN THERAPY

- Reassure the patient that starting insulin is not a personal "failure"; most patients with type 2 DM will eventually need insulin because of a decline in insulin production.
- As a rule, normalize fasting blood glucose levels before normalizing the levels throughout the remainder of the day ("fix the fasting first").
- With variable blood glucose readings, consider the following:
  - Absorption is reduced with increasing insulin doses; may try splitting the amount of each injection into two separate sites.
  - Site variability and absorption: fastest absorption from the abdominal wall, slowest from the leg and buttock, intermediate from the arm; may try pre-prandial regular or rapid-acting insulin injected in the abdominal wall and evening NPH into the leg or buttock.
  - To avoid deficient insulin absorption because of fibrosis, recommend rotating to a different site after 5 to 7 injections.
- Consider insulin degludec (Tresiba) if patient has severe nocturnal hypoglycemia on another basal insulin.
- If cost is a barrier, consider human insulins (regular, NPH, or 70/30). The overall hypoglycemia and A1c lowering is similar to analog insulins.
- Insulin pens are more convenient but since they contain 300 units/cartridge, the patient may have to use a new cartridge to complete a required dose, thus involving 2 injections. Insulin vials contain 1500 units, so they may be more cost-effective, but the patient must "draw up" the injection each time; this may be a concern with vision or dexterity issues.
- New insulins approved by the FDA will be classified as biologic or biosimilar and the generic name will have a four-letter suffix (e.g., Lyumjev [insulin lispro-aabc]). Their actions are similar to other insulins.
- Soliqua 100/33 is a combination of insulin glargine and lixisenatide (GLP-1 RA).
- Teach the patient what to do on sick days (see **ACUTE COMPLICATIONS OF DM, III,** later in this chapter).

H. With poorly controlled DM, consider the following
   1. Overeating (specifically, simple carbs)
   2. Inadequate exercise and/or activity
   3. Over-insulinization (usually in patients with marked "glucose bounces")
   4. Incorrect insulin injection (technique and/or sites; see **PRACTICE PEARLS FOR INSULIN THERAPY**)
   5. Overeating carbs at night in response to minor hypoglycemia symptoms
   6. Chronic ETOH use with an underlying hepatic disease
   7. Eating disorders
   8. Depression and/or anxiety disorders
I. Children and adolescents with Type 2 DM (differences from care of adults): lifestyle modifications are still a key component in the treatment.
   1. Nutrition
      (a) Provide a diet that decreases calories and avoids sugar-containing soft drinks but includes adequate nutrition for normal health and growth.
      (b) The diet should not be limited to the child but should also include other family members.

  (c) Suggestions to consider
   (i) Smaller portion sizes
   (ii) Substitute fruits and vegetables for carbohydrate-rich foods
   (iii) Replace soft drinks and juices with water or calorie-free liquids
   (iv) Eat out less often
 2. Weight goals
  (a) The decision for weight reduction or weight maintenance depends on the age of the patient, degree of obesity, and presence of other comorbidities.
  (b) Initially, recommend that the patient and family maintain the current weight (e.g., for 1 to 2 mo). After this is done, they can then begin changes for weight loss, depending on patient's age: prepuberty 0.5 kg/mo and after puberty up to 0.5 to 1 kg/wk.
  (c) The weight loss goal is BMI < 85th percentile.
 3. Physical activity
  (a) Initially, decrease the amount of sedentary time (e.g., watching TV, playing video or computer games).
  (b) The ADA recommends at least 60 min/day of moderate to intense aerobic activity and bone-strengthening activities at least 3 times a wk.
  (c) Children with BMI ≥ 95th percentile should primarily perform nonweight-bearing activities (e.g., swimming, biking, short walks).
 4. Pharmacological therapy
  (a) Only insulin and metformin are FDA-approved for use in children.
  (b) Recommend multivitamin daily if taking metformin because of possible impaired absorption of B12 and/or folic acid.
J. *Referral to endocrinologist* with
 1. *Concurrent illness (e.g., infection or dehydration requiring hospitalization), DKA*
 2. *Recurrent hypoglycemia or unable to obtain glycemic control*

ACUTE COMPLICATIONS OF DM

I. Hyperglycemia
 A. DKA (diabetic ketoacidosis)
  1. Definition: characterized by metabolic acidosis, ketosis, and hyperglycemia due to insulin deficiency
  2. Risk factors
   (a) Omission of insulin (type 1 or 2 DM)
   (b) New-onset DM, especially type 1 (20%–25% of DKA cases)
   (c) Infection (30%–40% of DKA cases)
   (d) Acute pancreatitis
   (e) Acute MI or CVA
   (f) Medications (e.g., clozapine or olanzapine; cocaine; lithium)
  3. Signs and symptoms: develop rapidly over 24 hr
   (a) Polyuria, polydipsia
   (b) Kussmaul respirations
   (c) Abdominal pain
   (d) Dehydration
   (e) May have a fruity odor to breath
   (f) Altered LOC

● = *non-urgent referral*

    4. Lab values

        (a) pH < 7.30, anion gap > 17 and/or low CO_2

        (b) Glucose > 500 to 800 mg/dL

        (c) Serum bicarbonate ≤ 15 mEq/L

▲   5. Treatment: ***emergency transfer to ED; DKA is a medical emergency***

  B. Hyperosmolar hyperglycemic state (HHS)

    1. Definition: severe hyperglycemia in the absence of ketosis

    2. Risk factors

        (a) Inadequate insulin or noncompliance (21%–41% of HHS cases)

        (b) Accompanying infection (32%–60% HHS cases): pneumonia, UTI, or sepsis

        (c) Acute illness

        (d) Type 2 DM (> 35% are previously undiagnosed)

        (e) Older than 50 yr of age

        (f) Diuretic or SGLT2 therapy

        (g) Nursing home residents

    3. Signs and symptoms: develop more insidiously

        (a) Polyuria, polydipsia; significant dehydration

        (b) Weight loss

        (c) Weakness

        (d) Hypotension

        (e) Altered LOC, possible coma

    4. Lab values

        (a) pH > 7.30

        (b) Glucose > 600 mg/dL and often ≥ 1000 mg/dL

        (c) Serum bicarbonate > 20 mEq/L

        (d) Osmolality > 320 mOsm

▲ C. Treatment: ***emergency transfer to ED; HHS is a medical emergency, with a mortality rate of 12%–42%***

II. Hypoglycemia

  A. Definition: blood glucose levels low enough to cause signs and symptoms or to have the potential to cause harm; in general, the BG is < 70 mg/dL

  B. Possible causes (not exclusive)

    1. Increase in the insulin dose or some noninsulin oral agents (i.e., sulfonylureas, meglitinides)

    2. Decrease or delay in food intake; gastroparesis

    3. Increase in exercise levels

    4. Alcohol ingestion (inhibits hepatic gluconeogenesis)

    5. Concomitant liver or renal disease (~ 80% of endogenous glucose release is by the liver and ~ 20% by the kidneys)

    6. Tight glucose control (i.e., A1c < 6.5%)

  C. Repeated episodes of hypoglycemia, even if not acutely symptomatic, may be linked to higher CV risk and all-cause mortality.

  D. Treatment of hypoglycemia

    1. Ingest 15 g rapid-acting carbohydrate (see Table 15.6), recheck glucose in 15 min and if still < 70 mg/dL, repeat 15 g of rapid-acting carbohydrate.

    2. If patient is unable to swallow or is unconscious from suspected hypoglycemia, give glucagon 1 mg IM.

▲ = *urgent referral*

TABLE 15.6 ■ **Treatment of Hypoglycemia**

Type of Hypoglycemia	Symptoms	Treatment
Mild	Hunger Tremors and palpitations Sweating	Give 10–15 g of simple carbohydrates* Should respond in 10–15 min
Moderate	As above plus: H/A Mood changes, irritability Drowsiness, decreased attentiveness	May require a second dose of simple carbohydrates The patient may have more difficulty treating hypoglycemia independently
Severe	Unresponsiveness Unconsciousness Convulsions	No oral carbohydrate Glucagon 1 mg IM or SC in the deltoid or anterior thigh (0.5 mg if < 5 yr of age) ***Transfer to the ED after emergency treatment***

* Each of the following foods gives ~ 10–15 g of carbohydrate:
- 4 oz (120 mL) fruit juice
- 8 Life Saver candies
- 1 tbsp honey or Karo syrup
- 2 tsp sugar or raisins
- 3 glucose tablets or gels
Do **not** use candy bar, ice cream, or other fatty foods that delay glucose absorption and contribute to weight gain.

3. Compare the onset of hypoglycemia with the insulin used, to determine if the dose needs to be adjusted (often reduced by 10%–20%, depending on degree of hypoglycemia).

4. With gastroparesis, consider delaying mealtime insulin until after patient has eaten or change to regular insulin (slower onset than rapid-acting insulin).

E. Prevention of hypoglycemia is a priority because of safety concerns.
   1. Eat meals and snacks on time.
   2. Take insulin as directed at appropriate times; make adjustments for decreased or delayed food intake.
   3. Take special care when sleeping late.
      (a) May need to decrease the evening NPH dose by 10%–15% if sleeping more than 45 min later than usual.
      (b) May require advancing the entire day's schedule.
   4. Make adjustments for increased activity or exercise.
      (a) Avoid exercising alone.
      (b) SMBG is essential: encourage patient to follow recommended adjustments (see Table 15.3).
      (c) If symptomatic hypoglycemia occurs during exercise, stop and eat a snack.

F. Special problems related to hypoglycemia
   1. Hypoglycemia unawareness
      (a) Severe hypoglycemia without warning: patients with low A1c and repeated episodes of recent hypoglycemia are most vulnerable
      (b) *Inability to recognize blood glucose levels < 55 mg/dL: referral to an endocrinologist, but in the meantime, raise target glucose levels to 100 to 150 mg/dL*

● = *non-urgent referral;* ▲ = *urgent referral*

fasting and before meals; consider changing from sulfonylurea or glitinide (if taking them) to other medications less likely to cause hypoglycemia.

  2. Elderly patients: glycemic goals can be higher because of safety risks (e.g., falls, syncope).

    (a) A1c < 8% with limited life expectancy or multiple comorbidities (ADA)

    (b) A1c 7.5%–9% with multisystem diseases or dementia or in a nursing facility (European DM Working Group for Older People)

  3. End-stage renal disease

    (a) With eGFR < 60 mL/min, A1c goal is < 8%.

    (b) With eGFR 10 to 50 mL/min, insulin dose should be reduced by 25%.

III. Sick day management guidelines when taking insulin—to help prevent hypoglycemia, significant hyperglycemia, and DKA.

  A. Monitoring

    1. Check blood glucose levels q2–4hr, and check urine ketones with every void when the blood glucose is over 250 to 300 mg/dL, especially if patient feels unwell.

    2. The patient or parent/caregiver should call the health care provider when preprandial blood glucose levels remain > 250 mg/dL or urine has moderate-to-large ketones.

  B. Insulin and diet

    1. Do *not* stop insulin despite N/V or inability to eat (although the dose may need to be temporarily adjusted to lower the risk of hypoglycemia).

      (a) Take usual dose of NPH or glargine or detemir insulin.

      (b) With hyperglycemia, additional doses of rapid-acting or short-acting insulin should be given, depending on the amount of ketones in the urine

        (i) With none or small amount, give 0.05 to 0.1 units/kg every 2 to 4 hr prn

        (ii) With moderate-to-large amount, give 0.1 to 0.2 units/kg.

    2. If no N/V but decreased activity (e.g., bed rest)

      (a) Decrease calorie intake by one-third.

      (b) Adjust insulin as previously mentioned (B.1., above).

    3. If the patient is having N/V or is unable to eat

      (a) Use short-acting insulin only.

      (b) Meal plan

        (i) Give ice cold, sugar-containing liquids such as soft drinks, fruit juices, sweetened tea: 4 to 6 oz (120 to 180 mL) each hour for adults or adolescents, 2 to 4 oz (60 to 120 mL) each hour for children.

        (ii) When tolerated, add soft carbohydrate foods.

    4. Some clinicians teach patients to replace usual carbohydrate calories with "sick day" foods (Box 15.1).

  ▲ C. *Seek medical attention immediately when*

    1. *Fever is > 100 °F*

    2. *Diarrhea persists beyond 4 hr*

    3. *The patient is vomiting and unable to take fluids for > 2 to 4 hr*

    4. *Blood glucose levels remain > 250 mg/dL despite insulin adjustments*

    5. *Moderate-to-large ketones appear in urine*

    6. *The patient experiences severe abdominal pain or other unexplained symptoms or has mental clouding*

    7. *Illness Persists for > 24 hr*

BOX 15.1 ■ Foods Allowed on Sick Days

Choose one of these foods for every **fruit** on your meal plan (10 g of carbohydrate each):
½ c regular ginger ale
½ c Kool-Aid
1 c Gatorade
½ c regular lemonade
1 Popsicle
½ c soft drink, 7-Up
¼ c regular gelatin
¼ c grape juice
⅓ c apple juice
¼ c cranberry juice
2 tsp syrup, sugar

Choose one of these foods for every **milk** product on your meal plan (12 g of carbohydrate each):
½ c regular cocoa
¾ c cream soup
1 c whole milk
⅓ c tapioca pudding
¼ c vanilla pudding
¼ c custard
1 tbsp sugar

Remember, you are taking sweetened drinks and foods because you cannot eat other foods!

Choose one of these foods for every **starch** product on your meal plan (15 g of carbohydrate each):
½ c cooked cereal
¼ c regular pudding
½ c ice cream
1 c cream soup
1 c chicken noodle soup
¼ c sherbet
⅓ c regular gelatin
1 tbsp jelly
½ c instant breakfast
5 vanilla wafers
6 saltine crackers
1 c milk

CHRONIC COMPLICATIONS OF DM

I. DM foot ulcer
   A. Results from decreased sensation and microvascular circulation; neuropathy is a contributing factor because injury is not found until damage has occurred.
   B. Description
      1. Painless ulcers usually noted on the plantar surface of the foot (commonly over metatarsal heads, heels, or sites of poorly fitting shoes)
         (a) Grade 1: superficial, involving full skin thickness but not underlying tissues
         (b) Grade 2: deep, penetrating down to the ligaments/muscle but no bone involvement or abscess
         (c) Grade 3: deep, with cellulitis or abscess formation; often with osteomyelitis
         (d) Grade 4: localized gangrene
         (e) Grade 5: extensive gangrene of the entire foot
      2. Feet may be warm or cool to touch; usually diminished pedal pulses.
      3. Paresthesias in part or all of the affected extremity
   C. Treatment
      1. Aggressive control of DM
▲   2. ***Referral to a vascular surgeon if the vascular status of the limb is compromised***
      3. Grades 1 and 2
         (a) Extensive debridement, good local wound care, and relief of pressure on the ulcer
         (b) If infection is present (obvious purulent drainage or redness/swelling or warmth around the ulcer): culture ulcer base after debridement and treat according to C&S results. If unable to obtain a culture
            (i) Mild infection: cephalexin or dicloxacillin; give amoxicillin/clavulanate if the patient has had antibiotics in the previous month
            (ii) Moderate infection (e.g., deeper or with redness over 2 cm but NO systemic signs such as fever): start with amoxicillin/clavulanate and add MRSA coverage if needed (e.g., TMP/SMX or doxycycline).

▲ = *urgent referral*

        (c) *Referral to a wound specialist, surgeon or podiatrist if the ulcer is not improv-*
           ing after 3 to 4 wk of above therapy.
    4. Grade 3: *referral to a surgeon or wound care specialist or podiatrist after obtaining*
       ABI and bilateral venous Doppler (to check circulation) and bone scan (to check for
       osteomyelitis). Consider empiric antibiotics if indicated (see 3b, above).
    5. Grades 4 and 5: *urgent referral to ED for hospital admission and treatment*

II. Increased incidence of NAFLD (see Chapter 9, **Liver Disease, NAFLD**) and increased risk of colon cancer

III. Nephropathy
  A. Leading cause of end-stage renal disease; 20 + yr after DM diagnosed
    1. Type 1 DM: reported in 30%–40% of patients
    2. Type 2 DM: 15%–20% of patients
  B. Screening/evaluation (*do not* use diagnosis of DM nephropathy *without* protein in urine)
    1. Yearly urine for albuminuria (albumin-to-creatinine ratio [ACR])
    2. If positive, repeat the test twice in a 3 to 6 mo period; if two or three tests are positive for severely increased albuminuria, begin treatment.
      (a) Moderately increased: 30 to 300 mg/g
      (b) Severely increased: > 300 mg/g
    3. Sudden *decrease* in insulin requirements can indicate renal compromise.
    4. If the ACR > 30 mg/g or the eGFR < 60 mL/min, assess these tests twice a year to monitor for progression of CKD.
  C. Treatment
    1. At the time of initial diagnosis, R/O other causes of renal disease (e.g., obstructive uropathy, infection).
    2. Aggressive glycemic control
    3. For treatment of severely increased albuminuria, begin ACE or ARB at usual doses (see Table 8.16); HTN does *not* need to be present.
    4. Aggressively monitor and treat HTN (BP goal is < 140/90 mmHg; if tolerated, can be < 130/80 mmHg).
    5. Treat dyslipidemia (see Chapter 8, **DYSLIPIDEMIA**).
    6. *Consider referral to a nephrologist or DM specialist with uncertainty about the cause of kidney disease, anemia, secondary hyperparathyroidism, resistant HTN, or eGFR <30 mL/min.*
    7. Promptly treat UTIs; repeat UA after treatment.

IV. Neuropathy
  A. Types
    1. Peripheral
      (a) Insidious onset, symmetric distribution, progressive course
      (b) Often affects the feet first, although can occur in hands
        (i) Small fiber damage: pain and dysesthesias (unpleasant burning and tingling sensations, electric shock sensations)
        (ii) Large fiber damage: numbness and loss of protective sensation; this is a risk factor for diabetic foot ulcers and also poor balance and falls
      (c) Consider other causes for the neuropathy (e.g., vitamin B12 deficiency, hypothyroidism, toxins [alcohol], malignancies).
    2. Autonomic
      (a) GI: may have GERD, gastroparesis (consider with early satiety, N/V, bloating, and postprandial abdominal fullness), diarrhea, constipation, or incontinence.

● = *non-urgent referral;* ▲ = *urgent referral*

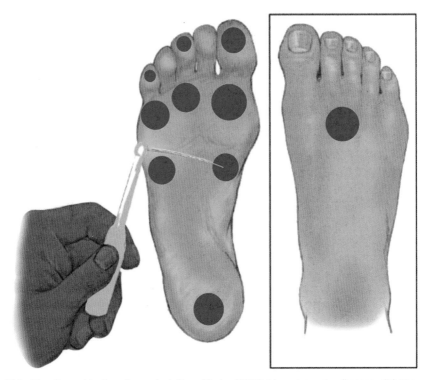

Fig. 15.4 Monofilament testing sites on feet. (From Mosby. (1998). *Managing major diseases: diabetes mellitus and hypertension*. New York: Elsevier.)

    (b) GU: may have neurogenic bladder, sexual dysfunction.

    (c) CV: may have resting tachycardia, exercise intolerance, orthostatic hypotension.

B. Screening/evaluation

    1. Yearly foot examinations

        (a) To identify loss of protective sense rather than early neuropathy: 10 g monofilament (see Fig. 15.4) and vibration perception with 128 Hz tuning fork at the big toes

        (b) Assess skin integrity of feet, especially between toes and under metatarsal heads, at least annually; note the presence of redness, increased warmth, or callus formation.

    2. EMG, if indicated

    3. Obtain ankle-brachial index (see Chapter 8, Table 8.19) if patient is experiencing claudication or with a venous filling time of > 20 sec; to evaluate venous filling time:

        (a) With the patient supine, identify a prominent pedal vein; elevate the leg to 45 degrees for 1 min until the vein collapses.

        (b) Have the patient sit up with the leg hanging over the examination table and note the time until the pedal vein bulges.

C. Treatment

    1. The main components are: control of blood glucose levels, lifestyle management (e.g., diet and exercise), foot care to prevent complications, and control of the pain; although there is no cure, symptoms can be improved with pharmacological and non-pharmacological therapies (see later in this section).

2. Stress realistic goals (e.g., 30%–50% reduction in symptoms).
3. Educate patient on DM foot care.
    (a) Daily checking the feet for changes in the skin (e.g., cracks or wounds)
    (b) Consider using an emollient cream (without alcohol) or petroleum jelly on the feet to prevent dry skin.
    (c) Visual examination of the feet with each visit (e.g., every 3 to 4 mo) and annual comprehensive foot exam
4. Pain/paresthesias: one or more of the following may help (change if not helping after 3 to 4 wk; antidepressant plus anticonvulsant may be more effective than one alone)
    (a) Antidepressants
        (i) Nortriptyline 10 to 25 mg hs; increase the dose q2wk to 75 mg or until the dose is not tolerated (*not* to be used in the elderly or patients with cardiac disease). May also be given with pregabalin or gabapentin, but NOT with duloxetine.
        (ii) Duloxetine 60 to 120 mg hs; may be taken with pregabalin or gabapentin.
    (b) Anticonvulsants
        (i) Pregabalin 50 mg bid, slowly increase to 300 mg daily total (150 mg bid or 100 mg tid); may be taken with nortriptyline or duloxetine but NOT with gabapentin.
        (ii) Gabapentin 300 to 3600 mg daily in three divided doses; may be taken with nortriptyline or duloxetine. May also be taken just at hs for nocturnal pain.
    (c) Others
        (i) Tramadol or alpha-lipoic acid (ALA) may be beneficial as well. ALA is an OTC dietary supplement and is usually taken once daily.
        (ii) Some studies have shown benefit from therapy with electrical stimulation and magnetic field treatment.
        (iii) Moderate aerobic exercise, resistance exercises, and balance training have been shown to decrease symptoms (evaluate by P.T. to receive an appropriate exercise program for patient).
5. Muscle pain
    (a) NSAIDs
        (i) Avoid with eGFR ≤ 60 mL/min.
        (ii) Use cautiously with eGFR 60 to 89 mL/min plus other conditions such as HF, cirrhosis, or diuretic use.
    (b) Physical therapy
    (c) Muscle relaxants
    (d) Avoid alcohol (may aggravate the development of neuropathy)
6. GI problems
    (a) Small, frequent meals
    (b) Avoid fats
    (c) ● ***Referral to a GI doctor, with continued symptoms***
V. Retinopathy
    A. Leading cause of impaired vision in adults 25 to 74 yr of age; much of the visual loss can be prevented by timely identification and treatment
    1. Type 1: begins 3 to 5 yr after diagnosis
    2. Type 2: 50%–80% patients have it 20 yr after diagnosis

---

● = *non-urgent referral*

    3. Additional risk factors for retinopathy include chronic hyperglycemia, DM kidney disease, HTN, and dyslipidemia.

B. Screening/evaluation: *annual* dilated eye examination with an ophthalmologist or optometrist
    1. All patients with type 1 DM of ≥ 5 yr duration
    2. All type 2 DM patients
    3. Early in the first trimester for any pregnant woman with known DM (pregnancy is associated with rapid progression of DM retinopathy)

C. Treatment
    1. Usually laser surgery
    2. Optimal glycemic control reduces incidence and progression.
    3. Treat HTN and dyslipidemia.
    4. Retinopathy is not a contraindication to ASA therapy for cardio-protection (ASA does not increase risk of retinal hemorrhage).

Thyroid Disorders

PRACTICE PEARLS FOR THYROID

- Screen asymptomatic patients who may be at increased risk for hypothyroidism.
  - Presence of goiter
  - History of autoimmune disease
  - Previous radioactive iodine therapy
  - Previous head or neck radiation
  - Family history of thyroid disease
  - Taking medications that may impair thyroid function (e.g., lithium, amiodarone)
- If the patient has unexplainable urticaria, check for thyroid dysfunction.
- Laboratory tests (Table 15.7)
  - Serum thyroid-stimulating hormone (TSH) is the primary test; if TSH is abnormal, repeat TSH along with free thyroxine (T4); consider checking free T3 if the TSH is low (indicating possible hyperthyroidism).
  - Serum T4: many factors may alter serum T4 measurements, including acute illness, high estrogen states and hormone replacement therapy, acute psychiatric problems, kidney and liver disorders, certain drugs, and biotin (B vitamin found in hair and skin vitamins).
  - If thyroid dysfunction is suspected, also check lipid panel, basic metabolic profile, and CBC levels and obtain an ECG.
- Thyroid medications *work best when taken alone* (at least 2 hrs apart from other meds). If this is not possible, be consistent with when it is taken and the thyroid dosage can be adjusted accordingly.
- With a thyroid nodule > 1 cm (by palpation and/or imaging): perform history and examination and obtain TSH and thyroid U/S; if TSH is low, obtain free T4 and free T3 and a thyroid radionuclide scan.
  - U/S features associated with increased risk of thyroid cancer include: hypoechoic, microcalcifications, irregular margins, incomplete halo, and nodule is taller than wide.
  - *"Hot" (functioning) nodule: hyperthyroidism (subclinical with normal FT4 and FT3 levels, overt with high FT4 and/or FT3 levels); referral to an endocrinologist*
  - ▲ *"Cold" (nonfunctional) nodule: referral urgently to surgeon or ENT for fine-needle aspiration (FNA). A "cold" nodule is a more serious finding.*
- FNA is preferable to distinguish between benign and cancerous thyroid nodules.

= non-urgent referral; ▲ *= urgent referral*

TABLE 15.7 ■ Laboratory Findings in Thyroid Disorders

Condition	TSH	Free T4 (FT4)	Free T3 (FT3)
Primary hypothyroidism (thyroid disease)	↑	↓	N/A
Secondary hypothyroidism (pituitary/hypothalamus disease)	↓ or N	↓	N/A
Hyperthyroidism	↓	↑*	↑*

* Some patients may have only the FT3 ↑ with a normal FT4.

GOITER

I. Signs and symptoms
   A. The thyroid may be multinodular; it may be very large and compress the trachea.
   B. It is related to inadequate iodine in the diet.
   C. It is often associated with other signs and symptoms of hyperthyroidism.
II. Diagnostic tests
   A. TSH and free T4 may indicate overactive or underactive thyroid function.
   B. Thyroid ultrasound
   C. Consider thyroid radioactive uptake and scan (nuclear scan).
● III. *Referral to endocrinologist*

HYPERTHYROIDISM

I. Definition: excessive amount of thyroid hormone, which can be caused by
   A. Graves' disease – autoimmune disorder. It is more common in women 20 to 60 yr of age.
   B. Toxic multinodular goiter—enlarged thyroid gland (goiter) occurs because of a need (e.g., puberty, iodine deficiency, viral infection); as TSH levels rise, the thyroid enlarges and as the underlying condition resolves and the TSH levels return to normal, the goiter resolves as well. It is more common in older patients.
   C. Can also occur with excessive intake of thyroid hormone medications.
II. Signs and symptoms
   A. Thyroid: firm, smooth, or nodular goiter (up to 50% of patients will not have an enlarged thyroid)
   B. General
      1. Hyperactivity, nervousness
      2. Anxiety, fatigue
      3. Weight loss (unintentional)
      4. Increased perspiration, heat intolerance
      5. Thinning scalp hair
   C. Eyes
      1. Stare and lid lag
      2. May have exophthalmos (with Graves' disease)
   D. Cardiac
      1. Tachycardia or atrial fib; palpitations
      2. Angina, HTN

● = *non–urgent referral*

    E. Neurologic
      1. Fine tremor of hands, tongue, or closed eye lids
      2. Hyperreflexia
      3. Proximal muscle weakness
    F. Genitourinary
      1. Female: amenorrhea or oligomenorrhea
      2. Male: gynecomastia and/or erectile dysfunction
    G. Musculoskeletal: decreased BMD and increased risk of fractures
III. Diagnostic tests
    A. TSH very low
    B. Increased free T4 and free T3
    C. If TSH is low but the free T4 and T3 are normal, consider subclinical hyperthyroidism; obtain thyroid radioactive uptake and scan (nuclear scan)
    D. Obtain thyroid U/S with palpable nodules
IV. Treatment
    A. *If lab results are abnormal, obtain thyroid radioactive uptake and scan (nuclear scan) and referral to endocrinologist;* do not order a scan if the patient is pregnant or breastfeeding.
    B. Atenolol 25 to 100 mg daily can help to control symptoms (while waiting to see an endocrinologist).

HYPOTHYROIDISM

    I. Possible causes (in most patients, it is a permanent condition requiring lifelong therapy)
      A. Autoimmune disease of thyroid
      B. Post thyroidectomy
      C. After treatment for hyperthyroidism (including post radiation to neck)
      D. Medications
    II. Signs and symptoms
      A. General
        1. Weakness, fatigue, lethargy
        2. Cold intolerance
        3. Mild weight gain or difficulty losing weight
        4. Depression; confusion (in elderly patients, this may be the only sign)
      B. Integumentary
        1. Dry skin and/or hair
        2. Hair loss, including loss of the lateral third of eyebrows
        3. May have brittle nails
      C. Cardiac: bradycardia, possible cardiac enlargement
      D. Genitourinary: amenorrhea, menorrhagia, infertility
      E. Gastrointestinal: constipation
      F. Metabolic
        1. Complains of feeling cold easily
        2. Hypercholesterolemia
        3. Elevated CK
        4. Hyponatremia
        5. Macrocytic anemia
      G. Neurological: slow DTRs (e.g., patellar and ankle jerk), slow speech

---

● = *non-urgent referral*

III. Diagnostic tests: elevated TSH and low free T4
   A. If the patient has signs and symptoms but normal lab results, consider depression.
   B. With elevated TSH but normal free T4, consider subclinical hypothyroidism.
      1. With TSH $\geq$ 10 units/L: treat with levothyroxine to normalize TSH and decrease the risk of progression to overt hypothyroidism.
      2. With TSH 4.5 to 10 units/L: routine treatment is controversial; consider levothyroxine with symptoms suggesting hypothyroidism.
IV. Treatment
   A. Levothyroxine (T4) is the medication of choice; it is best to take the same tablet consistently because potency can vary between brands and generics.
      1. Start with 25 to 50 mcg daily and recheck TSH in 2 mo. Increase the dose by 12.5 to 50 mcg daily, q2mo until TSH normalizes (average maintenance dose in adults is approximately 1.6 mcg/kg/d). Then recheck lab (usually just TSH) yearly and prn.
      2. If at any time, the dose becomes too high (the TSH will below), decrease the dose by 12.5 to 50 mcg and recheck TSH q2mo until TSH again normalizes.
   B. Consider brand name Synthroid if unable to correct TSH with generic levothyroxine.
   C. Either medication is most effective when taken on an empty stomach with no other medications; if unable to take on an empty stomach, be consistent with when it is taken.
   D. Some patients may be taking desiccated thyroid USP (e.g., Armour Thyroid), which is a combination of T4 and T3 hormones.
      1. Consider using if patient has not felt well on just T4 since thyroidectomy or radioiodine ablative therapy or who has a low or low normal free T3.
      2. It is not recommended in patients with cardiovascular disease (more prone to arrhythmias), older patients, or pregnant women.
      3. Thyroid USP metabolism may be erratic.
         (a) 60 mg thyroid USP = 100 mcg levothyroxine in potency
         (b) Adjust doses by 15 mg.
   E. Discourage overreplacement with medication, which can cause subclinical or overt hyperthyroidism.

THYROID CANCER

I. Signs and symptoms
   A. Enlarged thyroid or a painless, hard nodule that is progressively enlarging
   B. Palpable lymph nodes, dysphagia, or hoarseness
II. Diagnostic findings
   A. Normal thyroid function tests (TSH and free T4)
   B. Thyroid U/S
   C. Thyroid nuclear scan
      1. *"Hot" nodule: evaluate for hyperthyroidism and referral to an endocrinologist. referral to an endocrinologist*
      2. *"Cold" nodule: obtain a diagnostic thyroid U/S and referral urgently to ENT for FNA. A "cold" nodule is a more serious finding and would be more often seen with thyroid cancer.*

● *= non–urgent referral;* ▲ *= urgent referral*

CHAPTER 16

Pediatric Conditions

For details regarding complete history and physical examination, see Chapter 2.

Generalized Conditions

DEHYDRATION

   I. Definition: fluid loss at a rate greater than it can be replaced

  II. Risk factors for infants and children

     A. Inability to verbalize thirst

     B. Increased frequency of gastroenteritis

     C. Greater fluid loss with fevers and burns, due to higher body surface area (BSA)

 III. Clinical assessment

     A. Evaluate degree of fluid volume loss and severity (see Table 16.1)

     B. Determine cause of fluid loss

        1. Vomiting or diarrhea (or both)

        2. Insensible volume loss (e.g., fevers/burns)

        3. Urine (glucosuria or diabetes insipidus)

 IV. Diagnostic testing

     A. Urinalysis: SG > 1.015 indicates dehydration

     B. Electrolytes (see Chapter 4, **CHEMISTRIES, V** and **VI**)

        1. Hypernatremia (serum Na > 150 mEq/L) from diarrhea

        2. Hyponatremia (serum Na < 130 mEq/L) from vomiting

        3. Hypokalemia from diarrhea

     C. CBC: elevation of WBC without fever can indicate dehydration

   V. Treatment

     A. Rehydrate slowly but consistently with spoon, syringe, or cup, q15–30min (see Table 9.2); *close follow-up for first 24 hr*

     B. Mild dehydration

        1. Rehydrate with 10 mL/kg of appropriate formula or liquids

        2. Replace each fluid loss or give 1–2 tbsp of fluids q15–30min

        3. Avoid whole milk, simple sugars, and fluids and foods high in fat

     C. Moderate dehydration can be managed at home if child and parent are cooperative with aggressive with rehydration.

▲ **VI.** *Transfer to ED if the infant/child*

     A. *Will not or cannot cooperate or tolerate fluids*

     B. *Is lethargic, difficult in arouse or obviously in distress*

     C. *Cannot keep fluids down or has not taken in liquids in > 4 hr*

     D. *Vomits blood or has bloody diarrhea*

     E. *Has not urinated or had wet diapers in 6–8 hr*

▲ = *urgent referral*

TABLE 16.1 ■ Clinical Signs and Treatment of Dehydration in Children

Type of Sign	Mild	Moderate	Severe
Activity/mental status	Normal	Lethargic, irritable, restless	Listlessness to coma state
Color	Normal-pale	Cool, pale-grayish	Mottled and cool extremities, cyanosis
Eyes	Normal, tears present	Diminished or no tear production	Deeply sunken with tears absent
Thirst	Normal to slightly increased	Moderately increased	Very thirsty but may be too lethargic to take liquids
Urine output	Normal to mildly decreased (< 1–2 diapers qd)	Oliguric (1 diaper qd or < 1 mL/kg/h) Specific gravity > 1.030	Anuria Specific gravity > 1.015
Fontanelle	Flat	Slightly depressed	Sunken fontanelle
Mucous membrane	Slightly dry lips with decreased, thickened saliva	Very dry lips and oral mucosa with very little saliva	Cracked lips and dry oral mucosa
Skin turgor and elasticity	Normal to slight decrease	Marked decrease	Tenting
Pulse	Normal to slightly increased	Increased	Tachycardic at rest but may become bradycardic as dehydration worsens
Capillary refill	< 1.5 s	1.5–3 s	> 3 s
Blood pressure	Normal	Normal to slightly decreased	Decreased
Weight loss	5%	10%	15%
Respirations	Normal	Deep and slightly increased	Deep and increased

FAILURE TO THRIVE

I. Description
   A. Children *who fail to gain weight or suddenly slow the growth rate* and fall below the 2nd percentile on growth charts, or drop more than 2 SD on the growth curve without an obvious cause.
   B. This can cause a delay in growth and development (see Table 2.1).
   C. Causes include
      1. Inadequate intake of milk/formula (plant-based milk substitutes lack nutrients needed for growth) or solid foods
      2. Inability to absorb nutrients
      3. Increase in loss of nutrients
      4. Increase in nutrient needs
   D. Suspicion for child neglect
      1. Caregiver does not provide adequate nutrition for physical growth and development
      2. Caregiver preventing access to food
      3. Caregiver failure to prevent overnutrition leading to obesity

II. HPI: inquire about the following
   A. Any physical or genetic abnormalities (e.g., cleft palate, CF, protein allergy, growth hormone deficiency, chronic infections)
   B. Any issues with bonding between the child and/or caregiver
      1. Which primary caregiver is in control of meals and feeding?
      2. Do they understand how to feed the infant?
      3. Can the caregiver provide an adequate diet for age?
      4. Where is the child fed (in family setting, high chair)?
      5. Are there any meal time distractions?
      6. Are there strong likes/dislikes with food and does this cause struggles with meals?
   C. Detailed feeding and dietary history
      1. When did feeding difficulties begin (i.e., from birth, sudden onset later in infancy/childhood) and were they eating well and maintaining weight prior to this?
      2. Is there any spitting up, vomiting, or stooling issues? What are meal times and are they regular; are there any special dietary considerations?
      3. Can the infant get through a feeding without tiring?
      4. If breastfed: how often, how long, suck strength; is sucking stimulating milk let-down?
      5. If formula fed: how much formula/day, how is formula prepared, is anything added to formula, does caregiver hold bottle or prop it up?
      6. What sort of sugar products are offered, either at or before meal times?
      7. Has there been any stress in the household or any noticeable reason for any decrease in appetite?
   D. Is there any financial difficulty in obtaining foods, especially if the child is on a special or restricted diet?
III. Signs and symptoms (other than small body size and slow growth rate)
   A. Irritability at meal times or when food is offered
   B. GERD after meals, still appears hungry after eating; increased gas
   C. Disinterest in surroundings; avoidance of eye contact or poor interaction/socialization with caregivers/peers
IV. Physical exam
   A. Observe overall appearance of child and caregiver and interaction with caregiver
      1. Does the infant/child have a wasting appearance and little body fat deposition?
      2. Does the caregiver appear nurturing toward the infant/child?
   B. HEENT
      1. Abnormal shape of head (e.g., microcephaly or macrocephaly)
      2. Fontanelles (may have delayed closure due to thyroid dysfunction or vitamin D deficiency)
      3. Eyes
         (a) Cataracts (infection); papilledema (increased ICP)
         (b) Shortened palpebral fissures (fetal alcohol syndrome)
      4. Oropharynx
         (a) Hard or soft palate deformity(s)
         (b) Stomatitis (vitamin deficiency or Crohn's disease); cheilosis (vitamin B2, B6, B3 deficiency)
         (c) Delayed tooth eruption (could indicate delayed bone growth) or numerous cavities
         (d) Tongue deformity
         (e) Drooling (oral-motor disorder)
      5. Neck: thyroid enlargement with tachycardia/tachypnea or thyroid insufficiency with bradycardia/hypotension

C. Chest
1. Heart murmurs (congenital heart deformity)
2. Crackles, lung hyperexpansion (asthma, CF)
D. Abdomen/GU
1. Distention, hyperactive bowel sounds (malabsorption)
2. Enlarged liver/spleen (liver disease, cancer, glycogen storage)
3. Delayed development of penis/testicles (see Chapter 2, GENITOURINARY SYSTEM; and Box 2.1)
4. Rectal fissures/fistulae
5. Diarrhea (infection, malabsorption, lactose deficiency)
6. Vomiting (GERD, obstruction)
E. Neurological
1. DTRs (abnormal due to CP)
2. Hypotonia, spasticity (may indicate oral-motor disorders)
3. Poor suck reflex (oral-motor disorders, neurological disorders)
F. Musculoskeletal
1. Clubbing of fingers/toes (hypoxia from heart/lung disorders)
2. Edema from protein deficiency(s)
G. Skin
1. Excessive scaling skin (possible zinc deficiency)
2. Candidiasis (immune deficiency of some type)
3. Untreated excessive diaper rash (possible neglect); bruising in low impact areas (possible abuse)
4. Pallor (may indicate anemia)
V. Diagnostic testing
A. CBC (anemia or other blood disorders); CRP and ESR (inflammatory conditions or malignancy)
B. Urinalysis (glucosuria, protein or carbohydrate loss), urine culture (chronic infections)
C. CXR to evaluate heart/lung appearance
D. Stool cultures (if any diarrhea) for blood and O&P
E. Sweat test (if concerns for CF)
VI. Treatment
A. Speech therapy consultation for swallowing dysfunction
B. Dietician consultation
C. Closely monitor weekly weights.
D. For toddlers, encourage more *high-calorie frequent feedings* and more *high-protein snacks in between meals.*
1. Add infant formula powder to breast milk; can add rice cereal to formula.
2. Offer solid foods before offering drinks for meals.
3. Add high-calorie snack foods such as rice, cheese, puddings, or dried fruits; no high sugar drinks or snacks (e.g., Kool-aid, candy, or cookies).
4. No snacks 1 hr before meals
5. Add multivitamin (if age appropriate).
E. It's alright for the child to eat the same foods every day; *it's the calories that count.*
F. Do not fight with child over foods. Praise for eating well, and do not punish if child does not eat well.
● **VII. *Referral to a pediatrician if unable to gain weight or developmentally delayed***

_____

● *= non-urgent referral*

FEVER

I. Description
- A. Fever is any body temperature $\geq 38.3°C$ ($101°F$)
  - 1. Fever should be evaluated if
    - (a) Occurs at least once a day and persists > 8 days
    - (b) Sudden elevation in temperature > $38.9°C$ ($102°F$) that is difficult to control
    - (c) Development of new localized symptoms related to fever
    - (d) Persistent fever in the presence of underlying medical problems (e.g., heart disease, lung disease, immunocompromised)
  - 2. Child with a *simple febrile seizure* lasting < 15 min with no recurrence in 24 hr
    - (a) A febrile seizure does not mean that the child has a seizure disorder.
    - (b) Most common between the ages of 6 mo of age and 5 yr of age
    - (c) May occur with sustained elevated temperature (e.g., $\geq 39.4°C$ [$103°F$]), after immunizations, or with viral illnesses
    - (d) A thorough history and physical and neurological exam should be performed to determine need for further follow-up.
    - (e) ***All infants and children should be evaluated by neurologist if***
      - (i) ***The seizure lasts > 15 min or recurs within 24 hr***
      - (ii) ***The patient does not return to baseline activity within 30 min***
      - (iii) ***With any change in mental status***
II. Causes of fevers
- A. Bacterial infections (e.g., UTI, pneumonia, strep throat, otitis media)
- B. Infections related to animal or tick exposure (e.g., cat scratch, brucellosis, RMSF)
- C. Viral infection (e.g., COVID, flu, Kawasaki)
- D. Teething
- E. May see low-grade fever after immunizations (usually < $38.9°C$ [$102°F$]) especially if multiple immunizations given at once
- F. Cancer (e.g., blood or lymph most common) or hyperthyroidism
III. HPI
- A. How was the temperature taken? When did the fever start (e.g., hours or days ago)?
- B. How long does fever last with or without treatment? Does fever respond to treatment and what treatment has been used?
- C. Is the fever associated with any other symptoms (e.g., skin rash, N/V, H/A)?
- D. Is there a pattern to the fever? How does the fever effect the child's behaviors?
- E. Are there any other children or adults experiencing similar symptom?
- F. Any weight loss (DM, cancer), change in gait or mobility (osteomyelitis, idiopathic arthritis), urinary frequency (UTI), N/V/D (viral, bacterial)?
- G. Any recent known or possible animal (cat scratch disease)/tick (RMSF)/mosquito exposures (West Nile virus)?
- H. What medications does the child take and have there been any changes in medications?
IV. Physical examination
- A. Overall appearance
  - 1. Active, ill appearing, interactive or withdrawn
  - 2. Temperature (exam more pertinent if child currently has a fever), pulse rate (tachycardia is normal with fevers; bradycardia may indicate more severe disease)
  - 3. Evaluate growth chart and weight for any losses (could be related to cancers, IBD)
- B. HEENT, evaluate for

= non–urgent referral; ■ *= not to be missed*

1. Eyes/ears
   (a) Conjunctivitis (Kawasaki disease) or conjunctival hemorrhage (endocarditis)
   (b) Ear pulling (otitis media)
2. Sinus tenderness (rhinosinusitis)
3. Mouth
   (a) Ulcers (usually viral)
   (b) Tonsillar swelling with exudate (strep pharyngitis, mononucleosis)
   (c) Evaluate teeth for abscess(s), pain with "tapping"; gingival swelling and redness

C. Chest for crackles (pneumonia), murmurs (infective endocarditis), or rub (pericarditis)
D. Abdomen: palpate for pain and/or enlarged liver (e.g., hepatitis) or spleen (e.g., cat scratch disease)
E. Musculoskeletal system for injuries over bony areas or bone tenderness, joint swelling, or effusion; DTRs will be overactive with hyperthyroidism
F. GU
   1. Females: external genitalia looking for ulcers, vaginal discharge or trauma; consider pelvic exam on sexually active or abused females (consider PID with + CMT); examine rectal area for abscess/fissures
   2. Males: testicular tenderness, swelling or pain; unusual lesions or ulcers on penis; urethral discharge; examine rectal area for abscess/fissures
G. Lymph node: swelling, pain (or lack of), and location (e.g., neck, axillary, and inguinal)

V. Diagnostic testing
A. CBC
   1. Elevated WBCs with increased neutrophils: bacterial infection
   2. Decreased WBCs with increased lymphocytes: viral infection, pertussis
   3. Greatly elevated WBCs with lymphadenopathy: suspect leukemia or lymphoma
B. Elevated ESR and CRP indicates inflammatory process (if elevated with negative RF, ANA: suspect malignancy)
C. Urinalysis positive for leukocyte esterase, nitrite, and bacteria: obtain urine culture and consider urinary infection
D. Influenza, COVID-19, rapid strep
E. CXR (e.g., TB, pneumonia)

VI. Treatment
A. Nonpharmacological treatment
   1. Fever < 39°C (102.2°F) should only be treated if the child is uncomfortable or could become dehydrated; do not give antipyretics, keep child quiet and resting.
   2. Keep the child well hydrated (see Table 9.2 for oral rehydration solution) and monitor for dehydration (Table 16.1).
   3. Keep the environment comfortable and do not "bundle up" the infant or child; remove any excess clothing and use a lightweight sheet to cover the child.
   4. Tepid sponge water bath with both the parent and the child sitting in tub (caution the parent *not* to leave the infant or child alone in the bath; do not put alcohol in water).
B. Pharmacological treatment
   1. *Identify and manage the cause of fever.*
   2. Give antipyretics to make the child more comfortable.
      (a) If fever is not under control with one product in 4–6 hr, consider switching to another product; keep track of doses of medication to *prevent overdosing.*
      (b) DO NOT give acetaminophen and ibuprofen at the same time and caution if alternating doses; *this increases the chances of overdosing the child* and benefit of lowering fever is negligible.

   (c) Acetaminophen weight-based dosing (see Appendix C)
    (i) Infants > 3 mo of age to children < 12 yr of age: 10–15 mg/kg/*dose* q4–6h prn; do not exceed *75 mg/kg/day*
    (ii) Children ≥ 12 yr of age: 350–650 mg q4–6h; do not exceed *75 mg/kg/day*
   (d) Ibuprofen weight-directed dosing (see Appendix D)
    (i) Infants ≥ 6 mo of age to children < 12 yr of age: 5–10 mg/kg/*dose* every 6–8 hr prn; do not exceed *40 mg/kg/day*
    (ii) Children ≥ 12 yr of age: 200–400 mg q4–6h as needed; do not exceed *40 mg/kg/day*
   (e) Aspirin is not the drug of choice because of association with Reye syndrome, bleeding disorders, and hypersensitivity.
   (f) Give antipyretics for shortest amount of time; if fever is still present after 3–5 days, speak with medical provider.
  3. Antipyretic medication precautions
   (a) Acetaminophen
    (i) Monitor liver function if the child is taking barbiturates, carbamazepine, isoniazid, rifampin, or sulfinpyrazone.
    (ii) Some acetaminophen preparations contain aspartame; infants and children with phenylketonuria should not take these preparations.
   (b) Ibuprofen should be given with food and monitor for gastritis.

▲ C. *Urgent referral to ED*
  1. *Infants < 3 mo of age*
  2. *Fever > 40°C (104°F) and unable to lower fever*
  3. *The child appears ill, drowsy, dehydrated, nonresponsive, or has a seizure (see I. A. 2 above on febrile seizures)*

Upper Respiratory Tract Conditions

ALLERGIC RHINITIS

 I. Description: allergic response to substances that have been inhaled; can be seasonal or perennial; most common offenders are pollens, grasses, trees, and animal dander
  A. Less common in children under 2 yr of age
  B. If < 2 yr of age and symptom persist, consider cause being repeated viral infections (usually seen in children with multiple exposures from daycare).
  C. More common in children who are older and have had repeated exposure to outdoor/indoor allergens
 II. Signs and symptoms
  A. Red, itchy, and watery eyes; occasional periorbital swelling; dark circles under eyes ("allergic shiners")
  B. Stuffy, runny nose (clear rhinorrhea), sneezing, H/A
  C. Blue to pink boggy nasal turbinates with white exudate
  D. Allergic "salute," and persistent "gaping mouth"
  E. Mouth breathing and snoring; dry cough
  F. Sore throat with lymphoid hyperplasia of the posterior pharynx

▲ = *urgent referral*

III. Diagnostic testing: nasal swabs or CBC for eosinophils
IV. Treatment: involves distancing from the allergen when possible *plus*
  A. Nonpharmacological treatment
    1. Air purifiers and dust filters
    2. Air conditioner in house, especially where sleeping, keep windows closed
    3. Remove pets from house or at least from sleeping areas.
  B. Pharmacological treatment
    1. Second-generation oral antihistamine: one of the following either daily or prn
      (a) Cetirizine (Zyrtec)
        (i) > 2–5 yr of age: 2–5 mg
        (ii) ≥ 6 yr of age: 10 mg
      (b) Desloratadine (Clarinex)
        (i) 6–11 yr of age: 2.5 mg
        (ii) > 12 yr of age: 5 mg
      (c) Fexofenadine (Allegra)
        (i) 2–11 yr of age: 30 mg *bid*
        (ii) ≥ 12 yr of age: 60 mg *bid*
      (d) Levocetirizine (Xyzal)
        (i) 6–11 yr of age: 2.5 mg
        (ii) ≥ 12 yr of age: 5 mg
      (e) Loratadine (Claritin)
        (i) > 2 yr of age: 5 mg
        (ii) ≥ 6 yr of age 10 mg
    2. Intranasal steroids (use in each nostril)
      (a) Beclomethasone (Beconase AQ) 6–12 yr of age: 1–2 sprays bid
      (b) Budesonide nasal (Rhinocort Allergy Spray OTC) > 6 yr of age: 1–2 sprays daily
      (c) Ciclesonide (Omnaris) > 6 yr of age: 1–2 sprays daily
      (d) Fluticasone (Flonase Sensimist OTC)
        (i) 2–11 yr of age: 1 spray daily
        (ii) ≥ 12 yr of age: 1–2 sprays daily
      (e) Mometasone furoate (Nasonex)
        (i) 2–11 yr of age: 1 spray daily
        (ii) ≥ 12 yr of age: 2 sprays daily
      (f) Triamcinolone nasal (Nasacort Allergy OTC)
        (i) > 2–5 yr of age: 1 spray daily
        (ii) ≥ 6 yr of age: 1–2 sprays daily
    3. Intranasal antihistamine
      (a) Azelastine nasal
        (i) 5–11 yr of age: 1 spray bid
        (ii) > 12 yr of age: 1–2 sprays bid
      (b) Azelastine/fluticasone (Dymista) > 6 yr of age: 1 spray bid
      (c) Ipratropium bromide (Atrovent Nasal) ≥ 5 yr of age: 2 sprays qid; may use for up to 14 days
      (d) Olopatadine (Patanase)
        (i) 6–11 yr of age: 1 spray bid
        (ii) > 12 yr of age: 2 sprays bid
    4. Ophthalmic mast cell stabilizers for itching eyes related to allergies
      (a) Cetirizine (Zerviate) ≥ 2 yr of age: 1 gtt in eye(s) bid
      (b) Epinastine (generic) ≥ 2 yr of age: 1 gtt in eye(s) bid

       (c) Ketotifen: (Zaditor OTC) > 3 yr of age: 1 gtt in eye(s) q12h

       (d) Olopatadine ophthalmic (Pataday Once Daily Relief OTC) ≥ 2 yr of age: 1 gtt in eye(s) daily

    5. Leukotriene antagonist: Montelukast (Singulair)

       (a) 12–23 mo of age: 4 mg granule pkt q hs

       (b) 2–5 yr of age: 4 mg chewable q hs

       (c) 6–14 yr of age: 5 mg tab q hs; ≥ 15 yr of age: 10 mg hs

    6. Cromolyn sodium (OTC), in any age child: 1 spray each nostril 3–4 times a day (onset takes ~ 2–4 wk, so start ideally at least 1 mo before known exposure); it is not a steroid and has no systemic uptake or effects.

  C. Follow-up

    1. Monitor for hearing decrease or loss with long-term chronic allergic rhinitis.

    2. Nosebleeds may be caused by lack of humidity in the environment or chronic use of nasal steroids.

    3. If symptoms are severe and unrelieved with conventional treatment and child is > 16 yr of age, may consider annual IM steroid injection at the lowest effective dose.

    4. Evaluate the environment for dust and mold, do not let pets sleep with the child, remove carpets, use allergen-proof pillow covers, and wash bed linens weekly.

  V. *Referral to allergist if symptoms become unmanageable, especially if child < 2 yr of age*

BACTERIAL SINUSITIS, ACUTE

  I. Description: a *secondary* bacterial infection occurring in one or more of the paranasal sinuses; usually occurs after viral illness and can be a common problem in children as sinus cavities mature.

  II. Signs and symptoms persist without improvement for more than 10 days or initial symptoms improve but then worsen ("double sickening").

    A. Cough (can be productive or dry) and usually worsens at night

    B. Nasal congestion with discharge which can be serous, mucoid, or purulent

    C. Fever < 39°C (102.2°F) is usually present at beginning of illness and then resolves within a few days, it may recur or worsen again in 7 days at a higher temperature.

    D. H/A and facial pain (for older children)

    E. Sore throat and may have halitosis

    F. Purulent PND noted and may be associated with vomiting.

  III. Treatment for symptom control

    A. Normal saline nasal spray/irrigation frequently (e.g., 8–10 times daily) (see Chapter 6, PRACTICE PEARLS FOR ENT)

    B. Analgesics prn for pain: acetaminophen or ibuprofen (see Appendices C and D)

    C. Humidifier in the room and warm steamy showers 2–3 times daily

    D. Antibiotic treatment for *mild consistent* symptoms is 10 days

      1. Amoxicillin/clavulanate (Augmentin) 45–90 mg/kg/day ÷ q12h depending on child's risk factors (consider higher dose if immunocompromised or with recent antibiotic use)

      2. Ceftriaxone (Rocephin) 50 mg/kg IM daily up to 3 days (especially if child is vomiting), then can start/resume oral medications

      3. Cefpodoxime (generic) > 2 mo to 12 yr of age: 10 mg/kg/day ÷ q12h

      4. Cefdinir (Omnicef) > 6 mo of age: 14 mg/kg/day ÷ q12h or q24h

---

● = *non-urgent referral*

   E. Treatment failure is considered to be no improvement or worsening of symptoms within 72 hr of treatment
      1. Consider switching to different classification (see above antibiotics for dosing) of antibiotic, pathogen may be resistant to current regimen
         (a) Amoxicillin/clavulanate (Augmentin) 90 mg/kg/day ÷ q12h
         (b) Cefpodoxime (generic) > 2 mo of age: 10 mg/kg/day ÷ q12h
         (c) Cefdinir (Omnicef) > 6 mo of age: 14 mg/kg/day ÷ q12h
      2. Consider other causes of symptoms (FO in nose, structural abnormality, immunocompromised state)
   F. Follow up in 3–5 days after initial therapy and/or any change in treatment plan
IV. *Referral*
   A. *ENT if symptoms not improving*
   B. *Urgent transfer to ED*
      1. *Redness and swelling of eyelids and periorbital area and no proptosis or pain with EOM: consider periorbital cellulitis*
      2. *Pain with eye movement, conjunctival swelling, periorbital swelling, and erythema with H/A: consider orbital cellulitis*
      3. *Fever, H/A, nuchal rigidity, confusion/lethargy: consider meningitis*
      4. *Headache, fever, and change in the mental status, drowsiness, muscle weakness: consider brain abscess*

INFLUENZA

I. Description
   A. Highly contagious viral illness that has rapid onset; incubation is about 1–2 days.
   B. Easily spreads through schools and daycares, especially if individuals are not immunized and do not practice good hand and facial hygiene.
   C. Spread by droplets from normal respiratory activity, coughing, sneezing, and hand contact with the infected individual or inanimate objects.
II. Signs and symptoms
   A. *Sudden* high fever (can be > 39°C [102.2°F])
   B. *Cough*, sore throat, watery runny nose
   C. *Myalgia*, facial pain, and H/A; occasionally N/V/D
   D. Children may become dehydrated, have tachypnea, tachycardia.
   E. Numerous complications are associated with influenza.
      1. Otitis media
      2. Respiratory infections (viral pneumonia, croup)
      3. Secondary bacterial infections (bacterial pneumonia, orbital cellulitis, peritonsillar abscess)
III. Diagnostic testing: nasal swab for flu A & B
IV. Pharmacological treatment; best if started within 48 hr of symptoms; not approved for COVID-19
   A. Acetaminophen or ibuprofen prn for fever (see Appendices C and D)
   B. Oseltamivir (Tamiflu) 1–12 yr of age: *bid* for 5 days
      1. ≤ 15 kg: 30 mg
      2. 15–23 kg: 45 mg
      3. 23–40 kg: 60 mg
      4. > 40 kg: 75 mg

▨ = *not to be missed;* ● = *non-urgent referral;* ▲ = *urgent referral*

    C. Zanamivir: (Relenza) > 7 yr of age: 10 mg two inhalations *bid* for 5 days; patients; not recommended for asthma patients

    D. Baloxavir: (Xofluza) *single dose,* ≥ 12 yr of age

       1. < 80 kg: 40 mg

       2. ≥ 80 kg: 80 mg

V. Prophylactic treatment for 10–14 days or longer

    A. Oseltamivir: (Tamiflu) > 13 yr of age: 75 mg *once daily*

    B. Zanamivir: (Relenza) ≥ 5 yr of age: 10 mg two inhalations *once daily* for 10 days or up to 28 days if community outbreak

    C. Baloxavir: (Xofluza) single dose, ≥ 12 yr of age

       1. < 80 kg: 40 mg

       2. ≥ 80 kg: 80 mg

MONONUCLEOSIS

    I. Cause: Epstein-Barr virus (EBV) infection contracted through contact with oral or nasal secretions; most common in adolescents and young adults; 4–7 wk incubation period; usually self-limiting

  II. Signs and symptoms

    A. Gradual onset of low-grade fever, chills, malaise, and fatigue (which may persist up to 4 mo)

    B. Followed by recurring fever (up to 38.9°C [102°F]); primarily posterior cervical lymphadenopathy (can also be in the anterior cervical, inguinal, and axillary nodes)

    C. Sore throat with difficulty swallowing; tonsils are enlarged with grayish-white exudates; palatal enanthem

    D. H/A, nausea, petechial rash

    E. Abdominal pain, possible splenomegaly with increased risk for splenic rupture, hepatomegaly

 III. Diagnostic testing

    A. Monospot (may not be positive during the first 10 days of symptoms)

    B. CBC (may show decreased platelets and increased lymphocytes)

    C. AST/ALT (may be elevated)

    D. Consider abdominal U/S to evaluate for hepatosplenomegaly or if symptoms not resolving

 IV. Nonpharmacological treatment is primarily supportive

    A. Bed rest, antipyretics (acetaminophen), and analgesics (NSAIDs) for fever and discomfort (see Appendices C and D)

    B. Good hand hygiene, avoid sharing drinking or eating utensils or toothbrushes

    C. Hard candy or throat lozenges and saltwater gargles

    D. Encourage hydration (see Table 9.2)

  V. Pharmacological treatment

    A. May consider mouth rinse ("magic mouthwash") to decrease pain and help improve oral intake (see Chapter 6, PRACTICE PEARLS FOR ENT).

    B. If the tonsils and pharynx are *severely* swollen and the possibility of a compromised airway is present, consider oral prednisone: start with 30–50 mg daily and taper over 10–14 days, based on age.

    C. Antibiotics are not recommended and may cause a maculopapular rash if given without a bacterial cause (especially ampicillin and amoxicillin).

    D. Test for strep pharyngitis if symptoms are worsening or not improving in 3 days.

VI. Return to activity
   A. Return to school when afebrile and other symptoms resolved.
   B. No strenuous activities, contact sports or heavy lifting for minimum of 4 wk.
   C. Return to activity should be gradual and full performance may be delayed up to
      > 3 mo due to lingering fatigue.
   D. Follow up in office prior to resuming activities to make sure spleen has returned to
      normal.
   E. If splenomegaly is noted, consider U/S prior to return to sports or heavy lifting.
▲ VII. *Referral to ED with any symptoms of airway obstruction or dehydration*

OTITIS EXTERNA (SWIMMER'S EAR)

   I. Description: inflammation of the EAC or auricle with redness, pain, and discharge
  II. Causes
   A. Increased moisture (which disrupts normal flora of the canal) due to swimming in
      fresh or chlorinated water
   B. Chronic use of ear plugs or hearing aids
   C. Traumatic removal of packed cerumen to the canal
 III. Signs and symptoms
   A. Ear pain, feeling of fullness
   B. Localized tenderness to external ear especially with movement of ear or jaw
   C. May have discharge from ear that is yellowish/green and odorous
   D. Itching without pain to ear (may indicate fungal infection)
  IV. Physical exam
   A. *Physical exam of the affected ear(s) is usually painful.*
   B. Ear canal is visibly swollen, red with exudate at opening; tenderness with pressing
      against the tragus (cardinal sign) or pulling the pinna up.
   C. If visualized, TM may be red but without fluid behind the TM.
   V. Diagnostics: need for *good* visualization of TM, *provider* should remove debris in canal if
      at all possible
   A. Removal of ear canal debris will enhance topical medication absorption.
   B. Debris can be removed with either gentle suction, curette, or Q-tip through otoscope.
   C. Can place an ear wick in canal to try to remove thin secretions initially and then place
      new wick in canal for topical medications.
   D. *Do not flush the canal unless TM is visualized* (in case of perforation).
  VI. Treatment with *intact TM*
   A. Mild infection with some discomfort, pruritus, and minimal edema; hearing de-
      creased and no fever
      1. Use acetic acid (plain) or hydrocortisone/acetic acid otic > 3 yr of age: 3–5 gtts
         q4–6h with ear wick for 24 hr and then q6–8h for 5–7 days
      2. No water exposure until healed; if water exposure unavoidable, use cotton ball
         saturated with petroleum jelly inserted into ear canal during exposure; follow pre-
         ventive plan (see D., below)
      3. Pain relief prn with acetaminophen 10–15 mg/kg tid or ibuprofen 10 mg/kg tid
      4. Follow up in 7 days, unless resolved
   B. Moderate infection with increased pain, partial occlusion of canal, and pain with
      movement of pinna/tragus; decreased hearing and itching

---

▲ = *urgent referral;* ■ = *not to be missed*

    1. Treat with topical antibiotic/steroid drops for 7 days

      (a) Ciprofloxacin/hydrocortisone (CiproHC) otic, > 1 yr of age: 3 gtts q12h *(use with intact TM)*

      (b) Neomycin/polymyxin B/hydrocortisone (Cortisporin) otic, > 2 yr of age: 3 gtts 3–4 times daily for *10 days (use with intact TM)*

      (c) Ofloxacin (Floxin) otic

        (i) > 6 mo of age: 5 gtts daily *(can use if suspect perforated TM)*

        (ii) ≥ 13 yr of age: 10 gtts daily

      (d) Ciprofloxacin/dexamethasone (Ciprodex) otic, > 6 mo of age: 4 gtts bid *(use with intact TM)*

    2. No water exposure until healed; if water exposure unavoidable, use cotton ball saturated with petroleum jelly inserted into ear canal during exposure; follow preventive plan (see D, below)

    3. Pain relief prn with acetaminophen or ibuprofen (see Appendices C and D)

    4. Follow up in 2–5 days, depending on symptoms

  C. Severe infection with intense pain with complete canal occlusion, fever, lymphadenopathy, and severe pain with any movement of pinna/tragus

    1. Treat with topical antibiotics/steroids (see B, 1, above), ear wick placement, and oral antibiotics if needed (see **OTITIS MEDIA, I.** F, 5) for 7 days

    2. *Follow up in office in 24 hr*

    3. No water exposure until healed; if water exposure unavoidable, use cotton ball saturated with petroleum jelly inserted into *ear canal* during exposure; follow preventive plan (see D, below)

    4. Pain relief prn with acetaminophen or ibuprofen (see Appendices C and D)

  D. Prevention

    1. If involved in water sports, use earplugs, shake water from ears, or use blow dryer on lowest setting to ears after water exposure (safe distance is considered about 12 inches from ear).

    2. After each water exposure, instill a few drops of one of the following in both ears:

      (a) Mix rubbing alcohol and vinegar in 1:1 ratio

      (b) Acetic acid otic if > 3 yr of age: 3–5 gtts after each water exposure

    3. Hearing aids (if used) should be removed each night and cleaned according to the manufacturer's directions.

    4. Discourage cleaning ears with "anything smaller than the elbow."

▲ **VII.** *Emergent referral to ED if not improving in 24–48 hr or infection is spreading to surrounding skin*

OTITIS MEDIA (OM)

  I. Acute otitis (AOM)

    A. Description: inflammation or infection of the middle ear with purulent effusion

    B. Causes

      1. Bacterial/viral

        (a) *Streptococcus pneumoniae, Haemophilus influenzae, Moraxella catarrhalis*

        (b) RSV, adenovirus, influenza

      2. Environmental

        (a) Exposure to other sick children (i.e., daycare, school, or siblings)

▲ = *urgent referral*

        (b) Passive exposure to smoke
        (c) Sleeping with a bottle

C. Signs and symptoms
   1. *Nonsevere* illness
        (a) Mild otalgia
        (b) Fever < 39°C (< 102.2°F) in the past 24 hr
        (c) Preverbal child may pull at ears or hair near the ear to signify pain.
        (d) Decreased appetite, fussiness, and possibly V/D
        (e) May have H/A, sinus congestion, and runny nose
   2. *Severe* illness
        (a) Moderate-to-severe otalgia with otorrhea (if TM has perforated)
        (b) Fever ≥ 39°C (≥ 102.2°F) in the past 24 hr
        (c) Child may cry inconsolably; pull or rub at ear
        (d) Hearing loss or decrease in hearing
   3. Examination of TM
        (a) Moderate to severe bulging from fluid (indicates inflammation and effusion and is the hallmark sign of AOM)
        (b) TM color can vary from white to yellow (usually indicates purulence) or reddish brown to hemorrhagic (usually indicates inflammation) or gray to blue (can indicate OME)
        (c) Impaired mobility (with insufflation) and possible perforation (especially if drainage present)
        (d) Bullae may be present.

D. Diagnostic testing: otoscopy to visualize TM and/or pneumatic otoscopy or tympanometer for TM mobility

E. Diagnosis can be made if the patient has
   1. Bulging of TM and/or perforation with purulent discharge
   2. Marked redness of TM
   3. Middle ear effusion (MEE)
   4. Fever and ear pain

F. Treatment
   1. Consider conservative treatment with pain management if patient < 2 yr of age and
        (a) Has mild symptoms; does not appear ill and has been healthy prior to illness
        (b) Has no otorrhea and TM is intact
        (c) Any fever is < 38.9°C (< 102°F)
   2. Pain control with acetaminophen or ibuprofen (see Appendices C and D).
   3. Closely follow up with the parent to monitor pain and overall symptoms; if no improvement in 48–72 hr, start antibiotics (typically AOM will resolve or improve within 24–48 hr).
   4. Antibiotics can be used in patients
        (a) < 6 mo of age
        (b) 6 mo to 2 yr of age with unilateral/bilateral AOM and mild symptoms
        (c) ≥ 2 yr of age
           (i) If patient appears ill, with unilateral or bilateral AOM
           (ii) Fever ≥ 39°C (≥ 102.2°F) with severe otalgia and/or otorrhea for > 48 hr
   5. Antibiotic treatment
        (a) *First-line* treatment if no hx of recurrent AOM, *no* antibiotics within last 30 days, and and/no purulent conjunctivitis: amoxicillin 90 mg/kg/day ÷ bid
           (i) ≥ 2 yr of age: give for 5–7 days
           (ii) < 2 yr of age: give 10 days

      (b) *Second-line* treatment if there is hx of recurrent AOM, has had antibiotics within the last 30 days, with perforated TM and/or purulent conjunctivitis, and no PCN allergy: amoxicillin/clavulanate 90 mg/kg/day ÷ bid for 10 days

      (c) *Alternative to PCN antibiotics* (can be used with treatment failure or allergy); give the oral medications for 5–10 days

         (i) Cefdinir (Omnicef) 14 mg/kg/day ÷ bid *or*

        (ii) Cefpodoxime (Vantin) 10 mg/kg/day ÷ bid *or*

       (iii) Cefuroxime suspension (Ceftin) 30 mg/kg/day ÷ bid *or*

       (iv) Ceftriaxone (Rocephin) 50 mg/kg IM daily for 1–3 days ; max dose 1 gm/day

      (d) Alternatives for patients *allergic to both PCN and cephalosporins* or with treatment failures

         (i) Azithromycin (Zmax) 10 mg/kg on day 1 and 5 mg/kg days 2–5 *or*

        (ii) Clarithromycin (Biaxin) 15 mg/kg/day ÷ bid for 10 days *or*

       (iii) Clindamycin (Cleocin) 20–30 mg/kg/day ÷ tid for 5–10 days

  G. Follow-up

     1. In 48–72 hr, if symptoms have not improved, consider treatment failure and switch antibiotics and continue for 10 days

     2. In 8–12 wk after treatment to reassess TM and hearing

  H. ***Referral to pediatric ENT specialist if unresolved and/or <2 mo of age and noted decreased hearing***

II. AOM complicated by perforated TM

  A. Usually heals within 4–6 wk

  B. Initiate oral antibiotic treatment with perforation and hx of recurrent AOM; *give for 10 days.*

     1. Amoxicillin 90 mg/kg/day ÷ bid *or*

     2. Amoxicillin/clavulanate (Augmentin) 90 mg/kg/day ÷ bid

     3. Can use alternative antibiotic if allergy present to PCN (see AOM, above).

     4. Topical antibiotic drops *are not recommended* for perforation unless there are tympanostomy tubes (TT) present (see III, A, below).

     5. *Do not use analgesic ear drops with TT or with perforation.*

  C. Keep all water out of the ear until TM heals, using a cotton ball saturated with petrolatum before hair washing; no swimming or other water exposure until healed; do not use ear plugs and parent should refrain from cleaning ear canal with a Q-tip.

  D. Follow up in office in 8–12 wk.

  E. ***Referral to an audiologist or ENT with any concern about hearing loss or recurrent perforation.***

III. AOM with tympanostomy tubes (TT)

  A. Treatment: provider may need to clean debris out of ear(s) and place ear wick(s)

     1. Ciprofloxacin/dexamethasone otic (Ciprodex), > 6 mo of age: 4 gtts q12h for 5–7 days

     2. Ofloxacin otic (Floxin), > 1–12 yr of age: 5 gtts q12h for 10 days

     3. Ciprofloxacin/fluocinolone (Otovel), > 6 mo of age: 5 gtts q12h for 7 days

     4. No water exposure while under treatment; use a cotton ball saturated with petrolatum and gently insert into the outer auricular opening while showering/hair washing.

     5. *Do not use analgesic ear drops with TT.*

     6. Can use acetaminophen or ibuprofen for discomfort (see Appendices C and D).

     7. Follow up in 1 wk; if drainage is still present, start oral antibiotic (see AOM Treatment, above); follow up again in 2 wk or sooner if not resolving.

  B. ***Referral to ENT for persistent AOM with TT that does not respond to treatment***

● = *non-urgent referral*

IV. Otitis media with effusion (OME)

    A. Description: middle ear effusion *without acute signs of infection,* usually occurring after AOM as an inflammatory response or with eustachian tube dysfunction; usually resolves without treatment in < 3 mo

    B. Signs and symptoms

        1. Decreased hearing, hearing loss, and fullness or pain in ears

        2. Speech and language delays and poor school performance

        3. Tinnitus and problems with balance (e.g., falling, stumbling)

        4. Opaque and retracted TM with limited mobility

        5. Observable air-fluid levels

    C. Diagnostic testing

        1. Usually tympanometry and pneumatic otoscopy to follow improvement

        2. Hearing testing for initial diagnosis, especially if high risk for delay in speech development

    D. Treatment

        1. Reevaluate with persistent otitis media with effusion (OME) (with low-risk children) q3mo or until effusion resolves.

        2. Avoid exposure to smoking.

        3. Maintain immunizations, especially pneumococcal vaccine, in children > 2 yr of age.

        4. Antibiotics, steroids, antihistamines, or decongestants and autoinflation have not been shown to improve outcomes; intranasal steroids may be used if there is an allergic rhinitis component.

    E. *Referral to ENT*

        1. *Structural damage to TM*

        2. *If there is > 40 dB hearing loss*

        3. *Hearing loss of 21–39 dB if < 3 yr of age or with speech delay*

PHARYNGITIS

  I. *Bacterial* signs and symptoms

    A. Moderately ill-appearing patient with a complaint of abrupt-onset H/A and sore throat

    B. Tonsillar exudate

    C. Tender anterior cervical lymphadenopathy

    D. Fever

    E. Absence of *viral* symptoms

        1. Mildly to moderately ill; low-grade fever

        2. Conjunctivitis, coryza, and cough; hoarseness

        3. Preauricular lymphadenopathy

    F. Sore throat, mouth or lip ulcers, diarrhea

    G. May have scarlatina rash: a blanchable red rash, with a *fine sandpaper feel,* on the face and torso

    H. Often has a petechial appearance on the soft palate with inflamed uvula; a bright red tongue with white coating (strawberry tongue)

    I. May have abdominal pain, N/V

  II. Diagnostic testing

= non-urgent referral

    A. Rapid strep test; consider throat culture for all patients < 16 yr of age.

    B. Consider CBC; if negative leukocytosis, consider monospot test (if symptoms have been present at least 10 days).

III. Treatment considerations for bacterial causes

    A. If unable to obtain rapid strep test (and patient has bacterial symptoms listed in A, above): treat as bacterial infection with antibiotics while awaiting the throat culture report.

    B. If two or three of the above symptoms are present and patient does not appear that ill, culture first and if positive, treat with antibiotics.

IV. Antibiotic treatment

    A. Penicillin (first-line choice)

       1. Amoxicillin 50 mg/kg/day ÷ q12h for 10 days   *or*

       2. Penicillin VK 2–3 times a day for 10 days   *or*

         (a) ≤ 27 kg: 250 mg

         (b) > 27 kg: 500 mg

       3. Penicillin G benzathine (Bicillin LA)

         (a) ≤ 27 kg: 600,000 units IM *once*

         (b) > 27 kg: 1.2 million units IM *once*

    B. Cephalosporins

       1. Cephalexin (Keflex) for 10 days   *or*

         (a) > 1 yr of age: 40 mg/kg/day q12h

         (b) ≥ 15 yr of age: 500 mg bid

       2. Cefuroxime (Ceftin) for 10 days   *or*

         (a) 3 mo to 12 yr of age: 20 mg/kg/day ÷ q12h

         (b) ≥ 13 yr of age: 250 mg bid

       3. Cefdinir (Omnicef) for 5–10 days   *or*

         (a) > 6 mo to 12 yr of age: 14 mg/kg/day ÷ q12h

         (b) > 13 yr of age: 300 mg bid

       4. Cefpodoxime (Vantin)

         (a) 2 mo to 11 yr of age: 5–10 mg/kg/day ÷ q12h

         (b) > 12 yr of age: 100 mg q12h for *5–10 days*

    C. Macrolides

       1. Azithromycin (Zmax) > 2 yr of age: 12 mg/kg/day followed by 6 mg/kg/day *for 2–5 days* (growing resistance rates)   *or*

       2. Clarithromycin (Biaxin) > 6 mo of age: 7.5–15 mg/kg/day q12h for *10 days*

    D. Clindamycin (Cleocin) 7 mg/kg/dose tid for *10 days*

V. Follow up in office in 48 hr, and if symptoms not improving, consider switching to a different antibiotic.

VI. Symptomatic treatment for pharyngitis

    A. Comfort measures

       1. Saltwater gargles for children > 6 yr of age

       2. Increase fluids (either hot or cold) and encourage soft foods

       3. Throat lozenges or hard candy for children > 5 yr of age

       4. Rest

    B. Acetaminophen or ibuprofen for pain or fever (see Appendices C and D)

    C. No sharing utensils or drinks; discourage mouth-to-mouth contact; encourage covering mouth when coughing.

    D. Discard toothbrush immediately and buy two new toothbrushes; use one for 48 hr, then discard.

VII. After care: can return to school after on antibiotic therapy for 24 hr and/or when fever resolves.

VIII. *Referral to ENT*
    A. *If tonsils are chronically enlarged and affecting child's sleep pattern*
    B. *With chronic pharyngitis (> 6 episodes/yr)*

Lower Respiratory Tract Conditions

BRONCHIOLITIS

    I. Description: an acute infection primarily seen in children < 2 yr of age; commonly caused by viral illness (e.g., RSV)

    II. *Transfer emergently to ED via ambulance with severe bronchiolitis*
        A. *Appears acutely ill with difficulty breathing and worsening respiratory distress*
        B. *Hypoxia (e.g., pulse ox < 95%), nasal flaring, grunting, apneic episodes*
        C. *Lethargy but arousable*
        D. *Unable to keep fluids down*
        E. *Cyanosis*
        F. While awaiting ambulance:
           1. O_2 supplementation
           2. Nasal suction, if indicated
           3. Keep environment quiet and allow parents to hold infant/child

    III. *Nonsevere* bronchiolitis
        A. Signs and symptoms
           1. Low-grade fever, rhinorrhea
           2. Cough with wheezing and crackles; mild tachypnea and intercostal retractions
           3. May have associated OM
           4. Mild dehydration with dry mucus membranes (see Table 16.1)
        B. Treatment is supportive
           1. Increase humidity and fluid intake
           2. Nasal suction
           3. Rest; acetaminophen *or* ibuprofen for discomfort (see Appendices C and D)
           4. Consider trial of levalbuterol (Xopenex) nebulized solution 0.31–0.63 mg/3 mL tid *or* albuterol nebulized solution 0.63–2.5 mg/3 mL tid

    IV. Prevention
        A. Good handwashing and cleaning of environment
        B. No smoking
        C. Flu vaccine for ages > 6 mo of age
        D. Avoidance of individuals with URIs

    V. Prophylaxis for premature newborns or those with bronchopulmonary dysplasia: consider palivizumab (Synagis)

COMMUNITY-ACQUIRED PNEUMONIA

    I. *Atypical:* usually caused by *Mycoplasma pneumoniae* or *Chlamydia pneumoniae*
        A. Seen more often in children > 5 yr of age, with a more gradual onset
        B. Signs/symptoms usually begin with
           1. Low-grade fever with fatigue, malaise, and general achy feeling
           2. Cough that is nonproductive and gradually worsens; wheezing
           3. H/A, sore throat, photophobia, conjunctivitis, rash
           4. May have ear pain and bulla seen on TM, malaise, myalgia

---

● *= non-urgent referral;* ■ *= not to be missed;* ▲ *= urgent referral*

5. Physical exam findings may include
   (a) Nasal flaring and retractions
   (b) Tachypnea and hypoxia
   (c) Crackles, decreased breath sounds, bronchial breath sounds
   (d) Egophony, bronchophony, whispered pectoriloquy
   (e) Dullness to percussion

C. Diagnostic tests
   1. WBC usually normal or slightly elevated (< 15,000/μL); increased platelets
   2. Increased ESR
   3. CXR may show lobar or segmental infiltrates but not localization of pneumonia.

D. Treatment (*uncomplicated* atypical pneumonia)
   1. Supportive care
      (a) Increase in fluid intake and ORS (see Table 9.2)
      (b) Humidification, rest
      (c) Acetaminophen or ibuprofen for fever or discomfort (see Appendices C and D)
   2. Antibiotic treatment for 10 days (except azithromycin)
      (a) Azithromycin (Zmax) 10 mg/kg on day 1 then 5 mg/kg on days 2–5   *or*
      (b) Clarithromycin (Biaxin) 15 mg/kg/day ÷ q12h   *or*
      (c) Doxycycline 2–4 mg/kg/day ÷ bid in children > 8 yr of age   *or*
      (d) Erythromycin 40–50 mg/kg/day ÷ qid

E. Follow-up should occur in office within 24–48 hr; if not improving, consider switching antibiotic and follow-up again in 24–48 hr.

▲ F. *Urgent referral to ED if hypoxic (< 95% pulse ox), obvious respiratory distress, worsening symptoms in office or at home, dehydration, toxic appearance*

II. *Bacterial*: commonly caused by *S. pneumonia*
A. Can be seen in children of any age, at any time of year, usually after a URI
B. Signs/symptoms
   1. Child appears ill with abrupt onset of
      (a) Fever < 38.5°C (< 101.3°F)
      (b) Nonproductive cough
      (c) Constitutional symptoms with malaise, decreased appetite, fatigue
   2. Physical exam
      (a) Decreased breath sounds and crackles over involved area; may have chest pain over same area
      (b) Mild tachypnea and mild retractions with some SOB
      (c) Hypoxia (< 95% pulse ox), with grunting and retractions
      (d) Egophony, bronchophony, whispered pectoriloquy
      (e) Dullness to percussion

C. Diagnostic testing
   1. WBC elevated (can be > 15,000/μL)
   2. CXR may show lobar/segmental consolidation with alveolar infiltrates and localized area of pneumonia.
   3. ESR/CRP may be elevated.

D. Treatment for *uncomplicated* pneumonia in children > 6 mo of age
   1. Supportive therapy
      (a) Increase in fluid intake and ORS (see Table 9.2)
      (b) Humidification and rest
      (c) Acetaminophen or ibuprofen for fever or discomfort (see Appendices C and D)

▲ = *urgent referral*

    2. Antibiotic therapy for 5–7 days
      (a) Amoxicillin 90 mg/kg/day ÷ bid/tid   *or*
      (b) Amoxicillin/clavulanate (Augmentin) 90 mg/kg/day ÷ bid   *or*
      (c) Cefdinir (Omnicef) 14 mg/kg/day ÷ q12h   *or*
      (d) Clindamycin (Cleocin) 30–40 mg/kg/day ÷ tid/qid   *or*
      (e) Azithromycin (Zmax) 10 mg/kg on day 1 then 5 mg/kg/day on days 2–5
      (f) If patient is unable to tolerate oral medications or fluids, can give ceftriaxone 50–75 mg/kg IM *once* and then start oral antibiotics.
    3. Follow-up should occur in office in 24–48 hr; if not improving, consider changing antibiotic and follow-up again in 24–48 hr

▲   E. ***Urgent referral to ED***
     1. ***If infant < 6 mo of age***
     2. ***With hypoxia (< 95% pulse ox), obvious respiratory distress, worsening symptoms in office or at home, dehydration, or toxic appearance***

III. *Viral*: commonly seen after URI, RSV, or influenza
  A. It is seen more often in children < 5 yr of age, is more common in the winter months, and has a gradual onset.
  B. Signs/symptoms
    1. Clear rhinorrhea, nasal congestion, nonproductive cough, wheezing
    2. Conjunctivitis, sore throat, dehydration
    3. May see generalized rash
    4. Physical exam
      (a) Not acutely ill appearing
      (b) Diffuse and typically bilateral wheezes/crackles
      (c) Retractions, tachypnea
  C. Diagnostic tests
    1. WBC normal or very slightly elevated (much less than bacterial pneumonia)
    2. COVID and Flu testing
  D. Treatment
    1. Supportive care
      (a) With increase in fluid intake and ORS (see Table 9.2)
      (b) Humidification, rest
      (c) Acetaminophen or ibuprofen for fever or discomfort (see Appendices C and D)
    2. If test positive for
      (a) Influenza A or B: treat with oseltamivir (Tamiflu; see **INFLUENZA** treatment)
      (b) Covid-19
        (i) Supportive care with antipyretics (see Appendices C and D); maintain hydration and rest
        (ii) Isolation at home for 10–14 days
        (iii) If immunocompromised patient, consider hospitalization
        (iv) With outpatient treatment and ≥ 12 yr of age with comorbidities, consider monoclonal antibodies
    3. Consider nebulizer with either albuterol or levalbuterol tid.
    4. May need supplemental oxygen to keep pulse ox > 92%.
    5. Nasal suctioning with bulb may relieve some congestion.
  E. Follow up in office in 24 hr and if not improving, consider hospitalization.

▲ = *urgent referral*

F. *Urgent referral to ED if*
    (a) *Hypoxic (< 92% pulse ox), obvious respiratory distress*
    (b) *Dehydration*
    (c) *Change in mental status*

CROUP

I. Description: a viral illness that affects the larynx and trachea (may extend to the bronchi) of children between 6 mo and 6 yr of age; commonly occurs during fall and early winter
II. Signs and symptoms
   A. Typical illness begins as a URI infection with low-grade fever but within 1–2 days, the child has hoarseness, barky cough, and stridor.
   B. The *hallmark sign* is stridor: harsh, high-pitched sound produced by a partially obstructed upper airway.
   C. Respiratory symptoms typically worsen at night; resolve within 3–7 days.
   D. *Mild* croup
      1. Barky cough; hoarse cry
      2. No audible stridor at rest but has stridor if active
      3. None or very mild intercostal retractions
   E. *Moderate* croup
      1. Stridor with rest, mild retractions, and little or no agitation
      2. Decreased air entry and cyanosis
      3. The child does not appear toxic
   F. *Severe croup*
      1. *Significant stridor at rest (stridor that "improves" may actually be a sign of worsening obstruction)*
      2. *Decreased airway entry, cyanosis, intercostal retractions with in-drawing of the sternum*
      3. *Anxious, agitated, or fatigued*
      4. *Pulse ox < 92% with tripod self-position to ease breathing*
III. Diagnostic testing *if not acutely ill*
   A. Lateral neck X-ray to check for "steeple sign" of epiglottis
   B. CXR usually shows hyperinflation and mild infiltrates
IV. Treatment
   A. Treatment for *mild-to-moderate* croup in office is based on severity of symptoms.
      1. All symptomatic patients should receive steroids (can be either a or b).
         (a) Dexamethasone *once in office*
            (i) Oral dexamethasone 0.6 mg/kg (maximum dose 10 mg) in a cherry-flavored syrup as a *single dose* (the IM preparation [4 mg/mL] can be given mixed in syrup at 0.6 mg/kg)   *or*
            (ii) Dexamethasone 0.6 mg/kg IM single dose   *or*
         (b) Prednisolone (Prelone, Pediapred) 1–2 mg/kg/day PO in office and continue *daily dose for 3–5 days*
      2. Nebulized medications
         (a) Nebulized racemic epinephrine 0.05 mg/kg diluted in 3 mL normal saline or premixed tubule of 0.5 mL given once over a 15-min period of time

---

■ = *not to be missed;* ▲ = *urgent referral*

      (b) Nebulized budesonide (Pulmicort) 0.25 mg/2 mL bid (not as effective for immediate results) for 3–5 days; give first dose in office

3. Keep child calm and quiet, allow to sit with parent if possible.
4. *Cool mist* humidifier
5. Increase oral intake with cool beverages or ice pops (see Table 9.2).
6. Fever reduction with either acetaminophen or ibuprofen (see Appendices C and D)

B. Discharge criteria for mild croup after office treatment: return of a more normal respiratory rate and normal pulse ox, with no dyspnea

1. No stridor at rest, good color, and air exchange
2. Can tolerate fluids by mouth
3. Improved behaviors and normal mental status
4. Parents are capable of caring for child at home and understand instructions.
    (a) Instruction to parents to go to ED if symptoms recur or get worse.
    (b) Acetaminophen or ibuprofen routinely until fever or discomfort improve (see Appendices C and D).
    (c) Cool mist humidifier near face; if stridor recurs, immediately go to the bathroom and turn on hot water and sit with the child in the room until symptoms improve; if symptoms do not improve, go to ED.
5. Rest and try to keep the child quiet.
6. Increase oral fluids to prevent dehydration (see Table 9.2).
7. Nebulized budesonide (Pulmicort) 0.25 mg/2 mL bid at home for 3–5 days
8. Follow up in *24 hr* by phone or return to office.

▲ C. *Transfer to ED via ambulance with severe croup symptoms (see II. F, above); start treatments before transport if available.*

1. Work slowly and do not frighten the child, as this will make the symptoms worse.
2. Oxygen via cannula or mask (depends on what the child will tolerate)
3. Nebulized racemic epinephrine 0.05 mg/kg/dose (2.25% solution) diluted in 3 mL normal saline or premixed tubule of 0.5 mL given over 15 min
4. Oral dexamethasone 0.6 mg/kg up to maximum dose of 10 mg, as *a single dose* (made by mixing the IM preparation [4 mg/mL] in a cherry-flavored syrup) or dexamethasone 0.6 mg/kg IM *once*

EPIGLOTTITIS

   I. Description: acute inflammation and edema of epiglottis and surrounding structures

  II. Signs and symptoms: usually begins with fever 39°C up to 40.6°C (102.2°F up to 105°F), stridor, and labored breathing, which can rapidly progress to respiratory distress/failure; other presenting signs are

    A. *The child appears quite ill with restlessness, irritability, and anxiety.*
    B. *Drooling, dysphagia, and respiratory distress (hallmarks of epiglottitis)*
    C. *Sore throat and muffled voice (not hoarse)*
    D. *Minimal cough but significant retractions*
    E. *Tripod sitting position with mouth open to facilitate breathing; refusing to lie down*

▲ III. *Treatment is emergent transfer to ED via ambulance. DO NOT ATTEMPT VISUALIZATION of throat without intubation equipment readily available.*

■ = *not to be missed;* ▲ = *urgent referral*

Cardiac Conditions

HEART MURMURS (SEE CHAPTER 8, HEART MURMURS and TABLE 8.12)

I. Description
   A. Innocent murmurs (Still's murmur) are common findings in infants and children and occur with normal flow patterns and no structural defects in the heart or vessels; usually systolic murmur; more common > 2 yr of age.
   B. Pathological murmurs occur *with* structural or valvular defects and are usually diastolic or combined systolic/diastolic murmur; more common < 1 yr of age.

II. HPI
   A. What was the prenatal and birth history? Any complications related to birth process?
   B. Any FH of heart disease or congenital abnormalities or hypertrophic cardiomyopathy? Has anyone in the family died of heart conditions before 45 yr of age?
   C. Has their growth been maintained? Any issues with failure to thrive?
   D. Inability to feed with breast/bottle or eat regular foods without becoming fatigued or SOB?
   E. Have they experienced respiratory problems (e.g., cyanosis, syncope, DOE), and under what conditions?
   F. What has been the child's normal activity level (are they able to keep up with peers)?
   G. Has the child ever been identified as having a "heart murmur" in the past and was any testing done? What was the outcome? What documentation is there regarding type of murmur?

III. Physical exam
   A. VS should be compared to age-related normal.
   B. Child's overall appearance, including color and respiratory effort with activity
   C. Examine neck for any bruits, abnormal pulsations.
   D. Chest
      1. Inspect chest for abnormalities in sternum and contour of chest.
      2. Palpate over the heart for any thrills, pulsations and PMI.
      3. Auscultate lungs for crackles or wheezing.
   E. Heart
      1. Auscultate in all four areas (see Fig. 1.6), preferably with bell and diaphragm and with patient *sitting, lying, and standing* (if murmur disappears with standing, it is most likely *not* pathological in > 2 yr of age) (see Chapter 8, HEART MURMURS, and Table 8.12).
         (a) S_1: occurs with closure of AV valves and is best heard over the mitral and tricuspid areas; identified as QRS on ECG
         (b) S_2: occurs with closure of semilunar valves and is best heard over aortic and pulmonic valve areas
         (c) S_3: occurs in rapid filling stage in early diastole
            (i) Heard in hyperdynamic states (illness, stress, volume overload)
            (ii) Best heard in mitral and tricuspid area using the bell of stethoscope
            (iii) Ken---tuc---"*ky*"
         (d) S_4: occurs with atrial contraction phase in late diastole
            (i) Always pathological
            (ii) Best heard over aortic and pulmonic areas with bell of stethoscope
            (iii) "*Ten*"---nes---see
      2. If systolic murmur noted during acute illness, with no prior hx of murmur, recheck when patient has recovered.

　　F. Palpate peripheral pulses (see Fig. 1.7) and capillary refill.
　　G. Palpate abdomen for liver size, ascites.
IV. Diagnostic testing is usually performed by pediatric cardiologist and may include
　　A. ECG
　　B. CBC, TSH
　　C. Echocardiogram
V. Treatment: *Referral to pediatric cardiologist (no strenuous physical activity until cleared by the specialist)*
　　A. *First-time murmur without adequate explanation*
　　B. *Grade ≥ 3; intensity of murmur increases in sitting/standing*
　　C. *Holosystolic, harsh, or blowing quality murmur*
　　D. *Any diastolic murmur*
　　E. *Any hx of syncope, DOE, inability to keep up with peers in activities; change in pulses*

HYPERTENSION

I. Description:
　　A. Normal BP (see Table 2.3).
　　　　1. Primary HTN: usually occurs in child > 6 yr of age; no identifiable cause but may be due to
　　　　　　(a) Obesity
　　　　　　(b) Family history
　　　　2. Secondary HTN: usually occurs from underlying condition
　　　　　　(a) Renal disease(s)
　　　　　　(b) Hyperthyroidism, DM, Cushing syndrome, pheochromocytoma
　　　　　　(c) Anxiety, stimulants (e.g., caffeine), corticosteroids, OCs, smoking
　　　　　　(d) Cardiac abnormalities
　　B. Screening
　　　　1. Start at 3 yr of age with other vital signs at time of presentation; if HTN noted, check BP in all extremities to rule out coarctation.
　　　　2. Take a minimum of three readings on different visits (when the child is not ill) to determine if HTN is present.
　　C. Stages (see Table 2.3)
　　　　1. Elevated BP
　　　　　　(a) 1 to < 13 yr of age: BP between ≥ 90th and ≤ 95th percentile *or* 120/80 to < 95th percentile (whichever is lower)
　　　　　　(b) ≥ 13 yr of age: BP 120–129/<80 mmHg
　　　　2. Stage 1 HTN
　　　　　　(a) 1 to < 13 yr of age: systolic or diastolic pressures are ≥ 95th percentile *or* < 95th percentile + 12 mmHg or 130–139/80–89
　　　　　　(b) ≥ 13 yr of age: 130–139/80–89
　　　　3. Stage 2 HTN
　　　　　　(a) 1 to < 13 yr of age: systolic and diastolic ≥ 95th percentile + 12 mmHg or ≥ 140/90 mmHg
　　　　　　(b) ≥ 13 yr of age: ≥ 140/90
II. Signs and symptoms: typically asymptomatic, but could have H/A, blurred vision, irritability, nosebleeds, and poor school performance

---

■ = *not to be missed;* ● = *non-urgent referral*

III. Diagnostic testing > 6 yr of age
    A. CBC, CMP, lipid profile, TSH, U/A, and urine protein/creatinine ratio
    B. Consider CXR, renal U/S
    C. ECG/Echocardiogram
    D. Consider sleep study for OSA with obesity, history of snoring, or daytime sleepiness
    E. Consider ophthalmology evaluation with Stage 2 HTN
IV. Treatment for essential HTN

▲   A. *Emergent transfer to ED with hypertensive crisis with any symptoms such as headache, dizziness, or chest pain, confusion, SOB, vision changes*
    B. Lifestyle changes for elevated BP and/or Stage 1 HTN *without* target organ damage is the *first-line* therapy for all overweight/obese and/or sedentary children.
       1. Decrease weight by at least 5%–10%.
       2. Regular exercise (~ 150 min/wk)
       3. Decrease sedentary activity (< 2 hr/day).
       4. Improve dietary choices and recommendation to follow DASH diet (see Table 8.14), which includes more fruits and vegetables and decrease in sodium intake.
       5. Avoid or stop smoking; no alcohol or stimulant drinks (energy drinks or drugs, both OTC and illegal).
       6. Treat any underlying dyslipidemia or DM.
    C. Preparticipation sports requirements
       1. Has elevated BP or Stage 1 HTN (e.g., 130–139/80–89) with good control, is not symptomatic; no restrictions
       2. If participant has Stage 2 HTN (e.g., ≥ 140/ ≥ 90); may not participate until BP well controlled and cleared by pediatric cardiologist
  V. *Referral to a pediatric cardiologist as soon as possible*
       1. *For initial evaluation of Stage 1 or higher BP and then co-manage; referral within 1 wk if BP > 99th percentile plus 5 mmHg*
       2. *With secondary HTN*

Abdominal Conditions

COLIC

I. Description
    A. Inconsolable, paroxysmal crying for no apparent reason for ≥ 3 hr/day for ≥ 3 days/wk in < 3 mo of age infant that is otherwise healthy and well fed
    B. Crying has a sudden onset without trigger and abrupt ending that occurs mainly in the evening hours.
    C. Sound of crying is dysphonic (e.g., louder, higher in pitch, and variable).
    D. Hypertonia features (e.g., flushed facies, circumoral pallor, stiffening and tightening of fingers and arms, arching of back)
    E. Parent(s) are unable to console infant, crying may decrease but does not abate.
II. HPI
    A. Feeding habits
       1. Formula or breast fed?
       2. How often during the day/night and how much formula/breast feeding does baby take?

▲ = *urgent referral ;* ● = *non-urgent referral*

      3. Positioning during feeding and after feeding, consoling positions; any difficulty with feeding either with the baby or parental difficulty in feeding baby?

      4. Mother's diet (attention to special diets) and water/liquid intake (how much and what liquids?)

      5. Vomiting (if so how much and how often, is it related to feeding?)

  B. Timing of crying (mornings or evenings), duration of cries (how long does crying last?), and sound of crying

  C. Precipitating (after meals or after sleeping) or relieving factors (Ask: What do you do when they cry?)

  D. Prenatal/perinatal history/postnatal (any illness or infections)

  E. Has growth and developmental curve been normal to date?

  F. Psychological environment

      1. Parents'/siblings' interaction with infant

      2. Parents' feelings regarding crying and any guilt

III. Physical examination (see Chapter 2, Focused Examinations)

  A. Observe parent and baby interaction at rest and with crying, if possible.

  B. Is the baby sensitive to surrounding noises or touch?

  C. At each office visit, complete/review growth chart.

  D. Assess skin turgor and subcutaneous fat; evaluate any suspicious bruises or infections, difficulty with movement of extremity.

  E. HEENT

      1. Assess fontanels, asymmetry of head and tone of muscles.

      2. Assess eyes for vision abnormalities and strabismus.

      3. Assess ears for any infection and for position (see Fig. 2.2).

      4. Oral exam

         (a) Ulcers or thrush

         (b) Tongue-tie which could lead to sucking problems

         (c) Uvula movement/position, signs of infection

  F. Cardiovascular system for tachycardia, bradycardia, or HF

  G. Abdominal exam for bowel sounds, pain with palpation and firmness

  H. Genital area for rashes, ulcers on urinary meatus or vaginal opening, penis for any swelling due to "hair tourniquet," or anal fissures

IV. Diagnostic testing is not usually required unless positive findings on exam.

V. Treatment is individualized.

  A. *Reassurance* for parents

  B. Consider change in type of feedings with a trial of Alimentum, Nutramigen, or Pregestimil; results will usually be seen in about 2–3 days.

  C. Consider changing timing of feedings, amount of feeding.

  D. Change position for feeding, and increase number of times "burped."

  E. Soothing techniques

      1. Use of pacifier and/or change type of nipple or bottle

      2. Consider change in mother's diet (e.g., no milk, nuts, wheat, or eggs).

      3. Holding or carrying, rhythmic motions (e.g., rocking, swinging)

      4. Warm bath

      5. Gently rubbing abdomen

      6. Using sound (e.g., music of any type, pulsed music, white noise)

VI. Treatments of *no* probable value

  A. Medications (OTC or Rx)

      1. Simethicone

      2. Dicyclomine

      3. PPIs or H2 blockers
      4. Probiotics, sucrose, or lactose
   B. Herbal remedies
      1. Fennel seed
      2. Herbal teas
      3. Gripe water
      4. Fiber-enriched formula or soy milk formula
   C. Homeopathic remedies (some may contain toxic ingredients such as ethanol or pro-pylene glycol that aren't displayed on label)
   D. Manipulation or acupuncture
VII. Follow-up in office in 2–3 days after changing formula and monitor weight monthly until this subsides.

CONSTIPATION

  I. Definition
   A. Infrequent passing of stools ($\leq$ 2/wk) for a minimum of 8 wk
   B. Pain, especially with large size stool
   C. Excessive straining with eventual passage of stool
   D. Not uncommon in infants and children
 II. Causes
   A. Painful stooling which may cause withholding of stool
      1. Anal fissuring, hemorrhoids or ulcers
      2. Sexual abuse
      3. Improper toilet training
   B. Change in living conditions which may affect stooling routine
      1. Traveling which causes a change in routine and diet
      2. Moving to new area with schools, friends
      3. Family stressors
      4. Change in diet
         (a) Switch from formula/breast milk to cow's milk
         (b) Low fiber diet and decreased intake of water
         (c) Increased intake of fruit juices or caffeinated beverages
   C. Medical conditions
      1. CF, Hirschsprung disease (HD), CP
      2. Hypothyroidism, DM, spinal cord dysfunction
      3. Depression, mental retardation, behavioral problems
III. HPI
   A. Did infant have meconium stool > 48 hr after birth (suggestive of HD)?
   B. When did constipation issues start: with infancy, change in milk/diet, toilet training or other precipitating event?
   C. What problem(s) does patient have with stooling: pain (may suggest functional), large, hard stools (may suggest withholding), pellets (may suggest functional) or blood (may suggest anal fissures)?
   D. Are stains present in under garments (may suggest fecal incontinence)?
   E. What type of foods does the patient like or eat frequently? Is there fiber in the diet and adequate amount of water? Are there foods that the patient will not eat?
   F. What has been tried in the past and how did it work? What amount of time was spent on these changes?
   G. Is there a FH of constipation?

IV. Signs and symptoms
  A. Patient's overall appearance (active, happy, flaccid, interactive)
  B. Growth chart and current weight
  C. Abdominal distention
  D. Palpable stool mass or mass in suprapubic area
  E. Anal area
    1. Absent cremasteric reflex and anal wink (suggests neurologic disease)
    2. Increased anal tone may suggest HD
    3. Anal fissuring, abnormal placement of anal orifice
  F. Skin changes in lumbosacral region (dimpling, hair shafts and deviation of gluteal cleft)
  G. DRE indicated for
    1. Infants with constipation
    2. Infants/children with continued symptoms unresolved after treatment
■ **V.** *Alarm signs*
■   A. *History of late meconium passage* (> 48 hr after birth)
■   B. *Fever, V/D, weight loss, or poor weight gain (failure to thrive)*
■   C. *Severe abdominal distention especially without bowel sounds*
■   D. *Rectal bleeding* (unless anal fissure noted)
VI. Diagnostics if indicated
  A. CBC, CMP
  B. TSH, lead level
  C. U/A and C&S
  D. Celiac screening
VII. Treatment should be initiated early on to prevent stool withholding, functional constipation, and future complications. *The goal is stooling daily or every other day.*
  A. 4 mo to 1 yr of age
    1. Usually caused from dietary changes.
    2. Should include 2–4 ounces daily of juices/purees that contain sorbitol (e.g., apple, pear or prune).
    3. Increase fiber with multigrain or barley cereal.
    4. Switch to pureed peas or prunes for vegetables.
    5. If hard stool is present in rectum, consider digital stimulation with lubricated rectal thermometer; *beware, tolerance to this procedure can occur.*
    6. If constipation becomes more chronic, further evaluation is needed.
  B. > 1 yr of age without pain or other issues (e.g., bleeding or withholding)
    1. Toilet training is pivotal to preventing constipation.
    2. If treatment is needed
      (a) Increase fiber to ≥ 3 g/serving (see Appendix A).
      (b) Increase fluid intake to 32–64 ounces/day.
      (c) Consider 5–10 sugar-free gummy bears (these contain sorbitol), providing child can chew and swallow without difficulty.
  C. Older children with stool withholding issues, pain, or anal fissures
      (a) Polyethylene glycol 3350 (PEG) start with 2–4 tsp daily and may increase or decrease by 1–2 tsp daily as needed; do not dissolve in carbonated drinks.
      (b) Lactulose 1 mL/kg 1–2 times daily
      (c) Magnesium hydroxide (milk of magnesia) 1–3 mL/kg daily
      (d) Increase fiber foods (see Appendix A) and/or use bulking laxative (e.g., Fibercon, Metamucil or Citrucel) daily.

_____

■ = *not to be missed*

  (e) Increase water intake to 32–64 ounces/day.

  (f) Treat anal fissures with petroleum jelly after bowel movements.

VIII. *Referral to pediatric gastroenterologist*

  A. **Urgently** *for any infant/child that has alarm signs* (see **V.** above)

  B. **Nonurgent** *for any infant/child that does not respond to any of the above treatments or has chronic relapses.*

ENCOPRESIS

I. Description

  A. *Retentive encopresis (functional constipation)*: may be caused by pain with BM that leads to withholding stool, which causes the colon to enlarge from backup of stool and eventually a decreased sensation to defecate. As the stool backs up, liquid stool will seep around impaction and cause involuntary leakage.

  1. Usually seen in > 4 yr of age, already be toilet trained, with no identifiable pathologic reason for constipation

  2. Rome IV criteria: two of the following at least once weekly for 1 mo

  (a) $\lesssim 2$ stools in toilet/week

  (b) One episode of incontinence/week

  (c) Past history of retentive posturing or excessive volitional stool retention

  (d) Past history of painful or hard stools

  (e) Presence of large diameter stools that can obstruct the toilet

  3. Signs/symptoms

  (a) Stool leakage with or without knowledge of event

  (b) Stools are hard, dry, and large with increased straining while defecating.

  (c) ***Weight loss or slow weight gain, anorexia, abdominal pain with distention***

  (d) Abdominal mass in LLQ with palpation with or without pain

  (e) Anal fissures, dermatitis at anal opening

  (f) ***Abnormal sphincter tone (anal wink)***

  (i) Increased tone may indicate Hirschsprung disease.

  (ii) Decreased tone may indicate neurologic defect.

  (g) DRE (usually not required for obvious constipation) may show large amount of stool in rectal vault.

  4. Diagnostic testing is usually not recommended if no pathologic findings. May consider abdominal U/S or X-ray to determine if there is a large amount of stool in colon.

  5. Treatment for children > 5 yr of age

  (a) *Disimpaction*

  (i) Oral: polyethylene glycol 3350 (Miralax) 1–1.5 g/kg/day (~½ to 1 capful) for 3–6 days (should expect large stool within 12–24 hr); can be dissolved in water, juice, or milk; *do not dissolve in carbonated drinks*

  (ii) If no stooling in 6 days, consider sodium phosphate enema (Fleet saline enema); *5–12 yr of age:* 66 mL; *≥ 12 yr of age:* 133 mL enema

  (b) *Maintenance therapy* includes pharmacological (osmotic/lubricant laxatives) and lifestyle changes (see (c), below) to achieve daily or every-other-day soft stools.

  (i) Polyethylene glycol 3350 (Miralax) 1–4 tsp daily (can be dissolved in water, juice, or milk)

▲ = *urgent referral;* ● = *non-urgent referral;* ■ = *not to be missed*

  (ii) Lactulose or sorbitol: *6–11 yr of age*: 1 mL/kg 1–2 times daily; ≥ *12 yr of age*: 15–30 mL 1–2 times daily; can use for 1–3 mo and then prn

  (iii) Magnesium hydroxide (milk of magnesia): *6–11 yr of age*: 1–3 mL/kg daily; > *12 yr of age*: 15–30 mL daily or can be used prn for constipation

 (c) Lifestyle changes

  (i) Increase fiber in diet (see Appendix A for high-fiber foods) and consider stool softeners daily.

  (ii) Increase fluid intake and decrease caffeine/energy drinks (may cause mild dehydration).

  (iii) Encourage regular exercise (e.g., biking, walking, running).

 (d) Educate family on toileting protocols while regular stooling is established

  (i) Follow a routine of toilet sitting after a meal for 5–15 min.

  (ii) Routine should be maintained even with deviation in family routine (e.g., vacations).

  (iii) Use positive reinforcements with rewards that are age appropriate.

  (iv) Ensure that child can sit comfortably on stool with feet touching floor (or may need to use a stool for foot support).

  (v) This process may take several months to establish a habit and relapse is common; decrease medications as stooling habits improve but monitor closely.

 (e) Stimulant laxatives for acute constipation or relapse of maintenance program

  (i) Increase polyethylene glycol 3350 to 2–4 tsp daily or bid for 1–3 days until resolution then resume previous maintenance dose

  (ii) Senna tablets (Senokot regular strength or Ex-lax maximum strength): > 6 yr of age: 1–2 tabs at hs prn

  (iii) Bisacodyl (Dulcolax): > *6–11 yr of age*: 1 tab at hs; ≥ *12 yr of age*: 1–3 tab at hs prn

  (iv) Glycerin rectal supp (Fleet liquid glycerin suppository) > 6 yr of age: 1 supp rectally daily prn

 ● 6. ***Referral to pediatric gastroenterologist with continued problems at any age***

B. *Nonretentive encopresis*: passage of stools are normal but occur at inappropriate places; the child usually has behavioral problems such as avoidance of toileting or oppositional defiance, or a history of sexual/physical abuse.

 1. The child refuses to sit on toilet but will defecate in underwear or other inappropriate places.

 2. Refuses to take medications

 3. No symptoms of constipation

 4. Stools are normal in shape and consistency.

 5. Treatment for children > 6 yr of age

  (a) Pharmacological treatment is not recommended.

  (b) Behavioral therapy is recommended.

  (c) Do not use stool softeners or laxatives unless child is constipated (see **CONSTIPATION** for treatments).

  (d) Do not make a fuss over inappropriate stooling.

  (e) Clean up mess and change out of soiled underwear as soon as it happens without emotional harassment.

  (f) Use rewards when child stools in appropriate places.

  (g) Relapse is common.

● = *non-urgent referral*

GASTROENTERITIS

I. Description: self-limited occurrence of diarrhea (> 3 loose or watery stools in 24 hr) with/ without fever, vomiting, myalgia, and abdominal pain; usually transmitted via fecal-oral route, commonly caused by

    A. Viral infection: norovirus and rotavirus are seen more often in the fall and winter; adenovirus is more often in the summer

    B. Bacterial: usually *Escherichia coli or Salmonella*, and occurs more often in the summer in children > 2 yr of age

       1. Usually has blood or mucus in stool, abdominal pain with stooling, and high fever (> 40°C [> 104°F])

       2. May have seizures, small-volume stools, and acute abdominal pain

    C. Parasites (Giardia, *Cryptosporidium*) are ingested from streams or river water; seen more frequently in children > 2 yr of age.

    D. Antibiotics, which could cause *Clostridioides difficile* diarrhea (see Chapter 9, **DIARRHEA, VIII**; and Table 9.4)

    E. Traveler's diarrhea (see Chapter 9, **DIARRHEA, VII**; and Table 9.4)

II. Signs and symptoms

    A. Acute-onset profuse watery diarrhea, vomiting with abdominal pain/cramping

       1. Vomiting may last up to 2 days.

       2. Diarrhea may last up to 7 days; if diarrhea lasts > 7 days, this may be sign of bacterial or systemic disease.

       3. No blood or mucus in stool

    B. Dehydration signs (see Table 16.1) and weight loss; increase in thirst

    C. Fever, myalgias, headache, anorexia

III. Consider diagnostic testing with known outbreaks or recurrent diarrhea.

    A. CBC for anemia, dehydration, parasitic infection (e.g., elevated eosinophilia)

    B. CMP for electrolyte imbalance (hypernatremia common finding)

    C. COVID-19 testing if exposure to individuals with COVID-19

    D. Stool for O&P, culture, and *C. difficile*, fecal leukocytes (if suspect bacterial causes)

    E. Urinalysis for infection

IV. Treatment for *mild-to-moderate* dehydration

    A. Hydration and nutrition

       1. Initially start with very small amounts of fluids given frequently.

          (a) Rehydration formulas (see Table 9.2) or 1/2 strength apple juice

             (i) < 2 yr of age: ~ 500 mL/day

             (ii) 2–10 yr of age: ~ 1000 mL/day

             (iii) > 10 yr of age: ~ 2000 mL/day

          (b) Start with 1 tsp every 5–10 min as tolerated and gradually increase as tolerated.

       2. Decrease whole milk for 48 hr; may use diluted skim milk or lactose-free formula.

       3. Return to normal diet as soon as possible; if breastfeeding, try to increase number of feedings.

    B. Probiotics daily for at least 1 mo may help.

    C. No antimotility drugs but consider antiemetic if vomiting is severe.

    D. Follow up in office in 24 hr.

    E. Return to school when

       1. Stools episodes are < 2 times child's normal pattern

       2. Stools are contained in diaper and/or child is toilet trained without accidents

       3. No vomiting/diarrhea for 48 hr

    F. Encourage Rotavirus vaccine.

V. *Referral*
  A. *Urgent referral to ED*
  1. *Severe dehydration due to inability to drink or keep fluids*
  2. *Neurological symptoms and possible seizures*
  3. *Sustained fever > 39°C (102.2°F) for > 24 hr*
  4. *Projectile vomiting, or bloody or mucus stools*
  5. *Large volume diarrhea > 7 days*
  6. *Parent/caregiver is unable to care for child at home.*
  B. *Pediatric gastroenterologist for continued chronic problems with diarrhea*

GASTROESOPHAGEAL REFLUX DISEASE (GERD)

  I. Uncomplicated GERD in *infants*
  A. Commonly caused by delay in neurological maturation or diminished or reduced sphincter pressure and esophageal clearance
  B. Is seen frequently in premature and full-term infants and usually resolves by 12 mo of age
  C. Parents usually c/o baby frequently spitting up (both after and between meals) with mild irritability, but no weight loss and infant feeds well and appears happy.
  D. Conservative measures (if no concerning signs, see **V.** below)
  1. Avoid overfeeding and keep infant upright after feedings for 20–30 min.
  2. Thicken feedings with oat infant cereal (1 tbsp/1 oz of formula or breast milk).
  3. Omit cow's milk or soy milk in *diet of infant and mother (if breastfeeding)* for at least 2 wk to see if this is the cause. Consider using hypoallergenic formula (e.g., Enfamil Nutramigen or Similac Alimentum).
  4. Avoid of any type of smoking around infant.
  E. Gastric acid suppression *is not* recommended for mild GERD.
  F. With more significant symptoms (e.g., *irritability, weight loss, refusing to eat*), start a trial of medications and give 30 min before meal; should be tried for 4–8 wk
  1. Famotidine (Pepcid): 3–12 mo of age: 1–2 mg/kg/dose ÷ bid
  2. Nizatidine (Axid): 6 mo to 11 yr of age: 5–10 mg/kg/day ÷ bid
  3. Lansoprazole (Prevacid) > 3 mo of age (> 30 kg): 1–2 mg/kg/d once daily, 30 min before a meal
  II. Uncomplicated GERD in *children and adolescents*
  A. Signs and symptoms (may be seen into adulthood)
  1. Intermittent reflux, heartburn, emesis after meals, and "wet burps"
  2. Decreased food intake and food aversion
  3. Chronic sore throat, hoarseness
  4. Nausea, dysphagia, localized upper abdominal pain
  5. Chest pain or "chest pounding" (i.e., seen in younger children unable to verbalize pain)
  B. Child may not be verbal enough to identify symptoms but parent may notice
  1. Change in food selections from prior preferences
  2. Nocturnal coughing (may indicate asthma)
  3. *Weight loss (may indicate underlying metabolic disease)*
  4. *Chronic or recurrent pneumonia or OM*

■ *= not to be missed;* ● *= non-urgent referral;* ▲ *= urgent referral*

C. Symptoms may be aggravated by
   1. Foods (e.g., spicy/fried, large meals, and eating late in evening)
   2. Social stressors (e.g., school problems, anxiety, depression)
   3. Occult or known medical problems (e.g., asthma, prematurity, constipation)
III. Diagnostic testing
   A. CBC to check for anemia or changes in WBC
   B. CMP to check for metabolic dysfunction
   C. *Helicobacter pylori*
   D. U/A for occult infection
   E. Endoscopy to confirm esophagitis or ulcers
IV. Treatment
   A. Lifestyle modification
      1. Weight loss (if obese)
      2. Elevate head of bed
      3. Dietary modifications in meal times and amounts
      4. Refrain from foods known to aggravate GERD (see Boxes 9.1 and 9.2)
      5. No smoking (for child or secondhand smoke)
   B. PPI pharmacological therapy for children > 1 yr of age should be given 30 min before meal *once daily* for 4–8 wk; more effective than H2RA but has more potential side effects. Do not exceed adult dosage.
      1. Omeprazole (Prilosec): dosage based on weight
         (a) 10–20 kg: 10 mg
         (b) >· 20 kg: 20 mg
      2. Esomeprazole (Nexium)
         (a) 1–11 yr of age: 10 mg
         (b) ≥ 12 yr of age: 20 mg
      3. Lansoprazole (Prevacid)
         (a) 1–11 yr of age (< 30 kg): 15 mg; > 30 kg: 30 mg
         (b) ≥ 12 yr of age: 15 mg
      4. Dexlansoprazole (Dexilant) ≥ 12 yr of age: 30 mg
      5. Rabeprazole (Aciphex) ≥ 12 yr of age: 20 mg
   C. Discontinuation of PPI
      1. Should not be stopped suddenly
      2. Taper off slowly or by starting H2RAs daily with PPI for 2 wk then continue H2RA for 2 wk, then can stop medications.
   D. H2RAs have rapid onset but are only effective about 10 hr; can be used routinely or prn for 2–8 wk; have fewer side effects than PPIs. Do not exceed adult dose.
      1. Famotidine (Pecid)
         (a) < 3 mo of age: 0.5 mg/kg dose qd; 3–12 mo: 1–2 mg/kg ÷ bid
         (b) > 16 yr of age: 20 mg bid
      2. Nizatidine (Axid)
         (a) 6 mo of age: 5–10 mg/kg ÷ bid
         (b) > 12 yr of age: 150 mg bid
   V. *Referral to pediatric gastroenterologist if concerning signs are present.*
      1. *Urgent*
         (a) *Abdominal pain/distention*
         (b) *Bloody emesis, bilious or forceful emesis*

▦ = not to be missed; ◖ = non-urgent referral; ▲ = urgent referral

    (c) *Recurrent vomiting*
    (d) *Chronic cough or recurrent pneumonia*
    (e) *FUO, failure to thrive (FTT); weight loss*
    (f) *Neurologic signs with seizures or genetic anomalies*
  2. *Nonurgent after 8 wk of treatment if not improving or dysphagia is worsening.*

INTUSSUSCEPTION

I. Description: telescoping of one bowel segment into another; most commonly seen abdominal emergency in child < 2 yr of age

II. Signs and symptoms

  A. *Sudden, acute abdominal pain with inconsolable crying; vomiting that becomes bilious with time*

  B. *Colicky, abdominal pain characterized by drawing up knees and stiffening legs*

  C. *Bloody or "currant jelly" stools several hours after the onset of pain*

  D. *Sausage-shaped mass in the right upper quadrant*

  E. *Fever, lethargy, and shock-like state*

III. *Referral emergently to ED*

PYLORIC STENOSIS

I. Description: hypertrophy of the pyloric sphincter, leading to obstruction

II. Signs and symptoms are not present at birth, but usually start at about 4–8 wk of age.

  A. Nonbilious emesis with vomiting after feeding, which progressively worsens and becomes projectile; even trial of small frequent feedings worsens vomiting.

  B. May be dehydrated with obvious weight loss

  C. Appears hungry after emesis

  D. Has a visible peristaltic wave traversing the epigastrium left to right and a palpable "pyloric olive" sized mass to the right of the umbilicus just below the liver edge (more prominent after vomiting)

  E. Will be lethargic and irritable with progression of stenosis

III. Diagnostic testing if symptoms are not severe

  A. Abdominal ultrasound (best test) or UGI

  B. CMP may show metabolic alkalosis and electrolyte imbalance with decreased K^+ and Na^+

IV. *Referral*

  A. *Emergent referral to ED if dehydration is noted*

  B. *Urgent to a surgeon if stable*

Genitourinary Tract Conditions

CRYPTORCHIDISM (UNDESCENDED TESTICLE)

I. Definition: undescended or hidden testis not in scrotum and has not descended by 4 mo of age; usually unilateral; can reascend between 4 and 8 yr of age and require surgical intervention

II. Signs and symptoms

■ = *not to be missed;* ● = *non-urgent referral;* ▲ = *urgent referral*

A. Have the child sit in "tailor fashion" and observe testicles while the child is at rest.
  1. Both testicles should be seen and can be palpated.
  2. If not, note unilateral or bilateral absence of testicle(s).
B. Undescended testicle must be distinguished from retractile testis.
C. Undescended testicle increases risk of testicular cancer as an adult if not corrected early in child's life.
III. Diagnostic testing: scrotal U/S
IV. *Referral to*
  A. *Pediatric urologist for unilateral undescended testis by age 6 mo*
  B. *Pediatric endocrinologist or genetics specialist for bilateral undescended testes*

ENURESIS

I. Description
  A. Intermittent involuntary urinary incontinence usually at night but can occur during the daytime at least twice weekly in children > 5 yr of age
    1. Primary enuresis: child was never dry
      (a) Maturational delays, genetic causes
      (b) Detrusor overactivity, small bladder capacity
      (c) Disturbed sleep
      (d) Nocturnal polyuria caused from decrease in ADH
    2. Secondary enuresis: child was dry (for at least 6 mo) and now is incontinent of urine, usually due to stressful events in life (e.g., birth of sibling, bullying, parental discourse at home)
  B. Daytime continence: usually achieved by 18–28 mo of age
  C. Nighttime continence: usually achieved by 6 yr of age
II. HPI
  A. FH of enuresis (either nighttime or daytime)
  B. Question regarding potential for sexual abuse or illness related to timing of onset of enuresis.
  C. When does incontinence occur (e.g., only at night or during daytime or both)?
  D. Have there been periods of dryness and how long did these periods last?
  E. Stooling history and any associated fecal incontinence
  F. What has been tried and how effective was intervention?
  G. How has the problem affected the child and family?
  H. PMH of sleep apnea, DM, UTI or other medical/neurological conditions
III. Physical examination is usually negative, but evaluation is important
  A. Swollen tonsils or snoring may indicate OSA and may worsen night time enuresis
  B. Abdominal examination for stool mass in lower quadrants
  C. Genitalia for growth and development and any abnormal masses in the genital area
  D. Anal opening for any fissures/excoriation (looking for pin worm) and sphincter control
  E. Musculoskeletal growth
IV. Diagnostic testing
  A. Urinalysis (e.g., for infection)
  B. Ultrasound of the bladder for emptying dysfunction
V. Treatment
  A. Nonpharmacological treatment

● = *non-urgent referral*

1. Supportive attitude for parents and child with the understanding that usually the child will outgrow the condition; *do not punish the child for incontinence.*
2. Educate the parents and child how to strengthen the bladder muscle by urinating on schedule during the day and gradually lengthening time between urination times.
3. Discourage diapers at night because this may decrease the motivation to get up and urinate.
4. Keep a calendar of dry nights.
5. *Nighttime alarms* may be as helpful as medications; there are commercial products available that will awaken child on a schedule; safer option if parents are comfortable with situation at home.
6. Decrease liquid intake after 6 PM and avoid caffeine and high-sugar food and liquids before bed.
7. Void before sleeping and anytime child awakens at night.

B. Pharmacological treatment (if a quicker solution is required)
1. *Oral* desmopressin (DDAVP) acts as antidiuretic and is preferred route.
   (a) >6 yr of age: 0.2 mg approximately 1 hr before bedtime for 7 days and increase to 0.4 mg if needed.
   (b) If effective in 1–2 wk, continue therapy for up to 3 mo; if no response, incontinence may be related to small bladder capacity, consider enuresis alarm.
   (c) Taper medication slowly by reducing dose by half over 2–3 wk to decrease chance of relapse.
   (d) Do not give if gastroenteritis or fevers are present.
   (e) *Intranasal may increase the risk of water intoxication and is not recommended.*
2. Evaluate monthly until improvement; try to wean off medications q3–6 mo.

VI. *Referral to pediatric urologist for further evaluation*
   A. *If no improvement in symptoms after 6 mo*
   B. *Daytime incontinence*
   C. *Continual incontinence; weak stream*
   D. *Excessive thirst (not DM)*
   E. *Proteinuria*
   F. *N/V, weight loss*

URINARY TRACT INFECTION

I. *Uncomplicated* UTI in child > 2 yr of age
   A. Limited to the *lower urinary tract* in child with no underlying medical problems, anatomic or physiologic abnormalities.
   B. Usually caused by
      1. *E coli* and poor hygiene in the younger child
      2. Enterococcus species (especially with urinary procedures or catheters)
      3. *S. saprophyticus* in young, sexually active girls
   C. Signs and symptoms
      1. The most common in *infants and children < 2 yr of age*
         (a) Fever ≤39°C (≤102.2°F) <24 hr
         (b) Irritability
         (c) Poor feeding, increased spitting up or vomiting
         (d) Foul-smelling urine

■ *= not to be missed;* ● *= non-urgent referral*

   2. Most common in *children > 2 yr of age*
      (a) Dysuria, frequency, urgency, hematuria
      (b) Fever ≤ 39°C (≤ 102.2°F) for > 24 hr
      (c) Incontinence in previously continent child
      (d) Abdominal pain and or low back pain
   3. Most common in *adolescent*; ask about sexual activity, and/or use of condoms or spermicides
      (a) Suprapubic pain
      (b) Urinary frequency and dysuria
      (c) Flank pain and/or low back pain
      (d) Vaginal discharge
II. *Complicated* UTI in child > 2 yr of age
   A. Usually involves *upper urinary tract*
   B. Causes
      1. Usually related to *Enterococcus* species and *E. coli* species
      2. Urinary tract or neurologic dysfunction requiring intermittent catheterization
   C. Signs and symptoms most consistent with pyelonephritis
      1. Usually same as lower urinary tract but more acute in nature
      2. *Fever* ≥ 39°C (102.2°F) with chills and *flank pain*
      3. N/V, abdominal pain, CVA tenderness
      4. Hematuria
III. Diagnostic testing
   A. Urinalysis (see Table 4.1) obtained by
      1. *Clean catch*, with parent's assistance if needed, for potty-trained children or adolescents
      2. *Pediatric bag* (empty immediately into specimen collection bottle)
      3. *Catheter-obtained* specimen if not potty trained and immediate specimen is needed
   B. Testing results that may indicate UTI
      1. Urine dipstick test (approximately 88% sensitive): positive leukocyte esterase, nitrites
      2. Centrifuged microscopy: considered positive with pyuria (≥ 5 WBC/hpf) and/or bacteriuria (any amount)
      3. Urine culture is the gold standard for UTI; considered positive if
         (a) Clean-catch specimen: ≥ 100,000 CFU/mL of any bacteria
         (b) Catheterized specimen: ≥ 50,000 CFU/mL of any bacteria; if growth between 10,000 and 50,000 CFU/mL is present, repeat test and if > 10,000 CFU/mL and presence of pyuria on dipstick, then treat for UTI
         (c) Suprapubic specimen: ≥ 1000 CFU/mL of any bacterial growth
IV. Treatment
   ▲ A. **Urgent transfer to ED if the patient is *< 3 mo of age* or appears toxic, is not feeding or taking fluids, has vomiting, or has fever > 37.8°C (100°F) with evidence of recent UTI**
   B. Nonpharmacological treatment
      1. Increase fluid intake; decrease carbonated/caffeinated drink and juice intake.
      2. Cranberry juice at hs; may not be beneficial but not harmful.
      3. Avoid bubble baths.
      4. Encourage all-cotton underwear and removal of wet clothing and swimsuits immediately after use.

▲ = *urgent referral*

5. Good perineal hygiene, clean well after stooling and change diapers/pull-ups frequently.
6. If sexually active, encourage condom use.

C. Pharmacological treatment
1. Length of treatment
   (a) Uncomplicated UTI (immunocompetent and afebrile): 3–5 days
   (b) Complicated or recurrent UTI: 7–10 days
2. Antibiotics: ideally guided by C/S results, but if not available, consider one of the following
   (a) Cefuroxime (Ceftin) 15–30 mg/kg/day ÷ bid
   (b) Cefpodoxime (Vantin) 5–10 mg/kg/day ÷ bid
   (c) Cefixime (Suprax) 4–8 mg/kg *once* daily
   (d) Cefdinir (Omnicef) 14 mg/kg *once* daily
   (e) If low risk for *E. coli* species resistance in community and no renal involvement consider: cephalexin (Keflex) 50–100 mg/kg/day ÷ q12h
   (f) If considering *S. saprophyticus*: TMP-SMX (Bactrim) 4–6 mg/kg/day (of trimethoprim) ÷ bid
3. For fever or pain, see Appendices C and D.

D. Follow-up in 24–48 hr
1. If improving, no further testing is needed.
2. If no improvement but not worsening, repeat urine C&S.

E. *Referral*
1. *To a urologist*
   (a) *First UTI in boys and second UTI in girls; consider renal/bladder ultrasound: if normal, a referral may not be necessary unless recurrent UTI*
   (b) *All children with gross hematuria*
   (c) *All children ≤ 2 yr of age with complicated UTI should be referred to urologist after initiation of treatment.*
2. *To a nephrologist with*
   (a) *Renal abnormality or impaired function*
   (b) *Increased BP*
   (c) *Any type of known bowel/bladder dysfunction*

Gynecological Conditions

LABIAL ADHESIONS

I. Description
A. Not seen in newborns because of increased circulating maternal estrogen
B. Most common between 2 and 6 yr of age, after circulating estrogen hormones from birth have started to decline.
C. Cause may be unknown or may be from chronic inflammation (e.g., bubble baths, harsh soaps, over cleaning after diaper changes) or other types of recurrent trauma (child sexual abuse).

II. Signs and symptoms
A. Urinary dribbling, recurrent vulvovaginitis, or recurrent UTIs

---

● = *non-urgent referral*

B. Adhesion of the labia minora is usually seen in upper or lower one-third of the vaginal opening; vaginal opening may not be visualized but urethral opening should be visible, even if it is very small.

C. The skin involving labial minora can be pinkish-red to pale pink.

III. Diagnostic testing with ultrasound should be considered if genital anomalies, masses, or fusion of the labia majora are present; these may be indicative of absence of the uterus or of ambiguous sexual organs.

IV. Treatment

A. ***Do not forcefully try to separate the labia.***

B. Watchful waiting is recommended unless symptoms interfere with urination; this may resolve spontaneously when estrogen levels increase at puberty.

C. If treatment is indicated
1. Apply topical estradiol cream 0.01% to labial adhesion along thin white line twice daily for 2–8 wk, until the adhesion starts to resolve; *gently* apply with fingertip.
2. If estradiol cream fails, can use betamethasone cream 0.05% topically bid for 4–6 wk; *gently* apply with fingertip.
3. Frequency of application can be decreased as the adhesion resolves.

D. Once the labia separate, use emollient cream (e.g., A&D ointment or Aquaphor) 3–5 times daily for several months to allow healing and prevent recurrence.

V. ***Referral to a pediatrician or pediatric gynecologist if adhesions do not resolve or recur.***

VULVOVAGINITIS

I. Description: inflammation to the vulvar area that can involve the entire perineal area; most common genital condition in prepubertal children

II. Common causes

A. Poor perineal hygiene, improper wiping after BM, and tight clothing

B. Irritation from bubble baths; dirt or sand from sandbox imbedding in the folds of the labia or groin

C. Insertion of foreign objects into the vagina

D. Hypoestrogenic state, atopic dermatitis, lichen sclerosis

E. Viral and bacterial infections

F. Sexual abuse

G. Pinworms, scabies, or lice

III. Signs and symptoms

A. Burning, itching, vaginal discharge, bleeding, dysuria

B. Labia may be excoriated and red with rash, ulcers or bruising.

C. Vaginal discharge
1. Foul odor with greenish discharge or recurrent infection: suspect a foreign object or bacterial infection
2. White thickened discharge without odor: suspect *Candida*
3. Yellow color with excoriations: suspect secondary skin infection from scratching (*Staphylococcus or Streptococcus* species)

IV. Diagnostic testing should include the following

A. STI testing with NAAT swab or urine for GC/CT/Trichomoniasis

B. Anaerobic and aerobic culture for specific bacteria or *Candida* (*Candida* is rare in children unless they are immunocompromised)

C. Swab for *Streptococcus pyogenes* (group A *streptococcus*) infection

---

■ = ***not to be missed;*** ● = ***non-urgent referral***

    D. Urinalysis for occult infection (may need to obtain a catheter specimen to avoid discharge contamination)
- V. Nonpharmacological treatment
  - A. Proper hygiene
    1. Teach child to void with knees apart facing stool (if able) to reduce reflux of urine into vagina
    2. Wiping front to back and rinsing after voiding/stooling
    3. Use hair dryer on lowest setting at least 12″ from perineal area after exposure to water
    4. Avoidance of all irritants (e.g., bubble baths, scented soaps)
  - B. Sitz baths with cool water to ease itching and pain
  - C. All-cotton, loose-fitting clothing; do not leave wet clothing or bathing suits on for any length of time
  - D. Nonmedicated ointment to protect the vulvar skin (e.g., Vaseline, zinc oxide)
- VI. Pharmacological treatment
  - A. May need OTC hydrocortisone cream to relieve itching and decrease irritation.
  - B. Consider antibiotic treatment, especially if there is purulent vaginal discharge or no resolution of symptoms (could be caused by bacterial infection)
    1. Cephalexin (Keflex) 40 mg/kg ÷ bid for 10–14 days
    2. Amoxicillin 50 mg/kg ÷ bid for 10–14 days
    3. Azithromycin (Zmax) 12 mg/kg day 1, then 6 mg/kg days 2–4
- **VII. *Referral to a pediatric gynecologist for further evaluation, possibly under anesthesia, to identify the cause.***

Hematopoietic System Conditions

IRON-DEFICIENCY ANEMIA (SEE CHAPTER 4, ANEMIA, VII)

- I. Description: the most common nutritional deficiency found in infants and children usually due to
  - A. Inability to meet iron needs secondary to rapid growth
  - B. Poor intake of iron-fortified foods/formulas
  - C. Intake of whole cow's milk before 12 mo of age or over consumption of cow's milk (> 20 oz/day) after 12 mo of age (causes microscopic blood loss from the GI tract)
- II. HPI
  - A. Is the child formula or breastfed?
    1. What type of formula and how much in 24 hr?
    2. How many times a day does the infant breast feed and for how long?
  - B. If breastfed, have they ever been given iron-fortified cereals or high iron foods? Did infant start on iron supplementation at 6 mo of age while breastfeeding?
  - C. Any multivitamins or iron supplements given? If so, which ones and for how long?
  - D. Does the child drink whole milk, goat's milk, or plant-based milk? At what age did parent switch to whole milk or milk supplements? How many ounces daily?
  - E. Is the child eating any meat products or iron-fortified foods? Does the child eat a vegetarian diet and how strictly is that followed (iron from plants is poorly absorbed as compared to meat-based products)?
  - F. Any history of anemia for the child or in the family? Any FH of sickle cell anemia (SCA), Thalassemia, or G6PD (i.e., genetic error in metabolism that increases RBC breakdown)?

● = *non-urgent referral*

III. Signs and symptoms
    A. Pica; irritability, tachycardia
    B. Pallor, fatigue, blue sclera
    C. Refusing solid foods, poor feeding habits, and anorexia
    D. Delayed mental and physical development if anemia persists
    E. Increased number of infections
IV. Diagnostic testing
    A. Screening Hgb (consider ferritin if anemia suspected) can be considered at 9 mo of age, between 12 and 24 mo of age, and between 11 and 15 yr of age. Test is positive for iron deficiency anemia if
        1. < 5 yr of age: ferritin < 15 μg/L; Hgb < 11.0 g/dL
        2. 5 to < 12 yr of age: ferritin < 15 μg/L; Hgb < 11.5 g/dL
    B. Lead level testing at 12 and 24 mo of age or if lead exposure is suspected
    C. If anemic, consider additional testing: CBC, reticulocyte count, blood smear (also, ferritin, if not previously done with Hgb)
V. Treatment (see Chapter 4, **ANEMIA, VII**)
    A. Infant
        1. Breastfed: start supplementation at 6 mo of age with 1 mg/kg/day of oral iron until intake of iron foods is adequate to maintain iron levels (see Appendix A for list of iron-fortified foods).
        2. Formula-fed: start iron-fortified foods at 4–6 mo of age and continue until 12 mo of age (see Appendix A for list of iron-fortified foods).
        3. Avoid whole milk if < 12 mo of age; whole milk is irritating to the colon and causes microscopic chronic blood loss.
    B. Toddler/children: if not encouraged to eat iron-fortified foods (see Appendix A), should be given supplemental iron in multivitamin or oral iron supplements.
        1. *Iron from food intake*
           (a) 1–3 yr of age: about 7 mg/day
           (b) 3–9 yr of age: about 10 mg/day
           (c) 9–13 yr of age: about 8 mg/day
        2. *Iron supplements* are given for 3–6 mo; give between meals and with water or orange juice; do not give with milk or milk products.
           (a) Ferrous sulfate 3 mg/kg/day 2–3 times a day
           (b) Ferrous gluconate 3–6 mg/kg/day 2–3 times a day
           (c) If child can chew multivitamins, start children's multivitamin with iron daily.
        3. Limit whole milk in toddlers < 3 yr of age to about 20 oz daily.
    C. Adolescents: monitor closely due to self-induced dietary restrictions; history of anemia; heavy, irregular menstrual cycles. Rapid growth at this age will deplete iron stores faster than replacement can occur.
        1. Supplementation should provide about 60–300 mg elemental iron; give for 3 mo
           (a) Multivitamins with iron (e.g., Flintstones with iron) bid
           (b) Oral iron products 1–2 tabs daily
               (i) Ferrous sulfate 65–130 mg of elemental iron
              (ii) Ferrous gluconate 300 mg of elemental iron
        2. Iron is best absorbed on an empty stomach given with orange juice (e.g., vitamin C enhances absorption of iron).
        3. Decreased uptake with antacids, milk products, or caffeinated beverages.
    D. Follow-up Hgb and ferritin should be done 3 mo after starting supplement.

●   **VI.** *Referral to hematologist if anemia does not improve with adequate iron replacement.*

Musculoskeletal System Conditions

LIMPING CHILD

I. Description: Asymmetrical jerky, clumsy gait while walking or running
II. Possible causes of limp by age
   A. < 3 yr of age
      1. Infection/osteomyelitis/septic arthritis (e.g., hip, knee, or foot/ankle)
      2. Occult trauma (e.g., physical abuse) or toddlers' fracture
      3. Developmental dysplasia of hip (DDH)
      4. Malignancy (e.g., sarcoma, leukemia)
      5. Toe-walking (e.g., cerebral palsy [CP] with tight Achilles tendon) and leg length discrepancy (e.g., hip or knee dysplasia)
      6. Neuromuscular disease (e.g., CP, muscular dystrophy)
   B. > 3–10 yr of age
      1. Infection/osteomyelitis (e.g., hip, knee, or foot/ankle)
      2. Legg-Calve-Perthes disease (LCP)
      3. Juvenile RA (JRA)
      4. Trauma (innocent or abuse)
      5. Malignancy
      6. Foot deformity and torsion variances with hip/knee/foot
      7. Back pain/injury/inflammation
      8. Leg length discrepancy
   C. > 10 yr of age
      1. Avascular necrosis of femoral head secondary to trauma
      2. Overuse injury (e.g., sports injury to soft tissues or Osgood-Schlatter disease)
      3. Juvenile rheumatoid arthritis (JRA)
      4. Neuromuscular disease (e.g., CP, muscular dystrophy)
      5. Gonococcal septic infections
      6. Slipped capital femoral epiphysis (SCFE); more common in overweight boys
      7. Trauma secondary to abuse (e.g., at home or school)
      8. Malignancy
III. HPI
   A. How long has the limp been present?
      1. Recent limp could indicate acute infection.
      2. Chronic limp could indicate overuse injury or systemic disease.
   B. Any known trauma that could cause the limp?
   C. Any past or current fevers and how long did the fever last? Is it resolved with antipyretic?
   D. Type of pain with limp
      1. Constant, localized pain that worsens with activity is usually fracture.
      2. Intermittent or migrating pain
         (a) JRA
         (b) Legg-Calve-Perthes
         (c) Slipped capital femoral epiphysis
         (d) Osgood-Schlatter

● = *non-urgent referral*

3. Referred pain (e.g., pain in knee is sometimes referred from the hip)
4. Nocturnal pain could indicate neoplastic process.
5. Bilateral pain may indicate viral illness.
6. Gait preference (e.g., will only crawl or knee walk because of pain below the knee)
7. Lateral thigh pain could indicate lumbar injury.

IV. Physical examination
   A. Always examine and palpate the joint above and below the painful site and compare to opposite side.
   B. Observe gait with child wearing minimal clothing and on a flat surface, to determine type of gait abnormality.
      1. Normal gait
         (a) < 7 yr of age: gait has a shorter stride and faster cadence
         (b) > 7 yr of age: gait is smoother and has rhythmic cadence (adult gait)
      2. Antalgic gait
         (a) Short-stepping to avoid painful extremity
         (b) Refusing to walk to prevent pain
      3. Short-limb gait noted with toe-walking.
      4. Trendelenburg gait is seen when child shifts weight over affected hip to balance the center of gravity; causes no pain.
      5. Spastic or scissoring gait occurs with weakened quad muscles and hamstring tightness or hypertonic hip adductors.
   C. Inspect skin for any open wounds, bruising, swelling, heat, or redness.
   D. Palpate entire affected extremity; check ROM and strength (look for any atrophic or weak areas).
   E. Test for leg length discrepancy
      1. Galeazzi test
      2. Assess gluteal folds
   F. Test for sacroiliac pain with FABER test.
   G. Palpate abdomen for mass or infection.
   H. Inspect/palpate GU for testicular torsions.
   I. Test sensation and reflexes on both sides.
   J. Evaluate neurological development.

V. Diagnostic tests
   A. CBC (looking for anemia, increased WBC and platelet), ESR/CRP (looking for inflammation), LDH/alkaline phosphatase (looking for malignancy), ANA (looking for rheumatic disease)
   B. Ultrasound of painful joint (checking for hip/knee effusion)
   C. X-ray of painful joint(s)
      1. Frog-leg for suspected diagnosis of Developmental Dysplasia of Hip, Legg-Calve-Perthes, Slipped Capital Femoral Epiphysis
      2. Specific joint for occult fracture (may need to get opposing joint for comparison)
   D. MRI of painful joint(s) for evaluation of osteomyelitis and stress fractures

VI. *Referral*
   ▲ A. *Urgent referral to ED if symptoms are acute and child is in distress.*
   ● B. *Referral to orthopedist or neurologist for more chronic conditions.*

▲ = *urgent referral;* ● = *non-urgent referral*

OSGOOD-SCHLATTER DISEASE

    I. Description: painful, self-limiting injury noted at the tibial tubercle (anterior knee) with swelling involving the patellar tendon where it attaches to the tibia; usually starts in adolescence and is *associated with overuse activity* (e.g., heavy sports involvement)

    II. Signs and symptoms

        A. Most commonly unilateral knee pain with swelling and tenderness below the patella

            1. Exacerbated with strenuous activity (e.g., running, jumping, kneeling)

            2. May limit preferred activity

        B. Pain is relieved with rest.

        C. Symptoms develop over time (i.e., not acute) and no permanent disability.

        D. Most symptoms will completely resolve after the bone stops growing or if causative activity stops.

        E. May have swelling over the patellar tendon indefinitely due to callous formation, but no pain.

    III. Treatment

        A. Conservative treatment after strenuous activity using ice for 20–30 min, 2–3 times daily

        B. NSAIDs for pain relief (may not shorten the course)

        C. Consider wearing neoprene knee support or protective pad over knee.

        D. Quadriceps and hamstring stretching exercises may reduce tension on the tibial tubercle.

        E. Physical therapy for strengthening exercises for the quadriceps and to improve hamstring suppleness

    IV. *Referral*

        A. *Urgent pediatric orthopedist with antalgic gait, swelling with redness/heat, or if fever develops.*

        B. *Pediatric orthopedist or sports medicine specialist if the symptoms are not improving.*

SCOLIOSIS

    I. Description: a spinal deformity with a lateral curvature of the spine combined with vertebral rotation; usually painless and can cause disability if severe; if slight, the child may not think anything is wrong and may only notice that clothing does not fit correctly.

    II. Screening: early screening physical examinations should start in the fifth to seventh grades (10–12 yr of age in girls and 13–14 yr of age in boys)

        A. Maintain privacy, use good lighting, and for optimal results, use an inclinometer/scoliometer to determine the amount of angle present.

        B. Have the child stand in front of you with minimal clothing and observe the posture and physical proportions. The child's head should align over the sacrum; observe the shoulder height, scapula position and prominence, waistline symmetry, and levelness of the pelvis.

            1. Deviation represents curvature, especially with asymmetry of the scapula, waistline, or rib humps

            2. A tall, thin person may have Marfan syndrome if scoliosis occurs with long sweeping right thoracic curve and left lumbar curve, pectus excavatum, and arm span greater than height.

▲ = *urgent referral;* ● = *non-urgent referral*

C. The Adam's forward-bending test with the child standing is a good test to determine vertebral rotation:
 1. Have the child bend forward at the waist while standing with feet together, knees straight, and arms hanging free; view the child's back from the side and back; a visible rib hump is caused by convexity of ribs and suggests vertebral rotation.
 2. Inspect the chest for deformity in the rib cage or sternum.
D. *Full spinal X-rays* are needed to confirm scoliosis using Cobb angle test for degree of angle and to denote where the curvature(s) is located (most common is the right thoracic curve)
E. *Referral to a pediatric orthopedist with any of the following:*
 1. *School, or office screening shows angle of trunk rotation ≥ 7 degree curve noted with scoliometer*
 2. *New onset of curvature*
 3. *Worsening curvature ≥ 5 degree per yr with scoliometer*

Neurological Conditions

ATTENTION-DEFICIT HYPERACTIVITY DISORDER (ADHD)/ATTENTION-DEFICIT DISORDER (ADD)

 I. Description: defined by developmentally inappropriate degrees of inattention, impulsiveness, and hyperactivity. These symptoms affect the child's entire life.
 A. Parental reports of child's behavior and symptoms for at least 6 mo that occur often; onset before 12 yr of age with inattentiveness, hyperactiveness, or impulsiveness; must occur in at least two settings and affect their ability to function at home, in school and in social settings.
 B. If the child exhibits at least two of the following, recommend standardized testing with a psychologist trained in this type of testing.
  1. Often fails to finish projects and homework; does not pay attention to detail and makes simple mistakes on school or work
  2. Needs a lot of supervision for completion of projects, cannot stay seated, and talks excessively
  3. Has difficulty concentrating on tasks; difficulty organizing tasks; loses things necessary for completion of tasks
  4. Easily distracted by extraneous stimuli and forgetful of scheduled daily activities
  5. Is always on the "go" and often acts before thinking; goes from one activity to another rapidly
  6. Oftentimes interrupts or intrudes into others' personal space
  7. Often does not seem to listen when spoken to directly
  8. Unable to take part in leisure activities
 II. Diagnostic testing includes
 A. CBC, TSH, and lead screening
 B. Psychological testing
 III. Education points to review with parents
 A. Behavioral modification techniques (first-line treatment for preschool children)
 B. Encourage firm, realistic, and environmental limits
 C. Review routines for medications and attendance at appointments.
 D. Medications may be needed if behavioral therapy sessions do not correct the behaviors.

● = *non-urgent referral*

E. Citric acid and vitamin C significantly impair the absorption of stimulants; *do not* eat products containing these agents 1 hr before or after medication (e.g., citrus fruit and juice, toaster pastries, most carbonated beverages, granola/breakfast bars, high-vitamin cereals, oral suspension medicines).

F. All children on medications with diagnosis of ADHD/ADD should be involved in behavioral therapy and routine counseling.

G. All children on medications should be reevaluated on a routine basis using an ADHD-specific rating scale to evaluate their progress.

H. Refer for special education, if needed.

IV. Pharmacological treatment
   A. When to start medications
     1. Psychological testing confirms ADHD/ADD
     2. Child is at least 6 yr of age
     3. Parents and school accept the responsibility in monitoring and giving medication.
     4. Child has no underlying medical or psychological problems.
     5. No perceived problem in household regarding substance abuse
   B. Amphetamine/dextroamphetamine stimulant class (all are Schedule II)
     1. Adderall and Adderall XR
     2. Vyvanse
     3. Dexedrine
   C. Methylphenidate stimulant class (may be better for preschool children) (all are Schedule II)
     1. Focalin and Focalin XR
     2. Concerta
     3. Ritalin
     4. Daytrana transdermal
   D. Nonstimulants
     1. Atomoxetine (Strattera)
     2. Viloxazine (Qelbree)
   E. Alpha-2-adrenergic agonists (used with poor response to stimulants/nonstimulants)
     1. Guanfacine (Intuniv)
     2. Clonidine

  ● V. *Referral to a psychologist for testing of child and counseling (both individual and family) or psychiatrist for further evaluation or treatment and comanagement*

MIGRAINE HEADACHE (ALSO SEE CHAPTER 12, HEADACHES, V, B)

I. Description
   A. Acute onset, occurs episodically and lasts 2–72 hr without treatment and occurs about 8 times/mo
     1. Pain is usually bilateral, worsens with activity, and is throbbing in nature.
     2. Pain is usually shorter duration than adults, but at least 2 hr.
     3. <10% have an aura
     4. May have N/V, photophobia, or phonophobia
     5. Common to have first-degree relative with migraine headache history

---

● = *non-urgent referral*

     6. Incidence
       (a) < 12 yr of age: can be seen in boys and girls equally
       (b) > 12 yr of age: girls > boys 3:1
  B. Chronic migraine
    1. Most common in 12–14 yr of age
    2. Occurs ≥ 15 days/mo

II. Signs and symptoms
  A. Early symptoms (prodrome)
    1. Fatigue; pallor and dark areas around eyes
    2. Changes in behavior (e.g., irritability, euphoria)
    3. Neck stiffness; frequent yawning
    4. Bowel/bladder changes
  B. Aura phase (if applicable)
    1. Visual changes (may see things that aren't there)
    2. Scotoma and changes in visual fields (e.g., jagged lines, crescent shapes)
    3. Sensory symptoms with tingling in body/extremities
    4. Motor symptoms with one-sided weakness or ataxia
  C. Headache phase
    1. Young preverbal children may have pallor, sudden decrease in activity, or vomiting.
    2. Young children may have frontal pain and teens may have bitemporal pain.
    3. N/V and photophobia; nasal congestion or rhinorrhea; fullness in ears
    4. Child wants a quiet dark room and to sleep.
  D. Postheadache
    1. May feel increased fatigue and increased thirst and hunger
    2. Ocular pain, brain fogginess

III. Diagnostic testing
  A. MRI if indicated
    1. Worsening H/A, visual changes; pain awakens child at night
    2. Neurological symptoms of ataxia, numbness, or tingling
  B. Laboratory testing for any systemic complaint (e.g., fever, fatigue)

IV. Nonpharmacological treatment
  A. Lifestyle changes for acute onset or preventative migraine headache
    1. Consistent sleep times, for at least 8 hr a night
    2. Regularly scheduled meals and between-meal snacks; decrease caffeine and high-sugar-content foods/drinks
    3. Adequate fluid intake to prevent dehydration, especially with high-intensity sports/activity
    4. Avoid triggers (see Table 12.1).
    5. Keep headache diary to try to pinpoint triggers.
    6. Screen for depression and anxiety.
    7. Allow time in dark, quiet room when H/A occurs, use rescue medications as quickly as possible to prevent H/A continuing.
  B. Pharmacological *treatment* for acute migraine (for infrequent attacks at onset of symptoms)
    1. *Step one* for > 5 yr of age
      (a) Acetaminophen 15 mg/kg/dose and may repeat once in 2–4 hr *or*
      (b) Ibuprofen 10 mg/kg/dose and may repeat once in 4–6 hr *or*
      (c) Naproxen 5 mg/kg and can repeat in 8 hr; *can add*
      (d) Antiemetic: promethazine 0.25–0.5 mg/kg per dose (good safety profile)

2. *Step two*
   (a) *> 6 yr of age* (< 50 kg)
      (i) Sumatriptan (Imitrex) 3–6 mg *SC* or 5 mg *nasal spray* may repeat in 1–2 hr
      (ii) Rizatriptan (Maxalt) < 40 kg: 5 mg tab or ODT; > 40 kg: 10 mg tab or ODT; *one time only* (decrease dose if taking propranolol)
   (b) *> 12–17 yr of age*
      (i) Almotriptan 6.25–12.5 mg tab; may repeat in 2 hr
      (ii) Zolmitriptan (Zomig) 2.5 mg nasal spray; may repeat in 2 hr
      (iii) Sumatriptan/naproxen (Treximet) 10/60 mg tab *one time only*
3. *Step three*: can combine a triptan with promethazine 0.25–0.5 mg/kg/dose; tab/IM *one time only*

C. Pharmacological *prevention* (daily medications to decrease number of attacks; these are not abortive medications)
   1. Cyproheptadine (Periactin) 2–8 mg hs (monitor for weight gain)
   2. Propranolol (Inderal) 1 mg/kg/day ÷ tid (monitor BP, HR; avoid with depression or asthma) or atenolol (Tenormin) 0.3 mg/kg once daily
   3. Amitriptyline 0.25–0.5 mg/kg *or* nortriptyline 0.25 mg to 1 mg/kg at hs (obtain baseline and annual ECG [if higher doses are taken] and monitor for weight gain, dry mouth, and dizziness)
   4. Topiramate 25 mg at hs (for children > 12 yr of age); monitor for weight loss and cognitive slowing
   5. Riboflavin (vitamin B2) 25–400 mg daily (will turn urine bright yellow; not harmful)
   6. Magnesium oxide 15 mg/kg/day ÷ tid
   7. Melatonin 3 mg/kg/dose at hs

● **V.** *Referral to pediatric neurologist who specializes in headache treatment if unable to control either acute or chronic migraine pain.*

CHAPTER 17

Psychiatric Conditions

INITIAL OFFICE VISIT

I. Nurse practitioners must be constantly aware that as many as 50% of patients who are seen in a primary care setting may have psychiatric symptoms and that depression is common with many comorbid conditions (e.g., DM, CV disease, CVA, chronic pain, COPD, cancer). Many patients may be unable to accurately describe physical symptoms or attribute them to psychological issues/stressors that occur over a period of time; family interviews may be necessary to determine the symptoms and behavioral changes.

II. History: in addition to the typical questions asked during a routine history, questions that at times seem too personal but provide essential information may need to be asked. Patients and families are often guarded in their answers because of embarrassment or fear of judgment. Reassure the patient of confidentiality and of the importance of the questions, and then note the following regarding the CNS to rule out an organic disease:
   A. H/A: recent onset or change
   B. Vision: recent deterioration, blurring, or spots in vision; hallucinations
   C. Hearing: recent deterioration or changes related to sound (e.g., tinnitus, hearing voices)
   D. Speech: any recent difficulty or change (e.g., muffled, garbled, uncontrollable speech); Does the patient ramble on or focus on the topic? Does the patient swear, joke, or mimic another's words or actions (where this is not usual behavior for the patient)?
   E. Writing: any recent difficulty or change from previous functioning
   F. Memory: recent changes in both long-term and short-term memory
   G. Gait: recent change (e.g., shuffling, ataxia, waddling, dragging a limb)
   H. Dexterity: inability to grab objects, clumsiness
   I. Sensation: any unusual sensations (e.g., things crawling on the skin, brief burning pain, pins and needles)
   J. Strength: recent weakness in any limb, asymmetric grip strength
   K. Consciousness: history of blackouts or periods of time that cannot be accounted for
   L. Body movements: uncontrollable body movements (e.g., tongue biting, seizures, athetoid movements)
   M. Substance use: use of drugs or alcohol for relief of symptoms, anxiety, or nervousness; use of OTC or herbal products
   N. Family history (FH) of any psychiatric conditions or substance abuse

III. Mental status interview: *be alert for cues that something is not quite right* (e.g., inappropriate clothes, facial expression, verbal utterances, body language).
   A. Is the patient's affect inappropriate (e.g., laughing at sad events, weeping when others are happy)?
   B. During the history and physical examination, a mental status interview and evaluation for depression should be conducted.
   C. Use standardized instruments such as PHQ-2 and PHQ-9 (see Chapter 3, Fig. 3.1; also see www.phqscreeners.com/pdfs/02_PHQ-9/English.pdf).

IV. Diagnostic tests: relevant tests for a psychiatric disorder should include the following:
  A. CBC with differential, ESR
  B. CMP, vitamin B12 level
  C. TSH (with depressive or anxiety disorders)
  D. EEG (with seizures or sleep apnea)
  E. ECG (as baseline, for elderly patients and patients taking heart medications or tricyclic antidepressant [e.g., amitriptyline])
  F. Urinalysis (especially with elderly patients) and urine HCG (when appropriate)
  G. Urine drug screen

ANXIETY

  I. Description: anxiety is a normal reaction if it is aroused by realistic danger, if the reaction is appropriate to the threat, and if the anxiety disappears when the threat ceases. Anxiety that exceeds this definition is outside the patient's voluntary control and often renders the patient unable to function. Anxiety is among the most disabling diseases and frequently is a comorbid illness with depression, substance abuse, psychiatric disorders, and medical conditions
  II. Classification of anxiety disorders: the most common are generalized anxiety disorder (GAD), panic disorder, and posttraumatic stress disorder (PTSD)
  III. Signs/symptoms and treatment (according to the DSM-5 criteria)
  A. GAD
    1. Diagnosis/signs and symptoms
      (a) GAD is ruled out if the patient answers "no" to "Do you worry excessively about minor matters?"
      (b) Excessive and persistent worrying about a number of things occurring most days for ≥6 mo. The patient has difficulty controlling the worry (e.g., frequently thinking about "what if").
      (c) Associated with ≥3 of the following (only 1 is required in pediatrics):
        (i) Restlessness or feeling keyed up or on edge
        (ii) Fatigued easily
        (iii) Difficulty concentrating or remembering (e.g., "mind going blank")
        (iv) Irritability
        (v) Muscle tension
        (vi) Sleep disturbance
      (d) The symptoms cause significant distress or impairment in patient's life (e.g., may lead to difficulty making decisions).
      (e) The disturbance is *not* the result of a substance (e.g., excessive caffeine use or drug abuse) or other medical condition (e.g., hyperthyroidism).
    2. Treatment
      (a) The best option is an individualized plan combining the following: cognitive behavioral therapy, medications, long-term follow-up:
        (i) Some anxiety may be helpful, so a goal should be to make it manageable.
        (ii) Consider asking, "What can you do to make it lower, when you leave today?"
      (b) Pharmacological therapy
        (i) First line: SSRI or SNRI (see Table 17.1); if ineffective after a 4-wk trial, try a second medication before trying second-line medication.
        (ii) Second line: TCA (imipramine: see Table 17.1) or benzodiazepine or buspirone (Table 17.2). If using buspirone, increase dose q2 wk until maximum effective dose (safer than benzodiazepines)

Text continued on page 5

TABLE 17.1 ■ Common Antidepressants

	Starting Dose	Maintenance Dose	Sedation	Sexual Dysfunction*	Anticholinergic Effect	Approved Uses
Selective Serotonin Reuptake Inhibitors (SSRIs)						
Citalopram (Celexa)**	20mg qd	20–40	0	0/+++	0	Depression
Escitalopram (Lexapro)**	10mg qd	10–20	0	0/+++	0	GAD Depression
Fluoxetine (Prozac)**	20mg AM	10–80	0/+	0/+++	0	Depression Panic disorder OCD
Fluvoxamine (Luvox)	50mg hs	100–300	++	+/++	0	OCD
Paroxetine (Paxil)	20mg qd 10mg qd	10–60 12.5–62.5	++	++++	0/+	Depression OCD PTSD GAD
(Paxil CR)	25mg qd 12.5mg qd (panic)	Up to 62.5 Up to 75				
Sertraline (Zoloft)	50mg qd 25mg qd (panic and PTSD)	50–200	0	+++	0	Depression OCD Panic disorder PTSD
Serotonin Norepinephrine Reuptake Inhibitors (SNRIs)						
Desvenlafaxine (Pristiq)	50mg qd	100	+	+	0	Depression
Duloxetine (Cymbalta)	30–60mg qd	120	0	0/+	0	GAD Depression
Levomilnacipran (Fetzima)	20mg qd	120		0		Depression
Milnacipran (Savella)	25–50mg bid	100mg bid				Depression (off-label use)
Venlafaxine (Effexor) (Effexor XR)	37.5mg bid 37.5–75mg qd	75–225	0	+++	0	Depression GAD (XR only) Panic disorder

Continued

TABLE 17.1 ■ Common Antidepressants—cont'd

	Starting Dose	Maintenance Dose	Sedation	Sexual Dysfunction*	Anticholinergic Effect	Approved Uses
Tricyclic Antidepressants (TCAs)						
Amitriptyline (Elavil)	25 mg hs to 25 mg tid	40–150	++++	++	++++	Depression
Desipramine (Norpramin)	25 mg hs to 25 mg tid	50–300	+	+	+	Depression
Doxepin (Adapin, Sinequan)	75 mg hs or 25 mg tid	75–300	+++	++/+++	++/+++	Depression
Imipramine (Tofranil)	75 mg hs	50–200	++	++	++/+++	Depression
Nortriptyline (Aventyl, Pamelor)	25 mg hs to 25 mg tid	50–150	++	++	++	Depression
Miscellaneous						
Bupropion (Wellbutrin, Wellbutrin SR and XL)	100 mg bid 150 mg qd (XL only)	400–450	0	0	0	Depression SADD (XL only) ADHD (adult)
Mirtazapine (Remeron, Remeron SolTab)	15 mg hs	15–45	+++	0	+	Depression
Trazodone (Desyrel)	50 mg tid	50–400	++++	0	+	Depression
Vilazodone (Viibryd)**	10 mg qd	40	+	+/++	0	Depression
Vortioxetine (Trintellix)**	10 mg qd	20	0	0	0	Depression

0, none; +, slight; ++, moderate; +++, high; ++++, very high.

* Consider these options to help with sexual dysfunction, especially when it is a side effect of antidepressants: *Ginkgo biloba* 60–240 mg daily; bupropion SR 150 mg daily; Viagra 50–100 mg taken 1 hr before intercourse.

** Associated with low incidence of weight gain

TABLE 17.2 ■ **Common Anxiolytics**

Drug	Dosage Range (mg qd)	Half-Life of the Parent Drug (hr)
Benzodiazepines*		
Alprazolam (Xanax)	General: 0.25–4 Panic: 1.5–10	12–15
Chlordiazepoxide (Librium, Mitran)	5–100	30–100
Clonazepam (Klonopin)	1.5–4	18–50
Clorazepate (Tranxene)	7.5–60	36–200
Diazepam (Valium, Zetran)	4–40	50–100
Lorazepam (Ativan)	0.5–6	10–14
Oxazepam (Serax)	30–120	5–15
Miscellaneous		
Buspirone (Buspar)	15–60 (not for prn use)	48–72
Hydroxyzine (Atarax, Vistaril, others)	50–400	n/a

* Benzodiazepines have the potential for addiction.

    (iii) Consider propranolol 10 mg or hydroxyzine (Vistaril) 10 mg before anxiety-producing events (e.g., giving a talk or speaking in public).

    (iv) Gabapentin can help with anxiety (100 mg tid and titrate as needed); caution about possible dizziness for 1–2 wk, especially with head position changes.

    (v) With insomnia due to "mind racing," try hydroxyzine, imipramine, clomipramine, or amitriptyline at hs.

(c) Cautions with benzodiazepine use

    (i) FDA now requires boxed warnings, including abuse, dependence, and withdrawal.

    (ii) When benzodiazepines are started, there should be a plan in place for stopping them.

    (iii) Limit their use to the lowest dose, for the shortest time needed (e.g., for anxiety until SSRI or SNRI kicks in).

    (iv) Longer acting options (e.g., clonazepam) are probably better than alprazolam, which is faster acting but can cause rebound anxiety when it is wearing off.

    (v) *If using a benzodiazepine for a few weeks or more, taper to stop the medication. The longer the benzodiazepine is used, the slower the taper needs to be (maybe even over mo). Consider decreasing the dose by 25% the first week and then 10% each week after that.*

    (vi) Reassure the patient that withdrawal symptoms (e.g., anxiety, insomnia, sweating) are usually mild and short acting with a taper; the taper can be slowed if needed.

(d) Nonpharmacological therapy

    (i) Break-down overwhelming things into small, manageable steps; make a list, starting with easier steps.

■ = *not to be missed*

      (ii) Set boundaries on social media use and checking emails.

      (iii) Have the patient pick a 'worry time' (e.g., 30 min, from 5:00 PM to 5:30 PM [not near hs]), when they allow worry; any other time of the day, they put it off until the "worry time." At the end of the designated time, do something physical (e.g., cooking, working out).

      (iv) Progressive muscle relaxation, especially at hs, and diaphragmatic breathing (there are phone apps to guide this). Some patients like information on what is going on; explain "When you start getting anxious, the frontal part of your brain that makes decisions shuts down. Deep breathing for a few minutes 'turns the brain back on'."

   (e) Discourage ETOH and drug use (i.e., marijuana, illegal drugs) to help with anxiety; these can cause rebound anxiety, worsen any depression, and lead to addiction problems.

  3. Follow up in office

    (a) q2 wk while initiating therapy.

    (b) q3–4 mo while on maintenance therapy.

    (c) Continue medications for at least 6–12 mo.

    (d) If tapering off medications, follow up q3 mo until stable.

    (e) Follow up annually for evaluation of relapse of GAD.

  4. ***Referral to psychologist, psychiatrist, or psychiatric NP for management if the GAD is not controlled.***

B. Panic disorder

  1. Diagnosis: recurrent unexpected episodes of panic attacks

    (a) Discrete episodes of sudden-onset intense fear lasting minutes to an hour.

    (b) Often associated with

      (i) Chest pain, palpitations, tachycardia

      (ii) Shortness of breath, choking sensation

      (iii) Dizziness, trembling, or shaking

      (iv) Fear of "going crazy" or of dying

  2. Treatment

    (a) First line: cognitive behavioral therapy (CBT is an approach to help individuals recognize that feelings [emotions], thoughts, and behavior are connected; intervening on any of them affects the others. Behavioral interventions are the easiest to try to change.)

      (i) Relate a panic attack to a smoke alarm that sounds with smoke from burning food; it is a false protective alarm.

      (ii) Reassure the patient that it only lasts about 10 min and it will pass.

      (iii) Encourage diaphragmatic breathing (there are phone apps to help with this).

    (b) Pharmacological therapy

      (i) Patient is often given an SSRI or SNRI (see Table 17.1); paroxetine and venlafaxine are commonly used. The medication is ideally in addition to the CBT.

      (ii) Hydroxyzine 10 mg at the start of a panic attack may "break" it.

      (iii) Consider a benzodiazepine for the *first few weeks* until SSRI starts working (see Table 17.2; also **III., A.,** 2 c, earlier in chapter); taper benzodiazepine 10% per week to limit withdrawal symptoms and recurrent panic.

  3. ***Referral to a psychiatrist or psychiatric NP for management if not controlled.***

● = ***non-urgent referral***

C. PTSD
1. Description: results from the complex effects of psychological trauma (e.g., military combat, natural disasters, rape, abusive situations). It is characterized by
   (a) Recurrent thoughts, nightmares, and flashbacks
   (b) Avoiding reminders of the trauma
   (c) Hypervigilance and sleep disturbances
2. Treatment
   (a) *If considering this condition, refer to a psychiatrist or psychiatric NP because of the difficulty in diagnosis and complexity in management.*
   (b) SSRI or venlafaxine can be started until the patient can see the specialist; also consider prazosin 1 mg hs and titrate to 3–15 mg as tolerated for nightmares (do not stop this medication cold turkey).
   (c) Do not give benzodiazepines; there is no evidence they help PTSD and they may worsen recovery.
   (d) Avoid atypical antipsychotics - not much evidence they help. (see Table 17.3)

BIPOLAR DISORDER

I. Description: a chronic condition characterized by episodes of mania or hypomania and depression (specific criteria can be found in the DSM-5) and requiring long-term, continuous treatment
   A. There is likely a significant genetic component.
   B. Predisposing factors include FH of bipolar disorder or schizophrenia and personal history of drug or ETOH abuse.

II. Signs and symptoms
   A. Manic episodes last at least 1 wk and involve clinically significant changes in mood, behavior, energy, sleep, and cognition; examples include the following:
      1. Inability to sit still; intense overactivity in both body and mind
      2. Pressured speech pattern (often loud, inappropriate; often jumps from one subject to another)
      3. Mood lability (e.g., irritability, euphoria, suspiciousness)
      4. Cognitive abnormalities (e.g., poor concentration, racing thoughts, grandiosity, manipulativeness); psychosis with delusions and hallucinations; sleeplessness
      5. Hypersexuality and increase in risk-taking behaviors
      6. May be too hyperactive to eat or drink, causing fluid depletion and weight loss
   B. Episodes of major depression, hypersomnia, and weight gain follow manic episodes.
   C. If considering bipolar disorder, may screen the patient using a Mood Disorder Questionnaire (a good example can be found at www.integration.samhsa.gov/images/res/MDQ.pdf). This allows the patient to note their behaviors but also family history.

III. Treatment
   A. When interviewing the patient, talk in a calm, nonjudgmental manner.
   B. Best treated with mood stabilizer (i.e., atypical antipsychotic [see Table 17.3], which is indicated for both mania and depression phases); obtain baseline CMP and lipids.
   C. Monitor patient for development of extrapyramidal symptoms or tardive dyskinesia (see **V.** and **VI.**, following).
   D. Encourage patient to get at least 7–8 hr sleep each night, and to avoid caffeine and/or watching TV late at night.
   E. Encourage patient to see a professional counselor; place referral if necessary.
IV. *Referral to a psychiatrist or psychiatric NP if no improvement with medication.*

● = *non-urgent referral*

PRACTICE PEARLS FOR ATYPICAL ANTIPSYCHOTICS

- Uses
  - They are used for many conditions, including schizophrenia, as augmentation treatment for depression, as mood stabilizer for bipolar D/O.
  - They are not indicated for insomnia treatment (they do not help).
  - Use with dementia patients ONLY if they pose a danger to self or have disabling delusions and/or hallucinations. These meds are associated with an increased risk of CVA.
- Many of these medications can cause weight gain, dyslipidemia, or DM; monitor FBG (or A1c) and lipid levels when starting med, at 3 mo, and then at least yearly.
- Melatonin 3 mg daily has been shown to minimize the weight gain and metabolic effects associated with these medications.
- Also, note that high-dose first-generation antipsychotic agents are more likely to cause extrapyramidal symptoms and tardive dyskinesia (see V. and VI. respectively, following), although either can happen with the atypical agents as well.

TABLE 17.3 ■ Common Antipsychotics

Drug	Oral Dosage Range (Adult; mg qd)	Sedation	Extrapyramidal Side Effects	Weight Gain	Anticholinergic Effects
First Generation (Neuroleptics or Conventional Antipsychotics)					
Chlorpromazine (Thorazine)	30–800	+++	++	+++	++
Fluphenazine (Prolixin)	1–40	+	++++	+	+
Haloperidol (Haldol)	2–100 IM	0/+	++++	+	+
Thioridazine (Mellaril)	150–800	+++	+	++	+++
Second Generation (Atypical Antipsychotics)*					
Aripiprazole (Abilify)	5–30	+	0/+	+	0/+
Asenapine (Saphris, Secuado)	10–20	++	+/++	+	+
Brexpiprazole (Rexulti)	2–4	+	0	++	0/+
Cariprazine (Vraylar)	1.5–6	+/++	++	+	0/+
Clozapine† (Clozaril)	12.5–900 (usually 100–150)	+++	0/+	+++	+++
Iloperidone (Fanapt)	6–24	++	+	0	+
Lumateperone (Caplyta)	42	+	+	+	+
Lurasidone (Latuda)	20–120	+/++	++	+	0
Olanzapine (Zyprexa)	5–20	++	+	+++	++
Paliperidone (Invega)	3–12	+++	+++		0/+
Quetiapine (Seroquel)	50–800	++	0/+	+++	0/+
Risperidone (Risperdal)	4–16	+	+++	+++	0/+
Ziprasidone (Geodon)	40–160	++	+	+	+

0, none; +, slight; ++, moderate; +++, high.
* See **PRACTICE PEARLS FOR ATYPICAL ANTIPSYCHOTICS**.
† Monitor WBC count with differential weekly while the patient is undergoing therapy and for 4 wk after discontinuation.

V. Extrapyramidal symptoms (EPS)
  A. Description: *abnormal movements (see C., below) associated with the use of antipsychotic medication,* especially antipsychotics/neuroleptics (Table 17.3); patients with EPS are often at higher risk for developing tardive dyskinesia (see **VI.**, below)
  B. Acute onset very soon after starting medication (vs TD, which occurs months or more after starting medication).
  C. Types of EPS
    1. Akathisia (most common EPS)
      (a) Symptoms usually occur after the first dose: feeling of motor restlessness, accompanied by an inability to sit or stand still (e.g., repeated leg crossing, weight shifting).
      (b) Treatment
        (i) Cautious decrease in the dose of the offending medication.
        (ii) If inadequate, try benzodiazepines or propranolol.
    2. Parkinsonism (not related to Parkinson disease); usually seen in typical (first generation) antipsychotics
      (a) Symptoms may not occur for several weeks after medication started: masklike faces, drooling, resting tremors, cogwheel rigidity, or shuffling gait
      (b) Treatment
        (i) If uncomfortable or disabling, control with benztropine 1–2 mg bid for a few wk to 2–3 mo; then, reevaluate if the patient requires further treatment.
        (ii) Occasional dose reduction, drug discontinuation, or change in antipsychotic medication if needed.
    3. Dystonias
      (a) Symptoms: involuntary contractions of major muscle groups (e.g., torticollis, retrocollis, opisthotonos, oculogyric crisis [e.g., tongue protruding, sustained eye movement looking up or laterally]). The spasms can be brief or last for several hours and occur several times daily or weekly
      (b) Treatment
        (i) Symptoms usually occur within 4 days of starting medication and have a rapid onset; they are very disturbing to patients.
        (ii) May use benztropine 1–2 mg PO or diphenhydramine 50 mg IM or IV.
        (iii) *Referral or transfer to ED immediately.*
  D. Evaluation for EPS
    1. Evaluate when starting an antipsychotic medication, weekly until medication dose has been stable for ≥2 wk, and then at least q6mo thereafter.
    2. Use the same format each time for consistency; a commonly used test is the Abnormal Involuntary Movement Scale (AIMS) found at www.cqaimh.org/pdf/tool_aims.pdf.
    3. There is no "right" score; comparison of scores provides information on the development of involuntary movements (i.e., TD: see next section).
VI. Tardive dyskinesia (TD)
  A. Description: *characteristic involuntary movements (see B., below)*
    1. They usually appear within the first 6 mo on a antipsychotic/neuroleptic medication (see Table 17.3) or metoclopramide or chlorpromazine.
    2. Symptoms commonly appear with first-generation antipsychotics or after decreasing the dose, changing to a less potent medication, or stopping the medication.

■ = *not to be missed*; ▲ = *urgent referral*

B. Onset is often insidious and is *usually irreversible*. *Symptoms include sucking or smacking lips, facial grimacing, lateral jaw movements, protruding and twisting movements of the tongue, torticollis, and choreoathetoid movements (i.e., rapid, purposeless, spontaneous) of the extremities or trunk.*

C. Patients on antipsychotic medications should be evaluated at least q6mo (see AIMS, under Evaluation for EPS, earlier in the chapter); *the patient with EPS during acute treatment* may be at greater risk for TD.

D. Treatment
  1. *Do not* add an anticholinergic, such as benztropine (can worsen TD).
  2. Change to an atypical antipsychotic (low risk for TD); remission of TD may occur after several months off the offending medication, but often is irreversible, despite stopping the medication.
  3. *Consider referral to a psychiatrist or psychiatric NP.*

COGNITIVE IMPAIRMENT/DEMENTIA

I. Description
  A. "Normal" aging: mainly mild changes in memory and rate of processing new information, but these are not progressive and do not affect daily function
  B. With mild cognitive impairment and dementia: memory impairment is the primary complaint; other cognitive or behavior changes may also be present.

II. Evaluation
  A. The initial appointment
    1. Discussion of and evaluation for memory changes is usually stressful and/or embarrassing to the patient (and sometimes to the family). Do not mention dementia at this visit; the patient and family should come back for a follow-up visit to discuss test results and the diagnosis can be explained at that time.
    2. Focus on the history; a family member or someone who knows the patient well should also be present to give a history of cognitive and behavioral changes because the patient may not think there is anything wrong or notice any problems.
    3. Medication history (prescription and OTC) is very important, as many drugs can cause mental status changes.
    4. Perform a physical examination, including neurological examination; the neuro exam focuses on
      (a) Focal deficits that may indicate prior strokes
      (b) Signs of Parkinson disease [e.g., tremors, cogwheel rigidity]
      (c) Other changes with gait and eye movements
    5. Assess cognitive function with a screening test (dementia is strongly suspected when history and mental status examination agree)
      (a) Initially with a Mini-Cog test, which includes a clock drawing test (Box 17.1) and recall of 3 unrelated words (without any cueing)
      (b) If this test is positive, further evaluation is indicated at the follow-up visit (see below).
    6. To rule out reversible causes of dementia
      (a) Lab tests: CBC, vitamin B12 level, TSH and free T_4, and chemistry panel; depending on patient's history and medical condition, consider serum ammonia and RPR or VDRL

■ = *not to be missed;* ● = *non-urgent referral*

BOX 17.1 ■ Clock Test

The clock test is used to differentiate normal elderly aging from dementia.

Instructions

Ask the patient to draw a clock and put numbers in their correct positions. Have the patient draw hands indicating:
- 10 min after 11

OR
- 20 min after 8

Scoring

Patient receives 1 point for each of these criteria:
- Draws closed circle
- Places numbers in sequence
- Correct spatial arrangement
- Includes clock hands
- Places hands in the correct position

Results

Any score <5 indicates the need for further evaluation.

    (b) Consider noncontrast CT or MRI of the brain (subdural hematoma, brain tumor, Cryptococcus); see Table 4.2.

    (c) If indicated, carotid Doppler studies; possibly echocardiogram.

B. Follow-up appointments (individualized, based on how recent is the diagnosis and the patient's condition)

  1. Further evaluation of cognitive function; possible assessments include

    (a) AD8 Dementia Screening Interview can be completed by an informant in person or over the phone if necessary; it takes about 3 min.

    (b) Montreal Cognitive Assessment (MoCA) takes about 10 min to administer and can be found at www.mocatest.org; it is available in multiple languages.

  2. Repeat the same cognitive test at least yearly (it is very important to consistently use the same test, to accurately determine decline).

C. *Consider early referral for formal neuropsychological testing if unsure of the diagnosis* (to help detect cognitive changes of various types of dementia).

III. Mild cognitive impairment (MCI)

A. Description: memory difficulties but able to function in daily life; there is increased risk for dementia

B. Signs and symptoms

  1. Impaired memory (primary complaint), which is upsetting to the patient

  2. May also have depression, anxiety, irritability, apathy

  3. NO problems with ADLs

  4. Mild problems with word skills (e.g., "word search"), which is upsetting to the patient

C. Evaluation is used to establish the severity of impairment and provide a baseline

  1. The criteria are not precise; it may be difficult to determine what is normal impairment for the patient or what may indicate dementia.

  2. See **II.**, Evaluation, discussed earlier.

● = *non-urgent referral*

D. Treatment
   1. *No* pharmacologic therapy or dietary agents have been shown to help memory or lessen the chance of developing dementia (e.g., the Prevagen manufacturer has had to take claims of improved memory and cognition off of the labels).
   2. Because dementia is becoming referred to as "type 3 DM," screen for and treat vascular risk factors (e.g., HTN, DM, lipids, smoking).
   3. *Consider referral for formal neuropsychological testing; may refer to specialist with experience in MCI management if needed.*
   4. Diagnosis of MCI can help the patient and family be proactive in decisions about the future (e.g., financial plans, making a will, designating DPOA).
   5. Tips for helping with memory
      (a) Keep a routine; always put items in the same place (e.g., car keys).
      (b) Organize information on a calendar or day planner.
      (c) Relate new information to things already known.
      (d) Get full night's sleep.
      (e) Social interaction and "brain games" (e.g., sudoku, crossword puzzles) do not hurt but there is little evidence that they help.

IV. Dementia (also called major neurocognitive disorder)
   A. Description: chronic, progressive, significant cognitive impairment (as compared to previous level of functioning) in at least 1 of the following areas:
      1. Learning and memory
      2. Language and speaking clearly
      3. Social cognition reasoning (e.g., difficulty coping with unexpected events)
      4. Handling complex tasks (e.g., balancing the checkbook)
      5. Executive functioning: decision-making abilities and the ability to carry out plans
      6. Spatial ability/orientation (e.g., getting lost in familiar places)
   B. It does eventually affect ADLs.
   C. Dementia must be distinguished from delirium and depression (Table 17.4).
   D. Common types (Table 17.5): Alzheimer disease, vascular dementia, dementia with Lewy bodies (DLB), and frontotemporal lobe dementia (FTLD). It also results from chronic alcoholism or repeated head injuries (e.g., professional boxers).

TABLE 17.4 ■ Disorders of Cognition

Disorders	Symptoms
Dementia	Insidious onset; slowly progressive Impairment of memory More common in elderly
Delirium	Abrupt onset (review medications for any recent changes) Inattention and clouding of the sensorium Perceptual disturbances, hallucinations Anxiety, drowsiness; fluctuations in level of consciousness
Depression	Variable onset (may occur along with dementia) Normal memory but may have poor attention; more likely to complain of memory loss than patient with dementia No hallucinations May have anxiety, hopelessness

---

● = *non-urgent referral*

TABLE 17.5 ■ Common Dementias (also known as Neurocognitive Disorders)

	AD	VaD	DLB	FTLD
Course	Insidious onset and gradual progression Rare to occur before 65 yr of age	Onset depends on extent of cerebrovascular event Stepwise deterioration ("plateaus" between events)	Insidious onset; usually progresses quickly (compared to other types) Symptoms may be intermittent early in the disease	Insidious onset and gradual progression Progressive atrophy of frontal and temporal lobes primarily; personality and behaviors most affected Tends to occur at younger age (patient in their 60s)
Signs and symptoms	Earliest S/S is selective memory impairment Executive dysfunction often present relatively early (e.g., less multitasking, less organized, poor insight; they offer alibis/explanations for deficits With progression, behavior disturbances, wandering, apathy, sleep disturbances; late stage: gait disturbance, dysphagia, and incontinence Rare visual hallucination	Abilities affected depend on area of brain affected; may have significant cognitive problems before dementia develops Personality and mood changes Often becomes incontinent and unable to carry-out ADLs Depression often present	Cognitive dysfunctions are often presenting symptoms (e.g., driving difficulties, getting lost, impaired job performance) Usually affects areas of brain involving thinking and movement; symptoms are similar to Parkinson (rigidity; slow, shuffling movements) and AD Falls and syncope are common Visual hallucinations are common (distinguishes it from AD)	Memory and orientation to time not affected in the early stages May become withdrawn; disinhibited (losing ability to restrain behavior, e.g., public urination, touching or kissing strangers); delusions/hallucinations are NOT typical Progressive aphasia ranges from speaking less to echoing others' speech to being mute Can develop rigid food preferences and inflexibility to changes in routine
Evaluation	Brain MRI to rule out other possible diagnoses	MRI brain will show chronic ischemic changes	No diagnostic tests (clinical diagnosis) Early in disease: problems with clock drawing test and serial 7s	Primary psychiatric disorder should be ruled out (e.g., bipolar disorder, schizophrenia) Brief cognitive assessments often normal (early stage)

Continued

TABLE 17.5 ■ Common Dementias (also known as Neurocognitive Disorders)— cont'd

	AD	VaD	DLB	FTLD
Treatment points		No benefit with statins or antiplatelet agents Reducing risk factors for CVD inconsistently shown to affect the course of VaD	PT and mobility aids may help parkinsonism Cholinesterase inhibitors may help **Nearly 50% patients have life-threatening adverse reactions to atypical antipsychotics; DO NOT prescribe them** Sedatives can make the movement symptoms worse	Cholinesterase inhibitors are NO help For behaviors, consider SSRI (e.g., paroxetine 10 mg 1–2×qd) or trazodone 25 mg qd More susceptible to EPS, so cautious use of atypical antipsychotics Family and staff will need to have coping strategies to work around behavior rather than trying to get the patient to change
Other	Most common type Associated with amyloid plaques and neurofibrillary tangles in brain Often occurs with VaD	Second most common type; often occurs with AD or DLB Also called "multi-infarct" dementia ("little strokes")	Caused by protein deposits in neurons called Lewy bodies; unknown why or how they form Frequently co-exists with AD and VaD	Also called Pick disease Up to 40% are familial

AD, Alzheimer dementia; VaD, vascular dementia; DLB, Lewy body dementia; FTLD, frontotemporal lobe dementia.

■ = *not to be missed*

E. Treatment (mainstay of management is symptomatic, as there is no cure).

1. *If changes occur within 6 mo (e.g., independent 6–12 mo ago and now needs help): urgent referral to a specialist* (possible causes: vascular disease, Hashimoto thyroiditis, Creutzfeldt-Jakob disease, CA, vasculitis, cerebral infection)

2. Follow up in office at least q6mo, to monitor the patient's physical and cognitive abilities and the caregiver's coping ability

   (a) Repeat cognitive testing q1yr (see **II., B.**, Evaluation, earlier in this chapter).

   (b) Evaluate functional status with questions about ADLs (e.g., bathing, dressing) and instrumental ADLs (e.g., shopping for and preparing food, managing money). (See Table 3.11: The Vulnerable Elders Survey.)

   (c) Encourage end-of-life planning while the patient still has some cognitive function for decision-making (including appointing a POA for health care, discussing long-term care options, meeting with a certified financial advisor).

3. Neuropsychiatric symptoms include agitation, aggression, delusions, hallucinations, wandering, depression, apathy, disinhibition, and sleep disturbances; they lead to greater functional impairment

   (a) General treatment/prevention for behavior problems

      (i) Redirection is first-line treatment.

      (ii) Minimize changes in daily routines and establish a calm nighttime routine.

      (iii) Speak slowly and in a normal tone of voice.

      (iv) Do not disagree with the patient, respect their opinion.

      (v) Encourage physical activity and exercise (e.g., daily walk); this helps prevent physical decline and improves behavior problems.

   (b) With *unprovoked behavior changes*, evaluate for infection (e.g., UTI, pneumonia), pain, medication effects (especially anticholinergic, e.g., used to treat sleep or bladder incontinence), fear, boredom, hunger, thirst.

   (c) With increased agitation or aggression

      (i) Check for factors such as pain, constipation, hunger, or boredom; check to see if the environment has become cluttered (see Fig. 17.1 for Pain Assessment in Advanced Dementia Scale).

      (ii) *If patient poses severe risk of harm to self or others, consider hospitalization (potentially in geriatric psychiatric unit).*

      (iii) Aromatherapy, music therapy, and pet therapy may be beneficial.

      (iv) Consider Nuedexta if patient also has pseudobulbar affect; it is used off-label for agitation/aggression associated with Alzheimer's.

   (d) With delusions/hallucinations

      (i) No treatment if not disturbing to the patient or family.

      (ii) Use antipsychotics (see Table 17.3) *only for disabling delusions and/or hallucinations or if a danger to self*; use one-third to one-half usual starting dose and taper off if no benefit after 4 wk; reevaluate continued need every 3–6 mo; highest risk of excess mortality with olanzapine and risperidone and lowest with quetiapine. *Do not use if patient has dementia with Lewy bodies because of potential life-threatening side effects.*

   (e) With *depression*, consider citalopram 10–20 mg daily.

   (f) Sleep disorder

      (i) Daytime agitation is not likely to improve until sleep disturbances are corrected.

      (ii) Nonpharmacologic strategies preferred (e.g., activity program, no daytime naps, avoid evening alcohol and caffeine).

◼ = *not to be missed;* ● = *non-urgent referral;* ▲ = *urgent referral*

Pain assessment in advanced dementia scale (PAINAD)

Instructions: Observe the patient for 5 minutes before scoring the patient's behaviors. Score the behaviors according to the following chart. The patient can be observed under different conditions (e.g., at rest, during a pleasant activity, during caregiving, after the administration of pain medication).

Behavior	0	1	2	Score
Breathing Independent of vocalization	• Normal	• Occasional labored breathing • Short period of hyperventilation	• Noisy labored breathing • Long period of hyperventilation • Cheyne-Stokes respirations	
Negative vocalization	• None	• Occasional moan or groan • Low-level speech with a negative or disapproving quality	• Repeated troubled calling out • Loud moaning or groaning • Crying	
Facial expression	• Smiling or inexpressive	• Sad • Frightened • Frown	• Facial grimacing	
Body language	• Relaxed	• Tense • Distressed pacing • Fidgeting	• Rigid • Fists clenched • Knees pulled up • Pulling or pushing away • Striking out	
Consolability	• No need to console	• Distracted or reassured by voice or touch	• Unable to console, distract, or reassure	
			TOTAL SCORE	

Scoring:
The total score ranges from 0–10 points. A possible interpretation of the scores is: 1–3 = mild pain; 4–6 = moderate pain; 7–10 = severe pain. These ranges are based on a standard 0–10 scale of pain, but have not been substantiated in the literature for this tool.

Fig. 17.1 The pain assessment in advanced dementia scale (PAINAD). Warden, V., Hurley, A. C., & Volicer, L. (2003). Development and psychometric evaluation of the Pain Assessment in Advanced Dementia (PAINAD) scale. *Journal of the American Medical Directors Association, 4*(1), 9–15.

   (iii) Keep environment dark during the night and bright during the day.
   (iv) Discontinue any medications that may cause insomnia or interfere with sleep.
   (v) Medications *not shown* consistently to be effective: antihistamines, anticonvulsants, antidepressants (including trazodone), antipsychotics, or melatonin.
4. Pharmacological therapies
   (a) Discuss pros/cons with patient and family, since medications can aid with behavior issues but are not proven to slow down the decline of the disease process and can cause problematic side effects; they also can be expensive.

 (b) There is no recommended duration of therapy and no clear evidence regarding discontinuing therapy.

 (c) Cholinesterase inhibitors: donepezil (Aricept), rivastigmine (Exelon, oral and patch), galantamine (Razadyne, Razadyne ER): used with mild-to-moderate AD, vascular dementia (VaD), dementia with Lewy bodies, or Parkinson disease

 (d) Memantine (Namenda): used with moderate-to-severe AD and VaD; little benefit with mild AD

 (e) Vitamin E 2000 IU daily may help delay functional decline in mild-to-moderate AD only, but does not have an effect on cognitive performance.

 (f) The following have shown no benefit: NSAIDs, estrogen, vitamin B, *Ginkgo biloba*, statins, omega-3 fatty acids

 (g) Do not prescribe aducanumab (Aduhelm) at this point; there is not adequate data on its benefit yet plus it can cause brain microhemorrhages or edema.

5. Encourage mental exercises such as crosswords, word-finding games, and puzzles; also encourage leisure activities the patient enjoys (e.g., drawing/painting, singing, needlework).

6. Safety issues

 (a) Ensure a safe environment (e.g., turn water heater to ≤120°F, provide good lighting and night lights, "unclutter" the house but do not move furniture, install grab bars in the bathroom). If needed, install stove cut-off switch and lock up matches and firearms.

 (b) Place locks on windows and doors (all people with dementia are at risk of wandering and becoming lost).

 (c) Discourage driving

  (i) Consider disabling or selling the vehicle.

  (ii) A form is available from the state Department of Revenue, called Driver Condition Report; the NP can complete this form and fax/return to Department of Revenue. They will notify the patient to come in for re-testing for their Driver's license (requiring both driving and written tests).

7. Miscellaneous

 (a) Use memory aids and cues (e.g., handwritten daily schedule, labeling rooms and drawer contents, medication organizers).

 (b) Continued involvement in social activities (e.g., church, senior citizen activities) as long as possible is important.

 (c) Encourage the patient and loved one(s) to take any planned trips in the near future (rather than putting them off); the patient's condition may decline sooner than expected (e.g., in <6 mo).

 (d) Inability to handle finances is inevitable with all patients; this should be addressed with the patient and family early after diagnosis when the patient is still able to make decisions.

 (e) When independent living is no longer safe, options other than nursing home placement may include live-in assistance (family or hired caregivers), adult daycare, respite, or residential care.

 (f) Encourage caregiver(s) to join a support group (can provide helpful suggestions and emotional support).

 (g) An excellent resource for providers and family members/caregivers alike is "Coach Broyles' Playbook for Alzheimer's Caregivers: A Practical Tips Guide" (www.alzheimersplaybook.com); to get the most help from it, it is best to have them read this early in the stages of dementia.

DEPRESSION

I. Dysthymic disorder

A. Description: depressed mood on most days for at least 2 yr; during the depression period, the patient also has at least 2 of the following:

1. Poor appetite or overeating
2. Insomnia or hypersomnia
3. Low energy or fatigue
4. Low self-esteem
5. Poor concentration/difficulty making decisions
6. Feelings of hopelessness

B. May have symptom-free periods, but not >2 mo at a time.

C. Treatment

1. Often has an early and insidious onset and is a chronic disorder; may have concomitant medical disorders.
2. Antidepressants have been effective in a majority of patients (Table 17.1).
3. Counseling has been found to be beneficial for some patients.

II. Major depression (adults)

A. Description: depression that lasts at least 2 wk and includes ≥5 of the following symptoms, with one symptom being either the first or second one:

1. Depressed mood most of the day nearly every day
2. Loss of interest or pleasure in usual activities (anhedonia)
3. Change in appetite or weight
4. Insomnia or increased need for sleep
5. Psychomotor agitation or retardation *(not merely restlessness but unable to sit still or feels slowed down)*
6. Fatigue or loss of energy
7. Feelings of worthlessness or excessive guilt
8. Poor concentration
9. Recurrent thoughts of death or suicide

B. Common physical symptoms

1. Exhaustion
2. Vague pain not related to any disease process and not reproducible
3. Lump in the throat, nausea; H/A
4. Sexual complaints

C. Treatment

1. Major depression is highly recurrent. Use standardized instruments such as PHQ-2 and PHQ-9 (see Fig. 3.1; also see www.phqscreeners.com/pdfs/02_PHQ-9/English.pdf) for help with treatment decisions and monitoring progress. For medications, see Table 17.1.
2. A primary consideration with elderly patients is to distinguish depression from other physical and mental diseases, especially dementia and delirium (see Table 17.4).
3. Remission is resolution of the depression, as noted by a depression rating scale less than or equal to the cut-off given for that specific scale (e.g., PHQ-9 defines remission as a score of ≤5); use the same rating scale each time for consistency.
4. Treatment may also be needed for anxiety; if two or more antidepressants have either not worked or made patient feel worse, consider the diagnosis may actually be bipolar disorder.

5. Cognitive therapy (counseling) can work as well as medications, even for severe depression, and is more effective in preventing relapse.
6. Medications should be started slowly, and the dose should be titrated up to the therapeutic level that resolves the symptoms (see **PRACTICE PEARLS FOR ANTIDEPRESSANTS**)
    (a) Titrate the dose until the patient answers "yes" to the following questions: Are you 100% better? Are you again doing activities and hobbies that you enjoy (i.e., enjoying life again)?
    (b) If the patient is no better on the top dose of medication, change to a different medication—consider change to a different class.
    (c) Using a single antidepressant does not lead to remission in most patients; thus, it is common to add a second antidepressant or a second-generation antipsychotic or lithium. There are no evidence-based guidelines for combining antidepressants.
7. Length of pharmacological therapy
    (a) There is considerable variation in the amount of time required for antidepressants to reach a therapeutic level: there may be improved energy after ~2 wk, but mood effects may take 6–8 wk (although venlafaxine often eases symptoms faster).
    (b) Follow up in 2–4 wk, then again in 2–4 wk, then in 1–2 mo, then as indicated. If little improvement in symptoms after 4–6 wk, consider increasing the dose or changing/adding additional medications.
    (c) The dose should be maintained at the therapeutic level for at least 1 yr; patients with recurrent depression may need medication for life.
    (d) *Recurrent depression may result from inappropriate prescription of medications at a dose too low for an inadequate trial period coupled with poor follow-up.*
8. Nonpharmacological therapy
    (a) Suggest relaxation techniques (e.g., progressive muscle relaxation, imagining a beautiful or peaceful place).
    (b) Recommend physical exercise at least 3–5 times a wk.
D. *Referral*
    1. *To a psychologist for counseling or cognitive behavioral therapy.*
    2. *To a psychiatrist or psychiatric NP if*
        (a) *No improvement or remission not achieved after adequate trial with 1–3 agents*
        (b) *Comorbidities suspected (e.g., psychosis, bipolar disorder, severe depression, or dysthymia plus acute depressive episode).*
    3. *To inpatient treatment or ED with suicidal/homicidal ideations.*
E. Patient and family education
    1. Duration of depression (6 mo to 2 yr)
    2. Chronicity and recurrences
    3. Disability and intensity associated with depression
    4. The patient does not choose to be depressed; at times, depression is associated with a chemical imbalance
    5. Expected side effects of the prescribed medications (particular side effects for each patient cannot be predicted but will be treated)

■ = *not to be missed;* ● = *non-urgent referral;* ▲ = *urgent referral*

F. Antidepressant withdrawal
  1. TCAs: occurs from 24 to 48 hr up to 2 wk after discontinuation
     (a) GI complaints with or without anxiety
     (b) Sleep disturbances, paradoxical mania
     (c) Movement disorders
  2. SSRIs: timing depends on which is used (half-life varies)
     (a) Dizziness, anxiety, paresthesias
     (b) Nausea
     (c) Insomnia, nightmares
  3. MAOIs: comparable to opiate and amphetamine withdrawal
     (a) Anxiety, paresthesias
     (b) H/A
     (c) Muscle weakness, shivering
     (d) Psychosis, delirium, hallucinations
  4. Treatment
     (a) Withhold medicine in case of mild symptoms as they are temporary *or*
     (b) Restart medicine and taper off over at least 2–4 wk; may take up to 2 mo. If symptoms recur, consider a low dose of medicine for several months and then retry tapering off.

III. Major depression (pediatrics)
  A. Signs and symptoms
    1. Children overall exhibit more separation anxiety, somatic disorders, auditory hallucinations, temper tantrums, and changes in behavior at home and school.
    2. Children in middle-to-late childhood have more dysphoria, low self-esteem, guilt, and hopelessness.
    3. Teens are more likely to have sleep and appetite problems (e.g., bulimia, anorexia), delusions, or OCD; they are at increased risk for high-risk behaviors (e.g., promiscuity, smoking, alcohol and drug abuse, suicide attempts).
    4. A high percentage of these patients have a comorbid psychiatric disorder (e.g., anxiety, substance abuse, ADHD, eating or learning disorder).
  B. Diagnostics
    1. Complete chemistry panel, TSH, CBC
    2. Urine hCG (females)
    3. Physical examination focus: identification of self-harming behaviors (e.g., scarring from cutting or suicide attempts), drug abuse (IV tracts), signs of injury (e.g., bruising from falls or physical abuse)
  C. Treatment
    ▲ 1. *Referral to ED with suicide thoughts or intent.*
    ● 2. *Referral to a pediatric psychiatrist or psychiatric NP for medication management.*
    ● 3. *Referral to/encourage counseling with a psychologist trained in pediatrics.*

IV. Seasonal affective depressive disorder (SADD)
  A. Description: symptoms occur late fall through late spring and include increased sleep, increased appetite with carb cravings, increased weight, irritability
  B. Treatment
    1. Light therapy: there are commercially available devices (*not* tanning beds)
    2. Medications (see Table 17.1)

● = *non-urgent referral;* ▲ = *urgent referral*

PRACTICE PEARLS FOR ANTIDEPRESSANTS (ALSO SEE TABLE 17.1)

- SSRIs are usually first-line treatment
  - SSRIs may cause hyponatremia, especially in elderly patients; check serum sodium before starting and recheck in 1 mo.
  - Paroxetine can decrease cognition in elderly patients and cause sedation; it is better for anxious, younger people; it may also cause weight gain.
  - Fluoxetine is not recommended for elderly patients because of its long half-life but is safe in children.
  - SSRIs may cause sexual dysfunction in up to 50% of patients; treat with a lower dose or change to a non-SSRI agent.
  - Citalopram: *do not use* at a dose >20 mg daily in adults >60 yr of age (potential risk for QT prolongation)
- With comorbid cardiac conditions, use sertraline (safe and effective with CV disease); mirtazapine or bupropion may also be used alone or in combination with sertraline.
- SNRIs
  - Venlafaxine has a rapid onset of action and is helpful for patients who need an immediate boost (e.g., no energy or interest in activities).
  - Duloxetine is used for pain management (including DM neuropathy) with/without depression.
  - Venlafaxine and desvenlafaxine (Pristiq) are helpful for depression with fatigue and/or exhaustion.
- Use bupropion (Wellbutrin) for patients who are depressed and also want to stop smoking.
- TCAs
  - Use cautiously in elderly patients because of anticholinergic side effects (e.g., dry mouth, constipation, pupil dilation [worsens glaucoma], increased heart rate, urinary retention); nortriptyline (Pamelor) works for depression without anticholinergic effects.
  - Tend to cause weight gain.
  - Amitriptyline has potent α-blocking properties, which can result in orthostatic hypotension; it may be beneficial in hypertensive, depressed patients.
  - Obtain baseline ECG before starting routine use of amitriptyline.
- Sleep problems
  - Amitriptyline and trazodone are the *most sedating* antidepressants; administer at hs; usual starting dose is amitriptyline 10–25 mg or trazodone 50 mg.
  - SSRIs, bupropion, and venlafaxine *may worsen* sleep, at least at the start of therapy; have the patient take them in the morning.
- Sexual dysfunction
  - Encourage patient to continue with the medication for 1–2 mo, to see if the sexual symptoms improve (anxiety/depression can lead to reduced libido, so treating the condition may help).
  - If the patient does not want to wait, consider decreasing the dose or change to another SSRI or SNRI.
  - Bupropion or mirtazapine have the least sexual dysfunction concerns.
- With resistant depression, try an SSRI plus bupropion or mirtazapine.
- *Never give* fluoxetine and amitriptyline to the same patient; amitriptyline is not metabolized and can become toxic.
- When changing medications
  - Do a "next day" switch within the same class *or* SSRI to SNRI (the exception is fluoxetine because of its long half-life—wait 4–7 days after stopping it).
  - Do "cross-tapering" when switching to a different class (titrate down the current medication over a 1–2 wk period or longer and titrate up the new medication at the same time).
- Mirtazapine can cause weight gain; this may be an advantage in elderly patients with weight loss or poor appetite. Consider using 7.5 mg hs for appetite enhancement/sleep, especially in elderly patients; doses >15 mg daily cause more sedation.

Continued

PRACTICE PEARLS FOR ANTIDEPRESSANTS (ALSO SEE TABLE 17.1)—CONT'D

- Be aware of the many other medications that can cause depression (e.g., propranolol, cimetidine, methyldopa, OCs, corticosteroids). Also, long-term ETOH or marijuana use and cocaine or methamphetamine withdrawal can cause depression.
- St. John's wort: there is no consistent evidence of effectiveness and it has many side effects and interactions with commonly used medications; for these reasons, *its use should be discouraged*

INSOMNIA

I. Definition: inability to sleep
   A. Can either be short-term (<1 mo; result of psychologic or physiologic stress) or chronic.
   B. Can be difficulty falling asleep (sleep onset), staying asleep (sleep maintenance), and/or sleep may not be restful (sleep quality).
II. Potential causes
   A. Psychiatric conditions
      1. Anxiety, PTSD
      2. Depression
   B. Chronic medical conditions
      1. OSA, pulmonary disease
      2. Cancer
      3. Endocrine D/O (e.g., menopause, DM, thyroid disease)
      4. GI problems (e.g., GERD, IBS)
      5. Ischemic heart disease, HF
      6. Dementia
      7. Pain
      8. RLS
      9. Rheumatic disease (e.g., arthritis, fibromyalgia)
      10. Urologic disease (e.g., BPH, nocturia)
   C. Medications
      1. Antidepressants (e.g., SSRIs and SNRIs)
      2. Calcium channel blockers, diuretics
      3. Bronchodilators (e.g., albuterol)
      4. CNS stimulants (e.g., appetite suppressants, caffeine)
      5. Glucocorticoids (sleep may be improved with lower dose and taking earlier in the day)
      6. OTC allergy, cold, and cough medications
      7. Sedatives and hypnotics
   D. Substance abuse (e.g., alcohol, illicit drugs, tobacco)
   E. Circadian rhythm changes
      1. Changing shifts at work or working overnights
      2. Aging (getting sleepier earlier in evening and waking earlier in morning; also, total sleep time decreases by average of about 30 min per decade starting in mid-life)
III. Evaluation
   A. Perform history (medical and psychological) and physical examination. Ask each patient, "Do your legs bother you at night?" to screen for RLS.

B. Perform detailed sleep history (have patient fill out a sleep diary for at least 2 wk; sample diaries are available online and from DME agencies)
   1. Is the sleep problem new? If not, for how long?
   2. Are they actually sleepy at bedtime? Do they go to sleep after they get in bed? Do they go to sleep easily then wake up in 2–3 hr?
   3. How often does the patient nap and/or doze during the day or evening?
   4. Are there consistent times to go to bed and to wake up?
   5. Do they watch TV, read, or use electronic device in bed?
C. Obtain sleep study for OSA if indicated.
D. Consider labs if indicated, such as CMP, CBC, TSH and free T4; possibly PSA.
E. Review medication list and stop possible offending medications, if possible.

IV. Treatment
A. Treat underlying known medical or psychological problems (this may correct the insomnia).
B. Begin nonpharmacological therapy
   1. Sleep hygiene
      (a) Use the bedroom for sleep and sex only.
      (b) Maintain a regular sleep–wake cycle without naps in the daytime.
      (c) Lie down to sleep only when feeling sleepy; leave the bed if unable to fall asleep within 20 min; stay in bed for only the hours actually sleeping (but not less than 5 hr in 24 hr).
      (d) Maintain a consistent sleep pattern (e.g., get up at the same time each morning, including weekends, regardless of the number of hours slept).
      (e) Exercise regularly, but not within 4 hr of bedtime.
      (f) Limit fluid intake and avoid large meals in the evening hours.
      (g) Limit overall caffeine, tobacco, and alcohol intake; no "night cap."
      (h) Light-emitting screens (smart phones, electronic devices, TV) stimulate the brain; it is better to read or work on puzzles if unable to sleep.
      (i) Environment "restructuring" (i.e., keep the environment dark during the night and bright during the day, reduce noise at night).
   2. Relaxation techniques may help patient to relax (e.g., imagining a calm, pleasant environment; meditation, yoga; progressive muscle relaxation from feet up to the face).
   3. Consider use of a journal to write down thoughts; then it can be "set aside" until morning.
C. Pharmacological therapy, if needed (most *insomnia meds* increase sleep by about 15–30 min)
   1. Nonprescription
      (a) Melatonin 3–6 mg
      (b) Avoid first-generation antihistamines (e.g., diphenhydramine)—limited benefit and can cause confusion and urinary retention, especially in elderly
   2. Antidepressants
      (a) Doxepin (Silenor) 3–6 mg (also, Sinequan, which is same generic, with off-label use for sleep)
      (b) Mirtazapine 15 mg (off-label use)
      (c) Trazodone 25–150 mg (off-label use)
   3. Benzodiazepines (*not recommended with elderly patients* due to increased fall risk)
      (a) Estazolam 0.5–1 mg, with maximum dose 1–2 mg (for sleep onset and maintenance)
      (b) Flurazepam (Dalmane) 15–30 mg (for sleep onset and maintenance)

(c) Lorazepam (Ativan) 0.25–1 mg, with maximum dose 4 mg (off-label use; may help sleep maintenance with anxiety)

(d) Oxazepam (Serax) 10 mg with maximum 30 mg (off-label use; may help with sleep onset)

(e) Temazepam (Restoril) 7.5 mg with maximum 30 mg (*for short-term treatment*; helps with sleep onset and maintenance); one of the better benzos for elderly if appropriately dosed

4. Nonbenzodiazepine hypnotics

(a) Eszopiclone (Lunesta) 1 mg with maximum 3 mg (for sleep onset and maintenance); *not limited to short-term use*

(b) Ramelteon (Rozerem) 8 mg (for sleep onset); *not limited to short-term use*

(c) Suvorexant (Belsomra) 10–20 mg (for sleep onset and maintenance); no rebound and no apparent withdrawal symptoms when stopping the medication

(d) Zaleplon (Sonata) 5–10 mg with maximum 20 mg (*for short-term treatment*; helps with sleep onset)

(e) Zolpidem (Ambien)

(i) Immediate-release 5–10 mg (for short-term treatment; helps with sleep onset)

(ii) Controlled release 6.25–12.5 mg (for sleep onset and maintenance); *not limited to short-term use*

5. If abuse or dependence is a concern, consider ramelteon or suvorexant.

V. *Referral to sleep specialist if unsure of cause of insomnia or if the nonpharmacological and pharmacological therapies have not been effective.*

SEROTONIN SYNDROME

I. Description

A. *A potentially life-threatening condition associated with alterations in cognition and behavior, autonomic nervous system function, and neuromuscular activity; currently, there are no guidelines for preventing serotonin syndrome.*

B. Thought to be caused by increased or excessive serotonin activity and may be related to taking more than one of the following concurrently:

1. SSRIs
2. SNRIs (e.g., venlafaxine, duloxetine, milnacipran)
3. TCAs (e.g., amitriptyline, imipramine, doxepin)
4. Atypical antidepressants (e.g., trazodone, mirtazapine, vilazodone, bupropion)
5. MAOIs (more often associated with adverse outcomes, including death)
6. Opioids (e.g., tramadol, meperidine, fentanyl, methadone)
7. "Triptans"
8. Some GI medications (e.g., metoclopramide, ondansetron, granisetron)
9. Valproate, carbamazepine
10. Buspirone
11. Lithium
12. Antihistamines, first generation (e.g., chlorpheniramine, diphenhydramine)
13. "Street drugs" (e.g., amphetamine, cocaine, LSD, MDMA [Ecstasy], bath salts)
14. Herbs/supplements (e.g., St. John's wort, L-tryptophan, dextromethorphan)

■ = *not to be missed;* ● = *non-urgent referral*

II. Signs and symptoms: suggested diagnosis based on taking at least one serotonergic medication *plus* having ONE of the following:
  A. Spontaneous clonus (with rigidity usually greater in lower extremities)
  B. Inducible clonus *plus* agitation or diaphoresis
  C. Ocular clonus *plus* agitation or diaphoresis
  C. Tremor *plus* hyperreflexia
  D. Hypertonia *plus* temp >100.5 °F *plus* ocular or inducible clonus
III. Treatment
  A. Mild cases: stop potential offending medications; usually self-limited with complete recovery within a few days
▲ B. *Emergency transfer to ED with more severe cases: treatment focuses on supporting respiratory and cardiovascular systems*

▲ = *urgent referral*

Food Sources for Selected Nutrients

Vitamin K	Iron	Potassium
Green Leafy Vegetables	**Meat and Meat Substitutes**	**Cereals**
Broccoli	Organ meats	Bran flakes
Brussels sprouts	All meats and poultry	Kellogg's All Bran
Cabbage	Egg yolk	Nabisco 100% Bran
Collard greens	Shellfish	Shredded Wheat
Cucumber peel	Tofu, soybeans	**Fruits**
Endive	**Fruits**	Apricots, dates, or peaches
Green scallions	Apricots, prunes	(dried or fresh)
Kale	Grapes	Avocado
Lettuce	Raisins	Banana
Mustard greens	**Vegetables**	Cantaloupe
Parsley	Broccoli	Orange, grapefruit, or tomato
Spinach	Brussels sprouts	(fruit or juice)
Turnip greens	Collard greens	Prunes and raisins
Watercress	Celery	Watermelon
Fats	Green leafy vegetables	**Vegetables**
Canola, salad, soybean,	Lettuce	Asparagus
and olive oils	**Miscellaneous**	Baked winter squash
Mayonnaise	Dried peas, beans	Beet greens
Margarine	Fortified cereals, including baby	Blackstrap molasses
Miscellaneous	cereals	Broccoli
Beans	Grains, wheat germ	Canned tomato sauce
Pickles	Legumes (including chickpeas)	Carrots
Sauerkraut	Potatoes	Chard
Soybeans	Peanuts	Chocolate, unsweetened
	Carob	Cooked white beans
	Molasses	Lima beans
		Miscellaneous
		Mushrooms
		Peanuts
		Peas, cooked
		Sardines, canned in oil
		Spinach, fresh
		Sunflower seeds
		White or sweet potato

High Fiber Foods*	Sodium	Calcium

Cooked Vegetables
Broccoli
Brussel sprouts
Carrots
Green beans
Peas
Potato (with skin)
Spinach
Squash
Zucchini
Breads and Grains
Bran muffins
Brown rice
Oatmeal (cooked)
Fruits and nuts
Almonds ($^1/_2$ c)
Apple (with skin)
Banana
Dates
Oranges
Peanuts ($^1/_2$ c)
Pears (with skin)
Prunes
Legumes
Baked beans (canned)
Kidney beans (canned)
Lima beans (canned)
Lentils (boiled)
	**Foods to Avoid on a Sodium-
	    Restricted Diet**
	
	Milk and Dairy Products
	Buttermilk, malted milk
	Many cheeses
	Meat and Meat Substitutes
	Any meat, fish, poultry that is smoked,
	    cured, salted, or canned (e.g., bacon,
	    dried beef, cold cuts, ham or turkey
	    ham, hot dogs, sausages)
	Bread and Grains
	Bread/rolls/crackers with salted tops
	Instant hot cereals
	Instant rice and pasta mixes
	Pancakes, waffles, muffins, biscuits, and
	    corn bread with salt, baking powder,
	    or self-rising flour or instant mixes
	Quick breads
	Regular bread crumbs, cracker crumbs
	Stuffing and casserole mixes
	Vegetables and Fruits
	Frozen vegetables in sauce
	Pickles, olives
	Regular canned vegetables, juices
	Sauerkraut, pickled vegetables
	Miscellaneous
	Regular ketchup, chili sauce, mustard,
	    horseradish; sauces: BBQ, soy,
	    teriyaki, Worcestershire, and steak
	Regular canned or dried soup, bouillon
	Salt in seasonings (e.g., garlic salt)
	Salted snack foods (e.g., chips, nuts,
	    pretzels, seeds, popcorn)
	Seasonings containing MSG
		Dairy Products
		(providing ≥200 mg/serving)
		Cheese: hard cheese, ricotta,
		    or cottage cheese
		Ice cream
		Milk (whole, 2%, or skim)
		Milkshakes
		Yogurt
		Meat and Meat Substitutes
		(providing ≥100 mg/serving)
		Clams
		Oysters
		Sardines and salmon (with bone)
		Shrimp
		Tofu
		Vegetables and Fruits
		(providing ≥90 mg/serving)
		Broccoli
		Kale, turnip greens
		Okra
		Orange juice (calcium fortified)
		Spinach
		Breads, Grains, Legumes
		(providing ≥90 mg/serving)
		Beans
		English muffin
		Fortified, ready-to-eat cereal
		Fortified bread
		Waffles

* Serving size 1 c or 1 medium fruit.

BRATY Diet:

The BRATY diet can be used for patients with nausea and vomiting. The food consistency depends on the age of the patient and personal preference; e.g., bananas can be fresh, mashed, or from baby food jar. The diet can be used up to 24 hr.

B: bananas
R: rice or rice cereal
A: apples, applesauce
T: toast, crackers (preferably dry)
Y: yogurt, live culture (preferably plain)

Predicted Peak Expiratory Flow Rate

Child and adolescent female (age 6–20 yr)

Height (in):	42	46	50	54	57	60	64	68	72
Age: 6	134	164	193	223	245	268	297	327	357
8	153	182	212	242	264	287	316	346	376
10	171	201	231	261	283	305	335	365	395
12	190	220	250	280	302	324	354	384	414
14	209	239	269	298	321	342	373	403	432
16	228	258	288	317	340	362	392	421	451
18	247	277	306	336	358	381	411	440	470
20	266	295	325	355	377	400	429	459	489

Child and adolescent male (age 6–20 yr)

Height (in):	44	48	52	56	60	64	68	72	76
Age: 6	99	146	194	241	289	336	384	431	479
8	119	166	214	261	309	356	404	451	499
10	139	186	234	281	329	376	424	471	519
12	159	206	254	301	349	396	444	491	539
14	178	226	274	321	369	416	464	511	559
16	198	246	293	341	389	436	484	531	579
18	218	266	313	361	408	456	503	551	599
20	238	286	333	381	428	476	523	571	618

Adult female (age 25–80 yr)

Height (in):	58	60	62	64	66	68	70	72	75
Age: 25	350	365	379	394	409	424	439	498	515
30	342	357	372	387	402	417	431	489	506
35	335	350	364	379	394	409	424	480	497
40	327	342	357	372	387	402	416	471	488
45	320	335	349	364	379	394	409	462	479
50	312	327	342	357	372	387	401	453	470
55	305	320	334	349	364	379	394	444	461
60	297	312	327	342	357	372	386	435	452
65	290	305	319	334	349	364	379	426	443
70	282	297	312	327	342	357	371	417	434

| 75 | 275 | 290 | 304 | 319 | 334 | 349 | 364 | 408 | 425 |
| 80 | 267 | 282 | 297 | 312 | 327 | 342 | 356 | 399 | 416 |

Adult male (age 25–80 yr)

Height (in):	63	65	67	69	71	73	75	77	80
Age: 25	492	520	549	578	606	635	664	692	701
30	481	510	538	567	596	624	653	682	689
35	471	499	528	557	585	614	643	671	677
40	460	489	517	546	575	603	632	661	665
45	450	478	507	536	564	593	622	650	652
50	439	468	496	525	554	582	611	640	640
55	429	457	486	515	543	572	601	629	628
60	418	447	475	504	533	561	590	619	615
65	408	436	465	494	522	551	580	608	603
70	397	426	454	483	512	540	569	598	591
75	387	415	444	473	501	530	559	587	578
80	376	405	433	462	491	519	548	577	566

How to calculate predicted expiratory peak flow:
- Have the patient blow into the peak flow meter three times, reset the meter prior to each attempt, and then calculate the average.
- Divide the patient's peak flow by the predicted peak flow; answer equals the percentage of expected normal peak flow rate.
- Example: the patient is a 10-year-old male and 52 inches tall. The expected normal peak flow would be 234. The patient's average peak flow today is 100; $100 \div 234 = 0.427$ (43% of normal). After nebulizer treatment with albuterol, the patient's peak flow is 200; $200 \div 234 = 0.85$ (85% of normal). An improvement is noted.
- Can be used as a guide to the patient's condition at the time of examination and after nebulizer treatment has been given to determine if beta$_2$ inhalers (SABA) would be beneficial as a treatment to decrease bronchospasm.

Acetaminophen Dosing Chart

Age*	Weight*	Suspension 1 tsp = 160 mg/5 mL**	Junior Strength Chewable Tablet 160 mg**
0–3 mo	6–11 lb (2–5 kg)	$^1/_4$ teaspoon (1.25 mL = 40 mg)	N/A
4–11 mo	12–17 lb (6–7 kg)	$^1/_2$ teaspoon (2.5 mL = 80 mg)	N/A
12–23 mo	18–23 lb (8–10 kg)	$^3/_4$ teaspoon (3.75 mL = 120 mg)	N/A
2–3 yr	24–35 lb (11–15 kg)	1 teaspoon (5 mL = 160 mg)	1 tab (160 mg)
4–5 yr	36–47 lb (16–21 kg)	1½ teaspoons (7.5 mL = 240 mg)	1.5 tabs (240 mg)
6–8 yr	48–59 lb (22–26 kg)	2 teaspoon (10 mL = 320 mg)	2 tab (320 mg)
9–10 yr	60–71 lb (27–32 kg)	$2^1/_2$ teaspoon (12.5 mL = 400 mg)	$2^1/_2$ tab (400 mg)
11–12 yr	72–95 lb (32–43 kg)	3 teaspoons (15 mL = 480 mg)	3 tab (480 mg)
>12 yr	96 + lb	Can use adult dosing	

Ensure that the caregiver has an accurate measuring device.
* Dosage should be calculated by weight and not age, 10–15 mg/kg/dose.
** May give q4–6hr prn; maximum daily dose is 75 mg/kg/d.

Ibuprofen Dosing Chart

Age*	Weight†	Infant Drops 50 mg/1.25 mL**	Children's Liquid 1 tsp = 100 mg/5 mL**	Chewable Tablet 1 tab = 100 mg**
6–11 mo	12–17 lb (5.4–8.1 kg)	1.25 mL (50 mg)	0.5 mL (50 mg)	N/A
12–23 mo	18–23 lb (8.2–10.8 kg)	$^1/_4$ teaspoon (1.8 mL = 75 mg)	$^3/_4$ teaspoon (3.75 mL = 75 mg)	N/A
2–3 yr	24–35 lb (10–16.3 kg)	N/A	1 teaspoon (5 mL = 100 mg)	1 tab (If child can chew medication)
4–5 yr	36–47 lb (16.4–21.7 kg)	N/A	$1^1/_2$ teaspoons (7.5 mL = 150 mg)	$1^1/_2$ tab
6–8 yr	48–59 lb (21.8–27.2 kg)	N/A	2 teaspoons (10 mL = 200 mg)	2 tab
9–10 yr	60–71 lb (27.3–32.6 kg)	N/A	$2^1/_2$ teaspoons (12.5 mL = 250 mg)	$2^1/_2$ tab
11 yr	72–95 lb (32.7–43.2 kg)	N/A	3 teaspoons (15 mL = 300 mg)	3 tab
> 12 yr	Can use adult dosing.			

Ensure that the caregiver has an accurate measuring device.
*Do not give to infants age < 6 mo of age.
**May give q6–8hr; maximum daily dose is 40 mg/kg/d.
†Dosage should be based on weight, 5–10 mg/kg/dose.

INDEX

Note: Page numbers followed by *f* indicate figures, *t* indicate tables, and *b* indicate boxes.